European Union
Biomedical and Health Research

The BIOMED 1 Programme

Edited by

A.-E. Baert, S.S. Baig, C. Bardoux, G.N. Fracchia, M. Hallen, O. Le Dour, M.C. Razquin, V. Thévenin, A. Vanvossel and M. Vidal

European Commission,
Directorate-General for Science, Research and Development,
Directorate for Life Sciences
Division for Medical and Health Research, Brussels

1995

IOS
Press

Ohmsha

Amsterdam, Oxford, Tokyo, Washington, DC

ISBN 90 5199 173 8 (IOS Press)
ISBN 4 274 90014 2 (Ohmsha)
Library of Congress Catalogue Card Number 94 - 075420
Publication no. EUR

Publisher
IOS Press
Van Diemenstraat 94
NL-1013 CN Amsterdam
Netherlands

Distributor in the UK and Ireland
IOS Press/Lavis Marketing
73 Lime Walk
Headington
Oxford OX3 7 AD
U.K.

Distributor in the USA and Canada
IOS Press, Inc.
P.O. Box 10558
Burke, VA 22009-0558
U.S.A.

Distributor in Japan
Ohmsha, Ltd.
3-1 Kanda Nishiki - Cho
Chiyoda - Ku
Tokyo 101
Japan

PRINTED IN THE NETHERLANDS

CONTENTS

I. DEVELOPMENT OF COORDINATED RESEARCH ON PREVENTION, CARE AND HEALTH SYSTEMS

I.1 DRUGS AND THE ADMINISTRATION OF MEDICINES

I.3 BIOMEDICAL TECHNOLOGY

I.4 HEALTH SERVICES RESEARCH

II. MAJOR HEALTH PROBLEMS AND DISEASES OF GREAT SOCIO-ECONOMIC IMPACT

II.1 AIDS RESEARCH

x

II.2 CANCER RESEARCH

II.3 RESEARCH ON CARDIOVASCULAR DISEASES

II.4 RESEARCH ON MENTAL ILLNESS AND NEUROLOGICAL DISEASES

II.5 THE AGEING PROCESS, AND AGE-RELATED HEALTH PROBLEMS AND HANDICAPS

III. HUMAN GENOME ANALYSIS

IV. RESEARCH ON BIOMEDICAL ETHICS

OTHER ACTIVITIES

"L'Europe ne se fera pas d'un coup...
...elle se fera par des réalisations concrètes"
Robert Schuman

INTRODUCTION - The Concept of Concerted Action

This volume contains the summaries of 400 research projects, involving more than 6,600 scientific teams, supported by the European Union within the Biomedical and Health Research Programme (abbreviated BIOMED 1). BIOMED 1 is a specific programme of the third framework programme for Community activities in the field of research and technological development (RTD) for the period 1990-1994. The time period indicated can be misleading; it means that the last year of budgetary commitments was 1994. As project contracts last usually three years, many will finish only end 1997 and thus in fact BIOMED 1 is operational until end 1997.

The cover of this book shows an anatomic map by Andreas VESALIUS (1514-1564) who by an experimental method transgressed the taboo of opening the human body and became the founder of modern anatomy. At the background is a map of Europe by Gerardus MERCATOR (1512-1594), founder of modern mathematical geography, who by projection developed a world globe which became of strategic importance for maritime and, later, aerial navigation.

Today medical research is confronted with similar challenges: information technology and molecular biology have given medicine new tools, ones that make it possible to "open" the human genome and map its "anatomy" and functions, as well as opening the brain and map its complex, interactive mechanisms. Yet today as in the past the taboo effect looms, and with it the danger that it will cloud the ethical issues, block constructive, rational debate and might hinder research and progress in medicine.

Linguistic, ethnic, conceptual and structural differences separated the European countries, yet in the Middle Ages and Renaissance they were somewhat united by a common language (Latin) and shared a common culture. The scholars of that time (Magisters) undertook European tours; they created a network of personal contacts and established a tradition of regular exchange of ideas and information among those interested in the natural sciences. This tradition was maintained through the exchange of letters, books, and periodicals.

When the conceptual fathers of Biomedical and Health Research at European level met during the period 1972-1978 they felt confronted with a dilemma: How can the Member States of the European Community retain their sovereignty in the area of medical research while jointly tackling today's health challenges, ones not readily met at national level?

Through the four Medical and Health Research Programmes (MHR1,2,3, and 4) and now through the first Biomedical and Health Research Programme (BIOMED 1), the answer has been *Concerted Action*. It means: support European networking, let national sources fund the research. Community funds for a concerted action thus represent only about 5% of the total project budget. They are meant to be a catalyst, to increase the leverage of national research efforts. Can it work?

Despite the social and economic importance of biomedical and health research it was not until 1978 that the Commission of the European Communities was authorized to promote coordination of research projects in the various countries in very limited and strictly defined areas of common interest. Since this "pilot" work proved successful and considerably improved the effectiveness of efforts made at national level in the fields chosen, the EC Member States and European Parliament showed both interest and confidence in this new form of EC action. As a result, on 9 September 1991 the Council of the Ministers of the Member States adopted a wider-ranging and more coherent research coordination programme in biomedicine and health (BIOMED 1). Since then, this programme has grown substantially both in size and content as reflected in this book. During 1994 European Parliament and Council adopted BIOMED 2 with a substantial budget increase of 150% from 133 to 336 million ECU (1994-1998).

Collaboration is not natural and spontaneous within the scientific community which rather believes in competition to ensure scientific progress. The concerted action approach used in EU Biomedical and Health Research has created a (begin of a) European medical research community. This approach has other immediate advantages: scientists who are not in direct competition for the same national resources will be more enclined to work together at a European scale. Moreover, by delegating network management to the EU Project Leaders, the Commission enables them to adapt creatively the form of their networks to specific research situations.

The Project Leader is the cornerstone of the concerted action system, as he is accountable vis-à-vis the Commission and is the only recipient of EU funds. "He is fully responsible for the operational definition of the project from mobilizing teams to disseminating results, for organizing the work and arranging the logistics of staff exchanges, often considered to be the strategic hub of concerted actions." (1)

Also important is the inclusion of industrial partners and potential users of research results in many concerted actions. This should accelerate the transfer of these results into new medical tools and health care practice. Nearly all concerted actions brought together researchers and clinicians, who are in fact the potential users. Such "interweaving" of research and clinical practice enabled operational results to be directly integrated into practice in de facto harmonized ways throughout Europe. This may be considered equivalent to "industrial" developments found in other contexts.

European diversity often appears as an obstacle to be overcome, yet with the appropriate tools, it provides a wonderful "laboratory" where parameters of interest vary from country to country and from region to region.

Concerted actions have certainly succeeded in bringing European scientists together to develop the necessary tools. A recent evaluation report[1] by the Centre de Sociologie et de l'Innovation (Ecole des Mines, Paris) highlights the heavy involvement of numerous teams and echoes the feeling of many participants that concerted action encouraged them to aim for higher goals.

It confirmed that, although the level of EC funding was modest, the biomedical research programme stands among the major EC research programmes when using the number of involved teams as an indicator and the only one which has adopted an original approach to financial support, namely the concerted actions, as its principal mode of implementation.

And results there are. In some cases, the result is the network itself, as when experts are too isolated to be effective and the concerted action breaks their isolation. Through other projects, European scientists have developed linguistically, culturally, and scientifically common instruments: methods, questionnaires, data bases, joint experiments... One project, for example, enabled nine primate centres to conduct vaccine trials in macaques in a manner that minimised the use of experimental animals and optimised the scientific output. Another made it possible to develop facilities, chemicals, and safe conditions for testing a new form of cancer treatment. More examples are provided in EURO ABSTRACTS[2].

The present inventory of BIOMED 1 illustrates the spectacular growth of the programmes since 1978: from 3 projects with 100 participants to 400 projects with 6,643 participating legal entities. In all research areas but one, the projects are concerted actions. A glance at the titles shows that many of these studies are not even imaginable without multinational, multidisciplinary collaboration.

The EC biomedical research programmes have undeniably reached a key stage in their evolution, mainly because of the high level of demand revealed by the numbers of applications for each call for proposals. The issues are many and multi-faceted, such as selection, monitoring, management, information dissemination and exploitation of results, but also survival of established networks. The major challenge lies in fact in defining EU research programmes and their integration with national ones.

The BIOMED 1 Programme (Area III), has integrated the Human Genome Analysis Programme with the shared-cost mechanism as implementation method (up to 50 % of the real costs supported by the EU). There is no doubt that the approach to biomedical research at European level should undergo a thorough review. Now that the BIOMED 2 programme (4th Framework Programme 1994-1998) allows all possible mechanisms to support biomedical and health research, the definition and role of concerted actions must be reviewed. Its originality and feasibility are at the same time its strength and weakness.

André-Emmanuel Baert, MD, PhD, Head of Medical Research Unit
Brussels, January 1995

[1] Research Networks built by the MHR4 Programme, by P. Larédo, B. Kahane, J.B. Meyer, D. Vinck, working with Evaluation Unit coordinator I. Karatzas, 1992, EUR 14700
[2] EUROABSTRACTS Vol. 32, no. 6, 1994, pp 367-379.

BIOMEDICAL AND HEALTH RESEARCH ACTIVITIES UNDER THE THIRD FRAMEWORK PROGRAMME (1990-1994)

ADMINISTRATIVE OVERVIEW
André-Emmanuel Baert

Presenting BIOMED 1

This First Biomedical and Health Research Programme is a specific programme under the Third Framework Programme (1990-1994). Its objectives are "to contribute to improving the efficacy of medical and health research and development in the Member States, in particular by better coordination of the Member States".

In later chapters, the Responsible Scientists for the various areas and sub-areas of the BIOMED 1 programme, together with the 400 Project Leaders, present the scientific content of their specific research project in progress. This overview will therefore simply provide, in tables, a brief outline of the implementation of the BIOMED 1 programme.

BIOMED 1 in a Nutshell

	BIOMEDICAL AND HEALTH RESEARCH PROGRAMME 1 RESEARCH AREAS	NUMBER OF	
		contracts	participants
I	DEVELOPMENT OF COORDINATED RESEARCH ON PREVENTION, CARE, AND HEALTH SYSTEMS		
I.1	Drugs and the administration of medicines	23	298
I.2	Risk factors and occupational medicine	27	323
I.3	Biomedical Technology	39	717
I.4	Health Services Research	28	339
	TOTAL Area I	117	1,677
II	MAJOR HEALTH PROBLEMS AND DISEASES OF GREAT SOCIO-ECONOMIC IMPACT		
II.1	AIDS	39	480
II.2	Cancer	57	1,404
II.3	Cardiovascular disease	40	1,383
II.4	Mental illness and neurological disease	45	532
II.5	The ageing process, age-related health problems and handicaps	46	860
	TOTAL Area II	227	4,659
III	HUMAN GENOME ANALYSIS TOTAL Area III	41	172
IV	RESEARCH ON BIOMEDICAL ETHICS TOTAL Area IV	15	135
TOTAL	Areas I+II+III+IV	400[1]	6,643

[1] See Post-Scriptum

In the above table showing the breakdown of the total number of projects among the research areas and sub-areas of BIOMED 1, it is important to realise that "number of participants" means the number of legal entities with which contracts were signed. Since each legal entity may include several participating research teams and each team more than one staff member working on the project,the actual number of scientists involved can be far greater.

A major purpose of this publication with more than 6,000 complete addresses and access by key words, is to offer the scientific community an agora for transnational exchange and retrieval of scientific expertise, that may lead to possible cross-fertilization between disciplines and utilization of "collective expertise" when urgent questions arise.

BIOMED 1 in Figures

	Number of contracts	EC contribution (ECU)	Average EC contribution per contract	Number of participating legal entities	Average number of participants per contract
1. Concerted Actions [1]	359	109 400 000	304 735	6 471	18
2. Shared cost (Area III)	41	24 000 000	585 366	172	4.2
3. PECO•	217	9 670 350	44 564	391	1.8
4. Fellowships•	113	6 470 784	57 264	226	2
5. Grants•	90	1 800 000	20 000	90+	n.a
6. APAS•	39	4 000 000	102 564	45+	n.a
TOTAL	**859**	**155 341 134**	**n.a.**	**7 395+**	**n.a**

[1] See Post-Scriptum.
• provisional figures for 1994
n.a: not available

What do these figures show?

First of all, BIOMED 1 represents over 155 million ECU redistributed to the Member States to stimulate biomedical and health research in the EU. This is more than the 131.67 million ECU initially approved for BIOMED 1 for two reasons: firstly, a one-year extension was approved, bringing the amount to 149 million ECU, and secondly, some BIOMED-linked activities are budgetarily part of other programmes: PECO (Cooperation in Science and Technology with Central and Eastern European Countries-see below) and the so-called "Activités de Préparation, d'Accompagnement et de Suivi" (APAS) in the fields of Pharmaceuticals (3 million ECU) and Homeopathy (1 million ECU), requested by the European Parliament.

In BIOMED 1, the emphasis is on international, multidisciplinary cooperation. Concerted Actions occupy an important place, accounting for about 90% of the research projects. The aim is to bring national resources together in order to reach a critical mass, on the assumption that in this way the scientific targets can be better hit.

The 41 projects of Area 3 of the programme, Human Genome Analysis, are funded on a shared-cost basis. Scientifically, Europe has made an impressive contribution to the worldwide Human Genome Project, partly thanks to EU support.

From analyzing the first two lines in the table the difference between a concerted action and shared cost contract becomes more clear. Generally speaking a concerted action has 18 participants with an average annual EU contribution of 100,000 ECU or mathematically 5,500 ECU per participant. A shared cost activity has 4 participants with an average annual EU contribution (up to 50% of real cost) of 200,000 ECU or about 50,000 ECU per participant. This difference in amounts per participant makes clear that concertation is about coordinating research while shared cost is about doing research jointly.

The link between the BIOMED 1 and PECO programmes further highlights the stress laid on international cooperation. PECO enables scientists and researchers from Central and Eastern Europe to participate in ongoing EU projects.

Another important feature of BIOMED 1 is its "multiplier effect". This applies both to the money and to the energies mobilised. A total of 400 networks operate under the programme. About twice as many contracts have been signed. BIOMED-related activities involve more than 7,000 legal entities, each of which may include one or several teams of participating researchers. For Concerted Actions, with their average of 18 participants per project and their specific modality of funding, the effect can be enormous. In budgetary terms, the multiplier effect calculated on the basis of 114 first-year interim reports was 14.1. An earlier evaluation report (Laredo et al.) estimated the multiplier effect at 25. "The strength of the administrative approach adopted - the delegation of the budget together with the responsibilities - is that it authorizes flexibility and, with it, the emergence of numerous organizational innovations which have enabled project leaders to progress towards their objectives with modest financial EU contribution compared with the human and technical resources mobilized (less than 4% of the teams' budget on average)."

Fellowships in BIOMED 1

The research fellowships activity (5% of the budget) is linked to the specific targets of the Biomedical and Health Research Programme. Research training is undertaken in order to enhance scientific skills and expertise. This activity also serves to facilitate technology transfer to the health care related industries.

Applicants seek to undertake, in a laboratory/hospital located within one of the participating countries, specific research in the field of Biomedicine and Health. The training activities do not take place in the applicant's country of citizenship or in the country in which the applicant normally resides.

The evaluation of the application is based on the scientific qualities of the project, the applicant, and the host institute.

The qualities of the project are judged from (1) the originality of the hypotheses presented and the significance of he questions asked, (2) the potential of the proposed work to provide new and important knowledge, and (3) knowledge and critical attitude as reflected in the literature reviewed.

The qualities of the host institute are judged from (1) its scientific standing as reflected in publications lists and (when applicable) reputation, (2) the quality of the project proposal, and (3) its commitment to provide guidance and practical facilities for realizing the project as reflected in letters of such commitment and (when applicable) past experiences.

The evaluation and selection of proposals proceed as follows:

- Verification of selection and scientific eligibility of proposals by Commission staff
- Confidential evaluation of the proposals by anonymous peer review and subsequently by panels of independent experts
- Initial ranking of proposals by the Commission services and the preparation of a draft shortlist of the proposals selected for funding
- Examination of the evaluation process, discussion of the results and opinion on the Commission's shortlist by representatives of the responsible Programme Committee
- Final selection by the Commission of shortlisted proposals and communication of the results of the evaluation and selection of the applicants.

During the BIOMED 1 programme 1,357 applications were received and 113 were funded with a total budget of 6,470,784 ECU.

Success rate of proposals submitted to BIOMED 1

The perceived likelihood of receiving funding is one of the criteria that potential project leaders will consider before putting a lot of effort into preparing project proposals. The work involved is frequently regarded as an administrative burden rather than a necessary step in the elaboration and focussed definition of the intended research activities.

In accordance with the Council Decision 91/505/EEC of 9 September 1991 adopting the first Biomedical and Health Research Programme, three separate calls for proposals were published in the "Official Jopurnal of the EC". The number of full proposals received is totalling 1635, after selection leading to 400 contracted projects or a "success rate" of 24.2 % (see chart below). The success rate of 24.2% is seemingly within national trends.

It must be noted that a major reason for projects not being selected is that, apart from the evident overall budgetary limitations, they are lacking a clearly defined European added value, they are a repetition of earlier research, or that the proposed joint experiment by the network is insufficiently formulated.

Calls for proposals and research contracts issued

	Date	Number of Proposals	Contracts
1st call	25.10.1991 closing 31.01.1992	730*	114
2nd call (Human Genome only)	10.12.1992 closing 29.01.1993	115	41
3rd call	10.12.1992 closing 26.02.1993	808	107 (1993) 114 (1994) 24 (1994)
		Total 1635	400 Success Rate 24.2%

* 730 full proposals out of 1898 Declarations of Intent.

Post-Scriptum

While going to press, three additional contracts for concerted actions (totalling 750,000 ECU and another 39 participating legal entities) have been concluded:

Contribution of the vestibular system to motion perception: a physio-pathological study
(5 participating legal entities)
Project leader:
Prof. Alain BERTHOZ
CNRS/LPPA/UMR C9950
15, rue de l'Ecole de Médecine
F-75270 Paris Cedex 06
Tel. +33/1/44.27.12.11; Fax +33/1/44.27.14.03

European therapeutic trial on isolated systolic hypertension in the elderly: Syst-Eur
(26 participating legal entities)
Project leader:
Prof. Robert FAGARD
U.Z. Gasthuisberg
Hypertensie
Herestraat 49
B-3000 Leuven
Tel. +32/16/34.57.67; Fax +32/16/34.57.63

Surgery and rehabilitation for cancers involving the larynx
(8 participating legal entities)
Project leader:
Dr. H.F. MAHIEU
Free University Hospital
Dept. of Otorhinolaryngology
De Boelelaan 1117
NL-1007 MB Amsterdam
Tel. +31/20/444.3690; fax 31/20/444.3688

Everybody wants coordination but nobody wants to be coordinated
(Saul Feldmann, NIH)
Prestige is a major obstacle to progress in medicine
(Tore Scherstén, Swedish MRC)

HISTORY OF MEDICAL RESEARCH AT EC LEVEL
André-Emmanuel Baert

Legal Basis

The Treaty of Rome (1957) which established the European Economic Community provided no explicit legal basis for research activities in medicine and public health. Initially, the scientific and technical activities of the Community were carried out on a sector-by-sector basis: industrial safety and hygiene under the European Coal and Steel Community; nuclear energy, biology and health protection under the European Atomic Energy Community; agricultural research under the European Economic Community. Not until 1974 did the Member States agree to interpret Article 235 of the Treaty of Rome in a manner that opened the way for a wide variety of Community research and development projects outside the nuclear field.

This interpretation became official policy only in 1987, with the Single European Act. Title VI, Research and Technological Development, states that the Community "shall encourage undertakings, including small and medium-sized undertakings, research centres and universities in their research and technological development activities". This includes research activities in medicine and health.

The Maastricht Treaty (1992) further strengthens this commitment. Title X Public Health, Article 129 extends the scope of EU support to research in public health, stating:
"Community action shall be directed towards the prevention of diseases, in particular the major health scourges, including drug dependence, by promoting research into their causes and their transmission, as well as health information and education.
Health protection requirements shall form a constituent part of the Community's other policies".

Title XV: Research and Technological Development, Article 130f states:

"1.   The Community shall have the objective of strengthening the scientific and technological bases of Community industry and encouraging it to become more competitive at international level, while promoting all the research activities deemed necessary by virtue of other Chapters of this Treaty.

2.   For this purpose the Community shall, throughout the Community, encourage undertakings, including small and medium-sized undertakings, research centres and universities in their research and technological development activities of high quality; it shall support their efforts to cooperate with one another, aiming, notably, at enabling undertakings to exploit the internal market potential to the full, in particular through the

opening up of national public contracts, the definition of common standards and the removal of legal and fiscal obstacles to that cooperation;

3.   All Community activities under this Treaty in the area of research and technological development, including demonstration projects, shall be decided on and implemented in accordance with the provisions of this Title".

Exploratory phase 1972-1978

But let us jump back in time. As early as 1965, the first ground was laid for developing a joint research and development policy with the creation of the Working Party on Scientific and Technical Research Policy (PREST), whose terms of reference were confirmed by the Council in 1967. In 1972, PREST recommended the establishment of a body for coordinating national scientific policies. This led to the emergence of the Scientific and Technical Research Committee (CREST), which acts as an advisor to the Commission and the Council, preparing their decisions in most sectors of science and technology. Among the then five specialised sub-committees of CREST was the Committee on Medical and Public Health Research (CRM - Comité de Recherche Médicale).

At that early stage, it was nearly decided not to engage Community efforts in joint medical research. National resources, both public and private (including the pharmaceutical industry), seemed adequate in this area. On the other hand, it was impossible to ignore the number of Nobel Prizes going to American researchers in biomedicine. Why was Europe not matching this performance? The answer appeared to lie in the "critical mass" that an organisation such as the National Institutes of Health in the United States could mobilise.

The CRM members finally agreed to the following: (1) the Community should support medical research projects aimed at prevention of illness and disability, early detection of disease, and rehabilitation; (2) common actions should be undertaken by or in association with the research organisations of the Member States; 3) the research topics should be of practical importance to the Community as a whole; the projects should produce Community added value, i.e. results beyond what could be achieved through research carried out separately in each Member State; (4) coordination of national policies should encourage national organisations to operate more coherently, laying the foundations for an effective scientific community; (5) it should be possible, in specific fields, to make comparisons and to establish cooperation in respect of research policies, within the limits of constraints on policy making in the Community resulting from the widely differing national situations.

CRM then launched into a series of exploratory and preparatory activities, creating specialized and ad hoc Working Groups, performing studies, organising workshops and seminars. These efforts were crowned in 1978, with the adoption by the Council of Ministers of the first Medical and Health Research Programme (MHR1).

Period of growth 1978-1994

MHR1 (1978-1981) included only 3 concerted action projects. Its budget totalled 1.09 million ECU for a three-year period. The target areas were (A) cellular ageing and decreased functional capacity of organs (EURAGE); (B) extracorporeal oxygenation (EUROXY); (C) registration of congenital abnormalities (EUROCAT). A novel mode of implementation was adopted, based on the dual need to maintain national sovereignty in the area of medical research while achieving a "critical mass" and Community added value through international, multidisciplinary collaboration. The term coined for this new form of implementation was "Concerted Action".

A Concerted Action (CA) is a research project carried out by a network of researchers. It is funded essentially by public and private sources in the participants' respective countries. The Community contribution covers only the additional cost of collaboration (about 5% of the total real costs). A Project Leader chosen by the network participants is the link between the Commission structures and the network. This scientist is responsible for how the research work is organized and how the concertation budget is spent.

The concerted action approach is outlined further in the "Explanatory Note" below. Initially, it was greeted with great skepticism: could such a (comparatively) small amount of money really increase the scope and leverage of European medical research? This is why only three "test" projects were conducted under MHR1. The test was conclusive: an evaluation[1] of the programme determined that it had succeeded in creating a close European collaboration and in improving the efficiency of national research efforts in the selected topics. It was therefore decided to pursue the endeavour: MHR1 was followed by MHR2, 3, and 4, followed in turn by the first Biomedical and Health Research Programme, BIOMED 1, presented in this inventory. BIOMED2 is already in view. The growth of this activity is testimony to the increasing interest it has aroused and to the growing confidence of the Member States in the concerted action method:

BIOMEDICAL and HEALTH RESEARCH at EC level 1978-1998

1978-81 MHR1	1.09 million ECU	3 concerted actions	100 teams
1980-83 MHR2	2.32 million ECU	7 concerted actions	230 teams
1982-86 MHR3	13.3 million ECU	34 concerted actions	1,200 teams
1987-91 MHR4	65.0 million ECU	135 concerted actions	4,540 teams
1990-94 BIOMED 1	133.0 million ECU	362 concerted actions and 41 shared cost projects	7,300 teams
1994-98 BIOMED 2	336.0 million ECU	*	*

* First call for proposals deadline 31 March 1995
  Second call for proposals deadline 15 June 1996 (provisional)

From the very beginning, it seemed desirable to allow non-Member States to be associated with CAs. Members of COST (European Cooperation in Scientific and Technical Research), i.e. Austria, Finland, Iceland, Norway, Sweden, Switzerland, and Turkey, may participate. More recently, concerted actions have included countries from Central and Eastern Europe (via the PECO Programme - PECO stands for Pays de l'Europe Centrale et Occidentale).

Agreements exist with Canada and Australia and there are contacts with the USA. Countries that do not have a full association agreement with the EU can participate on a project-by-project basis, but do not receive any Community funding.

Another important feature of these programmes is the participation of industry. Industrial partners are involved at various levels: as sources of funds, as providers of specialized products and materials, as network members. There is even one case of a Project Leader who belongs to a private company. This participation should accelerate transfer of research results into clinical practice.

The ongoing BIOMED 1 programme includes four target areas: (I) development of coordinated research on prevention, care, and health systems; (II) major health problems and diseases of great socioeconomic impact; (III) human genome analysis; (III) research on biomedical ethics. In all but Area III (where the Community contributes up to 50% of the total cost of the project), concerted action remains the mode of implementation. The research conducted under these four headings is outlined in the following chapters of this inventory.

Explanatory Note on the Method of Concerted Action

1. Who manages a Concerted Action?
- Commission Structures:
In the implementation of the Programme's objectives, the Commission is advised by a Programme Committee, which has been consecutively called Comité de Recherche Médicale (CRM) assisted by Comités d'Action Concertées (COMACs), Management and Coordination Advisory Committee (CGC - Comité de Gestion et de Coordination for MHR4 (1987-1991) and finally for BIOMED 1 (1990-1994) Committee of an Advisory Committee, in short CAN MED.
The CAN MED is composed of representatives of the Member States and chaired by the representative of the Commission.

In tribute to their input and continued devotion to the programme management the names of members of the programme committee over three points in time in the history of EU biomedical and health research are given at the end of this chapter.
CAN MED assisted the Commission Services in assessing selecting proposals, supervise and evaluate the projects, exchange information with other Research Groups, inform on national health research, appraise European priorities in the Programme's fields, and advise the Commission on continuation or termination of the research contracts.

- The Project Leader and Steering Group:
The Project Leader is responsible for managing the project and the concertation funds. He or she is assisted by a Project Management Group or a Steering Group composed of network participants selected by the network members. The Project Leader is the link between the Commission structures and the teams. Network structures may vary in time and from CA to CA, from a very centralised "star network" to one in which sub-project leaders operate on an equal basis.

2. Calls for Proposals and Proposal Selection

In the early programmes (MHR1, MHR2, MHR3), the Programme Committee initiated all CAs. For MHR4 and BIOMED 1 the policy was changed and calls for proposals were issued, inviting would-be project leaders to submit declarations of intent and full proposals. After confidential evaluation by independent experts, proposals were then evaluated by the Programme Committee before final selection by the Commission.

The general criteria for proposal selection were (1) scientific and technical excellence and novelty; (2) conformity with the scope and objectives of the work programme; (3) a precompetitive character; (4) scientific, technical, social and economic benefits; (5) a European dimension, Community added value; (6) transnational collaboration; (7) managerial capability of the Project Leader; (8) potential exploitation of results.

3. The Instruments of Concertation

The Commission delegates to the Project Leader the task of managing the scientific collaboration and the concertation budget, so that he can make the best of local situations and the CA's specific features. The Project Leader has seven "instruments of concertation" at his disposal:

(1) the scientific and administrative management of the project for building an managing the network, for instance, creation of a central secretariat ;

(2) PL missions to meet the participating teams;

(3) meetings, steering committees, seminars, training workshops, trainingships, etc.;

(4) short-term exchanges of staff between participating centres;

(5) exchanges of materials, reagents, instruments, cell cultures, specimens, animals, etc. among participants;

(6) central data handling, computing, statistical analysis, software for the project;

(7) joint publications in scientific journals and books, reports to national and international congresses, publication of a specific Newsletter.

Furthermore, a "centralized facility" can be established. Centralized facility is a unique general service tool for other concerted or shared cost actions supported by the Programme in order to enable standardization, joint experiments, data collection and analysis, with access to particular quality control products, experimental materials or specialized services. Community funding may cover up to 100% of the costs of services rendered by the centralized facility to the research centre, universities, undertakings and enterprises participating in shared cost and concerted actions.

4. Project Monitoring and Evaluation of BIOMED 1

Project Leaders are required to submit yearly activity reports and a final report at the end of the contract period. These must notably describe the progress made towards the project objectives, the methodologies used, any ethical/safety considerations, benefits of the CA and Community added value achieved, difficulties encountered, a list of CA publications, a process assessment (describing the use made of the different concertation instruments), and a cost statement. This makes it possible to detect problems and take action as the CA progresses.

The Commission Services prepare an Interim Programme Review, based on process criteria (number of publications, exchanges, patents, etc..), outcome criteria (progress made towards the overall objectives of the programme), and programme impact criteria (scientific achievements, "success stories", exploitation of results, etc.).

At the end of BIOMED 1 implementation in 1996-97, the European Commission will set up an independent panel of experts to evaluate the programme.

Evaluation Reports

1. Evaluation of the concerted actions of the Community's first Medical Research Programme 1978-1981
   Authors: Gordon Wolstenholme (Chairman), R. Akehurst, L. Cedard, V.P. Eijsvoogel, N. Tygstrup, von Manger-Koenig and A. Zanchetti (EUR 7330 - Research Evaluation Report No. 5, 1981)
2. Evaluation of the Community's Medical and Public Health Research Programmes (1980-1986)
   Authors: Lord Hunter (Chairman), Prof. E. Betz, Prof. K. Luft, Prof. C. Rosenfeld, Sir Gordon Wolstenholme (XII/850/85 - Research Evaluation Report No. 15, 1985)
3. Evaluation of the fourth Medical and Health Research Programme (1987-1991)
   Authors: A. Maynard (Chairman), D. Fredrickson, S. Garattini, H. Mäkela, R. Mattheis, M. Papadimitriou
   (EUR 13001 - Research Evaluation Report No. 44, 1990)
4. The Research Networks built by the MHR Programme
   Authors: P. Larédo, B. Kahane, J.B. Meyer, D. Vinck
   Evaluation Unit Coordinator: L. Karatzas (EUR 14700 - Research Evaluation, 1992)
5. Evaluation of the Programme Human Genome Analysis (1990-1991)
   Authors: W. Petterson (Chairman), W. Doerfler, B. Latour, D. Toniolo, H. Vanden Berghe (EUR 15706 Research Evaluation Report No. 59, 1994)
6. An assessment of progress in Human Genome Programmes worldwide. A support study for the evaluation of the EC Human Genome Analysis Programme. Author: B.R. Jordan (EUR 15412 Research Evaluation, 1994)

EU BIOMEDICAL AND HEALTH RESEARCH PROGRAMME COMMITTEES
(1972, 1982, 1994)

1. Comité de Recherche Medicale (C.R.M.) Constituent session of 11 December 1972

J.A.B. Gray	United Kingdom (Chairman)	**European Commission**
S. Halter	Belgium	M. Schuster
P. Lafontaine	Belgium	A. Bertinchamp
J.Chr. Siim	Denmark	R. Villecourt
C. Burg	France	P. Recht
J.L. Bader	France	D. Rabe (secretary)
Brieskorn	Germany	
Henneberg	Germany	
L. Donato	Italy	
F. Pocchiari	Italy	
G. Humphreys	Ireland	
H. Metz	Luxemburg	
A. Betz	Luxemburg	
M.A. Bleiker	Netherlands	
M.J. Hartgerink	Netherlands	
J.M.G. Wilson	United Kingdom	

2. Programme Committee 9-10 December 1982

A. Lafontaine	Belgium	D. Knook	Netherlands
P. Levaux	Belgium	R. St.J.Buxton	United Kingdom
P. de Schouwer	Belgium	R. Cunningham	United Kingdom
K. Krebs	Germany	Sir J. Gowans	United Kingdom
H. Stein	Germany	J. Lee	United Kingdom
P. Backer	Denmark		(MRC secretariat)
N. Rossing	Denmark	A. Carpi	COMAC-BIO
B. Sørensen	Denmark (Chairman)	G. Dean	COMAC-EPI
P. Lazar	France	D. Laurent	COMAC-EPI
C. Rumeau-Rouquette	France	R. Buxton	COMAC-HSR
C. Chirol	France		
G. Maniatis	Greece	**European Commission**	
G. Papaevangelou	Greece	A. Baert	
L. Donato	Italy	H. Balner	
F. Pocchiari	Italy	K. Gerbaulet (Secretary)	
G. Humphreys	Ireland	F. Van Hoeck (Director)	
J. Scott	Ireland	E. Levi	
M. Hartgerink	Netherlands	W. Skupinski	

3. CAN-MED - Committee of an Advisory Nature for Biomedical and Health Research
September 1994

G. Thiers	Belgium	M.X. Fitzgerald	Ireland
M.-C. Lenain	Belgium	G. D'Agnolo	Italy
N. Henry	Belgium	L. Amaducci	Italy
A. Cochez	Belgium	C. Dolcetti	Italy
P. Lange	Germany	E. Cosmi	Italy
H. Stein	Germany	D. Hansen-Koenig	Luxembourg
Ch. Schneider	Germany	R. Hemmer	Luxembourg
H. Lehmann	Germany	P. Decker	Luxembourg
Th. Zickgraf	Germany	C.H.C.M. Buys	Netherlands
J. Olsen	Denmark	J.W. Hartgerink	Netherlands
C. Hugod	Denmark	E.C. Klasen	Netherlands
J. Degett	Denmark	D. van Waarde	Netherlands
M. Bennum	Denmark	J.M. Ribeiro da Silva	Portugal
Ph. Lazar	France	J. Cunha-Vaz	Portugal
G. Tobelem	France	A. Fonseca	Portugal
C. Rumeau-		E. Rodriquez-Farré	Spain
Rouquette	France	L.E. Claveria Soria	Spain
Ch. Chirol	France		
D. Loukopoulos	Greece	M. Alvarez	Spain
N. Anagnou	Greece	L. Soldevilla	Spain
H. Fleischer	Greece	D. Evered	United Kingdom
J. Devlin	Ireland	P. Greenaway	United Kingdom
V. O'Gorman	Ireland	G. Breen	United Kingdom

European Commission

B. Hansen (Chairman)
W. Hunter
A.E. Baert (Secretary)

EEA/EFTA and COST Countries

J.P. Klein	Austria
E. Eksler	Austria
J. Huttunen	Finland
M. Lehto	Finland
G. Agnarsdottir	Iceland
E. Andresdottir	Iceland
A. Stordahl	Norway
P. Wium	Norway
T. Scherstén	Sweden
T. Aronsson	Sweden
I. Vallin	Sweden
H. Nalbant	Turkey

Past Chairmen

J.A.B. Gray
L. Donato
B. Sørensen
H. Stein
Ph. Lazar
F. Van Hoeck
H. Tent

Past Secretaries
D. Rabe
K. Gerbaulet
A.J.G. Dickens

Area I

DEVELOPMENT OF COORDINATED RESEARCH ON PREVENTION, CARE AND HEALTH SYSTEMS

I.1 DRUGS AND THE ADMINISTRATION OF MEDICINES

Introduction

This part of the programme had as an objective the improvement and evaluation of systems for studying quality efficacy and toxicity in the development of pharmaceuticals, over the shortest duration and at the lowest cost.

The identification of hurdles and bottlenecks which can delay the entire process of manufacturing and marketing pharmaceuticals in the EC was also mentioned as a goal. Research had to be encouraged into the monitoring and surveillance of drug prescribing practices, patient compliance and the incidence of adverse drug reactions. A few examples can be mentioned such as the successful concerted action on an international case-control study of toxic epidermal necrolysis and Sven Johnson Syndrome in relation to drug use. Also, action was started in the creation of a European Pharmacovigilance research group which is being extremely performant and eliciting interest and requests for participation from American scientists.

Among other successful research actions, we could mention the creation of a European network for the detection and monitoring of major drug allergies and the determination of European standards for the safe and effective use of phytomedicines.

These and other activities, including the APAS activity presented later in this volume have set the scene for a more structured pharmaceuticals research part of the programme which will be implemented from 1995 in the Fourth Framework Programme now under preparation. The objective of the future programme have been stated as follows: to develop the scientific and technical basis required for the evaluation of new drugs, notably for the treatment of neurological, mental, immunological and viral illnesses. New in vitro tests, cell lines and where necessary animal models, their validation and multi-centre clinical trials and drug safety checks will be included. This research will have to underpin the activities of the European Medicines Evaluation Agency, and will be conducted through collaboration between industry, research centres, hospitals, universities, and the authority responsible for verifying the efficacy, safety and quality of new drugs.

Dr. Giovanni N. Fracchia

DRUG TRANSPORT ACROSS THE BLOOD-BRAIN BARRIER (BBB): NEW EXPERIMENTAL STRATEGIES

Key words
Blood-brain barrier, drug transport, cell culture, microdialysis.

Objectives
The objective of this Concerted Action is to focus on harmonization and exploration of new experimental and often very specialized and sophisticated, methodology on BBB transport and metabolism of drugs (precompetitive!).

Relevant and reliable (*in-vitro* and *in-vivo*) methodology is to be considered of fundamental importance to obtain new insights in possibilities for enhanced and selective drug delivery to the brain. Every participating group has more or less complementary expertise in *in-vitro* and/or *in-vivo* techniques in the area of BBB research. Therefore the action focuses on two complementary aspects:

1 the harmonization and validation of an *in-vitro* endothelial/astrocyte cell culture model to study drug transport across the BBB.

2 the harmonization and validation of an *in-vivo* model to study transport across the BBB (brain microdialysis).

Project leader:
Dr. A.G. DE BOER
Division of Pharmacology,
Center for Drug Research,
University of Leiden,
P.O. Box 9503
NL 2300 RA Leiden
Phone: +31 71 276215
Fax: +31 71 276292
Contract number: CT921193

Participants:
Dr. A. MINN
Centre du Medicament;
Sci Pharmaceutiques &
Biologiques
FR 54000 Nancy
Phone: +33 83 322923
Fax: +33 83 321322

Prof. D.D. BREIMER
Centre for Bio-Phamaceutical
Sciences
NL 2300 RA Leiden
Phone: +31 71 3241111
Fax: +31 71 3243273

Dr M. HAMMARLUND-
UDENAES
Uppsala Univ; Dept. of
Bioharm & Pharmacokin
SE 75123 Uppsala
Phone: +46 18 174357
Fax: +46 18 174003

Dr. M. LEMAIRE
Sandoz; WSP/Bio-
pharmaceutical Dept.
CH 4002 Basel
Phone: +41 61 3241111
Fax: +41 61 3243273

Dr. R. CECCHELLI
Serlia; Pasteur Inst.
P.O. Box 245
FR 59019 Lille Cedex
Phone: +33 20 877754
Fax: +33 20 877906

Dr. Shandt KUMAR
Cristic Hospital; Tumour
Biology Laboratory
UK Manchester M20 9BX
Phone: +44 61 4663210

Prof. Lee L. RUBIN
Eisai London Res Lab;
Univ College London
UK London WC1E 6BT
Phone: +44 71 3807799
Fax: +44 71 3832091

Prof. N.J. ABBOTT
Univ of London,
King's College London,
Biomed. Sci. Div.
Strand
UK London WC2R 2LS
Phone: +44 71 87 32 672
Fax: +44 71 87 32 286

Dr. A. BARTMANN
Merz GmbH & Co.,
Postfach 111353
DE 6000 Frankfurt am Main
Phone: +49 69 15 03 478
Fax: +49 69 59 62 150

Dr. D.J. BEGLEY
Biomed. Science Div.,
Neuropep. Res. Lab.
Strand
UK London WC2R 2LS
Phone: +44 71 83 65 454
Fax: +44 71 87 32 286

Dr. P.O. COURAND
Inst. Cochin-Paris-France,
ICGM, UPR 415
22 rue Mechain
FR 75014 Paris
Phone: +33 1 40 51 64 15
Fax: +33 1 40 51 72 10

Dr. M. DELI
Inst. of Biophysics,
Biol. Res. Ctr.,
P.O. Box 521
HU 6701 Szeged
Phone: +36 62 43 22 32
Fax: +36 62 43 31 33

Dr. C. FRELIN
Inst. de Pharmacologie,
Moleculaire and Cellulaire,
UPR 411 CNRS
Rte de Luc. Sophia Antipolis
FR 06560 Valbonne
Phone: +33 93 95 77 55
Fax: +33 93 95 77 08

Prof. Dr. H.J. GALLA
Westfalische Wilhems Univ,
Inst. für Biochemie
Wilhelm-Klemm-Strasse 2
DE 4400 Munster
Phone: +49 251 83 32 01
Fax: +49 251 83 83 58

Dr. V. VAN HINSBERGH
IVVO-TNO Gaubius Lab.
P.O. Box 430
NL 2300 AL Leiden
Phone: +31 71 18 18 18
Fax: +31 71 18 19 04

Prof. F. JOO
Inst. of Biophysics,
Biol. Res. Ctr.,
Hungarian Academy
of Science
P.O. Box 521,
HU 6701 Szeged
Phone: +36 62 43 22 32
Fax: +36 62 43 31 33

Prof. J. KALUZA
Inst. of Neurologii,
Zaklad Neuropathologii
Ul Botaniczna 3
PL 31503 Krakow
Phone: +48 12 21 41 80
Fax: +48 12 21 39 76

Dr. L.C.M. DE LANGE
Leiden-Amsterdam
Ctr. Drug Res.,
Section of Pharmacology
P.O. Box 9503
NL 2300 RA Leiden
Phone: +33 71 27 63 30
Fax: +33 71 27 62 92

Dr. F. MIXICH
Dept. of Cell Biology,
Faculty of Medicine
4 Petru Rares Str.
RO 1100 Craiova
Phone: +40 94 12 24 58
Fax: +40 94 12 27 70

Prof. Z. NAGY
Semmelweis Medical Univ,
Stroke Centre
Balassa 6
HU 1083 Budapest
Phone: +361 21 00 339
Fax: +361 21 00 339

Dr. J. PAVLASEK
Slovak Academy of Sciences,
Inst. Normal & Pathol.
Physiology
Sienkiewiczova 1
SK 81371
Phone: +42 7 375 428
Fax: +42 7 368 516

Dr. P.A. REVEST
Univ of London,
Dept. of Physiology,
Queen Mary and
Westfield College
Mile End Road
UK London E1 4NS
Phone: + 44 71 98 26 376
Fax: + 44 81 98 30 467

Dr. D. SCHERMAN
UMR 133 CNRS/RPS,
Rhone-Poulenc-Rorer,
Dpt. Biotechnol.
13 quai Jules Guesde, BP 14
FR 94403 Vitry-sur-Seine
Phone: +33 1 45 73 78 47
Fax: +33 1 45 73 77 96

Prof. J.M. SCHERRMANN
INSERM U.26, Unite de
Neurotoxicologie
rue Faubourgh Saint-Dennis
FR 75475 Paris Cedex 10
Phone: +33 1 40 05 43 43
Fax: +33 1 40 34 40 64

Dr. W. SUTANTO
Ctr. Drug Res.,
P.O. Box 9503
NL 2300 RA Leiden
Phone: +31 71 27 62 11

Prof. Z. TRACZYK
School of Medicine in Lodz,
Inst. of Physiol. & Biochem-
istry, Dept. of Physiology
ul. Lindleya 3
PL 90 131 Lodz
Phone: +48 42 78 94 33

Drs. H.E. DE VRIES
Ctr. Drug Res.,
Section of Pharmacology
P.O. Box 9503
NL 2300 RA Leiden
Phone: +31 71 27 62 40

Dr. A. WULFROTH
Merz+Co., GmbH & Co.
Pharmacology
Postfach 111353
DE 6000 Frankfurt am Main

PAEDIATRIC EUROPEAN NETWORK FOR THE TREATMENT OF AIDS (PENTA)

Key words
HIV epidemic, HIV in children, AIDS treatment, PENTA, AZT, anti retroviral drugs.

Brief description
The problems raised by HIV epidemic in paediatrics are of increasing difficulty.
The number of infected infants is steadily growing. This increase is partly linked to a rise in the number of women contaminated through sexual contact.
The clinical presentation of HIV infection in children is variable in its natural history and has not yet been fully elucidated. The Centre for Disease Control (CDC, Atlanta) revised the case definition of AIDS in children in 1987 and is working on a second revision.
The European and French prospective studies of children born to seropositive mothers have recently shown that the transmission rate from mother to child is approximately 20%. The last analysis of French cohort shows that 98% of the infected children are symptomatic at 24 months of age (12% with neurological impairment) and that survival rate of these children is 80% at 70 months.

Therapeutic strategy improvements will depend on several factors:
1 The first strategy is to treat children very early to prevent diffusion of infection. Early diagnostic techniques have to be developed and standardized.
  In adults, with early or symptomatic HIV infection, the results of two placebo controlled trials with AZT decreased the progression to AIDS and ARC. The transposition of these results to children is hazardous and the risk of promoting drug resistance by prolonged use of a drug in asymptomatic children unknown.
2 The second improvement will come from a better definition of factors predictive of severe evolution of the disease. This factors are both clinical and virologic: the poor prognosis of neurodevelopmental involved, is well known. Improved techniques to quantify viral and immunologic load are also needed.
3 The development of new anti retroviral drugs allow the evaluation of combination therapy. Tolerance study of these new drugs alone or in association have to be carefully performed in children before proposing large protocols using combinations or alternate therapy.

Project Leader:
Professor Cl. GRISCELLI
Service d'Immuno-Hématologie Pédiatrique
Rue de Sèvres 149
FR 75015 Paris
Phone: +33 1 42 73 83 01
Fax: +33 1 42 73 28 96
Contract number: CT921303

Participants:

Dr. MECHINAUD-
LACROIX &
dr. RELIQUET
FR 44035 Nantes cedex

Dr. NICOLAS &
dr. HURET
FR 34059 Montpellier cedex

Dr. COURPOTIN
FR 75012 Paris cedex

Dr. VILMER
FR 75019 Paris

Dr. BLANCHE &
dr. DEBRE
FR 75015 Paris cedex

Dr. LEVY & dr. ALIMENTI
Phone: +32 2 535 4647

Dr. LEON LEAL
ES 41013 Sevilla

Dr. Delgado & dr. Aristegui
ES 48013 Bilbao

Dr. RUIZ CONTRERAS &
dr. RAMOS AMADOR
ES 28041 Madrid

Dra. DE JOSE GOMEZ
ES 28046 Madrid

Dra. FORTUNY
ES 08034 Barcelona

Dra. Echeverria LECUONA
ES 20014 San Sebastian

Dr. H. SCHERPBIER
NL 1105 AZ Amsterdam ZO

Dr. Alfredo GUARINO &
Tina CASTALDO
IT 80131 Napoli

Dr. Andrea DE MANZINI
IT 34100 Trieste

Dr. GUIDO CASTELLI
IT 00161 Roma

Dr. Monica CELLINI
IT 41100 Modena

Dr. Patrizia OSIMANI &
dr. Massimo VIGNINI
IT 60100 Ancona

Dr. CANOSA &
dr. Perez TAMARIT
ES 46009 Valencia

Dr. MUR-SIERRA
ES 08003 Barcelona

Dr. Martin FONTELOS &
dr. Mellado PENA
ES 28029 Madrid

Dr. Ciria CALAVIA
ES 07014 Palma de Mallorca

Dr. NADAL
CH 8032 Zurich

Dr. D. CASELLI
IT 27100 Pavia

Dr. A. PLEBANI
IT 20122 Milan

Dr. CLERICI-SCHOELLER
IT 20122 Milan

Dr. C. GIAQUINTO
IT 35128 Padova

Prof. P.A. TOVO
IT 10126 Torino

Dr. E. PALOMBO
IT 10126 Torino

Prof. M. DUSE
IT 25123 Brescia

Dr. A. LOY
IT 16148 Quarto Genova

Dr. A. DE MARIA
IT 16132 Genova

Dr. C. DAMMANN
DE 2000 Hamburg 20

Dr. HEEREN
DE 90419 Nürnberg 91

Dr. D. RICHTER
DE 4000 Dusseldorf

Prof. WAHN
DE 4000 Dusseldorf

Dr. U. WINTERGERST
DE 8000 Munich 2

Dr. G. NOTHEIS
DE 8000 Munich 2

Dr. K. BUTLER
IE Dublin 8

Dr. K. SLOPER
UK Southall UB3 1HW

Dr. V. NOVELLI
UK London WC1

Dr. D. GIBB
UK London WC1

Dr. J. EVANS
UK London W2 1NY

Dr. S. WALTERS
UK London W2 1NY

Dr. G. DAVIES
UK London SW17 0RE

Dr. M. CHARLAND
UK London SW17 0RE

Dr. J. MOK
UK Edinburgh EH10 5SB

Dr. A.B. BOHLIN
SE 14186 Huddinge

Dr. M. DELLA NEGRA
BR Sao Paulo

BIOLOGICALLY ACTIVE CONFORMATIONS OF ANGIOTENSIN AND ANALOGUES AND THE DESIGN-SYNTHESIS OF THERAPEUTICALLY USEFUL DRUGS AGAINST HYPERTENSION AND CARDIOVASCULAR DISEASES

Key words
Angiotensin II, conformation, non-peptide antagonists, hypertension, antihypertensives.

Objectives
This research is aiming at the design-synthesis of therapeutically useful drugs against Hypertension and Cardiovascular diseases on the basis of the angiotensin II receptor conformation we have recently suggested. Structure-activity and conformational studies on angiotensin II and analogues have supported the presence of a Tyr charge relay system mechanism for initiating activity. The obtained information is exploited to understand the ligand-receptor interaction and subsequently to design non-peptide mimetics with improved therapeutic potency.

Brief Description
Angiotensin II is an octapeptide hormone (ANGII:Asp-Arg-Val-Ile-His-Pro-Phe) which is implicated in blood pressure regulation and congestive heart failure. Blockade of the renin-angiotensin system is of primary importance in the treatment of hypertension. The development of angiotensin converting enzyme (ACE) inhibitors that suppress the metabolism of angiotensin I to angiotensin II proved to be an important step forward. A more selective approach has now been realised through the discovery and development of imidazole-based non-peptide AII receptor antagonists.

On the basis of structure-activity relationships (SAR), and fluorescence lifetime and two dimensional nuclear magnetic resonance (2D-NMR) spectroscopic investigations in receptor-simulating environments, a conformational model for angiotensin II (ANG II) has been developed. Using the ANGII conformational model as a basis, non-peptide mimetics of ANGII have been designed, and subsequently were synthesized. Some of these compounds have been shown to act as angiotensin receptor antagonists with potential application in the treatment of hypertension and congestive heart failure. Previously AII receptor antagonists have been modified peptides which suffer rapid metabolism to give inactive fragments when administered orally. As such these compounds constitute a new generation of antihypertensive agents that are likely to have a profound impact upon antihypertensive treatment regimes.

Project Leader:
Professor John M. MATSOUKAS
Department of Chemistry,
University of Patras
GR 261 10 Patras
Phone: +30 61 977180
Fax: +30 61 977118/991996
Contract number: CT920038

Participants:
Dr. B. RIDGE
Dept. of Chemistry; Univ of Exeter
UK Exeter EX4 4QD
Phone: +44 392 263232
Fax: +44 392 263434

Dr. T. MAVROMOUSTAKOS
Inst. of Organic and Pharmacentical Chemistry;
National Hellenic Research
GR Athens
Phone: +30 1 7253821
Fax: +30 1 7247913

Prof. G. MOORE
Dept. of Chemistry; Univ of Exeter
UK Exeter EX4 4QD
Phone: +44 392 263263
Fax: +44 392 263434

Prof. G. MOORE & Prof. HOLLENBERG &
Prof. HABIBI
Pharmacology and Therapeutics;
Univ of Calgary
US Alberta
Phone: +1 3 2833723

Prof. H. MAIA & Dr. M. RONTRIGUES
Dept. of Chemistry; Univ of Minho
PT Braga
Phone: +351 53604370
Fax: +351 53604371

EUROPEAN PHARMACOVIGILANCE RESEARCH GROUP

Key words
Pharmacovigilance, Pharmacoepidemiological research, New Active Substances (NAS's), Adverse Drug Reaction (ADR), Postmarketing Surveillance (PMS), Spontaneous Reporting Schemes (SRS's), Case-Control Studies, Meta-analyses.

Objectives
The European Pharmacovigilance Research Group has been established, within the European Economic Area, to investigate and develop methodologies for the transnational assessment of the safety of marketed medicinal products. Members of the Group include (at present) 21 scientists from 11 European countries.

The objectives of the Group are:

1 to investigate patterns of spontaneous adverse drug reactions (ADR) across Europe; to identify reasons for variations in reporting rates; to develop strategies for improving reporting rates; and to optimise approaches to ADR signal recognition and evaluation.

2 to investigate the potential for, and to undertake, transnational case-control studies across Europe, carried out to a common protocol; and to undertake systematic overview of independent studies.

3 to investigate the feasibility of transnational cohort studies; and to explore possibilities for assembling transnational cohorts of treated and controlled patients for longitudinal studies.

Project leader:
Professor M.D. RAWLINS
Wolfson Unit of Clinical Pharmacology,
University of Newcastle upon Tyne
Claremont Place
UK Newcastle upon Tyne NE2 4AA
Phone: +44 91 222 8041
Fax: +44 91 222 8882
Contract number: CT921556

Participants:

B. BEGAUD
Université de Bordeaux 2;
Service de Pharmacologie
Clinique; Hopital Pellegrin
FR 33 076 Bordeaux Cedex
Phone: +33 57 57 1560
Fax: +33 57 24 5889

B.E. WIHOLM
Medical Products Agency
P.O. Box 26
SE 751 03 Uppsala
Phone: +46 18 17 4644
Fax: +46 18 54 8566

B.H.Ch. STRICKER
Academic Hospital Dijkzigt;
Dept. of Int Med II
Dr. Molenwaterplein 40
NL 3015 GD Rotterdam
Phone: +31 10 4635944
Fax: +31 70 3405048

C.J. van BOXTEL
Academisch Ziekenhuis bij de
Univ van Amsterdam
Meibergdreef 9
NL 1105 AZ Amsterdam
Phone: +31 20 566 9111
Fax: +31 20 566 4440

D.H. LAWSON
Royal Infirmary
UK Glasgow G4 0SF
Phone: +44 41 552 3535
Fax: +44 41 552 8933

E. WEBER
Univ of Heidelberg
DE 69000 Heidelberg
Phone: +49 6221 56 8740
Fax: +49 6221 56 3724

F. GRAM
Odense Univ; Inst. Med Biol
DK 5000 Odense C
Phone: +45 66 15 8696
Fax: +45 66 13 3479

F. SJOQVIST
Karolinska Inst.; Huddinge Hospital
SE 141 86 Huddinge
Phone: +46 8 746 1000
Fax: +46 8 746 8821

F. TEIXEIRA
Inst. of Pharmacology & Exp Therapeutics;
Fac of Medicine
PT 3000 Coimbra
Phone: +351 39 28121
Fax: +351 39 23236

G. TOGNONI
Istituto Mario Negri
Via Eritrea 62
IT 20157 Milano
Phone: +39 2 390141
Fax: +39 2 33200049

Joan-Ramon LAPORTE
Unitat de Farmacologie Clinica;
Dept. de Farm 1 de Psiquiatria
PG de la Vall d'Hebron s/n
ES 08035 Barcelona
Phone: +34 28 30 29
Fax: +34 28 51 12

K. STRANDBERG
Medical Products Agency
P.O. Box 26
SE 751 03 Uppsala
Phone: +46 18 17 4600
Fax: +46 18 54 8566

M. LEWIS
MONICA Project Augsburg; Zentralklinikum
Stenglinstrasse 2
DE 8900 Auchsburg
Phone: +49 821 400 4373
Fax: +49 821 400 2838

M.J.S. LANGMAN
Univ of Birmingham; Queen Elizabeth Hospital
UK Birmingham B15 2TH
Phone: +49 21 472 1311
Fax: +49 21 627 2384

N. MOORE
Cente Régional de Pharmacovigilance;
Hopital de Bolsguillaume
P.O. Box 10
FR 76233 Boisguillaume
Phone: +33 35 08 83 30
Fax: +33 35 08 83 49

P. FLETCHER
IMS International York House
UK London WC1N 3BH
Phone: +44 71 242 0112
Fax: +44 71 895 1052

P.K. LUNDE
Univ of Oslo; Ulleval Hospital
Kirkern 166
NO Oslo
Phone: +47 2 119000
Fax: +47 2 119013

R. EDWARDS
WHO Collaborating Centre for International
Drug Motitoring
P.O. Box 26
SE 751 03 Uppsala
Phone: +46 18 17 4850
Fax: +46 18 54 8566

R.J. ROYER
Service de Pharmacologie et Toxicologie;
CHU Nancy
FR 34 54035 Nancy
Phone: +33 83 85 1758
Fax: +33 83 32 3344

S.M. WOOD
Medicines Conrol Agency; Market Towers
Nine Elms Lane 1
UK Vauxhall
Phone: +44 71 273 0400
Fax: +44 71 273 0675

THE IMPACT OF A SINGLE PHARMACEUTICAL MARKET ON HEALTH CARE SYSTEMS, CONSUMERS AND INDUSTRY (EUROPHARMA PROJECT)

Key words
Health care systems, pharmaceuticals, single European market.

Objectives
The CA aims at contributing to the building up of a common and agreed body of information and knowledge concerning the aspects of the European pharmaceutical scenery. Its main objectives are:

1 an outline of the foreseeable consequences of a single European market on the pharmaceutical industry located in Europe, considered as one of the most important competitors with U.S.A. and Japan on the global international market. The focus will be on the size and quality of the concentration process and on its consequences on employment.

2 an outline of the likely impacts of the unifications process on national health care systems and consumers through the identification of the peculiarities of each national health care system and the consequences of the harmonizing process (induced by the market) on pricing and reimbursement and hence on the public health care expenditure.

Project leader:
Dr. Franco ROSSI
Istituto di Economia Sanitaria
(Institute of Health Economics)
Via Petrarca 13
IT 20131 Milan
Phone: +39 2 4693460\4693512\460242
Fax: +39 2 48195851
Contract number: CT920431

Participants:

Dr. A. BRANDT
Inst. for Medical Informatics and Bostatistics
Bachtelenweg 3
CH 4125 Riehen
Phone: +41 61 673810
Fax: +41 61 673754

Dr. Carlo LUCIONI
Istituto di Economia Sanitaria
Via Boccaccio 14
IT 20123 Milano
Phone: +39 2 4693512
Fax: +39 2 48195851

Dr. Elias MOSIALOS
Univ of Patras; Dept. of Operational Research
GR Patras
Phone: +30 61 997231
Fax: +30 61 997231

Dr. Frans RUTTEN
Erasmus Univ; Medical Faculty
P.O. Box 1738
NL 3000 DR Rotterdam
Phone: +31 10 4087317
Fax: +31 10 4087738

Dr. Reiner LEIDL
Univ of Limburg; Dept. of Health Economics
P.O. Box 616
NL 6200 MD Maastricht
Phone: +31 43 881727
Fax: +31 43 670960

Mme Simone SANDIER
Credes
Rue Paul Cezanne 1
FR 75008 Paris
Phone: +33 1 40768200
Fax: +33 1 45635742

Prof. Antonio BRENNA
Istituto di Economia Sanitaria
Via Boccaccio 14
IT 20123 Milano
Phone: +39 2 4693512
Fax: +39 2 48195851

Prof. Antonio CORREIRA DE CAMPOS
Escola Nacional de Saude Publica
Av. Padre Cruz
PT 1699 Lisboa Codex
Phone: +351 1 7585599
Fax: +351 1 7582754

Prof. Christian Hald JANSEN
The Danish Inst. for Clinical Epidemiology
Svanemollevej 25
DK 2100 Copenhagen
Phone: +45 31 207777
Fax: +45 31 208010

Prof. Felix LOBO
Universidad de Madrid;
Catadratico de Economia Aplicada
Calle Madrid 126
ES 28903 Getafe Madrid
Phone: +34 1 6249500
Fax: +34 1 6249757

Prof. Jean HERMESSE
Dept. of Research and Development
121 Rue de la Loi
BE 1040 Bruxelles
Phone: +32 2 2274111
Fax: +32 2 2373300

Prof. M.F. DRUMMOND
Univ of York; Centre for Health Economics
UK York Y01 5DD
Phone: +44 904 430000
Fax: +44 904 433644

Prof. Peter OBERENDER
Universitat Bayreuth;
Lehrstuhl für Volkswirtschaftslere
P.O. Box 10 12 51
DE 8580 Bayreuth
Phone: +49 921 552880
Fax: +49 921 552886

INTERNATIONAL CASE/CONTROL STUDY OF TOXIC EPIDER-MAL NECROLYSIS AND STEVENS-JOHNSON SYNDROME

Key words

Skin diseases, Erythema multiforme, Stevens-Johnson syndrome, Epidermal necrolysis toxic, Drug hypersensitivity, Drug tolerance, Drug monitoring, Pharmacoepidemiology.

Objectives

Toxic epidermal necrolysis (TEN) and Stevens-Johnson syndrome (SJS) are the most severe forms of cutaneous adverse drug reactions. Both conditions are rare (1 case/million/year for TEN, 1-3 cases/million/year for SJS) but severe (the death rate reaches 30% for TEN).

The primary objective of this study was to quantify risk factors (drugs and other) for SJS and TEN by a formal epidemiologic study comparing the rates of exposure of patients and those of the general population.

The collection of 500 cases and 1,500 controls would allow the detection of relative risks above 5 for most drugs of interest, with prevalence above 0,3% (calculations made with risks alpha=0.05 and beta=0,2). The feasibility of collecting 500 cases in less than 5 years required a base population of more than 100 millions, i.e. an international study. Medical teams form France, Germany, Italy and Portugal are already participating to the study with a combined base population of 100-120 millions.

The realization of our project on an European basis will improve the knowledge of risk factors for so severe disorders and will help Drug Companies and official Agencies to make decisions on what to consider as an *unacceptable* rate of such adverse drug reactions when dealing with spontaneous reports on a newly marketed drug.

Project leader:
Professor J.C. ROUJEAU
Service de Dermatologie,
Hôpital Henri Mondor,
Université Paris XII
FR 94010 Creteil
Phone: +33 1 49 81 25 12
Fax: +33 1 49 81 25 02
Contract number: CT921320

Participants:
Neil SHEAR
Dermatology Division;
Sunnybrook Health Science Centre A3
2075 Bayview Av.
CA Toronto; Ontario MAN 3M5
Phone: +1 416 480 4905
Fax: +1 416 480 6025

Ariane AUQUIER
INSERM U351; Institut G. Roussy
Rue C. Desmoulins
FR 94805 Villeneuf Cedex
Phone: +33 1 4559 4114
Fax: +33 1 4678 7430

Sylvie BASTUJI-GARIN
Dépt. de Recherche en Santé Publique;
Faculte de Medicine
8 rue du Gal Sarrail
FR 94010 Creteil Cedex
Phone: +33 1 4981 3664
Fax: +33 1 4981 3697

Elisabeth BERTELOOT
Dermatologie Hopital Claude Huriez
FR 59037 Lille
Phone: +33 20 44 59 62
Fax: +33 20 44 59 16

Anicet CHASLERIE
Pharmacovigilance; faculté de medecine
FR 33076 Bordeaux Cedex
Phone: +33 56 98 16 07
Fax: +33 56 98 16 07

Nathalie CNUDDE
Dermatologie; Hôpital Ste. Marguerite
FR 13274 Marseille Cedex
Phone: +33 91 96 87 11
Fax: +33 91 75 13 93

Laurent MISERY
Dermatologie; Hôpital Edouard Herriot
FR 69374 Lyon Cedex
Phone: +33 78 53 81 11
Fax: +33 72 33 71 31

Bruno SASSOLAS
Dermatologie Chu. Augustin Morvan
FR 29609 Brest Cedex
Phone: +33 98 22 33 15
Fax: +33 98 22 33 82

Loïc VAILLANT
Dermatologie; Hôpital Trousseau
FR 37044 Tours Cedex
Phone: +33 47 47 46 25
Fax: +33 47 27 71 98

Susan BAUR
Universitäts Hautklinik
Hauptstrasse 7
DE 7800 Freiburg 1 BR
Phone: +49 761 270 6723
Fax: +49 761 270 6829

Francesco LOCATI & Luigi NALDI
Clinica Dermatologica; Università degli studi di
Milano; Ospedali Riuniti di Bergamo
Largo Barozzi 1.
IT 24100 Bergamo
Phone: +39 35 269 401
Fax: +39 35 253 070

Osvaldo CORRELA & Carmen LISBOA
Serviço de Dermatologica; Hospital S. Joao
PT 4200 Porto
Phone: +351 2 617 0976
Fax: +351 2 498 119

David KAUFMAN & Judith KELLY
S.E.U. Boston University School of Med
1371 Beacon Street
US Brooklone; MA 02146
Phone: +1 617 734 6006
Fax: +1 617 738 5119

Robert STERN
Dermatology; Harvard Medical School;
Beth Israel Hospital
330 Brookline Ave
US Boston Ma 02215
Phone: +1 617 735 3200
Fax: +1 617 735 4948

ANTIVIRAL THERAPY OF VIRAL HEPATITIS C

Key words
Hepatitis C, Epidemiology, Drug Therapy, Antiviral therapy, Laboratory
standardization.

Objectives
1 to standardize methodology for hepatitis C RNA measurement;
2 to harmonize diagnostic criteria for viral hepatitis C and endpoints of interferon trials;
3 to study the survival in compensated cirrhosis C (natural course);
4 to meta-analyze individual data from randomized controlled trials in viral hepatitis C
   for prognostic indices without and with interferon therapy, and incidence of serious
   side-effects;
5 to perform long term follow-up of sustained responders of IFN therapy to document
   potential reduction in livercirrhosis, liver failure and hepatic cancer;
6 to study the effect of repeated interferon therapy;
7 to evaluate combination therapy;
8 to confirm the efficacy of interferon in acute hepatitis C;
9 to further develop Eurohep central facilities for statistical analysis and reference
   reagents.

Brief description
Viral hepatitis, in particular chronic viral hepatitis due to hepatitis C, is an important
health problem in Europe. In the high-endemic countries like Greece, Italy, Spain and
Portugal there are at least 1 million virus carriers; in the low endemic countries of
North-Western Europe chronic viral hepatitis predominantly affects haemophiliacs and
other recipients of bloodproducts, drugaddicts, but 30% of virus carriers do not belong
to specific risk groups.
Chronic viral hepatitis progresses in about 25% to cirrhosis, and the majority of cirrho-
tics die from liver failure of hepatocellular carcinoma. The death rate from complications of cirrhosis is particularly high in cases of persistent active viral replication. Chronic viral hepatitis C is now amendable to treatment by alpha-interferon.
Numerous randomized controlled trials have documented that treatment with alpha-
interferon 3 mega Units 3 times a week lead to normalization of the serum enzyme alani-
neaminotransferase (ALT), a marker of liver inflammation, in about 60% of the patients.
However, remission after discontinuation of treatment is observed in only 10-25 percent
(4,8).
Current gaps in knowledge regarding antiviral therapy in viral hepatitis C include:
- is progression of liver disease related to serum markers of liver inflammation and/or
  to the degree of virus C replication?
- is biochemical and virological remission (normal ALT, negative HCV-RNA) after
  interferon therapy associated with inactive liver disease and prevention of cirrhosis,
  liver failure and hepatocellular carcinoma?
- which prognostic factors predict remission after interferon therapy?
- how often does a second course of interferon therapy induce sustained remission in
  patients with an early response, but relapse after a first course of interferon therapy?
- can combination therapy (interferon and ribavirin) induce biochemical and virological
  remission in patients not responding to an initial course of interferon therapy.

- can interferon therapy in acute viral hepatitis C prevent development of chronic viral hepatitis C?

To study these questions, the Eurohep group will collate individual data form prospective randomized controlled trials of antiviral therapy of viral hepatitis C, and analyze stored sera centrally with validated new methodology.

Project leader:
Professor S.W. SCHALM
Dept. Internal Medicine & Hepatogastroenterology,
University Hospital Dijkzigt
Dr. Molewaterplein 50-Ca326
NL 3015 GD Rotterdam
Phone: +31 10 463 59 42
Fax: +31 10 436 59 16
Contract number: CT920735

Participants:

Dr. A. ALBERTI (IT)
Dr. A. ELEFTHERIOU (CY)
Dr. A. MACELA (CS)
Dr. A.P. GEUBEL (BE)
Dr. B. EICHENTOPF (DE)
Dr. Ch. BRÉCHOT (FR)
Dr. Ch. TRÉPO (FR)
Dr. C. FÉRAY (FR)
Dr. D. SAMUEL (FR)
Dr. E. CHRISTENSEN (DK)
Dr. F. BONINO (IT)
Dr. F. DEGOS (FR)
Dr. F. NEVENS (BE)
Dr. F. ZAHM (CH)
Dr. G. FATTOVICH (IT)
Dr. G. GERKEN (DE)
Dr. G. GIUSTINA (IT)
Dr. G. SARACCO (IT)
Dr. G. TEUBER (DE)
Dr. G.E. KITIS (GR)
Dr. G.J.M. ALEXANDER (UK)
Dr. G.M. DUSHEIKO (UK)
Dr. H. RING-LARSEN (DK)
Dr. H.G.M. NIESTERS (NL)
Dr. H.T.M. CUYPERS (NL)
Dr. H.W. REESINK (NL)
Dr. I. CASTILLO (ES)
Dr. I. HOWE (UK)
Dr. J. MAIN (UK)
Dr. J. Van BINSBERGEN (NL)
Dr. J. WILBER (US)
Dr. J.A. ALBRECHT (US)
Dr. J.A. HELLINGS (NL)
Dr. J.A. QUIROGA (ES)
Dr. J.Ch. RYFF (CH)
Dr. J.E. HEGARTY (IE)
Dr. SANCHEZ-TAPIAS (ES)
Dr. J.T. BROUWER (NL)
Dr. K. KROGSGÅRD (US)

Dr. M. KUHNS (US)
Dr. M. PARDO (ES)
Dr. M. RANKI (FI)
Dr. M. URDEA (US)
Dr. M.F. BASSENDINE (UK)
Dr. M.R. BRUNETTO (IT)
Dr. N. BINDSLEV (DK)
Dr. N. OSNA (LT)
Dr. N.V. NAOUMOV (UK)
Dr. P. ALMASIO (IT)
Dr. P. BERANEK (UK)
Dr. P. HONKOOP (NL)
P. KRAGH-ANDERSEN (DK)
Dr. P. MARCELLIN (FR)
Dr. P. SCHLICHTING (DK)
Dr. P. SIMMONDS (UK)
Dr. P.N. LELIE (NL)
Dr. R. ESTEBAN MUR (ES)
Dr. R. NEUMANN (DE)
Dr. R. THOMSSEN (DE)
Dr. R. TUR KASPA (IS)
Dr. R.A. DE MAN (NL)
Dr. R.A. HEIJTINK (NL)
Dr. R.H. DECKER (US)
Dr. S. MAGRIN (IT)
Dr. V. CARREÑO (ES)
Dr. V. HILTBRUNNER (CH)
Dr. W. QUINT (NL)
Dr. W.J. HABETS (NL)
Dr. Z. SCHAFF (HU)
Prof. A. CRAXI (IT)
Prof. A. GOUDEAU (FR)
Prof. A.J. ZUCKERMAN (UK)
Prof. A. EDDLESTON (UK)
Prof. C.F. McCARTHY (IE)
Prof. Dr. K.H. MEYER zum
BÜSCHENFELDE (DE)
Prof. D. SHOUVAL (IS)
Prof. F.B. BIANCHI (IT)

Prof. G. HESS (DE)
Prof. G. LEROUX-ROELS (BE)
Prof. G. REALDI (IT)
Prof. H. BISMUTH (FR)
Prof. H.C. THOMAS (UK)
Prof. H.P. DIENES (DE)
Prof. J. DESMYTER (BE)
Prof. J. FEVERY (BE)
Prof. J.P. BENHAMOU (FR)
Prof. J.P. PASCAL (FR)
Prof. J.P. Vandenbroucke (NL)
Prof. J.P. VINEL (FR)
Prof. K. MADALINSKI (PL)
Prof. L. FASSATI (IT)
M. CARNEIRO DE MOURA (PT)
Prof. M. MANNS (DE)
Prof. M. RIZZETTO (IT)
Prof. O. PESCU (RO)
Prof. P.J. SCHEUER (UK)
Prof. P.L.M. JANSEN (NL)
Prof. R. MÜLLER (DE)
Prof. S.H. YAP (BE)
Prof. S.J. HADZIYANNIS (GR)
Prof. V. DESMET (BE)
Prof. W.H. GERLICH (DE)
W.F. CARMAN (UK)

HISTAMINE H₃ AGONISTS AND ANTAGONISTS AS DRUGS

Key words

Histamine receptors, H_3-agonists, Drug design, Drug synthesis, Molecular cloning, Radioligands, Neuropsychiatry, Gastroenterology, Neuroendocrinology.

Objectives

The main objective of the present program is to design two novel classes of drugs, the H_3-receptor agonists and antagonists, that could be used in therapeutics. We feel, however, that a rational design of such drugs will be facilitated by a letter knowledge of the molecular properties of the H_3-receptor(s), its (their) precise cellular localisation and physiological functions. Hence it is the multidisciplinary efforts of molecular biologists, biochemists, pharmacochemists, physiologists and pharmacologists toward this aim that we want to co-ordinate through the present program.

The partial objectives can be summarized as follows:
a H_3-receptor cloning;
b design, synthesis and initial biological testing of compounds with histamine H_3 agonist or antagonist activity;
c assessment of gastrointestinal effects;
d cardiovascular testing;
e behavioral testing;
f drug development from preclinical up to Phase II clinical assessment.

Project leader:
Professor J.C. SCHWARTZ
INSERM; Unité 109,
Centre Paul Broca
2 ter, rue d'Alésia
FR 75014 Paris
Phone: +33 1 45 89 89 07
Fax: +33 1 45 80 72 93
Contract number: CT921087

Participants:
Dr. J.M. ARRANG & Mr. G. DRUTEL &
Dr. M. GARBARG & Mrs. A. ROULEAU &
Dr. M. RUAT & J.TARDIVEL-LACOMBE &
Dr. E. TRAIFFORT
INSERM Unité 109, Centre Paul Broca
2 ter rue d'Alésia
FR 75014 Paris
Phone: +33 1 40 78 92 83
Fax: +33 1 45 80 72 93

Prof. C.R. GANELLIN & Ms. W. TERTIUK &
Ms. A. PIRIPITSI & Dr. J.A.D. CALDER &
Dr. K.S. WIBLEY & Dr. J.G. VINTER
Univ College London, Dept. of Chemistry,
Christopher Ingold Laboratories
UK London WC1H 0AJ
Phone: +44 71 380 7459
Fax: +44 71 380 7463

Prof. W. SCHUNACK & Dr. H. STARK &
Dr. K. KIEC-KONOWICZ & Ms. K. PURAND
& Ms. A. HÜLS & Mr. M. KRAUSE &
Mr. S. REIDEMEISTER &
Mr. M. NÜMBERG
Freie Univesität Berlin,
Inst. für Pharmazie
Königin-Luise-Straße 2+4
DE 14195 Berlin
Phone: +49 30 838 3278
Fax: +49 30 838 3854

Prof. H. TIMMERMAN & Dr. R. VOLLINGA
& Dr. F. JANSEN
Vrije Universiteit, Dept. of Pharcacochemistry
1083 De Boelelaan
NL 1081 HV Amsterdam
Phone: +31 20 548 4710
Fax: +31 20 646 1749

Prof. G. BERTACCINI & Prof. G. CORUZZI
& Prof. E. POLI & Dr. G. MORINI &
Dr. M. ADAMI & Dr. C. POZZOLI &
Dr. E. GAMBARELLI
Università degli Studi di Parma,
Istituto di Farmacologia, Ospedale Maggiore
Via Gramsci 14
IT 43100 Parma
Phone: +39 521 29 03 83
Fax: +39 521 29 40 89

Prof. G. SOLDANI & Dr. L. INTORRE
Università degli Studi di Pisa,
Istituto di Patologia Speciale e
Clinica Medica Veterinaria
Viale Delle Piagge 2
IT 56124 Pisa
Phone: +39 50 57 05 83
Fax: +39 50 54 35 49

Dr. U. KNIGGE & Dr. A. KJAER &
Dr. H. JORGENSEN & Dr. B. FLEMMING &
Mr. E.L. MADSEN & Mr. P. SOE-JENSEN &
Mr. M. ANTHONISEN & Dr. M. MOLLER &
Dr. P.J. LARSEN & Mrs. E. LARSEN &
Mr. J. BIDSTRUP & Dr. J. WARBERG
Univ of Copenhagen, Dept. of
Medical Physiology C, The Panum Inst.
Blegdamsvej 3C, Building 12
DK 2200 Copenhagen N
Phone: +45 35 32 75 17
Fax: +45 35 32 75 37

Prof. J. COSTENTIN & Mrs. C. PANISSAUD
Laboratoire de Pharmacodynamie et Physiologie,
UER de Médecine et Pharmacie
Avenue de l'Université, B.P. 97
FR 76800 Saint Etienne du Rouvray
Phone: +33 35 66 08 21
Fax: +33 35 66 44 13

Dr. J.M. LECOMTE & Dr. A. KRIKORIAN &
Mr. X. LIGNEAU & Dr. H. BERARD &
Dr. N. PELLOUX
Laboratoire Bioprojet
3 Avenue Pasteur
FR 92430 Marne la Coquette
Phone: +33 1 47 01 17 17
Fax: +33 1 47 01 20 72

Dr. M. BORGGREFE
Medizinische Klinik und Poliklinik;
Innere Medizin C; Westfalische
Wilhelms-Universität Munster
DE 48129 Munster
Phone: +49 25 18 21 45

Prof. Dr. A.J. CAMM
Dept. of Cardiological Sciences;
St. George's Hospital Medical School
Cranmer Terrace
UK London SW17 ORE
Phone: +44 81 76 77 141

Dr. R.N.W. HAUER
Univ Hospital of Utrecht; Heart Lung Inst.
NL 3508 GA Utrecht
Phone: +31 30 67 32 02

Prof H. KLEIN
Med. Akademie; Haus 3/5; Abt. Kardiologie
DE 39120 Magdeburg
Phone: +49 391 67 32 02

Prof. K.H. KUCK
Universitatsspital Eppendorf;
Kardiologische Abt.; 2 Med. Klinik
DE 2000 Hamburg 20
Phone: +49 40 47 17 41 25

Dr. S.G. PRIORI
Ctr di Fisiologia Clinica e Ipertensione;
Ist. di Clinica Medica Generale e Terapia
Medica II; Univ degli Studi Milano
IT 20122 Milan
Phone: +39 2 545 76 66

Prof. P.J. SCHWARTZ
Universita di Pavia; c/o Ist. di Clinica Medica
Generale e Terapia Medica;
Univ degli Studi di Milano
IT 20122 Milan
Phone: +39 2 545 76 66

Dr. P. TOUBOUL
Hopital Cardiovasculaire et Pneumologique
Louis Pradel
FR 69394 Lyon Cedex 03
Phone: +33 72 37 73 41

Dr. H.J.J. WELLENS
Academisch Ziekenhuis Maastricht;
Rijksuniversiteit Limburg
NL 6202 AZ Maastricht
Phone: +31 43 87 51 04

EUROPEAN NETWORK FOR DETECTION AND MONITORING OF MAJOR DRUG ALLERGIES (ENDA)

Key words
Drug allergies, anesthesia, antibiotics, sulfamides, pseudo-allergy, aspirin, non-steroideal anti inflammatory drugs, Ige antibodies, pharmacovigilance, cellular allergen stimulation assay, leukotrienes, leukocyte activation, T lymphocyte activation, T lymphocytes.

Brief description
It is proposed to create a European Network for the study of Drug Allergies (ENDA). Diagnostic and epidemiology of major drug allergies remains a difficult problem. Improvements and development of new diagnostic techniques, require a multicentric European effort. The first goal of the proposal is to pool within a European network the scientific resources and the clinical experience available in the field of drug allergy. As major allergies representing a first priority goal, from an epidemiological point of view, are:

a allergy to drugs (e.g. myorelaxants) and devices (e.g. latex) used in anesthesia;

b allergy to antibiotics and sulfamides;

c allergy and pseudo-allergy to aspirin and other non-steroideal anti inflammatory drugs (NSAIDS). In a first step, the participants to the project would complete the development and evaluate the diagnostic value of two new diagnostic tests:

1 A multidot strip, enabling to detect in a single procedure specific Ige antibodies directed against drugs used in anesthesia or against major antibiotics. This test is particularly suited for epidemiological studies (pharmacovigilance) and for preoperative screening of allergic patients (prevention).

2 A cellular allergen stimulation assay (CAST), based on the production of leukotrienes by leukocytes of allergic patients in contact with drug allergens. This test has the potential advantage to detect not only reactions based on Ige-mediated mechanisms, but also reactions based on other modes of leukocyte activation (e.g. pseudo-allergy to aspirin).

3 The development of easier cellular assays based on T lymphocyte activation. A majority of allergic reactions to drugs are due to interaction of the drug with specifically sensitized T lymphocytes. It seems to develop easier tests amenable to routine use, on the basis of early detection of T cell activation. The ENDA proposed network would provide the most competent scientific frame within Europe to handle problems of Pharmacovigilance related to allergic reactions to drugs, a field somewhat neglected up to now and in which individual, isolated efforts cannot lead to real progress.

Project leader:
Professor Alain DE WECK
Departamento De Alergología
Clínica Universitaria,
Universidad de Navarra
Avda. Pío XII 36
ES 31080 Pamplona
Phone: +34 48 25 54 00
Fax: +34 48 17 22 94
Contract number: CT931661

Participants:

Dr. B. PRZYBILLA
Dermatologische Klinik und
Poliklinik der Universität
Frauenlobstr. 9-11
DE 80337 München 2
Phone: +49 89 5169 4674
Fax: +49 89 5160 4551

Prof. Ag. D. VERVLOET
Hôpital Sainte-Marguerite, Clin de
Pneumo-Pathophysiologie et Allergologie
P.O. Box 29
FR 13277 Marseille Cedex 9
Phone: +33 91 75 17 70
Fax: +33 91 74 16 06

Prof. Ag. D.A. MONERET-VAUTRIN
Hôpital de Brabois, Serv de Méd,
Générale D
Route de Neufchâteau
FR 54511 Vandoeuvre Cedex
Phone: +33 83 15 33 93
Fax: +33 83 59 60 67

Prof. Dr. Alexander KAPP, Dr. W. CZECH
Universitäts-Hautklinik
Hauptstrasse 7
DE 79011 Freiburg
Phone: +49 761 270 6789
Fax: +49 761 270 6818

Prof. Dr. A. OEHLING
Clinica Universitaria,
Dep de Alergologia, Apartado 192
ES Pamplona
Phone: +34 48 25 54 00
Fax: +34 48 17 22 94

Prof. Dr. B. WÜTHRICH,
Dr. F.E. MALY
Universitätsspital Zürich,
Gloriastrasse 31
CH 8006 Zürich
Phone: +41 1255 30 78
Fax: +41 1255 44 31

Prof. Dr. Gianni MARONE
Università degli studi di
Napoli Federico II
Via S. Pansini 5
IT 80131 Napoli
Phone: +39 81 545 28 12

Prof. Dr. H. MERK
Univ of Köln, Dep of Dermatology
Josef Stelzmannstr. 9
DE 50931 Köln 41
Phone: +49 221 478 4540
Fax: +49 221 478 4549

Prof. Dr. Johannes RING,
Dr. D. VIELUF
Universitäts-Hautklinik
Martinistrasse 52
DE 20251 Hamburg 20
Phone: +49 40 4717 2630

Prof. Dr. W.J. PICHLER
Inst. of Clinical Immunology, Inselspital
CH 3010 Bern
Phone: +41 31 64 22 64
Fax: +41 31 25 57 35

Prof. M. BLANCA
Carlos Haya Hospital, Allergy Unit
ES Malaga
Phone: +34 52 30 44 00
Fax: +34 52 27 57 63

Prof. M. SANZ
Clinica Universitaria, Dep de Alergologia,
Apartado 192
ES Pamplona
Phone: +34 48 25 54 00
Fax: +34 48 17 22 94

EFFECTS OF GROUP AUDITING ON IMPROVING DRUG THERAPY IN PRIMARY CARE: A RANDOMIZED CONTROLLED TRIAL

Key words
Group auditing, drug therapy, primary care, elderly dependant, public services, private services, resource allocation.

Brief description
Objective of the project are to define a new protocol in order to integrate public and private activities that offer services for the elderly dependant, and to provide a better understanding of the difference in role and interests among public and private organizations operating in this field. The research presents innovative potential in terms of its approach because it uses a multidisciplinary one in order to consider a wider number of aspects involved in the research subject (such as: financial, medical, engineering and legal). It is also innovative in terms of its contents because till now there have been no attemps to integrate public and private services for the elderly into a single model. The model will provide a framework of reference for a better resource allocation.
Moreover it will facilitate the implementation of new initiatives at an European level.
The project will be divided into four phases:

Phase 1, of data gathering and comparative analisys, will include methodology, carachteristics of the elderly dependant and of the services available to them, and legislations/regulations.

Phase 2, of development of public/private integration scheme, will include organizational diagram, functional and space contents, operational policy, investment and management costs, public-private Integration scheme, cost financing and legal framework.

Phase 3, of implementation of the model of integration, will be carried out testing the model in the following areas: Italy, Denmark, U.K.

Phase 4, of conclusions, will point out relevance of the integration opportunities/problems in general and by country, redefinition of the model of integration, conclusions on public and private roles and interests; recommendations on how to amend the legal frameworks, applicability of the model in other EEC countries, identifications of key elements that condition applicability of the model.

Research duration will be 36 months and will employ 133 man/months.
Results of the research will be made available to the EEC and local Public Authorities.

Project leader:
Dr. Flora M. HAAIJER-RUSKAMP
Dept. of Health Sciences,
Northern Centre of Health Care
Antonius Deusinglaan 1
NL 9713 AV Groningen
Phone: +31 50 63 32 16
Fax: +31 50 63 24 06
Contract number: CT931377

Participants:

Dr. Cl. CRISCELLI
Società Italiana di Medicina Generale
Via Il Prato 66
IT 50123 Firenze
Phone: +39 55 28 40 30
Fax: +39 55 28 40 38

Dr. V.K. DIWAN
Karolinska Inst.
Dept of Int Health Care Research
P.O. Box 60 400
SE 10401 Stockholm
Phone: +46 8 72 86 924
Fax: +46 8 31 15 90

Mr. M. ANDREW
Univ of Oslo,
Dept of Pharmacotherapeutics
P.O. Box 1065 Blindern
NO 0316 Oslo 3
Phone: +47 22 11 9009
Fax: +47 22 11 9013

Prof. Dr. M. KOCHEN
Dept. Practice, Gothingen
Robert Kochstrasse 40
DE 37075 Gothingen
Phone: +49 551 39 26 38
Fax: +49 551 39 95 30

Dr. P. DENIG
Groninger Institute of Drugs Studies,
Noordelijk Centrum Gezondheidsvraagstukken,
University of Groningen
Ant. Deusinglaan 1
NL 9713 AV Groningen
Phone: +31 50 633 216
Fax: +31 50 632 406

Dr. I. MATHESON
Dept. of Pharmacotherapeutics,
University of Oslo
P.O. Box 1065 Blindern
NO 0316 Oslo 3
Phone: +47 22 119 009
Fax: +47 22 119 013

Dr. G. TOMSON & dr. R. WAHLSTROM
Dept. of International Health Care Research
(IHCAR),
Karolinska Institutet
PO Box 60 400
SE 10401 Stockholm
Phone: +46 8 7286 928
Fax: +46 8 311 590

DESIGN AND DEVELOPMENT OF THERAPEUTIC AND DIAGNOSTIC AGENTS FOR THE TREATMENT OF DISEASES OF THE LIVER AND BILIARY TRACT

Key words
Diseases of the liver, targeted drug therapy, liver disease, biliary tract, drug-liand complexes, cell-specific receptors, bile acid-drug complexes, asialoglycoproteins, sinusoidal carries, canalicular carriers, canalicular bile acid transporter, canalicular multispecific organic anion transporter, liver fibrosis, immunological liver disease, advanced fluorescence microscopy, video-image analysis, metabolite analysis.

Brief description
Nine European research groups are working together to develop the concepts and the agents for targeted drug therapy for the treatment of liver disease and diseases of the biliary tract.

Subarea 1   The development of drug-ligand complexes that can be targeted to a particular liver cell by means of cell-specific receptors or carriers. several have already been developed such as bile acid-drug complexes and asialoglycoproteins complexed to various drugs. The drugs of interest are labeled with fluorescent groups to study their destiny within the liver and within the cell. carriers and receptors have been shown to faithfully transport rather bulky complexes. This part of the study requires the synthesis of some of these fluorescent complexes.

Subarea 2   Information will be obtained from cloning and characterization of sinusoidal carriers that have already been cloned and canalicular carriers that will be cloned. candidates for the latter are the canalicular bile acid transporter, CBAT, and the canalicular multispecific organic anion transporter, CMOAT.

Subarea 3   Receptors and carriers on fat-storing cells and bile duct epithelial cells will be characterized. These cells play an important role in liver fibrosis and immunoligical liver disease. Transport and accumulation of drugs into these cells will be studied.

Subarea 4   Cells of interest will be exposed to drug-ligand complexes tagged with a fluorescent label. The uptake, intracellular processing, accumulation and secretion will be studied using the fluorescence microscopy unit.

Request: In all 4 subareas there is a need for advanced fluorescence microscopy and techniques for video-image analysis and metabolite analysis. The purpose of this request is to develop this as a centralized facility with a system of fellowships for use by the EUROTRANS group.

Project leader:
Professor P.L.M. JANSEN
Academic Medical Centre,
Div. Gastroentereology & Hepatology
P.O. Box 30 001
NL 9700 RB Groningen
Phone: +31 50 61 26 20
Fax: +31 50 69 67 91
Contract number: CT931436

Participants:
C. TIRIBELLI
Univ of Trieste, Liver Study Center
and Dep of Biochemistry
IT 34100 Trieste
Phone: +39 40 7764545
Fax: +39 40 910690

D.K.F. MEIJER
Univ Centre for Pharmacy,
Dep of Pharmacology and Therapeutics
Ant. Deusinglaan 2
NL 9713 AW Groningen
Phone: +31 50 633273
Fax: +31 50 633311

E. PETZINGER, K. ZIEGLER
Univ Giessen, Inst. of Pharmacology
and Toxicology
Frankfurter Str. 107
DE 6300 Giessen
Phone: +49 641 702 4950
Fax: +49 641 702 7390

F. KUIPERS
Univ of Groningen, Dep of Pediatrics
Bloemsingel 10
NL 9712 KZ Groningen
Phone: +31 50 632669
Fax: +31 50 632606

G. KURZ
Albert Ludwigs Univ Freiburg, Inst. für
Organische Chemie und Biochemie
Albertstr. 21
DE 7800 Freiburg
Phone: +49 761 203 2833
Fax: +49 761 203 2815

G.L. SOTTOCASA
Univ of Trieste, Dip di
Biochemicia Biofisica e Chimica
delle Macromole
IT 34100 Trieste
Phone: +39 40 5603680
Fax: +39 40 5603694

J. GRAF
Univ Hospital, Dept. of General
and Experimental Pathology
Waehringer Guertel 18-20
AT 1090 Vienna
Phone: +43 1 40400 5130
Fax: +43 1 40400 5126

J. REICHEN
Univ of Berne, Dep of Clin Pharmacology
Murtenstrasse 35
CH 3010 Berne
Phone: +41 31 643191
Fax: +41 31 254713

P.J. MEIER-ABT
Univ Hospital, Dept. of Medicine
Rämistrasse 100
CH 8091 Zürich
Phone: +41 1 2552068
Fax: +41 1 2554411

S. ERLINGER
Université Paris 7, Hôpital Beaujon
FR 92118 Clichy Cedex
Phone: +33 1 40875510
Fax: +33 1 47309440

W. STREMMEL
Univ Hospital of Düsseldorf,
Dep of Int Med
Moorenstr. 5
DE 4000 Düsseldorf
Phone: +49 211 3118944
Fax: +49 211 342229

DETERMINING EUROPEAN STANDARDS FOR THE SAFE AND EFFECTIVE USE OF PHYTOMEDICINES

Key words
Phytomedicines, pharmacovigilance.

Brief description
This project will convene the best available academic, medical and pharmacological expertise towards determining effective standards of safety and efficacy for phytomedicines in the European Community in the public interest.

There are three parts:

1 The ongoing publication of standards for the supply of phytomedicines; a Europe-wide pharmacovigilance programme for phytomedicines with associated validation studies fully integrated with existing national pharmacovigilance centres;

2 the establishment of an expert panel to set operational guidelines

3 and support for new clinical research, and for ethics committees.

Project leader:
Professor Fritz H. KEMPER
Inst. fur Pharmacologie und Toxicologie,
Univ. Munster/FRG
Domagkstrasse 12
DE 48149 Münster
Phone: +49 25 183 55 10
Fax: +49 25 183 55 24
Contract number: CT931238

Participants:

Dr. Catherine CHARVALA
Univ. of Athens,
Dept of Pharmacy
Ventouri Str 23
GR Athens 15561

Dr. Gunter MENG
Dr. Willmar Schwabe
GmbH & Co
Willmar Schwabestrasse 4
DE 7500 Karlsruhe 41

Dr. Nicola CRICHTON
Univ of Exeter, Dept. of
Math Stat and Oper Res,
Laver Building
North Park Road
UK Devon EX4 4QE

Dr. Ulrich SCHMIDT
Arbeits- und
Forschungsgemeinschaft für
Arneimittel-Sicherheit e.V.
Hermeskeiler Strasse 17
DE 5000 Köln 41

Mr. P. BRADLEY
British Herbal Med Ass
Imber Park Road 2
UK Surrey KT10 8JB

Mr. Simon MILLS
Centre for Complementary
Health Studies,
Univ of Exeter
UK Devon EX4 4PU

Prof. Dr. R.P. LABADIE
Rijksuniversiteit Utrecht
Ankermonde 41
NL 3434 GB Nieuwegein

Prof. Dr. W. DORSCH
Kinderkrankenhaus der
Univ Mainz
Langenbeckstrasse 1
DE 6500 Mainz

Prof. J.D. PHILLIPSON
Univ of London
Brunswick Square 29-39
UK London WC1N AX

Prof. Richard EISER
Univ of Exeter,
Dept of Psychology
UK Devon EX4 4QG

Prof. R. ANTON
Faculte de Pharmacie,
Univ Louis Pasteur
Route du Rhin 74
FR 76401 Illkirch

Dr. Desmond CORRIGAN
School of Parmacy
Shrewsbury Road 18
IE Dublin 4

Prof. Dr. H. SCHILCHER
Inst. für Pharmazeutische
Biologie, Freie Univ Berlin
Köningin Luisestrasse 2-4
DE 1000 Karlsruhe 41
Phone: +49 30 8383731
Fax: +49 30 8383729

IMPLICATION OF THE ENDOGENOUS OPIOID SYSTEM IN THE AETIOPATHOGENESIS OF AFFECTIVE DISORDERS AND DRUG DEPENDENCE

Possible therapeutic role of new inhibitors of enkephalin catabolism

Key words

Endogenous opioid system, affective disorders, drug dependence, opioid aganists, inhibitors of the enkephalin catabolism, blood-brain barrier, physical dependence, delta agonists, endogenous enkephalin system, depressive disorders, drug addiction, in vivo autoradiography, behavioral studies, self-stimulation, place conditioning.

Brief description

In the last few years, several delta selective opioid agonists and inhibitors of the enkephalin catabolism have been designed in our laboratory.

Being different from previous compounds, the new agonists (BUBU and BUBUC) and inhibitors (RB 101) are able to cross the blood-brain barrier and are thus active after systemic administration. This improvement in the pharmacokinetic properties represents a decisive step to evaluate their promising therapeutic perspectives. Recent studies show that RB 101 induces potent analgesic and behavioural responses. Interestingly, chronic administration of RB 101 does not induce the physical dependence classicaly associated to opiate administration, not tolerance to the analgesic activity, nor cross-tolerance to morphine. Therefore, the aim of this program is: first, to study the possible therapeutic application of these new delta agonists and inhibitors of enkephalin catabolism; and second, to evaluate the role of the endogenous enkephalin system, by using these new compounds, in the pathogenesis of the depressive disorders and drug addiction. Our research program will allow the harmonization of the chemical, biochemical and behavioral methodologies used in five different laboratories. Indeed, we dispose in our laboratory (INSERM U266-CNRS URA D1500, Paris, Professor ROQUES) of the chemical, biochemical (microdialysis) and molecular (in situ hybridization) equipment necessary for this project.

Biochemical studies concerning binding in vivo autoradiography will be performed in the Department of Pharmacology (Madrid, Professor FUENTES).

Furthermore, to study the antidepressant-like effects and the reinforcing properties it is necessary to use complex behavioral techniques that we do not have. We propose to cooperate with three laboratories that have a large experience in behavioral studies. The techniques developed in these laboratories, self-stimulation (Laboratory of Psychobiology, University of Louvain, Professor DE WITTE), place conditioning (Welsh School of Pharmacy, Professor SEWELL) and Cádiz, Professor MICO), will permit the biochemical and molecular results to correlated with the behavioral responses. The cooperation between several European laboratories, specialized in behavioral studies, mean that a competitive European group in this field will be obtained, able to compete with the well-established behavioral groups in USA.

Project leader:
Dr. Rafael MALDONADO
INSERM U 266, Pharmacochimie Moléculaire
Département de Chimie Organique
Avenue de l'Observatoire 4
FR 75270 Paris Cédex 06
Phone: +33 1 43 25 50 45
Fax: +33 1 43 26 69 18
Contract number: CT931721

Participants:
Dr. Bernard P. ROQUES
Inserm U266, Faculté de Pharmacie
Avenue de l'Observatoire
FR 75006 Paris
Phone: +33 1 43255045
Fax: +33 1 43266918

Dr. José A. FUENTES
Facultad de Farmacie,
Universidad Complutense de Madrid
Cludad Universitaria s/n
ES 28040 Madrid
Phone: +34 1 3941766
Fax: +34 1 3941742

Dr. Juan A. MICO
Facultad de Medicina,
Dep de Neurociencias
Plaza Fragela s/n
ES 11003 Cádiz
Phone: +34 56 228717
Fax: +34 56 223139

Dr. Philippe DE WITTE
Laboratoire de Psychobiologie
Croix du Sud 1
BE 1348 Louvain La Neuve
Phone: +32 10 474384
Fax: +32 10 474745

Dr. Robert D.E. SEWELL
Welsh School of Pharmacy
King Edward VII Avenue,
Cathays Park
UK Cardiff CF1 3XF
Phone: +44 222 874000
Fax: +44 222 874149

PHARMACOLOGY OF METABOTROPIC GLUTAMATE RECEPTORS: THEIR ROLE IN PHYSIOLOGY AND PATHOLOGY

Key words

Metabotropic glutamate receptors, ligands, receptors, second messengers, ischemia, epilepsy.

Brief description

A family of metabotropic glutamate receptors (mGluRs) has been recently descibed. However, no specific ligands are available for these receptors and their pharmacology and functional role remain to be defined.

The proposed research seeks to study the role of mGluR receptors in physiology and pathology. Different groups of scientists will participate to the project. Medicinal chemistry, molecular biology, biochemistry, physiology, pharmacology and experimental neurology techniques will be used.

Seven independent groups from five European countries will be involved. Functional properties of brain regions or neuronal populations expressing different pre- or post-synaptic mGluRs will be evaluated by localizing the neuronal populations expressing different mGluR subtypes and by measuring second messengers (IP3, cAMP, arachidonic acid) and neurotransmitter release in synaptosomes, neuronal primary cultures, brain slices and in vivo .

The modifications of intracellular cytosolic Ca2+ concentrations following activation of mGluRs will be determined in cerebellar granule cells in vitro using fluorescent dyes, such as fura-2, and an image analysis system.

In addition, the possible role of mGluRs in the induction and/or the maintenance of LTP of excitatory synaptic transmission will be investigated in rat hippocampal and visual cortex.

Preliminary experiments suggest the possibility of obtaining selective mGluR agonists using modified sulfate analogs of excitatory amino acids. Newly synthesized molecules will be tested for their potential activity as mGluR agonists or antagonists.

The ischemia- or epilepsy-induced changes of the pharmacological properties of these receptors will be tested by using biochemical assays and hybridization techniques.

We expect to clarify whether mGluRs play a role in these pathologies, and whether their activation or blockade might be protective against seizures or ischemic damage.

Newly designed molecular structures will be synthesized and studied in order to find selective agonists and/or antagonists for the different mGluR subtypes. Upon completion of the project, novel pharmacological tools will be available to the scientific community, as well as molecules which might be developed as drugs.

Project leader:
Professor Flavio MORONI
Dept. of Pharmacology,
University of Florence
Viale Morgagni 65
IT 50134 Florence
Phone: +39 55 423 74 11
Fax: +39 55 436 16 13
Contract number: CT931033

Participants:

Dr. José SANCHEZ-PRIETO
Universidad Complutense de Madrid
ES 28040 Madrid
Phone: +34 1 3943891
Fax: +34 1 3943824

Dr. Klaus REYMANN
Dep of Neurophysiology,
Inst. for Neurobiology
P.O. Box 18
DE 39008 Magdeburg
Phone: +49 391 674160
Fax: +49 391 674161

Dr. Max RECASENS
INSERM - Unité 254
Rue Auguste Broussonnet 300
FR 34059 Montpellier Cedex 1
Phone: +33 67 336975
Fax: +33 67 525601

Prof. David NICHOLLS
Univ of Dundee, Dept. of Biochemistry
UK Dundee DD1 4HN
Phone: +44 382 307780
Fax: +44 382 200894

Prof. Roberto PELLICCIARI
Università di Perugia, Istituto di Chimica
Farmaceutica e Tecnica Farmaceutica
Via del Liceo 1
IT 06123 Perugia
Phone: +39 75 46640
Fax: +39 75 5855124

Dr. Guido VANTINI
FIDIA S.p.A. Research Laboratories
Via Ponte della Fabbrica 3/A
IT 35031 Abano Terme (Padova)
Phone: +39 49 8232111
Fax: +39 49 810927

GENETIC AND BIOCHEMICAL DETERMINANTS OF ALCOHOL TOXICITY AND ADDICTION: THE ROLE OF ALCOHOL DEHYDROGENASE ISOZYMES

Key words
Alcohol toxicity, alcohol addiction, alcohol dehydrogenase, drug addiction, acetaldehyde, susceptibility to alcoholism, sigma-ADH gene.

Brief description
Alcoholism is the most widely spread drug addiction and dependence in Europe, and it is now clear that genetic factors are involved in the development of this illness. A limiting step in ethanol metabolism is its oxidation to acetaldehyde, which is mainly catalyzed by the enzyme alcohol dehydrogenase ADH). The objective of the present project is the search in the European population for specific ADH isozyme patterns and activities which could represent higher susceptibility to alcoholism and to ethanol related diseases such as hepatic diseases and carcinogenesis in the digestive tract. The study will focus on the liver enzyme, which is principal responsible for ethanol oxidation, and on stomach ADH, which may play a major role in the elimination of ingested ethanol (first-pass metabolism). In this regard an additional objective is the characterization of the recently reported gastric sigma-ADH isozyme at the protein, cDNA and gene levels. Liver and stomach biopsies and blood samples from patients with liver disease or gastrointestinal cancer will be collected in Barcelona, Bordeaux, Heidelberg and Stockholm. Biopsy samples will be analyzed for ADH activity and isozyme patterns, and blood samples will be used for genotyping studies by ycr. Statistical analys will be performed to correlate ADH data to alcoholism and to the severity of liver and gastrointestinal diseases. Gender and age of patients will be also considered. Gastric ADH results will be correlated with measures of first-pass metabolism. The possible inhibitory effect of common antiulcerous drugs, such as H2-receptor antagonists, on sigma-ADH will be determined.
Sequence analysis of sigma-ADH will be performed at the protein and CDNA levels, and its three dimensional structure will be estimated by computer-graphics. Kinetic properties will be related to structural features and structure-function relationship will be further investigated by site-directed mutagenesis. The structure and regulation of the sigma-ADH gene will be finally studied.

Project leader:
Dr. X. PARES
Departament de Bioquimica i
Biologia Molecular,
Facultat de Ciencies
Universitat Autonoma de
Barcelona,
Campus de Bellaterra
ES 08193 Cerdanyola del
Vallès
Phone: +34 3 581 12 56
Fax: +34 3 581 12 64
Contract number: CT931601

Participants:
Prof. Hans JÖRNVALL
Karolinska Inst,
Dept. of Chemistry I
SE 171 77 Stockholm
Phone: +46 87 28 7702
Fax: +46 83 37 462

Prof. Helmut K. SEITZ
Krankenhaus Salem,
Dept. of Internal Medicine
DE 69121 Heidelberg
Phone: +49 6221 483 201
Fax: +49 6221 483 494

Prof. Patrice COUZIGOU
Univ Bordeaux II,
Dept. of Biochemistry
and Molecular Biology
FR 33076 Bordeaux
Phone: +33 57 57 1010
Fax: +33 56 99 0380

OPTIMIZING OF CYCLOSPORIN IMMUNOSUPPRESSION: ROLE OF THE DIFFERENT CYCLOSPORIN RECEPTORS AND CD28 ACTIVATION PATHWAYS FOR ACTIVITY AND TOXICITY

Key words
Cyclosporin immunosuppression, CD28 activation, cyclosporin, transplantation, autoimmune disorders, cyclophilins, immunosuppression, nephrotoxicity, CD28 pathway.

Brief description
Cyclosporin (CsA) is a potent immunosuppressant used in clinical transplantation and autoimmune disorders. Cyclosporin binds to specific receptors, known as cyclophilins, and inhibits gene transcription, particularly interleukin-2, upon T-lymphocyte activation. The distribution, intracellu]ar location and role of the different cyclophilins inhibiting the transcriptional machinery is unknown.

The major limitations in clinical use of CsA immunosuppression are large inter-individual variability to the inhibitory effects of CsA and the narrow therapeutic range. The most common complication is nephrotoxicity.

The aim of the proposed investigation is to define the biological role of the cyclophilins and investigate the inter-individual variability of the response in patients.

1 Distribution of the recognized CsA-receptors, cyclophilin A,B and C in the body, cells and fluids, as well as the subcellular location of these proteins.

2 Inter-individual differences in the sensitivity of patients T-lymphocytes to the inhibitory effect of CsA to different modes of activation, especially the CsA resistant CD28 pathway.

3 Correlation of clinical efficacy and side effects in CsA treated patients with experimental parameters: levels of serum and or cellular cyclophilin A,B and C and with in vitro immunosuppressive activity on cultured lymphocytes.

4 Experimental investigations on the role of cyclophilins by over-expression or deletion of distinct cyclophilin gene both in cell lines and mice by homologous recomhination.

5 Exploration on the fine specificity of the cyclosporin-cyclophilin interaction, by using drug derivatives and cyclophilin mutants.

6 Investigations on the role of cycophilins in toxicity in both in vitro and in vivo models.

CsA immunosuppression allowed organ transplantation on a large scale.

The results from these investigations should provide criteria to select patients responding to CsA immunosuppression and predict nephrotoxicity.

It is predicted that the knowledge of cyclosporin receptors in patients and cells as well as of the in vitro sensitivity of the patient lymphocytes, might be useful criteria for the patient selection. The proposed parameters could he easily assessed by ELISA and in vitro proliferation assays in many centers.

The necessary tools eg. ELISA will be developed for a broader and commercial use.

The social and economic benefit of optimizing an immunosuppressive regimen is obvious, if the disaster of graft rejection and/or nephrotoxicity can be avoided in a transparent recipient.

Project leader:
Professor Geneviève SPIK
USTL Laboratoire de Chimie Biologique,
Unité Mixte de Recherche du CNRS n°111,
Bâtiment C9
FR 59655 Villeneuve d'Ascq Cédex
Phone: +33 20 43 48 83
Fax: +33 20 43 65 55
Contract number: CT931748

Participants:
Dr. Bernard HAENDLER
Schering AG
DE 13342 Berlin
Phone: +49 30 468 26 29
Fax: +49 30 469 16 70 7

Prof. Bernard RYFFEL
Inst. of Toxicology of the Swiss Federal,
Inst. of Technology and Univ of Zürich
Schorenstrasse 16
CH 8603 Schwerzenbach
Phone: +41 1 825 74 11
Fax: +41 1 825 04 76

Prof. Brian FOXWELL
Kennedy Inst. for Rheumatology, Sunley Div.
The Charing Cross Hosp
Lurgan Avenue Hammersmith 1
UK London W6 SLW
Phone: +44 81 741 8966
Fax: +44 81 563 0399

Prof. Jean-Paul DESSAINT
Service d'Immunologie, Centre
Hospitalier Universitaire
Place de Verdun 1
FR 59045 Lille Cedex
Phone: +33 20 44 55 72
Fax: +33 20 62 68 93

EUTERP (EUROPEAN TRIAL OF ESTROGEN/PROGESTERON REPLACEMENT TREATMENT IN POSTMENOPAUSE)

Key words
Hormone replacement treatment (HRT).

Brief description
EUTERP pilot study is a necessary preliminary study for an international controlled clinical trial aimed at evaluating the overall risk/benefit ratio of a long term preventive hormone replacement treatment (HRT) in post menopausal women. There is an urgent need for controlled studies to stop controverse on aspects of HRT (need of progestogens, the reduction of cardiovascular risk, the increased risk of breast cancer, the safety for women with atheromatous diseases, the effect on the quality of life). The pilot study main objectives are to compare and finally make a choice of a treatment to be used in a large scale study, to evaluate the safety of the treatment for women with specific risk factors for cardio-vascular diseases, and to constitute a network of doctors throughout Europe, able to work in large-scale field projects.
EUTERP pilot study is a controlled clinical trial, with a factorial design, comparing 2 estradiol routes (transdermal, oral) and 2 progestogens to a placebo. The sample size is 900 allowing a fair power to detect an effect on biological parameters. Post menopausal women between 55 and 60 years, including diabetic women, those with history of deep venous thrombosis, and those with other cardiovascular risk factors will be included. The investigators, 360 general practionners and gynaecologists will recruit each 2 to 5 women. The follow-up duration is 12 months, with 5 visits. Biological tests will be performed for each woman before entry and at the end of the study, and bone mass on a random subsample. Data will be collected using a telematic system, with an interactive quality control. The study will be closely monitored for safety, in particular for women at high risk for CVD. A special Committee will manage bleeding, with access to the code. It will advise the investigators to perform further investigations in women with bleeding.
All patients will be informed about the study by the local investigator and will be required to give informed consent to participation according to local ethical policy.
The investigators - monthly GPs - will be especially trained for the study and to cooperate in large transnational research projects.

Project leader:
Professor Jean-Pierre BOISSEL
University de Pharmacology Clinique
B.P. 3041
162 avenue Lacassagne
FR 69394 Lyon Cedex 03
Phone: +33 72 115 265
Fax: +33 78 31030
Contract number: CT931314

Participants:

Dr. J. STEVENSON
National Heart and Lung Institute,
Wynn Institute for Metabolic Research,
University of London
21 Wellington Road
UK London NW8 9SQ
Phone: +44 71 586 22 66
Fax: +44 71 586 31 23

Dr. F. BORRUTO
Dept. of Gynaecology, Vicolo Monachine,
University of Padova
IT 40 37 100 Verona
Phone: +39 49 8213 40 00
Fax: +39 49 875 08 60

Dr. B. PORNEL
Brussels Menopause Medical Center
505 Avenue Louise
BE 1050 Brussels
Phone: +32 2 647 07 53
Fax: +32 2 646 63 72

Dr. G.B. MELIS
Instituto di Ginecoligia Ostetricia e
Fisiopatologia Della Riproduzione Umana,
Università degli Studi di Cagliari
Via Ospedale 46
IT 09100 Cagliari
Phone: +39 70 65 27 97
Fax: +39 70 66 85 75

Dr. C. NETELENBOS
Free University Hospital,
Dept. of Endocrinology
P.O. Box 7057
NL 1007 MB Amsterdam
Phone: +31 20 548 75 33
Fax: +31 20 548 72 02

Dr. C. CHRISTIANSEN
Glostrup Hospital,
Dept. of Clinical Chemistry,
University of Copenhagen
DK 2600 Glostrup
Phone: +45 42 96 43 33
Fax: +45 44 68 42 20

Dr. E. DRAPPIER FAURE
Hopital Edouard Herriot, Pavillon L
Place d'Arsonval
FR 69437 Lyon Cedex 03
Phone: +33 72 34 48 28
Fax: +33 72 34 48 40

ADR SIGNAL ANALYSIS PROJECT (ASAP)

Key words
Adverse Drug Reactions (ADR), drug monitoring, pharmacovigilance, post-marketing surveillance, drug use, ADR signals, drug safety.

Brief description
This proposal aims to combine existing data from EC and other countries on adverse drug reactions, from the WHO Collaborating Centre for International Drug Monitoring, with drug denominators from IMS International. After examining the best ways to use the data with illustrative drug/ADR examples, the data bases will be used to evaluate contemporary drug problems and drug/ADR signals.

The data collected by both organizations on a routine basis will allow adverse drug reaction reports to be examined against a variety of drug use and demographic denominators. New drug/ADR signals can be easily evaluated over time, so that new perspectives on those signals should result.

Whilst the limitations of continuously collected ADR and drug use data are accepted, it is considered that the combined use may give new drug safety insights and allow for more focused studies.

Project leader:
Professor Ivor Ralph EDWARDS
WHO Collaborating Centre for
International Drug Monitoring
P.O. Box 26
SE 751 03 Uppsala
Phone: +46 18 17 48 50
Fax: +46 18 54 85 66
Contract number: CT941301

Participants:
Dr. J. SANDERSON
IMS International Ltd.
37 Queen Square
UK London WC1N 3BH
Phone: +44 71 2420 112
Fax: +44 71 8951 052

Prof. J.S. SCHOU
Dept. of Pharmacology, University
of Copenhagen, Panum Institute
Blegdamsvej 3
DK 2200 Copenhagen
Phone: +45 31 357 900
Fax: +45 31 395 068

THE USE OF THE EUROPEAN FORMULARY FOR GENERAL PRACTICE TO IMPROVE COST EFFECTIVE PRESCRIBING

Key words
Drug formulary, cost-effective prescribing, prescribing habits.

Brief description
Since 1988 50 general practitioners, clinical pharmacologists and pharmacists from 16 European countries have collaborated together to produce a formulary of drugs for patients common conditions which are necessary, safe and effective.

This formulary is now to be received by departments of general practice, clinical pharmacology and pharmacists and some individual GPs prior to final publication towards the end of 1993. The planned action is to select a sample of GPs from a number of European countries to see if they will use the formulary to improve costeffective prescribing.

Firstly, they will prescribe as they do now, and we will have a base line assessment of prescribing habits.

Then they will be given the European formulary and access to the appendix which explains the reasons for the choice of drugs.

The same number of prescriptions will then be collected again and we shall assess the changes introduced by contact with the formulary and its appendix.

We hope from this to improve cost-effective prescribing and ascertain how best to disseminate this information and knowledge throughout general practitioners in Europe.

Project leader:
Dr. David GREGORY
University of Newcastle upon Tyne,
Dept of Primary Health Care,
The Medical School
Framlington Place
UK Newcastle-upon-Tyne NE2 4HH
Phone: +44 91 222 60 00
Fax: +44 91 222 78 92
Contract number: CT941477

Participants:
Dr. George GRANT
Dept. of Health Care,
The Medical School
Framlingtyon Place
UK Newcastle upon Tyne NE2 4HH
Phone: +44 661 823 294
Fax: +44 91 222 7892

Dr. J.D. GILLEGHAN
Lothian Formulary Group,
Ladywell Medical Centre
Ladywell Road
UK Edinburgh EH12 7TB
Phone: +44 31 334 3602
Fax: +44 31 316 4816

Prof. Philip REILLY
Dept. of General Practice,
Queens University of Belfast,
Dunluce Health Centre
UK Belfast BT9 7HR
Phone: +44 232 240 884
Fax: +44 232 310 202

Dr. Luc BLONDEEL
Project Farmaka
J. Vervaenestraat 14
BE 9050 Gent
Phone: +32 2 238 2859
Fax: +32 2 230 3862

Dr. Daniele COEN
Instituto Mario Negri
Via Eritrea 62
IT 20157 Milano
Phone: +39 2 932 3200
Fax: +39 2 390 01916

Dr. Gaut GADEHOLT
Bjerkebakken 75 A
NO 0756 Oslo
Phone: +47 22 897 737
Fax: +47 22 897 799

Prof. Michael M. KOCHEN
Abt. Allgemeinmedizin der Universitat Gottingen
Robert-Koch-Strasse 40
DE 3400 Gottingen
Phone: +49 551 392 638
Fax: +49 551 399 530

Dr. Gerd GLEASKE
Oststrasse 53
DE 4000 Dusseldorf
Phone: +49 2241 108 330/285
Fax: +49 2241 108 325

Dr. Nicholas MOORE
CHU Rouen
BP 100
FR 76233 Boisguillaume cedex
Phone: +33 35 08 8330
Fax: +33 35 08 8349

Dr. P.G.M. Theo DE VRIES
Dept. of Pharmacology, University of Groningen
Bloemsingel 1
NL 9713 BZ Groningen
Phone: +31 50 632 808/810
Fax: +31 50 632 812

Dr. O.V. CLARKE
Dublin Regional Vocational Training Scheme
for General Practice, Corrigan House
Fenian Street
IE Dublin 2
Phone: +353 1 661 6049
Fax: +353 1 676 5791

Dr. J.M. ARNAU
Dept. of Farmacologica i de Psiquiatria,
Cuitat Sanitaria de la Vall d'Hebron
Pg. Vall d'Hebron s/n
ES 08035 Barcelona
Phone: +34 3 428 3029
Fax: +34 3 428 5112

Dr. Z. AZEREDO & mrs. M. PERAIRA
Hospital de Santa Maria
Rua Coelho da Rocha 155-4
PT 1300 Lisboa
Phone: +351 1 67 36 59
Fax: +351 1 52 14 24

DEVELOPMENT OF RECOMBINANT ORTHO- AND PARA-MYXOVIRUS VACCINES BY REVERSE GENETIC TECHNIQUE

Key words
Influenza and Sendai viruses, HEF antigen.

Brief description
The final goal of the proposed project concerns the development of recombinant ortho- and paramyxovirus vaccines. For that purpose, influenza and Sendai viruses will be modified using reverse genetic technique to change viral antigens or antigenic epitopes.

Therefore, a first important step is the identification and analysis of epitopes located on mumps virus HN and F antigens (participant 02). After expression in prokaryotic and eukaryotic cells, the entire or fragmented proteins will be purified and the immunological potential of all recombinant viruses developed.

Naturally occurring virus will be manipulated in two different ways:

1 Based on the high experience of participant (03), who analyzed the structure of the influenza C virus HEF antigen, the respective gene will modified by site-directed mutagenesis. Antigenic epitopes of the mumps virus genes HN and F will be inserted into this glycoprotein at those positions where the foreign insertion may not adversely affect the biological activities of this protein.

2 In another approach, participant (04), will replace parts of the HA protein from high growth influenza A or B virus with the respective ones from strains which are believed to cause a new epidemic. The resulting chimeras will exhibit growth characteristics of a high growth strain and will express the HA antigen of a new virus and paramyxoviruses will be developed.

Based on the influenza C virus strain of team (03), participant (04) will construct a viral vector which is able to express foreign genes. Helper cell lines expressing the viral capsid proteins should be very useful in the initial steps of viral rescue. For the construction of those cell lines, the great experience of team (01) can be used which has already established cell clones expressing up to three genes simultaneously. These cell clones are shown to support the replication and packaging of RNA from Sendai virus defective interfering particles (DIP). Furthermore, team (01) constructed Sendai viral replicons containing the termini of the viral genome and a reporter gene. Based on these constructs, recombinant viruses will be developed which are able to express foreign antigens in high amounts.

Project leader:
Dr. Wolgang J. NEUBERT
Max-Planck-Institut
für Biochemie,
Abteilung Virusforschung
Am Klopferspitz 18A
DE 82152 Martinsreid
Phone: +49 89 8578 2268
Fax: +49 89 8578 3777
Contract number: CT941600

Participants:
Prof. Pier E. VALENSIN
Università degli Studi,
Sezione di Microbiologia
Via Laterina 8
IT 53100 Siena
Phone: +39 577 280903
Fax: +39 577 42011

Prof. H. MEIER-EWERT
Institut für Medizinische
Mikrobiologie and Hygiene,
Abteilung für Vorilogie
Biedersteinerstrasse 29
DE 80802 München
Phone: +49 89 3849 3245
Fax: +49 89 3849 3243

Dr. James S. ROBERTSON
National Inst. for Biological
Standards and Control
UK Hertfordshire EN6 SQG
Phone: +44 707 654 753
Fax: +44 707 646 730

EARLY IDENTIFICATION FACTORS RESPONSIBLE FOR THE IN-TERINDIVIDUAL VARIABILITY IN DRUG METABOLISM IN MAN

Key words
Interindividual variability in drug metabolism, therapeutic response, pharmacokinetics, conjugation reactions, acetylation, cytochrome P-450, quantative drug interaction predictions.

Brief description
There is a general consensus in the scientific pharmacological community to consider the variability in drug metabolism as the primary factor in determining the variability in the tissue concentration of drugs, and therefore, in the therapeutic response.

The present project focuses on the interindividual variability in drug metabolism and in man.

This project focuses on the variability of the quantitatively more important enzymes catalyzing the oxidation and conjugation of drugs.

The approach to the study includes *in vivo* and *in vitro* tests all performed in man or in human tissues.

The subsidiarity of this project is evident, and our results including the protocols for in vitro assays and the in vivo kinetics, will be the starting point for others.

The objectives of the present proposal are:

A   To determine the extent of variation and to define the frequency distribution of the quantitatively more important conjugation reactions: the glucuronidation, the acetylation, the methylation and the sulphation in the human liver, intestine, kidney and lung. The enzyme activities will be measured with the phenotype and the genotype of the acetylation will also be studied in vivo in a population of patients before and after liver transplant. In vitro methods for predicting variability will be investigated.

B   To characterize the expression and the frequency distribution of sulphation and methylation in the blood components of 2 European ethnic groups residing in distant European areas and characterized by different social backgrounds: the Finnish and the Spanish.

C   To investigate the interindividual distribution of relevant forms of cytochrome P-450. The study will focus on the variability in the metabolism of clinically important drugs such as neuroleptics, antidepressants betablockers, antivirals and analgesics. The relationship between the expression of individual isoforms and the susceptibility to disease and ethnic differences will be studied. Methods for predicting specificity and variability of oxidation of new drugs will be studied.

D   To examine interindividual variability in pharmacokinetics with assessment of the variability in the rate of formation of pharmacologically active metabolites in vivo.

Statistical (population) methods will be applied to estimate the contribution of various factors. Strategies will be developed to scale quantitatively in vitro and in vivo data and estimate variability due to drug interactions including the use of Quantitative Drug Interaction Predictions (Q-DIPS).

Project leader:
Professor G.M. PACIFICI
Department of Biomedicine,
Medical School, University of Pisa
Via Roma 55
IT 56100 Pisa
Phone: +39 50 554851/66
Fax: +39 50 554929
Contract number: CT941622

Participants:

Prof. Cesare SIRTORI
Institute of Pharmacological
Sciences
Via Balzaretti 9
IT 20133 Milan
Phone: +39 2 2940 4672
Fax: +39 2 2940 4961

Prof. Mario FURLANUT
Dept. of Internal Medicine
and Medical Therapy
Piazza Botta 10
IT 27100 Pavia
Phone: +39 382 386360
Fax: +39 382 22741

Dr. Edoardo SPINA
Institute of Pharmacology
Piazza XX Settembre 4
IT 98122 Messina
Phone: +39 90 712 533
Fax: +39 90 661 090

Prof. Pierre KREMER
Service of Medical Chemistry
Domaine Universitaire du
Sart Tilman, B35
BE 4000 Liege 1
Phone: +32 41 562 471
Fax: +32 41 562 481

Prof. Pierre BECHTEL
Service of Clinical Pharma-
cology, Hopital Jean Minjoz
FR 25030 Besancon Cedex
Phone: +33 81 658 300
Fax: +33 81 669 499

Dr. Alain R. BOOBIS
Dept. of Clinical
Pharmocology, Royal Post-
graduate Medical School
Du Cane Road
UK London W12 ONN
Phone: +44 81 7403 221
Fax: +44 81 7493 439

Prof. G.T. TUCKER &
Dr. Martin S. LENNARD
University Dept. of Medicine
and Pharmacology,
Section of Pharmacology and
Therapeutics, The Royal
Hallamshire Hospital
Glossop Road
UK Sheffield S10 2JF
Phone: +44 742 766 222
Fax: +44 742 720 275

Prof. Malcom ROWLAND
Dept. of Pharmacy
UK Manchester M13 9PL
Phone: +44 61 2752 378
Fax: +44 61 2738 196

Dr. David BACK
Dept. of Pharmacology
and Therapeutics
Ashton Street P.O. Box 147
UK Liverpool L69 3BX
Phone: +44 51 7945 547
Fax: +44 51 7945 540

Prof. Ulrich KLOTZ &
Dr. Heyo K. KROEMER
Dr. Margarete Fischer-Bosh-
Institute
Auerbachstrasse 112
DE 7000 Stuttgart 50
Phone: +49 711 8101702/5
Fax: +49 711 859295

Prof. Julio BENITEZ
Dept. of Pharmacology,
Medical School
ES 06071 Badajoz
Phone: +34 24 275 459
Fax: +34 24 271 100

Prof. Folke SJOQVIST
Dept. of Clinical Pharma-
cology, Karolinska Institute,
Huddinge Hospital
SE 14186 Huddinge
Phone: +46 8 7461 166
Fax: +46 8 7468 821

M.INGELMAN-SUNDBERG
Dept. of Physiological Chem-
istry, Karolinska Institute
P.O. Box 60400
SE 10401 Stockholm
Phone: +46 8 7287 735
Fax: +46 8 338453

Prof. Anders RANE
Division of Clinical
Pharmocology,
University Hospital
SE 75185 Uppsala
Phone: +46 18 663 000
Fax: +46 18 519 237

Prof. Olavi PELKONEN
Dept. of Pharmacology and
toxicology,
University of Oulu
Kajaanintie 52D
FI 90220 Oulu gen
Phone: +358 81 332 133
Fax: +358 81 330 687

Dr. Thierry LEEMAN
Division of Clinical Pharma-
cology, Hospital Cantonel
Universitaire de Geneve
24 rue Micheli-du-Crest
CH 1211 Geneve 4
Phone: +41 22 3729 932/30
Fax: +41 22 7894 356

HEPATOCYTE CULTURE TECHNOLOGY: APPLICATION POSSIBILITIES IN A BIOARTIFICIAL LIVER DEVICE

Key words
Hepatocytes culture, bioartificial liver device, liver transplantation, liver metabolism, in vitro studies, pharmacotoxicology, metabolism of xenobiotics.

Brief description
The liver is an indispensable, complex organ. At present, neither a temporary replacement therapy for patients with liver failure exists (excepting organ transplantation), nor is there an acceptable model available for in vitro studies on liver metabolism that would be extremely useful for a variety of hepatological, pharmacological, and toxicological investigations. Many research activities have aimed at the construction of a bioartificial liver device with human and animal cells, but still fundamental questions as the suitability of carrier materials, the cell attachment and survival in long-term cultures remain to be answered. Until now standard techniques have failed to support the survival of liver cells in any kind of bioartificial device.

It will be the aim of the proposed concerted action to bring together four teams from three different European countries to exchange knowledge and to coordinate their research Work in biotechnology and hepatology. The purpose of the cooperation Will be the design of a bioreactor to be used as a bioartificial liver.

Each of these teams is actually involved in hepatological and/or bio-technological research programs and is therefore highly specialized in different technologies which are essential for the development of the bio-artificial liver device. This includes specialists in clinical hepatology, cell biology, hepatocyte culture, bioreactor usage, pharmacology and in the development of biomaterials and devices.

The project program includes meetings, to discuss the culture of hepatocytes and the approaches already been made to realize an artificial liver device. The different culture technologies Will be demonstrated at the individual laboratories and their suitability for the device will be studied: carrier materials for hepatocytes, already developed for other biomedical purposes, Will be exchanged and tested under the particular conditions of every team. The comparison of the different culture methods and reference materials will be the basis for a standardized and optimized hepatocyte culture. Finally the technology will be implicated in the design of a bioreactor for long-term hepatocyte culture, which may be usable both for temporary liver replacement and investigation of the metabolism of xenobiotics in the liver.

Project leader:
Dr. Ing. Heinrich PLANCK
Institut für Textil- und Verfahrenstechnik
Forschungsbereich Biomedizintechnik
Körschtalstrasse 26
DE 73770 Denkendorf
Phone: +49 711 3408 263
Fax: +49 711 3408 297
Contract number: CT941097

Participants:

Dr. M. DOSER
Institute of Textile Research and Chemical
Engineering, Div. of Biomedical Engineering
Körschtalstrasse 26 Körschtalstrasse 26
DE 73770 Denkendorf
Phone: +49 711 3408 263
Fax: +49 711 3408 416/297

Prof. J. FEVERY & prof. S.H. YAP
Dept. of Medicine, Universital Hospital
Gasthuisberg
BE 3000 Leuven
Phone: +32 16 33 2211
Fax: +32 16 34 4387

Dr. H.G. KOEBE & W. THASLER
Dept. of Surgery, Klinikum Grosshadern
Marchioninistrasse 15
DE 81377 Muenchen
Phone: +49 89 7095 3432
Fax: +49 89 7004 418

Prof. M.J. GOMEZ-LECHON &
Prof. J.V. CASTELL
Unida Hepatologia Experimental,
Hospital Universitario 'La Fe'
Avenida de Campanar 21
ES 46009 Valencia
Phone: +34 6 3868 748
Fax: +34 6 3868 718

ANTIGENICITY OF RECOMBINANTLY DERIVED PHARACEUTICALS IN MAN

Key words
Recombinant DNA technology, cytokines, hormones, therapeutic proteins, vaccines, antigenicity interferons, interleukines, naturally occurring antibodies.

Brief description
A number of cytokines, hormones and therapeutic proteins produced by recombinant DNA technology are at present under clinical evaluation or already have been marketed for shorter or longer periods.

Although produced in cells transformed with human genes, the products apparently are not completely identical to their natural counterparts, for example, some may not be glycosylated, at all.

The differences between the natural proteins and their r-DNA analogues are apparent from their pharmacokinetic behaviour, stability, biological activity and antigenicity.

Formation of antibodies have been reported for a number of recombinant DNA products such as interferon alpha, interferon beta, interleukine-2, GM-CSF, insulin, growth hormone and others.

Sometimes, these induced antibodies may cross-react with the native proteins present in man (for example, interferon-alpha). In some cases the formation of antibodies has resulted in diminished response to the products.

The long term consequences for the individuals which produce antibodies which neutralise the naturally produced proteins are unknown, but may be potentially severe.

For example, as it appears that man, generally speaking, has naturally occurring auto-antibodies against several of the cytokines described the eventual biological status may be even more difficult to predict as it can be expected that the levels of these autoantibodies might be changed subsequent to treatment with the recombinantly derived cytokines.

Thus, an analysis of factors influencing the formation of antibodies to recombinantly derived proteins and the eventual consequences can only be made via a large international study.

Project leader:
Dr. H. SCHELLEKENS
Diagnostic Centre SSDZ
Rainier de Graafweg 7
PO Box 5010
NL 2600 GA Delft
Phone: +31 15 60 30 50
Fax: +31 15 56 81 03
Contract number: CT941699

Participants:
Dr. D. POLLET
Innogenetics SA
Kronenburgstraat 45
BE 2000 Antwerpen
Phone: +32 32 523 711
Fax: +32 32 523 798

Dr. P.H. VAN DER MEIDE
TNO-Rijswijk
P.O. Box 5815
NL 2280 HV Rijswijk
Phone: +31 15 842 842
Fax: +31 15 843 998

Dr. P. VON WUSSOW
Abt. Immunologie und
Transfusionsmedizin,
Interferonlabor, Medizinische
Hochschule Hannover
Postfach 610180
DE 3000 Hannover 61
Phone: +49 511 532 3617
Fax: +49 511 532 5890

Dr. K. BERG
The Interferon Laboratory,
Int. Med. Microbiology,
The Panum Institute 22.3.19
Blegdamsvejen 3
DK 2200 Copenhagen
Phone: +45 3532 7690
Fax: +45 3532 7691

I.2 RISK FACTORS AND OCCUPATIONAL MEDICINE

Introduction

Research on risk factors and occupational medicine is aiming at improving the scientific knowledge needed to improve the occupational health of European workers by establishing safe work places and a safe environment.

The research projects carried out in this area, are dealing with the evaluation of the risk associated with the use of specific equipment (e.g. display screen equipment), with exposure to dangerous substances (e.g. solvents, diesels, organic acid metals, asbestos, etc.) and to virus and other infectious agents, bio-allergens, with an emphasis on susceptibility and hypersensitivity to specific risk. Epidemiological studies are aiming at identifying determinant of occupation - related disease, with an emphasis on pulmonary diseases, cancer (including non-common cancers), congenital pathologies, and fertility and at assessing environmental risk factors on morbidity or mortality.

Standardization and validation of methodology for in vitro toxicology research is being performed within a European network of laboratories.

Dr. Christiane Bardoux

SULPHATION OF INDUSTRIAL AND OTHER CHEMICALS IN MAN: SUSCEPTIBILITY TO CHEMICAL-INDUCED DISEASES

Key words
Sulphotransferase, Cancer, Occupational Disease, Carcinogens, Bioactivation.

Objectives
1 To provide the scientific knowledge base to facilitate assessment of the role of sulphotransferases in the toxicity of industrial chemicals.
2 To study the role of sulphation in carcinogenesis by alkyl aromatic hydrocarbons and
   aromatic amines, and to identify the specific ST isoforms involved in the bioactivation
   of these compounds in man.
3 To identify key structural features of the above groups of chemicals which determine
   their bioactivation by sulphation.
4 To assess the effects of disruption of endogenous compound sulphation by industrial
   chemicals, with particular reference to effects on key physiological systems such as
   the brain and the thyroid.
5 To investigate the use of safe marker compounds which can be used to assess sulphation capacity *in vivo* in man.
6 To determine the relationship between genetic variability in the expression of sulfo-
   transferases in the human population and susceptibility to occupation-related diseases,
   as well as to organ-specific toxicity, related to exposure to aromatic amines and alkyl
   aromatic hydrocarbons.

Brief description
Disease resulting from exposure to toxic chemicals in the workplace represents a significant burden on society, both from the moral and economic standpoints. Our ability to
reduce the incidence of such occupational illness is dependent on numerous factors including, in particular, legislation aimed at improving safety in the workplace. However, it
is of equal importance to understand the mechanisms controlling the processes of chemi-
cal-induced disease in order that we may more readily identify groups of compounds
which represent a particular risk, and also groups of individuals who may be at
increased risk of succumbing to the toxic effects of particular chemicals.
This project is designed to determine the role of the conjugating enzyme family, the
sulphotransferases (STs), in the bioactivation of precarcinogens, using two widely used
classes of compound which are known to be bioactivated following conjugation with
sulphate, namely aromatic amines and benzylic alcohols of polycyclic aromatic hydrocarbons. Particular study will be made of two potential target organs for such toxicity,
namely the brain and the thyroid.
The approach to be taken involves cloning of the cDNAs representing the STs involved
in these reactions, and the establishment of stable cell lines expressing these enzymes in
order to determine, using computer molecular modelling, the structural features of molecules which determine their bioactivation by this pathway. Molecular probes generated
by this molecular biological approach will be also be used to assess the location and the
tissue-specific and interindividual variation in ST expression. In parallel, safe drug
probes for sulphation will4 be developed in order to study this variability *in vivo*.
It is therefore the aim of this project to harness the expertise of the major groups working on sulphation within the EC to investigate, at the molecular level, the role of sulpha-

tion and STS in the bioactivation of industrial chemicals and in individual susceptibility to the toxicity of these compounds. This important information will, in addition to providing a substantial knowledge base for our understanding of the mechanisms of toxicity of such compounds, improve the reliability of evaluating risks associated with exposure to these chernicals.

The project will be performed through provision and exchange of data and materials, exchange of personnel, expert meetings and workshops. It will be managed by the Project Leader with the assistance of a core Organising Committee.

The project is scheduled to comprise 36 months of research.

Project leader:
Dr. Michael W.H. COUGHTRIE
Department of Biochemical Medicine,
University of Dundee,
Ninewells Hospital and Medical School
UK Dundee DDI 9SY
Phone: +44 382 632510
Fax: +44 382 644620
Contract number: CT920097

Participants:
Dr. Gian Maria PACIFICI
Dept. of Biomedicine, Med Sch, Univ of Pisa
Via Roma 55
IT 56100 Pisa
Phone: +39 50 554851
Fax: +39 50 554929

Dr. John H.N. MEERMAN
Sylvius Laboratories, Center für
Bio-Pharmaceutical Sciences
P.O. Box 9503
NL 2300 RA Leiden
Phone: +31 71 276227
Fax: +31 71 276292

Dr. Richard C. ROBERTS
Dept. of Med, Univ of Dundee
UK Dundee DD1 9SY
Phone: +44 382 23125
Fax: +44 382 23282

Prof. G.J. MULDER
Sylvius Laboratories, Center for
Bio-Pharmaceutical Sciences
P.O. Box 9503
NL 2300 RA Leiden
Phone: +31 71 276211
Fax: +31 71 276292

Prof. G.M.J. van KEMPEN
Dept. of Psychiatry, Univ of Leiden
P.O. Box 1251
NL 2340 BG Oegstgeest
Phone: +31 71 275246
Fax: +31 71 275240

Prof. Hansruedi GLATT
Inst. fur Toxicologie, Univ Mainz
Obere Zahlbacher Strasse 67
DE 6500 Mainz
Phone: +49 6131 233662
Fax: +49 6131 230506

Prof. Theo J. VISSER
Dept. of Int Med III,
Erasmus Univ
P.O. Box 1738
NL 3000 Dr. Rotterdam
Phone: +31 10 463 5463
Fax: +31 10 463 5430

EPIDEMIOLOGICAL SURVEYS ON CHRONIC OBSTRUCTIVE PULMONARY DISEASES (COPD) IN DIFFERENT EUROPEAN COUNTRIES: PREVALENCE RATES AND RELATIONSHIP TO HOST AND ENVIRONMENTAL RISK FACTORS

Key words
Lung Diseases, Obstructive EP, Asthma, Bronchitis, Pulmonary Emphysema, Epidemiological Methods, Risk Factors, Ageing, Occupational Exposure, Europe.

Objectives
The objectives of this research project within the framework of the BIOMED Programme are:
1 to realize an European protocol for parallel performances and analyses of epidemiological surveys on COPD;
2 to evaluate the rate of comparability among the different epidemiological surveys;
3 to identify the relevant information on the epidemiological determinants of COPD (in particular, occupational exposure and ageing) that are currently investigated in the existing studies and on the determinants (e.g. biologic and genetic markers) that are useful to collect in new epidemiological surveys to be carried out in other countries in Europe (these include markers of immuno-inflammatory response and of exposure to occupational and environmental agents);
4 to compare the prevalence rates of symptoms, diseases and lung function abnormalities collected in various European countries, after taking into account the effects of hostre-lated and environment-related risk factors;
5 to investigate the relationship between morbidity and mortality rates of COPD in the European countries.

Brief description
Respiratory diseases are among the leading causes of morbidity and mortality in many countries. Chronic bronchitis and emphysema are undoubtedly the major causes of death for the respiratory diseases, while asthma appears to account for less than 10% in men and for less than 20% in women. Further, mortality for respiratory diseases appears highly dependent on age. In spite of the evident public health implications of those observations and of the expected socio-economic impact, few epidemiological surveys on chronic obstructive pulmonary diseases morbidity have been carried out in Europe and no attempt has been made to exploit the existing ones from an European perspective.
The methodology will be that followed in other COST (European Cooperation in Science and Technology) Concerted Actions within the European Community; e.g. a collaborative work among different investigators through meetings, definition of standard protocols exchange of data and common statistical analyses.
This research proposal can achieve community added values:
a it can provide a better knowledge of the distribution of chronic respiratory disorders that is useful to ensure a safe environment for the whole European population;
b it can supply data on the relationship between chronic respiratory disorders and ageing throughout Europe;
c it can facilitate the comprehension of the causes of chronic respiratory disorders at each age and it can improve the utilisation of the acquired knowledge for prevention purposes;

d it can provide data on the relationship between external risk factors and health, especially for the most susceptible ages.

Project leader:
Professor C. GIUNTINI
Fisiopatologia Respiratoria,
Clinica Medica II Universita degli Studi di Pisa
Via Roma 67
IT 56126 Pisa
Phone: +39 50 59 27 12
Fax: +39 50 55 34 14
Contract number: CT920849

Participants:
Prof. Bert RIJCKEN
Epidemiology, State Univ of Groningen
Antonius Deusinglaan 1
NL Groningen
Phone: +31 50 632 860
Fax: +31 50 633 082

Prof. Amund GULSVIK
Thoracic Med, Univ of Bergen,
Haukeland Sykehus
NO 5021 Bergen
Phone: +47 5 97 40 70
Fax: +47 5 97 47 85

Prof. Francine KAUFFMANN
Inserm U.169, Recherches en Epidemiologie
16 Avenue Paul-Vaillant Couturier
FR 94807 Villejuif Cedex
Phone: +33 1 45 59 50 72
Fax: +33 1 45 59 51 69

Prof. Bo LUNDBACK
Med Div, National Inst of Occupational Health
PO Box 7654
SE 907 13 Umea
Phone: +46 90 166 607
Fax: +46 90 165 027

Prof. Peter BURNEY
United Med & Dental Schools
Lambeth Palace Road
UK London SE1 7EH
Phone: +44 71 928 9292
Fax: +44 71 928 1468

Prof. Helgo MAGNUSSEN
Pneumologie und Thoraxchirurgie,
Krankenhaus Grosshansdorf
Wohrendamm 80
DE 2070 Grosshansdorf
Phone: +49 41 02 60 10

Prof. Josep M. ANTO
Consorci d'Hospital de Barcelona,
Inst Municipal d'Investigacio Medica
P. Maritim 25-29
ES 08003 Barcelona
Phone: +34 3 300 75 62
Fax: +34 3 485 49 52

STANDARDIZATION AND VALIDATION OF THE USE OF PULMONARY EPITHELIAL CELLS FOR TOXICITY ASSESSMENT OF OCCUPATIONAL AGENTS AND DRUGS

Key words
Lung disease, Occupational, Environment, Drug, Alveolar epithelial cells, Bronchiolar cells, Cell culture, Toxicity, Carcinogenicity.

Objectives
1 Harmonize methodologies for valid *in vitro* research into risk factors involved in occupational lung disease and in adverse drug reactions in the lung.
2 Validate the use of primary cultures of pulmonary epithelial cells for the assessment of pulmonary toxicity caused by chemicals.

The concerted action consists of a European research network of 8 laboratories from academic and public research institutes with the following specific targets spread over a 3 year period.

Brief description
Target 1. To obtain, by ensuring that similar techniques are used by all participating teams and by the pooling of research efforts, a valid and uniform method for the preparation of rodent pulmonary epithelial cells in primary culture.
It is not always clear from published studies on isolated pulmonary epithelial cells whether the cells used by different investigators are comparable both quantitatively (yield per lung, purity of the preparation, etc.) and qualitatively (cellular integrity, ability to metabolize chemicals, etc.). The concerted action should allow the definition of commonly agreed standard operating procedures for the preparation and utilization of primary cultures of alveolar type 2 and nonciliated bronchiolar cells from laboratory animals.
Target 2. To validate the use of pulmonary epithelial cells in toxicology by assessing the effects of six model compounds using sensitive tests of cell injury and dysfunction.
Adverse effects of chemicals in the lung concern much more than cell death, but include changes in cellular metabolism, decreased cell defence against oxygen and other environmental stress, alterations in the metabolism of foreign chemicals and carcinogens, synthesis of new proteins, release of mediators of inflammation, etc. The participating laboratories have each developed specific expertise in one or more of these areas, so that they wilt be able to carry out tests on cells obtained by the other teams. Here again the pooling of research efforts, the centralization of some assays, the common quality control, and the rapid dissemination of results to all participating teams should provide a validated battery of useful endpoints of toxicity.
Target 3: To achieve a satisfactory procedure to prepare and use primary cultures of human pulmonary epithelial cells for the in vitro testing of chemicals.
Work on isolated human alveolar cells is only done in very few centers, including some of the participating laboratories; methods to obtain human bronchiolar epithelial cells have to a large extent still to be developed. These laboratories will pool their efforts to adapt the methodology developed for the rodent cells to human lung specimens, taking into account the need for standardization and quality control.

Target 4: To collect valid information on the response of human lung cells to six model compounds.

The human pulmonary epithelial cells will be exposed to the same compounds as those tested in the animal cells and the responses will be compared with the animal results. Through the pooling of data from different centers an attempt will be made to analyse possible relations between the response to chemicals and patient characteristics, such as e.g. sex, time since smoking cessation, residence area, occupation, levels of anti-oxidant systems and (genetic) profile of cytochrome-P450 enzymes.

Target 5: Drafting of sound recommendations for the use of primary lung cells in culture for testing drugs and occupational chemicals.

Project leader:
Dr. Benoit NEMERY
Laboratorium voor Pneumologie,
Katholieke Universiteit Leuven
Kapucijnenvoer 35
BE 3000 Leuven
Phone: +32 16 337167
Fax +32 16 337467
Contract number: CT921229

Participants:
Bruno VOSS
Berufsgenossenschaftliches Forschungsinstitut
für Abreitsmedizin
Gilsingstrasse 14
DE 4630 Bochum
Phone: +49 234 316271
Fax: +49 234 308601

Emilio GELPI
Dep de Neuroquimica, Consejo Superior de
Investigaciones Cientificas
Jordi Girona 18-26
ES 08034 Barcelona
Phone: +34 3 2040600
Fax: +34 3 2045904

Benoit WALLAERT
Inst Pasteur, Lab de Pathologie Respiratoire
Exp et de Pollution Atmospherique
P.O. Box 245
FR 59019 Lille
Phone: +33 20 877739
Fax: +33 20 877906

Martyn CLYNES
National Cell & Tissue Culture Centre,
Dublin City Univ
Glasnevin
IE Dublin 9
Phone: +353 1 7045700
Fax: +353 1 7045484

Roy J. RICHARDS
Dep of Biochemistry, Univ of Wales College of
Cardiff
P.O. Box 903
UK Cardiff CF1 1ST
Phone: +44 222 874125
Fax: +44 222 874116

David DINSDALE
Med Res Council, Toxicology Unit
Woodmansterne Road
UK Carshalton Surrey SM5 4EF
Phone: +44 81 6538000
Fax: +44 81 6426538

Per E. SCHWARZE
Dept of Environmental Medicine, Nat Inst of
Public Health
Geitsmyrveien 75
NO 0482 Oslo 4
Phone: +47 2 356020
Fax: +47 2 353605

IMMUNOGENETIC BASIS OF HYPERSENSITIVITY TO METALS: IDENTIFICATION OF SUSCEPTIBILITY MARKERS

Key words
Immunogenetic, metals, lung disease, hypersensitivity, susceptibility, HLA.

Objectives
1 To establish the immunogenetic basis of the association of chronic beryllium disease with HLA as a model of susceptibility to metal hypersensitivity;
2 To design and test protocols for multicentre genetic screening for hypersensitivity to metals;
3 To institute an inter-laboratory tissue and cell bank from metal-related hypersensitivity cases, to be used to analyse the interaction of genetic factors with environmental factors such as beryllium, zirconium, nickel, gold, platinum, cobalt, and other hapten-like chemicals, and to search for genetic markers of disease for the early identification of individuals at occupational risk.

Brief description
Occupational exposure to metals is associated with hypersensitivity-type chronic lung disorders. Beryllium, aluminium, titanium, zirconium and gold are the cause of granulomatous pneumonitis; tungsten, cadmium and cobalt of fibrogenic interstitial pneumonias; aluminium, platinum, chromium and cadmium of bronchial asthma.

Chronic beryllium disease is an excellent model whereby to assess the immunogenetic basis of hypersensitivity to metals. The disease is not strictly dependent from exposure levels, i.e. is not due to direct metals toxicity, is maintained by hypersensitive CD4' T cells at site of disease, i.e. is allergic in nature, and its low incidence suggests that individual susceptibility plays a role in pathogenesis. In the context that it has been possible to eliminate the risk of acute beryllium toxicity by adopting strict industrial hygiene standards, while it has not significantly reduced the incidence of the chronic granulomatous disease, the identification of immunogenetic markers associated with susceptibility to metal hypersensitivity may be critical to prevent exposure-associated risk.

Preliminary studies have shown that susceptibility to chronic beryllium disease is strongly associated with a single aminoacid (Glu 69-coding) variant of HLA-DP, a gene associated with chronic inflammatory disorders. Thus, the beryllium disease model may be instrumental to uncover genetic factors implicated in occupationrelated hypersensitivity to metals. Further, the model may be used to test the application and standardisation of protocols of molecular diagnosis and occupational epidemiology and prevention of metal-related hypersensitivity lung disorders.

Project leader:
Professor C. SALTINI
Istituto di Fisiologia e
Malattie dell'Apparato Respiratorio,
Università di Modena
Via del Pozzo 71
IT 41100 Modena
Phone: +39 59 379 558
Fax: +39 59 370 913
Contract number: CT920934

Participants:

Dr. Rosa SORRENTINO
Dipartimento di Biologia Cellulare
Via degli Apuli 1
IT 00186 Roma

Francesco SINIGAGLIA
Pharma Res Techn, F. Hoffman La Roche Ltd
CH 4002 Basel
Phone: +41 61 6919391

Robert LECHLER
Dept of Immunology, Hammersmith Hospital
Du Cane Road
UK London W12 ONN
Phone: +44 81 7403034

Oreste ACUTO
Lab d'Immunologie, Inst Pasteur
Rue du Dr. Roux
FR Paris
Phone: +33 1 43069835

Roland M. DUBOIS
Interstitial Lung Disease Unit,
Nat Heart & Lung Inst
Manresa Road
UK London SW3 6LR
Phone: +44 71 351 8327
Fax: +44 71 351 8331

William JONES-WILLIAMS
Dept of Tuberculosis and Chest Diseases,
Univ of Wales
Penarth
UK South Glamorgan CF6 1XX
Phone: +44 222 705187
Fax: +44 222 712284

Roland BUHL
Abteilung fur Pneumologie,
Zentrum der Inneren Medizin
Theodor Stern Kai 7
DE 6000 Frankfurt 70
Phone: +49 69 6301 7388
Fax: +49 69 6301 7391

Prof. Giorgio ASSENNATO
Associato di Igiene Industriale,
Inst di Med del Lavoro
Piazza Giulio Cesare
IT 70124 BARI
Phone: +39 80 5575451

Prof. Dario OLIVIERI
Univ di Parma-Ospedale Rasori
Via V. Raschi 8
IT 43100 Parma
Phone: +39 521 292615

Romiro AVILA
Dept de Pneumotisiologia, Ospital Pulido
Valent Alameda de linhas de tones
PT 1700 Lisboa
Phone: +351 1 7590541

OCCUPATIONAL CANCER AMONG EUROPEAN WORKERS

Key words
Occupational cancer, exposure assessment, pulp-paper industry, styrene, mercury, textile industry.

Brief description
Epidemiology has been the most important tool to identify occupational carcinogens since the early years of research in this field. New causes of occupational cancer are being suggested, related to old as well as new technologies. The relatively stable national populations in Europe since World War II, allow the investigation on possible adverse health consequences of a broad spectrum of industrial activities. Today in order to reach valid scientific judgments, epidemiological studies need to be larger than what was necessary in the past. These large numbers of exposed workers are not always available in single countries, and the need for collaborative research is indicated. Evaluation of fairly low levels of exposure requires, more than previously, accurate recording and interpretation of data on exposures in the workplace.

Previous Work
This type of collaborative research has been successfully coordinated by IARC since 1976, when a programme on occupational cancer risk in various industries was established on a international basis. In the past, multicentric international studies have been conducted on cancer risk among workers in the production of man-made mineral fibres, workers in the production and spraying of chlorophenoxy herbicides, welders, and workers exposed to vinyl chloride. All these studies included an epidemiological investigation on cancer mortality or incidence as well as an industrial hygiene investigation aimed to characterise exposure to relevant chemicals at individual or group level.

Work Programme
The proposed work programma builds upon this core resource, developing it to include new centres with yet scarce experience (which will particularly benefit from the collaboration) and concerns six areas of research under-investigated up to now and of importance both from the preventive and the scientific points of view. The work programme will cover, in a period of 36 months, the following tasks:
1 to assess occupational exposures qualitatively and quantitatively and to evaluate the cancer risks in: (i) workers of the pulp and paper industry; (ii) workers exposed to styrene (in the production of fibreglass reinforced plastics); (iii) workers exposed to mercury (in mines and mills); (iv) workers in the textile manufacturing industry. An ancillary task of these studies is to promote research on occupational cancer in European countries and centres with little previous experience in this field, by associating them in the investigations.
2 (i) to review and develop methods for exposure assessment, in particular in relation to the evaluation of past exposures in the workplace; (ii) to prepare a comprehensive review of occupational cancer in Europe.

Criteria for the selections of themes of research have been substantially based on the output of a workshop, jointly organised by the EC and the IARC a few years ago, on priorities, for epidemiological studies in occupational cancer.

Project leader:
Dr. R. SARACCI
International Agency for Research on Cancer
150, cours Albert-Thomas
FR 69372 Lyon
Phone: +33 72 73 84 85
Fax: + 33 72 73 85 75
Contract number: CT921110

Participants:
Dr. Alain BERGERET
Inst. Univ de Med du Travail
8 Avenue Rockefeller
FR 69373 Lyon Cedex 08
Phone: +33 78777158
Fax: +33 78777158

Dr. David COGGON
MRC Environmental Epidemiology Unit,
Univ of Southampton
UK Southampton S09 3XY
Phone: +44 703777624
Fax: +44 703704021

Dr. Franco MERLETTI
Cancer Epidemiology Unit, Univ of Torino
Via Santena 7
IT 10126 Torino
Phone: +39 11678872
Fax: +39 11635267

Dr. Jordi SUNYER
Dept. d'Epidemiologia, Inst. Municipal
d'Investigacio Medica
Passeig Maritim 25-29
ES 08003 Barcelona
Phone: +34 34851085
Fax: +34 34854952

Dr. Manolis KOGEVINAS
Unit of Analytical Epidemiology,
Int Agency for Res on Cancer
150 Cours Albert Thomas
FR 69372 Lyon Cedex 08
Phone: +33 72738485
Fax: +33 72738575

Dr. Paolo BOFFETTA
Unit of Analytical Epidemiology,
Int Agency for Res on Cancer
150 Cours Albert Thomas
FR 69372 Lyon Cedex 08
Phone: +33 72738485
Fax: +33 72738575

Dr. Pascal WILD
Service d'Epidemiologie, INRS
Avenue de Bourgogne
FR 54501 Vandoeuvre les Nancy
Phone: +33 83502000
Fax: +33 83502097

Prof. Dr. Salvador Massano CARDOSO
Inst. de Higiene e Medicina social,
Univ de Coimbra
PT 3049 Coimbra Cedex
Phone: +351 3929431
Fax: +351 3920484

EUROPEAN COMMISSION RESPIRATORY HEALTH SURVEY

Key words
Asthma prevalence, environment, risk factors.

Brief description
The European Commission Respiratory Health Survey is a survey of asthma prevalence
and risk factors in 38 centres in the European Community and cost countries and in
many other centres elsewhere in the world, including the USA, Canada, New Zealand,
Australia, India, the Middle East and North Africa. The study is exploiting the wide
variations in asthma prevalence and in the environment across Europe to identify the
most influential modifiable risk factors that determine areas of high prevalence. This will
help to determine the reasons behind the current epidemic of asthma that has been noted
in several European countries, and will lead to preventive strategies to deal effectively
will the epidemic.
So far the project has agreed and prepared a common protocol for identifying and assessing asthma in surveys and for recording risk factors. Using this protocol surveys have
now been completed of over 125 000 people and detailed tests have been completed on
over 25 000 people selected systematically from defined populations in the community.
The data have been collected using a standardised protocol and under central quality
control.
The current request is for a grant to check, collate and analyse the information collected
in this survey, to prepare a full report on the findings, and to ensure that the results are
widely understood and their implications discussed by those with responsibility for health
policy within the European Community. The study will provide the most comprehensive
information to date on the prevalence of asthma, the impact of important risk factors,
and the distribution of care for patients with asthma in the European community.
The high level of standardisation and the extensive quality control during the survey
ensure that this will remain a benchmark in studies of asthma and atopic disease for
many years to come. The wide variations between the populations studied make it a very
powerful study for identifying the important risk factors that determine high prevalence.

Project leader:
Dr. P.G.J. BURNEY
Dept. of Public Health Medicine
St Thomas's Hospital
Lambeth Palace Road
UK London SE1 7EH
Phone: +44 71 928 9292 Ext.3145
Fax: +44 71 928 1468
Contract number: CT931048

Participants:
T. GISLASON
Vifilsstadir Chest
Hospital
IS 210 Gadabaer

A. AL-FRAYH
King Khalid Univ Hospital
SA Riyadh

A. CAPELASTEGUI
Hospital de Galdakao
ES Galdakano (Viscaya)

A. GULSVIK
Universitet i Bergen,
Haukeland Sykehus
NO Bergen

A. MARQUES
Faculdade de Medicina
de Porto
PT Porto

A. TAYTARD
Hospitalier Regional de
Bordeaux; FR Pessac

B. HARRISON
West Norwich Hospital
UK Norwich, Norfolk

B. RIJCKEN
State Univ of Groningen
NL Groningen

C. FLOREY
Ninewells Hospital
Medical School
UK Dundee, Scotland

C. LOUREIRO
Faculdade de Medecina
de Coimbra
PT Coimbra

D. NOWAK
Krankenhaus Grosshansdorf
Wohrendamm
DE Grosshansdorf

F. NEUKIRCH
Inserm Unite 226, Faculte de
Medecine Xavier Bichat
FR Paris

G. BOMAN
Univ of Uppsala,
Akademiska Sjukuset
SE Uppsala

H. WICHMANN
Bergische Universitat
Wuppertal
DE Wuppertal

I. PIN
Service de Pneumologie, Chu
Albert Michallon
FR Grenoble

J. ANTO
Hospital del Mar
ES Barcelona

J. BOUSQUET
Hospital l'Aiguelongue
FR Montpellier

J. CASTILLO
Servicio de Neumologia
ES Seville

J. CRANE
Wellington Hospital
NZ Wellington South

J. MALDONADO
Hospital General Manuel
Lois
ES Huelva

J. MANFREDA
Respiratory Hospital
CA Winnipeg, Manitoba

J. PRICHARD
Trinity College Medical
School, St. James' Hospital
IE Dublin

J. ROVIRA
Servicio de Neumologia
ES Allbacete

J. STARK
Addenbrookes Hospital
UK Cambridge

K. MADHAN
Hamad Medical Corporation
QA Doha

L. ROSENHALL
Umea Univ Hospital
SE Umea

M. ABRAMSON
Monash Medical School,
Alfred Hospital
AU Prahran, Victoria

M. BUGIANI
Dispensario di Igiene Sociale
IT Torino

M. BURR
Llandough Hospital
UK Penarth, South
Glamorgan

N. AIT-KHALED
Hopital Beni-Mesous
DZ Algiers

N. NIELSEN
Bispebjerg Hospital
DK Copenhagen

N. PAPAGEORGIOU
Chest Diseases Hospital
(Sotiria)
GR Athens

P. PAOLETTI
CNR Inst. of Clinical
Physiology
IT Pisa

P. PLASCHKE
Univ of Goteborg,
Renstromska Sjukhuset
SE Goteborg

P. VERMEIRE
Universitaire Inst.elling
Antwerp
BE Wilrijk

R. AVILA
Hospital Pulido Valente
PT Lisboa

R. CHOWGULE
Bombay Hos & Med Cent,
New Marine Lines
IN Bombay

R. DAHL
Univ of Aarhus
DK Aarhus

R. DE MARCO
Instituto di Science Sanitarie
Applicate
IT Pavia

R. HALL
Ipswich Hospital
UK Ipswich

R. QUIROS
General Elorza 32, Oviedo
ES Asturias

S. BUIST
Oregon Health Sciences Univ
US Portland, Oregon

U. ACKERMAN-LIEBRICH
Univ of Basle
CH Basel

V. LO CASCIO
Ospedale Policlinico Borgo
Roma
IT Verona

W. POPP
Krankenhaus der Stadt
Wien-Lainz
AT Wien

OCCUPATIONAL EXPOSURES AND
CONGENITAL MALFORMATIONS

Key words
Teratogens, occupational exposures, birth defects.

Brief description
The attitude to have when a female worker becomes pregnant has long been a subject of concern among occupational physicians. Especially since, when the pregnancy is clinically recognized, exposure has already taken place during the first weeks, a period very sensitive to teratogens.

Thus, there is a need to identify teratogens (or more generally reprotoxic agents) in the workplace in order to protect women potentially exposed to them.

Risk factors known to date explain only a small proportion of birth defects and on the other hand several improvements can be made over published epidemiological studies which have looked specifically at occupational risk factors.

In this context, an international collaborative study on the role of occupational exposures in the etiology of birth defects, grouping several European registries will contribute significantly to the knowledge on this problem.

A multicentric casecontrol study using a detailed standardized procedure for assessment of occupational exposure and classification of birth defects will increase power and specificity, which were lacking in many studies published on the subject.

It will allow the identification of risk factors for birth defects present in the workplace and the quantification of the percentage of birth defects attributable to occupational factors in a variety of European populations.

It will also provide a wide detailed and standardized data base (in the order of 2000 subjects: 1000 cases of major birth defects and 1000 controls) which could be used to test specific hypotheses about new chemicals suspected of reprotoxic effects (ex.: glycol ethers).

Project leader:
Dr. S. CORDIER
INSERM, Unit 170,
Rech. Epidémiologiques et Statistiques
sur l'Environnement et la Santé
av. Paul Vailland Couturier 16
FR 94807 Villejuif Cédex 07
Phone: +33 1 45 59 50 34
Fax: +33 1 45 59 51 51
Contract number: CT931585

Participants:
Dr. Janine GOUJARD
INSERM U.149
FR Paris

Dr. Martina CORNEL
Univ of Groningen
NL Groningen

Dr. Ségolè AYME
INSERM SC11
FR Paris

Dr. Elis CALZOLARI
Istituto di Genetica Medica
IT Ferrara

Dr. Fabrizio BIANCHI
Istituto di Fisiologia Clinica
del CNR
IT Pisa

Dr. Robin KNILL-JONES
Univ of Glasgow
UK Glasgow

OCCUPATIONAL HAZARDS TO MALE REPRODUCTION

Key words
Environmental exposures, occupational risk factors, reproductive system, infertility, heritable disease.

Brief description
Suggestive evidence of a decline in quality of semen has accumulated during the last decade. Other lines of evidence indicate that the male reproductive system is highly sensitive to some environmental exposures. Nevertheless knowledge in this area is limited. The overall aim of this European Concerted Action is to identify and characterize common occupational risk factors to the male reproductive system. With the objective of preventing infertility and transmission of heritable disease to the offspring. This is to be achieved by combining biological and epidemiological research methods addressing greenhouse and agricultural workers with exposure to pesticides, reinforced plastic workers with exposure to styrene and lead exposed workers.

The basic study design combine 3 separate interview studies of time to pregnancy with 3 separate controlled longitudinal studies of semen quality and male germ cell genotoxicity. creation of cohorts and enrolment of volunteers takes place in 9 European countries, while laboratory analyses of biological specimens are centralized in 6 specialized laboratories.

The time to pregnancy studies comprize 3 cohorts of 500 current male worker and a control group of equal size. Data collection is by interview. The study utilizes experience from and shares researchers with the ongoing European Concerted Action on Infertility and Subfecundity.

Participants to the sperm studies are consecutively enrolled at time of new appointment to jobs involving one of the 3 exposures of interest during a 2 year period. Semen samples are collected before exposure and during 12 month follow-up. Each of the 3 study groups and one control group include 75 subjects. Outcome measures include semen quality determined by computerized video imaging techniques, sexual hormones, sperm chromatin structure assay and germ cell genotoxic damage to be determined by 3 new techniques.

The Concerted Action is to be conducted from 1/9 1993 to 1/7 1998 through collaborative efforts of 14 European research institutions. The proposed study will offer improvements and added value over national research programmes at the both qualitative and quantitative level.

Project leader:
Professor G. DANSCHER
The Steno Institute of Public Health,
Department of Neurotoxicology
C.F. Mollers Allé, Building 233/34
DK 8000 Aarhus C
Phone: +45 8942 1122
Fax: +45 8619 8664
Contract number: CT931186

Participants:

Dr. Helena TASKINEN,
Dr. Marja-Lüsa LINDBOHM
National Inst. of
Occupational Health
Topeliuksenkatu 41 a A
FI 00250 Helsinki
Phone: +358 0 474 71
Fax: +358 0 41 36 91

Dick HEEDERIK
Wageningen Agricultural
Univ
P.O. Box 238
NL 6700 AE Wageningen
Phone: +31 83 70 8 20 80
Fax: +31 83 70 8 27 82

Dr. Jaana LÄHDETIE
Dept. of Medical Genetics,
Inst. of Biomedicine,
Univ of Turku
Kiinamyllynk 10
FI 20520
Phone: +358 21 633 71
Fax: +358 21 331126

Dr. Marcello SPANO
Div. of Molecular Biology,
Biophysics and
Bioelectronics, CRE Casaccia
S.P. Anguillarese 301
IT 00060 Rome
Phone: +39 63 048 4737
Fax: +39 63 048 4630

Dr. Michael JOFFE
Academic Dept. of Public
Health, St Mary's Hospital
Medical School
Norfolk Place
UK London W2 1PG
Phone: +44 71 725 1496
Fax: +44 71 724 7349

Dr. Patrick THONNEAU
Hospital de Bicêtre, Sante
Publique Epidemiologie,
Reproduction Humaine U 292
Rue du General Leclerc 7B
FR 94275 Le Kremlin Bici
Tre Cedex
Phone: +33 1 45 21 22 96
Fax: +33 1 45 21 20 75

G.A. ZIELHUIS
Univ of Nijmegen,
Dept. of Epidemiology
P.O. Box 9101
NL 6500 HB Nijmegen
Phone: +31 80 619 132

Luigi BISANTI
Regione Lombardia,
Settore Sanita e Igiene,
Servizio di Epidemiologia
Via Stresa 24
IT 20125 Milano
Phone: +39 2 67 65 30 79
Fax: +39 2 67 65 31 28

Michel Van HOORNE
University Hospital of Gent,
Section for Environmental
and Occupational Health
De Pintelaan 185
BE 9000 Gent
Phone: +32 91 40 36 28

Prof. B. BARANSKI
Nofer Inst. of Occupational
Medicine,
Who Collaborating Centre
for Occupational Health
Teresy Str. 8
CT90 950 Lodz
Phone: +48 42 55 25 05
Fax: +48 42 34 83 31

Prof. G. LEHNERT
Dept. of Occupational and
Social Medicine,
University of
Erlangen-Nürnberg
Schillerstrasse 25/29
DE 91054 Erlangen
Phone: +49 131 23 784
Fax: +49 131 85 23 12

Prof. N. E. SKAKKEBAEK
University Dept. of
Growth and Reproduction,
Rigshospitalet
Blegdamsvej 9
DK 2100 Copenhagen East
Phone: +45 35 45 5085
Fax: +45 31 39 9054

Wim L.A.M. De KORT
Dept. of Occupational
Toxicology,
TNO Medical Biological
Laboratory
P.O. Box 45
NL 2280 AA Rijswijk
Phone: +31 15 842 842
Fax: +31 15 843 989

MOLECULAR EPIDEMIOLOGY OF DIESEL EXHAUST EXPOSURES

Key words
Diesel, mutagenic risks, carcinogenic risks, environmental pollution.

Brief description
This programme is designed to provide a means of assessing human exposure to diesel exhaust emissions at the molecular level and thus provide a better understanding of the mutagenic and carcinogenic risks associated with such exposure.

Automobile emissions constitute a major form of environmental pollution in the European Community.

The emissions contain numerous chemicals which are known to have toxic, mutagenic and carcinogenic properties. One result of environmental policy has been to make diesel-engined vehicles more attractive by differential fuel pricing (gasoline versus diesel).

However there are a number of serious concerns to this approach, not least the possible increase in the amount of particulate matter emitted from diesel exhausts.

Whilst particulates constitute only a small percentage of gasoline emissions ($<1\%$) they can account for as much as 30% for diesel emissions.

Diesel emissions are more carcinogenic than gasoline emissions in experimental animals, under inhalation exposure conditions, and are more mutagenic in in vitro test systems.

This programme is designed to provide a means of assessing human exposure to diesel exhaust emissions at the molecular level.

In this research programme, characteristic marker chemicals for diesel exhaust emissions such as 6-nitrobenzo(a)pyrene, 1-nitropyrene, 1-nitrochrysene, 3-nitrofluoranthene and 2-nitrofluorene will be examined since nitropolyciclics appear to be responsible for the majority of the mutagenicity. Immunological and physico-chemical methods will be developed to characterise the interactor products of these marker chemicals with biological molecules such as DNA and haemoglobin.

The relationship between DNA adducts and a surrogate dose monitor, such as haemoglobin adducts of these marker chemicals, will be examined with a view to establishing the relative contribution of individual chemicals in the diesel exhaust to react with biological molecules. Human molecular epidemiological studies will be performed on individuals more heavily exposed to diesel emissions than controls for comparative purposes.

In addition metabolites of nitro-PAH's will be sought in the urine of diesel exhaust-exposed persons. The biological parameters will also be compared to levels of exposure to diesel exhaust emissions.

In this programme, the combined research efforts of several expert groups in genetic toxicology and epidemiology will provide an excellent opportunity to address important environmental issues that are of general interest fo the European Community, viz the genotoxic risks associated with diesel exhaust exposure.

Project leader:
Dr. R. C. GARNER
The Jack Birch Unit for Environmental
Carcinogenesis, Univ. of York
Heslington
UK York Y01 5DD
Phone: +44 904 43 29 00
Fax: +44 904 42 39 54
Contract number: CT931309

Participants:
Dr. D. COGGAN
MRC Environmental Epidemiology Unit,
Southampton General Hospital
UK Southampton SO9 4XY
Phone: +44 703 777624
Fax: +44 703 704021

Prof. H-G. NEUMANN
Insitut fur Phamakologie und
Toxicologie, Der Universitat Wurzburg
Versbacher Strasse 9
DE 9700 Wurzburg
Phone: +49 9312011
Fax: +49 9312013446

Dr. R.A. BAAN
Dept. of Genetic Toxicology,
TNO Medical Biological Laboratory
P.O. Box 5815
NL 2280 HV Rijswijk
Phone: +31 15 843163
Fax: +31 15 843989

Dr. R.P. BOS
Dept. of Toxicology, Faculty of
Medical Sciences, Univ of Nijmegen
P.O. Box 9101
NL 6500 HB Nijmegen
Phone: +31 80 613550
Fax: +31 80 540576

RISK ASSESSMENT IN LYME BORRELIOSIS

Key words
Lyme borreliosis, exposure, treatment, tick.

Brief description
Lyme borreliosis is a Zoonotic disease caused by the spirochaete Borrelia burgdorferi and transmitted by ticks of the Ixodes ricinus species complex.

It has a world wide distribution, mainly in the northern hemisphere and many thousands of cases are thought to occur every year in Europe.

Symptoms can arise a long time after exposure and are very variable involving the skin, nervous system, heart and joints. The disease can be very seriously debilitating and in view of the many difficulties involved in diagnosis and treatment it is very important to determine the element of risk in relation to both exposure and treatment. In this concerted action risk assessment will be investigated as two separate, but interacting components.

1 The factors that contribute to a high risk of infection in tick habitat. Such factors include tick densities, tick hosts, spirochaete reservoir hosts, spirochaete serotypes and pathotypes, tick strains in relation to feeding behaviour and vector capability, the dynamics of the circulation of the spirochaete in nature and of transmission to humans and the pattern of human exposure to infection in high risk situations. Definition of the correct criteria, which may vary in different geographical areas, will allow the accurate and rapid assessment of risk in particular and different habitats and the recommendation of intervention strategies for control if necessary.

2 The decisions faced by clinicians and patients when infection is suspected must be based on validated criteria. The risk of infection following a tick bite will be assessed from data on transmission in relation to tick infection rates, engorgement periods, methods of tick removal, sero and pathotypes, and the relationship between infection and development of symptoms.

These data will be obtained from experimental, prospective and retrospective clinical studies and will be integrated wherever possible. A geographical basis for these studies will be maintained at all levels, so that should different pathotypes emerge from the study they can be characterised according to the various other parameters investigated.

Much of the relevant data have already been accumulated by the participants and integration of these and also new data on all the facets.

Project leader:
Dr. J. GRAY
Dept. of Environmental Resource,
University College Dublin
Belfield
IE Dublin 4
Phone: +353 1 706 77 39
Fax: +353 1 283 73 28
Contract number: CT931183

Participants:

Dr. A. ESTRADA-PENA
Unidad de Parasitologia,
Facultad de Veterinaria
C/Miguel Servet 177
ES 50013 Zaragoza
Phone: +34 76 414800
Fax: +34 76 591994

Dr. E. GUY
Medical Microbiology, PHL,
Singleton Hospital, Sgeti
UK Swanssea SA2 8QR
Phone: +44 792 205666
Fax: +44 792 202320

Dr. F. JONGEJAN
Dept. of Parasitology and
Tropical Veterinary Medicine
Univ of Utrecht
P.O. Box 80165
NL 3508 TD Utrecht
Phone: +31 30 532568
Fax: +31 30 540784

Dr. H. SMITH
Scottish Parasite Diagnosis
Laboratory, Bacteriology
Stobhill General Hospital
UK Glasgow G21 3UW
Phone: +44 41 5580111
Fax: +44 41 5585508

Dr. I.SAINT-GIRONS
Unité de Moleculaire et
Médicale,
Institut Pasteur
FR 5724 Paris Cedex
Phone: +33 1 45688366
Fax: +33 1 40613001

Dr. L. GERN
Institut de Zoologie
Chantemerle 22
CH 2000 Neuchâtel
Phone: +41 38 256434
Fax: +41 38 242695

Dr. M. CIMMINO
Dipartimento di Medicina
Interna, Università degli
Studi di Genova
Viale Benedetto XV 6
IT 16132 Genova
Phone: +39 10 3538905
Fax: +39 10 352324

Dr. O. KAHL
Institut für Amgewandte
Zoologie, Freie Universität
Berlin FB Biologie, WE 4
Haderslebener Str.9
DE 12163 Berlin 41
Phone: +49 30 8383918
Fax: +49 30 8383897

Dr. P. NUTTALL
Inst. of Virology and
Environmental Microbiology
Mansfield Road
UK Oxford OX1 3S
Phone: +44 865 512361
Fax: +44 865 59962

Dr. S. O'CONNELL
Dept. of Med. Microbiology,
Southampton General
Hospital
UK Southampton SO9 4XY
Phone: +44 703 796412
Fax: +44 703 774316

Dr. S. RIJPKEMA
National Institute of
Public Health and
Environmental Protection
A. van Leeuwenhoeklaan 9
NL 3720 BA Bilthoven
Phone: +31 30 749111
Fax: +31 30 292957

Prof. F. FRANDSEN
Dept. of Ecology and
Molecular Biology,
The Royal Veterinary and
Agricultural University
Bülowsvej 13
DK 1870 Frederiksberg C,
Copenhagen
Phone: +45 3528 2660
Fax: +45 3528 2670

Prof. G. GETTINBY
Dept. of Statistics and
Modelling Science,
Univ of Strathclyde,
Livingstone Tower
Richmond Street
UK Glasgow G1 1XH
Phone: +44 41 5524400
Fax: +44 41 5524711

Prof. G.STANEK
Hygiene Institut,
Unversität Wien
Kinderspitalgasse 15
AT 1095 Wien
Phone: +43 222 404900
Fax: +43 222 0490295

RELATION OF WORK-RELATED AND CULTURE-RELATED PATTERNS OF COLD EXPOSURE TO LARGE AND PARADOXICAL DIFFERENCES IN EXCESS WINTER MORTALITY WITHIN EUROPE

Key words
Mortality in winter, seasonal mortalities, cold-related mortality.

Brief description
All European countries experience large increases in mortality in winter, mainly from arterial thrombosis and respiratory disease.
Surprisingly, the increases are much larger in Italy, Greece and Britain than in countries with much colder winters, such as Finland.
Excess deaths in winter from arterial thrombosis have not changed, and excess deaths from respiratory disease have not always changed, in line with changes in home heating. This suggests an important role for outdoor activities. Experiments on volunteers have indicated possible mechanisms for a causal role of brief outdoor cold exposures, particularly on thrombotic deaths. Seasonal mortality is accordingly being covered in the new edition of Hunter's of Occupational Medicine.
We propose a Europe-wide study to determine associations of home and outdoor factors with cause-specific seasonal mortalities. We will obtain seasonal data on deaths from coronary thrombosis, cerebral thrombosis, respiratory disease, and all causes; over a five year period, for ages 50-59 and 65-74 years, and men and women, separately, in each of 8 regions of Europe with widely differing climates and cultures. Cold-related changes in each of these causes of death in the 32 sub groups will be correlated with night and day home heating and outdoor activities, using poisson analysis to adjust for age and gender effects. Key elements are:
- use of indices of cold-related mortality undistorted by heat induced mortality; commissioning of regional surveys of home heating and outdoor activities; inclusion of both pre-retirement and post-retirement age groups.

Since excess winter deaths in the Participating Countries total approximately 200,000 annually, the problem is large. As regards Community Added Value, the proposals provide an unusual opportunity to use diverse cultural patterns within Europe to obtain evidence of causes of a major source of mortality in all regions. Immediate benefit is expected through preventive advice, and lasting benefit from establishment of agreed procedures and working links by a Europe-wide consortium in this field.

Project leader:
Professor W.R. KEATINGE
Dept. of Physiology,
Queen Mary and Westfield College
Mile End Road
UK London E1 4NS
Phone: +44 71 982 63 65
Fax: +44 81 983 04 67
Contract number: CT931229

Participants:

Dr. G.C. DONALDSON
Dept. of Physiology, Basic
Medical Sciences, Queen
Mary & Westfield, College
Mile End Road
UK London E1 4NS
Phone: +44 71 982 6365
Fax: +44 81 983 0467

Dr. J.P. MACKENBACH
Faculteit der Geneeskunde en
Gezondheids-Wetenschappen
Erasmus Universiteit
Dr. Molenwaterplein 50
NL Rotterdam
Phone: +31 10 4087720
Fax: +31 10 4366831

Dr. K. KATSOUYANNI
Univ of Athens, School of
Medicine, Dept. of Hygiene
& Epidemiology
GR 11527 Athens (Goudi)
Phone: +30 1 7719725
Fax: +30 1 7704225

Dr. P. Van Der TORN
Environmental Health Office,
Municipal Health Service of
Rotterdam
P.O. Box 70032
NL 3000 LP Rotterdam
Phone: +31 10 411 6377
Fax: +31 10 404 8843

Dr. S. NAYHA
The Regional Inst. of
Occupational Health in Oulu
FI 90101 Oulu
Phone: +358 81 333 353
Fax: +358 81 333 343

Prof. I. VUORI
UKK Inst. for Health
Promotion Research
P.O. Box 30
FI 33501 Tampere
Phone: +358 31 282 9111
Fax: +358 31 282 9200

Prof. L. DARDANONI
Departimento di Igiene
e Microbiologia,
Universita di Palermo
Via del Vespro 133
IT 90127 Palermo
Phone: +39 91 6512318
Fax: +39 91 6553649

Prof. M. MARTINELLI,
Dr. E. CORDIOLI
Instituto di Patologia,
Speciale Medica e
Metodologia Clinica
dell'Universita degli Studi
di Bologna, Policl S
Via Massarenti 9
IT 40138 Bologna
Phone: +39 51 343723
Fax: +39 51 392486

Prof. M.G. MARMOT
Dept. of Community
Medicine,
University College
and Middlesex School
of Medicine
Gower Street 66-72
UK London WC1E 6EA
Phone: +44 71 387 7050
Fax: +44 71 380 7608

Dr. G. JENDRITZKY
Deutscher Wetterdienst
Stefan Maier Strasse 4
DE 7800 Freiburg 1
Phone: +49 761 28202 54
Fax: +49 761 28202 90

Prof. S. EVANS
Dept. of Clinical
Epidemiology,
Basic Medical Sciences
Building
Queen Mary & Westfield
College
Mile End Road
UK London E1 4NS
Phone: +44 71 982 6387
Fax: +44 81 983 0502

OCCUPATIONAL RISK FACTORS FOR SINONASAL CANCER: A REANALYSIS OF SEVERAL CASE-CONTROL STUDIES

Key words
Sinonasal cancer, risk factors, wood and leather industries, non-occupational and occupational factors, case control studies.

Brief description
Although many studies on the occupational causes of sinonasal cancer have been performed, most of them were national-based with a small number of cases. The proposed project is a combined reanalysis of several case-control studies.
The objective of the analysis of the common data set is to examine the risk of nasal cancer associated with known or suspected risk factors, with more specific occupations and exposures than was previously possible. This combined analysis would also allow to identify new risk factors and to generate new hypotheses.
This project is a part of a joint project involving IARC and INSERM Unit 88, each team having leadership roles in different analyses. Occupations and exposures related to wood and leather industries will be studied by IARC.
INSERM Unit 88 will take the lead on analysis related to other` non-occupational and occupational factors, which are of primary concern for the proposed project: textile dust, formaldehyde, occupational exposures in agriculture, tobacco smoking.

Scientific and technical description: At the present time, a common data set has been set up from seven casecontrol studies, six of them from European countries (Italy, Germany, the Netherlands and France).
The detailed work histories including job titles and dates of employment have been recoded with ILO (International Labour Office) code for occupation and ISIC (International Standard Industrial Classification, United Nations) code for industry.
Five other investigators from European countries, United States and Asian countries have agreed to supply their data. As a consequence, the definite common data set will include more than 1000 cases and 3000 controls.
The main parts of the project can be described as below: Analysis based on job titles: The objective of this part of the analysis is to get more precise estimations of odds-ratios for job titles and activity branches.
The analysis will be performed in two different ways: a systematic screening of occupations and industries, and specific analyses focussing on occupations and industries described as associated or possibly associated with sinonasal cancer in literature.
Analysis based on substances, with two approaches: Use of the larynx cancer job exposure matrix: The JEM we intend to use in the present project has been developed for a multicentric European study on occupational exposures associated with larynx cancer.
The job classification system is the ILO/ISIC classification. Exposure to formaldehyde, chromium and nickel may be estimated from this matrix.
A first step will be to complete the existing JEM with the ILO-ISIC combinations needed for this project.
Case by case evaluation: A case by case assessment by experts will be used for some substances: textile dust, and, if possible, formaldehyde and occupational exposures in agriculture.

Results: In addition to scientific results on occupational exposures for sinonasal cancer, this project could be positive for analysis of case control studies on occupational risk factors in European countries: improvements in comparability by promotion of comparable questionnaires and use of the same international code for occupations and industries; better validation and improvement of an European Job Exposure Matrix which can be used in future studies.

Project leader:
Ms. A. LECLERC
INSERM, Unit 88
Boulevard de l'Hôpital 91
FR 75634 PARIS Cédex 13
Phone: +33 1 45 84 63 74
Fax: +33 1 45 83 83 02
Contract number: CT931158

Participants:
Corrado MAGNANI
Cancer Epidemiology Unit
Via Santena 7
IT 10126 TORINO
Phone: +39 11 690 327
Fax: +39 11 635 267

Danièle LUCE
INSERM Unit 88
Boulevard de l'Hopital 91
FR 75634 Paris Cedex 13
Phone: +33 1 45 84 63 74
Fax: +33 1 45 83 02 02

Enzo MERLER
Centro per lo Studio e
la Prevenzione Oncologia,
USL 10/E, Epidemiology Unit,
Presidio di San Salvi
Via di San Salvi 12
IT 50136 Firenze

Franco BERRINO
Istituto Nazionale per lo
Studio e la Cura dei Tumori
Via Venezian 1
IT 20133 Milano
Phone: +39 2 239 04 60
Fax: +39 2 236 26 92

Lennart HARDELL
Dept. of Oncology,
Orebro Medical Center,
Regionsjukhuset
SE 107 85 Orebro

P. BOFFETA, P. DEMERSIARC
150 cours Albert Thomas
FR 69272 Lyon Cedex 08
Phone: +33 72 73 84 85
Fax: +33 72 73 85 75

Stefano BELLI and Pietro COMBA
Istituto Superiore di Sanita,
Laboratorio di Igiene Ambientale
Viale Regina Elena 299
IT 00161 Roma
Phone: +39 6 49 90 249
Fax: +39 6 44 40 064

Ulrich BOLM-AUDORFF
Hessen Ministry for Woman,
Work and Social Welfare,
Dept. Occupational Safety,
Div. Occupational Medicine
P.O. Box 3140
DE 6200 Wiesbaden 1
Phone: +49 611 81 73 669
Fax: +49 611 86 837

OCCUPATIONAL RISK FACTORS FOR RARE CANCERS OF UNKNOWN AETIOLOGY

Key words
Genetic and environmental risk factors, occupation-related diseases, cancer.

Brief description
The project is related to the work program in several ways: it seeks to identify risk factors in occupational medicine, and it studies the interaction between genetic and environmental risk factors for occupation-related diseases (I.2). It also uses European opportunities to investigate less common cancers (II.2). It is a study which cannot be done without European collaboration.

The objective is to look for new potential carcinogens in the workplace by examining diseases whose causes are presently unknown. Seven cancer sites have been selected for study since their general epidemiology suggests a possible occupational etiology, and they have not yet been carefully scrutinized in an epidemiologic study with a reasonable sample size.

Cancers of small intestine, gall bladder, thymus, bone, male breast, eye, and mycosis fungoides will be included In the study. At least 100 cases will enter each case-control study and at least 800 controls.

In the case-control study information on occupational exposures and potential confounders will be collected by face to face interviews using a structured questionnaire. The final development of a questionnaire for the exposure assessment will be done with the help of experienced, local hygienists and toxicologists. These principles have been used and evaluated in several other European studies in cancer epidemiology.

A study of p53 deactivation in tumor tissue will also be carried out. This is a frequent genetic change in human cancers. Interesting associations between an occupational exposure and cancer found by means of the questionnaire information will be explored further by analysing mutations in exons 5-8 by using PCR-amplification and DNA sequencing. Comparing exposures between persons with either activated or deactivated p53 tumor suppressor gene will tell us whether the exposure plays a role through deactivation or if it interacts with prior genetic damage.

Project leader:
Dr. E. LYNGE
Steno Institute of Public Health,
Dept of Epidemiology and Social Medicine
Hoegh-Guldbergsgade 8
DK 8000 AARHUS C
Phone: +45 8942 3075
Fax: +45 8613 1580
Contract number: CT931630

Participants:

Aivars STENGREVICS
Latvian Oncological Centre
Hippokrate Str. 4
LV 1079 Riga
Phone: +371 2 539 209

Carlos Alberto GONZALEZ
Institut De Recerca
Epidemiologica I Clinica
Jordi Joan 5
ES 08301 Mataro
Phone: +34 9 3790 55 13

Consol SERRA
Consorci Hospitalari
Del Parc Tauli
Pl. Parc Tauli s/n
ES 08208 Sabadell
Phone: +34 3 7231 010

Enzo MERLER
Center for Study and Cancer,
Via san Salvi 12
IT 50135 Florence
Phone: +39 055 5662691

Flora van LEEUWEN
The Netherlands Cancer Inst.
Plesmanlaan 121
NL 1013 CA Amsterdam
Phone: +31 2 0512 2483

Wolfgang AHRENS
Bremen Inst. for Prevention,
Research and Social Medicine
Grünenstrasse 120
DE 28199 Bremen
Phone: +49 42159 59656

Tiiu AARELEID
Inst. of Experimental and
Clinical Medicine
Hiiu 42
EE 0016 Tallin
Phone: +3722 514 334
Fax: +3725 248 260

Franco MERLETTI
Unversita' Degli Studi
di Torino
Via Santena 7
ES 10126 Torino
Phone: +39 11 678872

Gerard M.H. SWAEN
University of Limburg,
Dept. of Epidemiology
P.O. Box 616
NL 6200 MD Maastricht
Phone: +31 043 882386

Gun WINGREN
Department of
Occupational Medicine,
University Hospital
SE 582 85 Linköping
Phone: +46 1322 1441

H. AUTRUP, J. OLSEN,
H. KOLSTAD, S. SABROE
Steno Inst. of Public Health,
Dept. of Epidemiology and
Social Medicine
Hoegh-Guldbergsgade 8
DK 8000 Aarhus
Phone: +45 89 42 30 75

Janine BELL
Thames Cancer Registry
Cotswold Road 15
UK Sutton Surrey SM2 5PY
Phone: +44 081 642 7692

Lainonas JAZUKEVICIUS
Lithuanian Cancer Centre
Santariskiv 2
LT 2060 Vilnius
Phone: +370 2 778 587

Lorenzo SIMONATO
Unversita di Padova
Via Giustiniani 7
IT 35100 Padova
Phone: +39 049 8213890

Malcolm HARRINGTON
Inst. of Occupational Health,
University of Birmingham
Edgbaston
UK Birmingham B15 2TT
Phone: +44 21 414 6030

Maria M. MORALES
SUAREZ-VARELA
Hygiene and Environment
Health, Faculty of Pharmacy,
Valencia University
Av. Vicente A. Estelles s/n
ES 46100 Valencia
Phone: +34 6 3864 951

Mikael ERIKSSON
Dept. of Oncology,
University of Unea
SE 901 85
Phone: +46 9010 2855

Olov Lennart HARDELL
Dept. of Oncology,
Örebro Medical Center
SE 70185 Örebro
Phone: +46 1915 1546

Pascal GUENEL
INSERM Unité 88, Santé
Publique et Epidémiologie,
Sociale et Economique
Boulevard de l'Hoptital 91
FR 75634 Paris
Phone: +33 1 4077 9606

CONCERTED ACTION ON A MULTICENTRIC CASE REFERENCE STUDY ON MALIGNANT MESOTHELIOMA, ENVIRONMENTAL ASBESTOS EXPOSURE AND RISK FACTORS OTHER THAN ASBESTOS

Key words
Mesothelioma, asbestos, non-occupational exposure.

Brief description
Malignant mesothelioma is a rare disease and an indicator of exposure to asbestos fibers. The occurrence of mesothelioma following non-occupational asbestos exposure is a reason for concern and is the main focus of the study.

The rarity of the disease make a multicentric study necessary. None of the participating centers alone is able to collect a sufficient number of cases to identify the association.

The proposed Concerted Action refers to a multicentric population-based case-referent study which is being planned in some European countries in areas of relevant environmental (non occupational) asbestos exposure for exploring the association between mesotheliomas, environmental exposure to asbestos and other risk factors.

It will contribute to harmonizing criteria for selection of cases and controls and for exposure assessment in the participating countries.

Furthermore the concerted action will include common statistical analyses.

National studies will be population based and include histologically diagnosed cases of mesothelioma, incident in the period January 1994-December 1995. A sample of histological diagnoses will be verified by a panel of pathologists set up during the concerted action.

Assessment of exposure to occupational and environmental asbestos will be harmonized using a common questionnaire and defining criteria for the interpretation of occupational and residential histories.

A matrix will be developed to evaluate the likelihood of occupational exposure to asbestos and other risk factors.

Common criteria will be defined and applied also for: assessing exposure to asbestos from history of residences and distance from potential sources of pollution, assessing exposure to asbestos from various sources within the household, converting results of environmental determinations of asbestos, where available, into indicators of individual exposure.

Feasibility of the collection of biological samples for measuring lung burden of asbestos fibres in mesothelioma cases) will be evaluated at beginning of the concerted action. Specimens will be analyzed in laboratories with good expertise.

Project leader:
Dr. C. MAGNANI
Servizio di Epidemiologia dei Tumori,
Cancer Epidemiology Unit
Via Santena 7
IT 10126 Torino
Phone: +39 11 67 88 72
Fax: +39 11 663 52 67
Contract number: CT931297

Participants:

Athena LINOS
Inst. for Preventive Medicine,
Occupational and Environmental Health
Kifissias Avenue 227
GR 14561 Kifissias
Phone: +30 1 8064548
Fax: +30 1 6126170

Carlos A. GONZALEZ
Hospital de Mataro, Insitut de Recerca
Epidemiologica i Clinica IREC
Jordi Joan 5
ES 08301 Mataro
Phone: +34 3 7905513
Fax: +34 3 7906802

Dr. Elisabetta CHELLINI
Centro per lo Studio e
la Prevenzione Oncologia U.O.
di Epidemiologia
Via di San Salvi 12
IT 50136 Firenze
Phone: +39 55 5662644
Fax: +39 55 6774842

Dr. R. Van Den OEVER
National Confederation of
Christian Sickness Funds,
Medical Direction
Wetstrast 121
BE 1040 Brussels
Phone: +32 2 2374469
Fax: +32 2 2373300

Elsebeth LYNGE
Danish Cancer Registry,
Inst. of Cancer Epidemiology
Strandboulevarden 49
DK 2100 Copenhagen
Phone: +45 35268866
Fax: +45 35260090

Gunnar HILLERDAL
Univ of Uppsala, Dept. of
Lung Medicine - Lungkliniken,
Akademiska sjukhuset
SE 75185 Uppsala
Phone: +46 18 663000
Fax: +46 18 664086

Luc RAYMOND
Registre Genevois des Tumeurs
Blvd. de la Cluse 55
CH 1205 Genève
Phone: +41 22 3291011
Fax: +44 22 3282933

EXPOSURE TO SELECTED VIRUSES IN RESEARCH LABORATORIES (EVIL PROGRAMME)

Key words
Exposure of research personnel, viruses, research laboratories.

Brief description
The goal of this study is to evaluate exposure of research personnel to specific viruses including DNA viruses such as SV4O and polyoma virus, as well as retroviruses, such as avian leukosis/sarcoma viruses, reticuloendotheliosis viruses and murine leukaemia virus.

These biological agents are frequently handled in research laboratories, in particular in molecular biology, either for the study of the virus itself, as viral vectors, or as a contaminant of various biological specimens. Use or handling of viruses will be assessed through questionnaires and will be validated by determination of the serological profile of antibodies to specific viruses in various categories of research workers. In addition to immunological tests, which may not be very sensitive, new PCR techniques will be used for a few viruses. We shall proceed from simply knowing a given virus is being used in a laboratory to the demonstration of seroconversion with or without apparent clinical infection. It will provide an objective measure of the reality of contact of personnel with viruses being used in a given laboratory as well as well as quantification of exposure in groups exposed differently to viruses. Four groups will be distinguished:
- persons currently handling the virus;
- persons having handled the virus in the past but not currently working with it;
- persons not handling the virus themselves but working in the same laboratory as persons who do;
- persons not working in the laboratories but employed in the same research institution.

These groups will be selected in order to be comparable in terms of age, sex and educational level.

Project leader:
Dr. A. J. SASCO
International Agency for
Research on Cancer, Unit of
Analytical Epidemiology
150 cours Albert-Thomas
FR 69372 Lyon Cedex 08
Phone: +33 72 73 84 12
Fax: +33 72 73 85 75
Contract number: CT931347

Participants:
Dr. P.A. BURNS
The Jack Birch Unit of Environmental Carcinogenesis,
Univ of York
UK York Y01 5DD

Dr. S. BELLI
Istituto Superiore di Sanità
IT 00161 Rome

Dr. Van LEEUWEN
The Netherlands Cancer
Inst.,
Antoni van Leeuwenhoek
Huis
Plesmanlaan 121
NL 1066 CX Amsterdam

Mme. M. TIRMARCHE
Institut de protection et
de sureté nucléaire
P.O. Box 6
FR 92265 Fontenay-aux-Roses

Mme. S. BENHAMOU
INSERM U 351, Institut
Gustave Roussy
Rue Camille Desmoulins
FR 94805 Villejuif Cedex

M. Claude TEISSIER
Inspection d'Hygiène et
de Sécurité, CNRS
P.O. Box 20 CR
FR 67037 Strasbourg Cedex

Prof. A. AHLBOM
Dept. of Epidemiology,
Inst. of Environmental Medicine, Karolinska Inst.
P.O. Box 60208
SE 104 01 Stockholm

Prof. C. CHILVERS
Dept. of Public Health &
Epidemiology,
The Univ of Nottingham,
Medical School,
Queen's Med Centre
UK Nottingham NG7 2UH

A PILOT CASE CONTROL STUDY ON THE INFLUENCE OF MATERNAL AND PATERNAL OCCUPATIONAL EXPOSURE AND OF OTHER EXTERNAL FACTORS ON THE INCIDENCE OF CONGENITAL LEUKAEMIA

Key words
Congenital leukaemia, (occupational or environmental) factor.

Brief description
Congenital leukaemia is a very rare condition accounting for about 1% of all leukemias in childhood.

A hypothesis about factors in the pathogenetic process of congenital leukaemia presumes the influence of a very potent external (occupational or environmental) factor during the development of the haematopoietic system in utero.

In this pilot study the relationship with occupational or other exposures of the parents will be studied through a case control approach.

The collaboration with cytogenetic laboratories allows for a very rapid registration of cases. It also allows for identifying some genetic factors to be considered in order to increase the sensitivity in a more extensive case control study which will be carried out afterwards.

Project leader:
Dr. Ludwine CASTELEYN
Vlaamse Vereniging voor Informatie over
Kankerverwekkende en Mutagene Agentia VZW
Terkluizendreef 45
BE 1640 Sint-Genesius Rode
Phone: +32 23 80 14 10
Contract number: CT941014

Participants:
Dr. A. AVENTIN
Laboratio de Hematologia Hospital de la
Santa Creu de Saint Pau
Avgdda. St. Antonio M. Claret 167
ES 08025 Barcelona
Phone: +34 3 3473133
Fax: +34 3 4503290

Dr. A. CUNEO
Cattedra di Ematologia Universita di Ferrara
Corso Glovecca 203
IT 44100 Ferrara
Phone: +39 532212142

Dr. C. MECUCCI
Instituto di Ematologia Policlinico Monteluce
IT 06100 Perugia
Phone: +39 75 578 3808
Fax: +39 75 578 3691

Dr. C. SAN ROMAN & Dr. T. FERRO &
C.E. RAMON Y CAJAL
Servicio de Genetica Medica Ministerio
de Sanidad Y Seguridad Social
ES 28034 Madrid
Phone: +34 1 3368334
Fax: +34 1 3369016

Dr. D. LEROUX
Cytogenetic Laboratory, Faculté de
Medecine Université Joseph Fourier
FR 38700 La Tronch
Phone: +33 76 51 8000
Fax: +33 76 51 2477

Dr. J. KLAVEL
Unite Inserm U 170
16 Av. Paul-Vaillant-Couturier
FR 94807 Villejuif Cedex
Phone: +33 1 45 59 50 38
Fax: +33 1 45 59 51 51

Dr. K. van DAMME
Univ of Antwerpen, VVIKMA, Vlaamse Verg.
voor Informatie in-zake Kankerverwerkende
en/of Mutagene Agentia VZW
C/O Bd E. Jacqmain, 155
BE 1210 Bruxelles
Phone: +32 2 224 05 67
Fax: +32 2 224 05 61

Dr. A. Seniori COSTANTINI
C.S.P.O. Centro por le Studio e la Prevenzione
Oncologica U.O. Epidemiologia
Via di San Salvi 12
IT 50136 Firenze
Phone: +39 55 56 62 647
Fax: +39 55 67 74 89

Dr. K. ZANG
Institut for Humangenetic, Universität des
Saarlandes Universitätskliniken Bau 68
DE 6650 Homburg/Saar
Phone: +49 68 41166600

Dr. S. CASTEDO
Dept. of Medical Genetics Medical Faculty
of Porto, Hospital S. Joao
PT 4200 Porto
Phone: +351 2 590591
Fax: +351 2 5503940

Prof. Dr. A. HAGEMEIJER
Dept. of Cell Biology & Genetics Erasmus Univ
P.O. Box 1738
NL 3000 Dr. Rotterdam
Phone: +31 10 4087196
Fax: +31 10 4360225

Prof. Dr. B. de JONG
Dept. of Human Genetics, Univ of Groningen
Antonius Deusinglaan 4
NL 9713 AW Groningen
Phone: +31 50 632925
Fax: +31 50 632947

Prof. Dr. F. MITELMAN
Dept. of Clinical Genetics,
Univ Hospital Univ of Lund
SE 22185 Lund
Phone: +46 46 17 33 62
Fax: +46 46 13 10 61

Prof. Dr. H. van den BERGHE
Center for Human Genetics Univ of Leuven
Herestraat 49
BE 3000 Leuven
Phone: +32 16 34 58 77
Fax: +32 16 34 59 92

Prof. Dr. O.A. HAAS
St. Anna Children's Hospital
Kinderspitalgasse 6
AT 1090 Vienna
Phone: +43 1 40470/406
Fax: +43 1 4087230

Prof. Dr. R. BERGER
Centre Hayem Hopital St. Louis
1 Av. Claude Vellefaux
FR 75475 Parix Cedex 10
Phone: +33 142069531

Prof. E. SCHIFFELERS
Lambda, Laboratory for Mathematical Data
Analysis Facultés Universitaires
Rue de Bruxelles, 61
BE 5000 Namur
Phone: +32 81 640 388
Fax: +32 81 640 059

EUROPEAN PROGRAMME OF OCCUPATIONAL RISKS AND PREGNANCY OUTCOME (EUROPOP)

Key words
Pregnancy, preterm birth rate, abortion, growth retardation, working conditions.

Brief description
During the life time of the EEC there has been a significant increase in the number of women employed during pregnancy.

There is evidence from France that there is a relationship between heavy physical load during employment and preterm birth rate and there are other data which suggest that heavy physical load may be related to other deleterious perinatal outcomes such as abortion and intrauterine growth retardation.

In France, social policies related to work in pregnancy have been developed which are thought to have reduced the preterm birth rate in that country. Information about this area from other countries is lacking.

This concerted action will examine the relationship between working conditions and pregnancy outcome in Europe.

Cross sectional surveys of working conditions, the pregnancy outcomes of interest, i.e. preterm birth, intrauterine growth retardation and spontaneous abortion and their confounders will be undertaken and integrated into a stratified analysis.

The data will form a scientific basis for social policy on work during pregnancy in Europe.

Project leader:
Dr. Gian Carlo DI RENZO
European Association of
Perinatal Medicine
c/o Institute of Obstetrics
and Gynaecology,
Policlinico Monteluce
IT 06122 Perugia
Phone: +39 75 572 92 71
Fax: +39 75 572 92 71
Contract number: CT941041

Participants:
A. van ASSCHE
Dept. of Ob/Gyn,
Univ Hospital Leuven U.Z.
Gasthuisberg
Herestraat 49
BE 3000 Leuven

L. PEREIRA-LEITE
Hospital de S. Joao Servicio
de Obstetricia
PT 4200 Portugal

A. ANTSAKLIS
Dept. of Ob/Gyn, Div. MFM
Athens Univ
11 Lamsakou Street
GR 11528 Athens

A. GONZALES MERLO
Dept. of Ob/Gyn, Universidad Autonoma de Granada
Facultad de Medicina
ES Granada

A. GONZALES-GONZALES
Universidad Autonoma de
Madrid Facultad de Medicina
Avda. del Arzobisco Morcillo
ES 28029 Madrid

A. HUCH
Dept. of OB/Gyn,
Universitätsspital Zürich
Frauenklinikstrasse 10
CH 8091 Zürich

A. KURJAK
Dept. of Ob/Gyn - Ultrasonic
Inst. Univ of Zagreb
Sveti Duh 64
HR 4100 Zagreb

C. O'HERLIHY
Dept. of Ob/Gyn,
National Maternity Hospital,
Univ College of Dublin
Holles Street
IE Dublin 2

M. PAJNTAR
Dept. of Ob/Gyn, Research
Slajmerjeva 3
SI 6100 Ljublana

D.J. TAYLOR
Dept. of Ob/Gyn, School of
Medicine Sciences Bldg,
Leicester Royal Infirmary
P.O. Box 65
UK Leicester LE2 7LX

E. PAPIERNIK
Service de Gynecologie
Obstetrique-Baudelocque
123, Boulevard de Port Royal
FR 75679 Paris Cedex 14

E.V. COSMI
2nd Inst. of Ob/Gyn,
Univ La Sapienza,
Policlinico Umbert I
Viale Regina Elena 324
IT 00161 Roma

F. BRANCONI
Dept. of Ob/Gyn, Policlinico
Careggi, Univ of Florence
Viale Morgagni
IT 50100 Firenze

F. FACCHINETTI
Dept. of Ob/Gyn
Univ of Modena
Via del Pozzo 71
IT 41100 Modena

G. BREART
Epidemiology Research Unti
INSERM
123 Bd de Port Royal
FR 75014 Paris

G.H. BREBOROWICZ
Dept. of Perinatology, Univ
School of Medical Sciences
PL 60 535 Poznan

H. SINIMÄE
Tartu Univ Women's Clinic
36 Lossi Street
EE 2400 Tartu

H. van GEIJN
EC CAP Perinatal Surveil-
lance, Free Univ Hospital
P.O. Box 7057
NL 1007 MB Amsterdam

J. ARENDT
Centre Hospitalier
de Luxembourg
4, rue Barbie
LU 1210 Luxembourg

J. DUDENHAUSEN
Abt. für Geburtsmedizin,
Frauenklinik und Poliklinik
Freie Universität Berlin
DE 1000 Berlin 19

J. GARDOSI
Perinatal Research and
Monitoring Unit, Dept. of
Ob/Gyn, Faculty of Medi-
cine, Floor D, East Block
UK Nottingham NC7 2UH

J. MUNTEANU
Dept. of Ob/Gyn
Timisoara Univ of Medicine
and Pharmacology
Bvd.V. Babes, 12
RO 1900 Timisoara

J. STENCL
Dept. of Ob/Gyn,
Postgraduate Medical Inst.
Derer's Hospital
Limbova 5 - Kramere
SK 833 02 Bratislava

J.M. CARRERA
Dept. of Ob/Gyn,
Inst. Univ Dexeus
Passeig Bonanonva 67
ES 08017 Barcelona

J.M. THOULON
Dept. of Ob/Gyn Hotel Dieu
61 Quai Jules-Courmont
FR 69288 Lyon 02

K. MARSÀL
Dept. of OB/Gyn
Malmö General Hospital
SE 21401 Malmö

L. KOVACS
Dept. of Ob/Gyn
Albert Szent-Györgyi
Semmelweiss u 1
HU 6725 Szeged

L. SICHINAVA
2nd Moscow Medical Inst.
Dept. of Ob/Gyn
Shablovka Street 57-11
RU 113 162 CIS Moscow

M. BRINCAT
Dept. of Ob/Gyn, St. Luke's
Hospital Medical School
MT Malta

M. KEIRSE
Dept. of Obstetrics Leiden
Univ Hospital
NL 2300 RC Leiden

M. KUDELA
Dept. of Ob/Gyn
L.P. Pavlova 6
CZ 77600 Olomouc

M.J.SAUREL-CUBIZOLLES
INSERM
16 Av. P. Vaillant-Couturier
FR 94807 Villejuif Cedex

N. PATEL
Dept. of Ob/Gyn,
Ninewells Hospital
UK Dundee DD2 1UB

O.GÖKMEN
Maternity Hospital
Hamamönü
TR Ankara

R. ERKKOLA
Dept. of Ob/Gyn,
Univ Central Hospital
FI SF-20520 Turku

S. EIK-NES
National Center for Fetal
Medicine, Dept. of Ob/Gyn,
Trondheim Univ Hospital
NO 7006 Trondheim

T. WEBER
Dept. of Ob/Gyn,
Hvidovre Hospital
DK 2650 Hvidovre

T.K.A.B. ESKES
Dept. of Ob/Gyn,
Univ Hospital Nijmegen
P.O. Box 9101
NL 6500 Nijmegen

W. HOLZGREVE
Zentrum für Frauenheilkunde
Westfalen Wilhelms
Universitäts Münster
Albert Schweizer Strasse 33
DE 4400 Münster

W. KÜNZEL
Frauenklinik der
Justus-Liebig-Universität
Klinikstrasse 28
DE 6300 Giessen

EUROHAZCON: EUROPEAN COLLABORATIVE STUDY OF HAZARDOUS WASTE DISPOSAL IN LANDFILL SITES AND RISK OF CONGENITAL MALFORMATION

Key words
Waste landfill, congenital malformation, mutagenic effects, teratogenic effects.

Brief description
The aim of the project is to investigate whether residence near hazardous waste landfill sites is associated with an increased risk of congenital malformation. Landfill is a common means of disposal of hazardous waste. The health effects of residence near hazardous waste landfill sites are a subject of current concern to both public health professionals and the public.

Exposure to hazardous wastes could increase the risk of congenital malformation via either mutagenic (preconceptional) or teratogenic (postconceptional) effects. There is at present very little evidence on which to base the assessment of options for waste disposal for the future or on which to base information to the public. Waste disposal and its environmental health impact is a transnational problem in Europe. Individual reports of clusters of congenital malformations near hazardous waste sites are of limited value since it can be expected that some such clusters will be found by chance alone. There is thus a need for large studies using good quality congenital malformation data, and covering multiple waste sites. These conditions can be fulfilled in this collaborative study using existing population-based congenital malformation registers with multiple sources of information for high and unbiased case ascertainment and detailed diagnostic information.

The study design is a case-control study. Cases will be all malformed livebirths, stillbirths and induced abortions following prenatal diagnosis living within a defined geographical zone, registered on population-based registers held by the participating centres. Cases will include malformations diagnosed after the neonatal period, particularly important for the ascertainment of cardiac anomalies. Malformations will be classified into subgroups which reflect their mutagenic (eg Downs Syndrome) or teratogenic origin, and evidence of association with environmental exposures. Controls will be a random sample of normal births, with two controls per case, matched by year of birth. Account will be taken of possible confounding by maternal age and socioeconomic status. Distance of residence from the waste sites will be the surrogate exposure variable. Distance from multiple waste sites will be pooled in the statistical analysis to increase statistical power, and to give an overall estimate of effect.

Project leader:
Dr. Helen DOLK
London School of Hygiene and
Tropical Medicine,
Environmental Epidemiology Unit
Keppel Street
UK London WC1E 7HT
Phone: +44 71 92 72 415
Fax: +44 71 58 04 524
Contract number: CT941099

Participants:

Dr. M. CORNEL
Eurocat Dept. of Human Genetics,
Univ of Groningen
4 Ant. Deusinglaan
NL 9713 Groningen
Phone: +31 50 632952
Fax: +31 50 187268

Dr. D. STONE
Public Health Research Unit, Univ of Glasgow
1 Lilybank Gardens
UK Glasgow G12 8RZ
Phone: +44 041 339 3118/19
Fax: +44 041 337 2776

Dr. E. GARNE
Inst. of Genetics, Pediatric Dept., Odense Univ
JB Winslows Vej 17
DK 5000 Odense
Phone: +45 66 11 33 33
Fax: +45 66 13 28 54

Dr. J. CHAPPLE
Congenital Malformation Register Office,
Clinical Research Centre,
Northwick Park Hospital
Watford Road
UK Harrow, Middlesex HA 1 3UJ
Phone: +44 081 869 3527

Dr. K.N. MATEJA
Inst. of Public Health of the
Republik of Slovenia
Trubarjeva 2
SI 61000 Ljublijana
Phone: +38 61 123 245
Fax: +38 61 323 955

Dr. S. GARCIA-MINAUR
Registro de Anomalias Congenitas
de la Communidad Autonoma Vasca Clinica
Materno-Infantil, Hospital de Cruces
ES 48903 Baracaldo (Vizcaya)
Phone: +34 4 499 30 35
Fax: +34 4 499 30 35

Dr. V. NELEN
Provinciaal Instituut van Hygiene
Kronenburgstraat 45
BE 2000 Antwerpen
Phone: +32 3 238 51 29
Fax: +32 3 237 70 22

Dr. Y. GILLEROT
Institut de Morphologie Pathologique,
Dept. Genetique
Allee des Templiers 41
BE 6270 Loverval
Phone: +32 71 43 79 01
Fax: +32 71 47 15 20

F. BIANCHI
Instituto di Fisiologia, Clinica del CNR,
Univ di Pisa
Via Trieste 41
IT 56100 Pisa
Phone: +39 50 21 28 /25 771
Fax: +39 50 58 9038

Prof. R. TENCONI
Genetica Medica Dip Pediatrica
Via Giustiniani 3
IT 35128 Padova
Phone: +39 49 821 3513/3509
Fax: +39 49 821 3510/3509

OCCUPATIONAL CANCER RISK RELATED TO IRREVERSIBLE CENTRAL NERVOUS EFFECTS AFTER NEUROTOXIC SOLVENT EXPOSURE

Key words
Solvents, brain stem, CNS-lesions, neuro-endocrinological regulation, carcingens.

Brief description
Industrial chemicals represent more than 50% of established human carcino-gens, among them solvents known for their narcotic action.

Numerous publications on the prenarcotic action OE-solvents occurring at the workplace have raised suspicion of irreversible damage to the brain stem. The brain is essential in regulating adequate responses of the autonomous nervous system in relation to neoplastic growth after carcino-genic exposures. A long-term follow-up of persons/populations exposed to defined quantities OE-solvents or solvent-like organic chemicals has to address the acute risk of persistent CNS-lesions with related deficiencies and effects on neuro-endocrinological regulation, and to assess the long-term risk of decreased resistance against exogenous risk factors, such as carcinogens. Epidemiological studies usually do not cover a whole pathogenic process but identify associations between exposure to a risk factor, i.e. promotor, and outcome such as time of manifest occurrence of (latent) cancer.

Published results of pertinent studies indicate an increased risk OE-cancers such as melanoma, breast cancer, pancreatic and other gastro-intestinal cancers, thyroid cancer, kidney cancer, brain tumours, lymphoma and leukemias after solvent exposures specifically to styrene, benzene, vinylchloride and perchloroethylene. The variety of excess cancer incidences in such occupational cohorts indicates a role of the solvent at the level of promotion following pre-existing carcinogenesis. The required follow-up of previously diagnosed subgroups with lesions of the brain stem is a task or interdisciplinary concerted action with epidemiologic planning. The controlled approach used for the quantification of a hypothetic association requires access to large cohorts exposed to defined solvents for a sufficient period of time and a competent testing for irre-Versible damage of the brain stem.

This proposal is relevant to the area: *Risk factors in Occupational medicine*, as well as for etiological factors for less common cancers.

Plans are to allocate 500 persons exposed to neurotoxic solvents in 6 study centers for neuropsychological testing and to follon the subcohort.

Project leader:
Dr. Rainer FRENTZEL-BEYME
German Cancer Research
Centre Deutsches Krebsforschungszentrum
Im Neuenheimer Feld 280
DE 69120 Heidelberg
Phone: +49 622 1422378
Fax: +49 622 1409516
Contract number: CT941117

Participants:

Dr. Ch. EDLING
Dept. Occupational Medicine,
University Hospital
SE 75185 Uppsala
Phone: +46 18 51 99 78

Dr. K. EKBERG &
Prof. Dr. O. AXELSON
Dept. of Occupational
Medicine,
Faculty of Health Sciences
SE 581 85 Linköping
Phone: +46 13 14 58 31

Prof. Dr. J. KONIETZKO &
Dr. A. MUTTRAY
Institut für Arbeits- und
Sozialmedizin, Johannes-
Gutenberg-Universität Mainz
Obere Zahlbacher Str. 67
DE 55131 Mainz
Phone: +49 6131 17 32 35

Dr. P. ARLIEN-SOBORG
Hvidovre Hospital, Munici-
pality of Copenhagen,
Dept. of Neurology,
Univ. of Copenhagen
Kettegard Alle 30
DK 2650 Hvidovre
Phone: +45 31 47 39 41

Prof. Dr. A. MUTTI
Instituto di Clinica Medica
e Nefrologia, Cattedra di
Medicina Del Lavoro, Lab.
di Tossicologia Industriale,
Univ. degli Studi di Parma
IT Parma
Phone: +39 521 29 13 43

Dr. R. LUCCHINI &
Dr. S. PORRU
Opedali Civili Brescia,
Cattedra di Medicina del
Lavoro dell'Università degli
Studi di Brescia
IT Brescia
Phone: +39 30 39 49 02

Dr. M. PEPER
Psychologisches Institut, Abt.
Persönlichkeitspsychologie,
FS Neuropsychologie, Albert
Ludwigs-Universität Freiburg
Niemensstr. 10
DE 79085 Freiburg
Phone: +49 761 270 5310

Prof. A. SEATON
University of Aberdeen,
Environmental &
Occupational Medicine,
Medical School
Foresterhill
UK Aberdeen AB9 2ZD
Phone: +44 224 66 29 90

Dr. A. SPURGEON
Institute of Occupational
Health, University of
Birmingham
Edgbaston
UK Birmingham B15 2TT
Phone: +44 21 471 52 08

Prof. Dr. M. VANHOORNE
Vakgroep Maatschappelijke
Gezondheidskunde
Universitair Ziekenhuis
De Pintelaan 185 Blok A
BE 9000 Gent
Phone: +32 9 240 49 94

Prof. Dr. W. ZATONSKI
Cancer Control Office,
The Maria Sklodowska-Curie
Memorial Cancer Center
Wawelska Street 15
PL 00 973 Warszawa
Phone: +48 2 643 92 34

Prof. Dr. H. CHECKOWAY
School of Public Health and
Community Medicine,
University of Washington,
Dept. of Environmental
Health
US 98195 Seattle WA

Dr. C. SIN-ENG
Division of Occupational
Medicine, Dept. Community,
Occupational and Family
Medicine, National
University Hospital
Lower Kent Ridge Road
TH 0511 Singapore
Phone: +65 779 14 89

Prof. Dr. H. FENGSHENG
Institute of Occupational
Medicine, Chinese Academy
of Preventive Medicine
29 Nan Wei Road
CN 10050 Beijing
Phone: +861 301 4323

Dr. F. LABRECHE
Regional Occupational Health
Team, Hospital de
Sacre-Coeur de Montreal
75 De Port Royal est bureau
CA H3L Montreal

Dr. P. KHUNAWAT &
Dr. S. KONGPATANAKUL
Department of Preventive
Medicine, Dept. of Pharma-
cology, Faculty of Medicine
Siriraj Hospital, Mahidol
University
TH 10700 Bangkok

Dr. J. TU
Shanghai Cancer Institute,
Shanghai Cancer Registry
270 Dong Au Road
CN Shanghai

Prof. Dr. Y. WANG
Dept. Occupational Medicine,
Shanghai Institute of
Occupational Health of
Chemical Industry
369 Chengdu Road (N)
CN 20041 Shanghai

Prof. Dr. S.Z. XUE
Dept. of Occupational Health
Toxicology Program, School
of Public Health, Shanghai
Medical University
CN 200032 Shanghai

EPIDEMIOLOGY OF OCCUPATIONAL ASTHMA
AND EXPOSURE TO BIO-ALLERGENS

Key words
Respiratory allergy, asthma, occupational health, bio-allergens.

Brief description
The overall objectives of this concerted action are to identify, characterize and quantify workspace risk factors wich lead to respiratory allergy and asthma. The concerted action should lead to the development of scientific knowledge as a basis for occupational health programmes aimed at the prevention of the prevention of occupational allergic respiratory diseases.

The knowledge generated by the program could in the long term be used for standard setting purposes for bio-allergens and could support the implementation of recently developed EC regulations for biologic agents in general.

The proposal consist of the following elements:

A   development of validated and standardized techniques to measure bio-allergens wich make a cross-comparison possible between laboratories and over time;

B   applications of A in ongoing cross-sectional and longitudinal epidemiological studies in a number of European countries aimed at deriving valid and generalizable study results in order to study relationships between bio-allergen exposures and occupational asthma incidence.

The ongoing studies have similar cross-sectional design and comprise in total more than 3,000 workers. The advantage offered by the conserted action will be:

a   comparability of results of allergen qualification on the work place; and,

b   a pooled analyses can be undertaken for some of the measured endpoints such as serological parameters (specific antibodies) and skin prick test results in relation to the exposure.

The study has an important European dimension. Until now comparison of European studies in the area of occupational asthma has been difficult if not impossible. By combining and sharing knowledge on the identification of allergens, comparability can be obtained of exposure data, and prevalence and incidence rates over different countries and studies. The study ensures collaboration of the few European laboratories active in the important areas of exposure assesment of bioallergens and biological outcome measures.

Project leader:
Dr. D. HEEDERIK
Dept. of Epidemiology
and Public Health
Wageningen University
P.O. Box 238
NL 6700 AE Wageningen
Phone: +31 8370 82 012
Fax: +31 8370 82 782
Contract number: CT941446

Participants:
Dr. P. MALMBERG
National Inst. of Occcupatio-
nal Health Respiratory Div.
SE 171 84 Solna

Dr. K. VENABLES
Dept. of Occupational
Medicine, E. Kaye Building
UK London SW3 6LR

Dr. L. BERLIN &
Dr. L. LILLIENBERG
Occupational Medicine
SE 41266 Göteborg

Dr. T. VIRTANEN
Dept. of Clinical Micro-
biology, Univ of Kuopio
FI 70211 Kuopio

Dr. X. BAUER
Inst. of Occupational
Medicine, Dept. of
Allergology, Univ Bochum
DE 4630 Bochum

AN INVESTIGATION OF REGULATORY CIRCUITS IN THE DEVELOPMENT OF ALLERGIC DISEASE

Key words
Allergy, immunoglobuline, receptor interaction.

Objectives
The proposed research program will combine immunological, genetic-, protein- and cell engineering studies with environmental and clinical research. The studies aim at:

1 the identification of the structural requirements and amino acid residues contributing to the interaction of human immunoglobulin E (IgE) with its high- and low-affinity receptors.

2 the isolation of IgE-binding factors from the sera of atopic donors by affinity chromatography.

3 the development of new diagnostic predictors to monitor the onset and progress of allergies.

4 the design of novel therapeutic interventions for evaluation in vitro and pre-clinical studies.

Brief description
The team in Sheffield will initiate: large scale expression and purification of native IgE and C-terminally truncated recombinant IgE-derived (rFcε) peptides. The team in Bochum will monitor the levels of interleukin (IL)-4, IgE and CD23 in the serum of workers exposed to occupational allergens, A study will be initiated for the monitoring analysis and isolation of IgE-binding factors from the sera of newborns from parents with or without a history of atopy. The complementary role of the participating laboratories i.e. the input of basic research leading to the generation of recombinant ligand and receptor-derived peptides, or engineered cell-lines by the Sheffield team as tools for investigation in clinical research by the Bochum group, is clearly outlined.

Project leader:
Dr. Birgit HELM
Krebs Institute
Western Bank
P.O. Box 594
UK Sheffield S10 2UH
Phone: +44 74 27 68 555
Fax: +44 74 27 95 495
Contract number: CT941184

Participants:
Dr. W. KOENIG
Ruhr Universität Bochum,
Arbeitsgruppe für Infektabwehrmechanismen
Universitätsstrasse 150
DE 4630 Bochum 1
Phone: +49 234 7006860
Fax: +49 234 7094122

Dr. M. SUTER
Institute für Virologie, Veterinaermedizinische
Fakultät, Universität Zürich
Winterthurerstrasse 266a
CH 8057 Zürich
Phone: +41 1 365 1511
Fax: +41 1 363 0140

Dr. E.A. PADLAN
National Institutes of Health,
NIDDK, Building 5, Room 302
US Bethesda MD 20298
Phone: +1 301 402 1780
Fax: +1 301 496 0201

ADVERSE EFFECTS OF VISUAL UNITS (VDUS) WITH PARTICULAR REFERENCE TO EYE MOVEMENT CONTROL IN TEXT PROCESSING

Key words
Display screen equipment, headache, visual disturbances.

Brief description
Member States of the Community have implemented Regulations following the Council Directive of 29 May 1990 on minimum safety and health requirements for work with display screen equipment (VDUs). This was a response to the fact that large numbers of users report difficulties, such as headache, eye-strain and minor visual disturbances, when processing text on refreshed display screens.

It has been assumed that these adverse effects relate, in part, to the presence of flicker or visible (i.e. perceptible) instability.

However, modern displays are refreshed at frequencies well above traditional estimates of fusion and this has not led to a marked reduction in complaints.

This Concerted Action builds on recent research findings showing an association between aspects of eye movement control and pulsating illumination at frequencies of 100 Hz or above, when no flicker is visible.

Pulsation interferes with the normal suppressive effects which occur when a saccade is executed. Saccades fall short of their intended target and, from the subjects' perspective, there is degree of perceptual instability, which is quite independent of perceived *flicker*.

These small modifications to saccade control have a disproportionate effect on word-recognition because they reduce the probability that a word will be fixated at its optimal position.

Recent psycholinguistic research has demonstrated that shifts in the initial point of fixation of only one or two characters lead to large changes in the probability that a word will be refixated.

The Action aims to examine the nature of this effect in textprocessing and in particular the way it interacts with reading strategy, since there is evidence that professional typists are particularly intolerant of mislocations in the point of first fixation within the word.

The Action will also take the first steps towards linking the whole class of effects concerning eye movement control to reports of visual fatigue in specific work situations.

This better scientific understanding will be essential if future Guidelines are to be effective in reducing complaints.

Project leader:
Professor Alan KENNEDY
University of Dundee,
Dept. of Psychology
UK Dundee DD1 4HN
Phone: +44 38 223181
Fax: +44 38 229993
Contract number: CT941441

Participants:

Dr. A. HENDRIKS
Nijmegen Inst. for Cognition and Information
(NICI) Univ of Nijmegen
P.O. Box 9104
NL 6500 HE Nijmegen
Phone: +31 80 61 2620
Fax: +31 80 61 5938

Dr. BRYSBAERT
Laboratory of Experimental Psychology
Univ of Louvain
Tiensestraat 102
BE 3000 Louvain
Phone: +32 16 285964
Fax: +32 16 286099

Dr. C.M.M. de WEERT
Director, Nijmegen Inst. for Cognition and
Information (NICI) Univ of Nijmegen
P.O. Box 9104
NL 6500 HE Nijmegen
Phone: +31 80 61 2620
Fax: +31 80 61 5938

Dr. J.A.M. van GISBERGEN
Dept. of Medical Physics & Biophysics
Geert Grootplein N21
NL 6525 EZ Nijmegen
Phone: +31 80 519111
Fax: +31 80 540576

Dr. T. BACCINO
Psychology Dept., Univ of Dundee
Tayside
UK Dundee DD1 4HN
Phone: +44 382 23181
Fax: +44 382 29993

Dr. W.S. MURRAY
Psychology Dept., Univ of Dundee
Tayside
UK Dundee DD1 4HN
Phone: +44 382 23181
Fax: +44 382 29993

Prof. Dr. HELLER
Institut für Psychologie der RWTH
Jagerstr. 17/19
DE 5100 Aachen
Phone: +49 271 806012
Fax: +49 241 803995

Dr. A.J. WILKENS
Medical Research Council
Appleid Psychology Unit
15 Chauser Road
UK Cambridge
Phone: +44 223 355294
Fax: +44 223 359062

Dr. J. PYNTE
Centre de Recherche et Psychologie Cognitive
(CREPCO), URA 182, Université de Provence
29 Avenue Robert Schuman
FR 13621 Aix-en-Provence

Dr. M.T. SWANSTON
Dept. Psychology, Dundee Inst. of Technology
Bell Street
UK Dundee
Phone: +44 382 308000
Fax: +44 382 308877

Dr. R. RADACH
Institut für Psychologie der RWTH
Jagerstr. 17/19
DE 5100 Aachen
Phone: +49 241 806012
Fax: +49 241 803995

Prof. G. d'YDEWALLE
Laboratory of Experimental Psychology,
Univ of Louvain
Tiensestraat 102
BE 3000 Louvain
Phone: +32 16 285964
Fax: +32 16 286099

STUDY OF THE ROLE OF PERCEIVED JOB STRESS ON SICK LEAVE FROM WORK AND ON THE INCIDENCE OF CORONARY HEART DISEASE ACROSS EUROPE

Key words
Work-stress, epidemiological prospective studies, coronary heart disease.

Brief description
- Given the absence of concerted epidemiological research at the European level concerning the relation of self-perceived work-stress with seack leave.
- Given the rarity of epidemiological prospective studies concerning the relation of self--perceived work-stress and incidence of coronary heart disease.
- Given the existences since 12 years of an empiric approach based on a model whereby job-stress is assessed by way of a self administered questionnaire: the Karasek-Model. In this model four scales are computed: Job-Demand, Job-Control (or Job-Discretion), Job-support and Job-Security.

It is proposed to initiate a concerted action in 5 European countries (7 participating centers) with the following working hypotheses:
1 Between EC member states differences in perceived job-stress exist, independant of age, sex and job-title (ISCO 88).
2 There exists a direct association between perceived job-stress and sickness absence independant of other known determinants.
3 There exists a direct association between perceived job-stress and the incidence of coronary heart disease, independant of serum total cholesterol, serum HDL-cholesterol, arterial blood pressure, smoking habits and serum fibrinogen.

All three working hypotheses will be tested in male middle-aged populations (total = 44600) and the first two in female populations (total = 19000). Standardized and well validated methods will be used.
The answers to the three working hypotheses could lead to important recommendations for the prevention of sickness absences as well as for the prevention and/or management of job-stress in order to preserve health.
Input of the participating centers:

	BE(OI)	FR(O2)	BE(O3)	IT(O4)	ES(O5)	SE(O6)	SE(O7)	TOTAL
Males	12500	5000	12500	4000	2200	7500	900	44600
Females	2500	2500	2500	2000	2000	7500	-	19000
Total	15000	7500	15000	6000	4200	15000	900	63600

Project leader:
Professor Marcel KORNITZER
Laboratoire d'Epidemiologie et de Medicine Sociale,
Ecole de Santé Publique
Campus Erasme, Route de Lennik 808
BE 1070 Bruxelles
Phone: +32 2 555 40 89
Fax: +32 2 555 40 49
Contract number: CT941336

Participants:
Dr. L. WILHELMSEN
Dept. of Medicine,
Ostra Hospital Ck Plan 2
SE 41685 Göteborg
Phone: +46 31 37 40 81
Fax: +46 31 25 92 54

Dr. M. FERRARIO
Univ of Milan, Inst. of Occupational Health,
Clinica del Lavoro Devoto
Via S. Barnaba, 8
IT 20122 Milano
Phone: +39 2 546 44 57
Fax: +39 2 551 871 72

Dr. M. ROMON-ROUSSEAUX &
Dr. Ch. BOULENGHEZ
Laboratoire de Médicine du Travail
Faculté de Médecine
1 Place de Verdun
FR 59045 Lille Cedex
Phone: +33 20 62 69 65
Fax: +33 20 88 36 64

Dr. S. SANS
Pavello del Convent 20p U.D.
Hospital Sant Pau
167 Avenida San Antonio Claret
ES 08025 Barcelona
Phone: +34 3 456 36 12
Fax: +34 3 433 15 72

Dr. M. KOMPIER
NIPG, TNO
Postbus 124
NL 2300 AC Leiden

Dr. S.O. ISACSSON & Dr. P.O. OSTERGREN
Lunds Universiteit, Institutionen for
Klinisk Samhällsmedicin,
Dept. of Community Health Sciences
SE Malmö
Phone: +46 40 33 26 75
Fax: +46 40 33 62 15

Prof. G. de BACKER & Dr. P. GHEERAERT
Universiteit Gent, Faculteit Geneeskunde,
Vakgroep Maatschappelijke Gezondsheidkunde
de Pintelaan, 185
BE 9000 Gent
Phone: +32 92 40 36 27
Fax: +32 91 40 49 94

Dr. I. MAYNE
Faculté de Médecine, Ecole de Santé Publique,
Laboratoire d'Epidémiologie
et de Médecine Sociale
Campus Erasme, CP 595,
Route de Lennik 808
BE 1070 Bruxelles
Phone: +32 2 555 40 87
Fax: +32 2 555 40 49

MERCURY AS AN ACTIVATOR OF THE IMMUNE SYSTEM AND AN INDUCER OF AUTO-IMMUNE AND OTHER DISEASES IN GENETICALLY PREDISPOSED INDIVIDUALS

Key words
Mercury, autoimmune reactions, glomerulonephritis, dental amalgam, genetically predisposed.

Brief description
Background: The heavy metal mercury is toxic in high concentrations and can cause injuries in the nervous system and the kidneys.

Mercury can also induce autoimmune reactions with the synthesis of autoantibodies against DNA and the basement membrane of kidney glomeruli. The autoantibodies and the immune complexes formed will eventually cause glomerulonephritis.

Mercury released from dental amalgam: During the last years an increasing public health problem has been the large number of patients who attribute their manifold symtoms to mercury released from amalgam fillings.

It is clear that the amount of mercury released from the amalgam fillings cannot cause toxic symtoms. Therefore, the hypothesis that mercury released from these filling affect the immune system has gained acceptance.

It is now generally believed in large patients groups that the effect of mercury on the immune system is the cause of their multiple symtoms.

Recently, a considerable patient group consider that their symtoms are caused by exposure to electromagnetic fields from computer screens and electric wires. They also consider that the electromagnetic fields act by releasing mercury from amalgam fillings. Thus, these patient groups have identified a common cause of their symtoms.

Research project: Mercury and zink are unique molecules with regard to their ability to affect the immune system.

No other small molecules can induce polyclonal T-cell dependent activation of the immune system. It is not impossible that these molecules can cause a variety of symtoms in sensitive individuals.

Mercury can only activate the immune systems of certain mouse and the genetic control is to a large extent controlled by genes with the Major Histocompatibility Complex (MHC).

Hypothesis: We will test the hypothesis that mercury binds to molecules on antigenpresenting cells and transform molecules on these cells to superantigens capable of activating T-cells with a particular set of VB antigen-binding receptors.

Thus, variety of symptoms in patients who are genetically predisposed, because their T-cells have been selected in the thymus by endogeneous expression of MHC class I and II molecules to express certain antigen specificities.

Project leader:
Professor Göran MÖLLER
Stockholm University,
Dept of Immunology
SE 10 691 Stockholm
Phone: +46 8 15 78 82
Fax: +46 8 15 41 63
Contract number: CT941527

Participants:
Prof. Antonio COUTINHO
Unité d'Immunobiologie,
CNRS URA 359
25 rue du Docteur Roux
FR 75724 Paris cedex 15
Phone: +33 1 45 68 85 93
Fax: +33 1 45 68 89 21

Dr. Artur AGUAS
Center for Experimental
Cytology, Univ of Porto
Rua do Campo Alegro 823
PT 4100 Porto
Phone: +351 2 699 154
Fax: +351 2 699 157

PREVALENCE AND RISK FACTORS FOR OBSTRUCTIVE AIRWAY DISEASES IN FARMERS

Key words
Farmers, airway obstruction, occupation-related risk factors.

Brief description
Farmers have traditionally been described as having one of the most dangerous occupations. In many countries, respiratory disorders, especially airway obstruction, are the most frequently occurring occupational diseases in this population.

Since, on the other hand, occupational asthma and occupational bronchitis are potentially preventable conditions, we suggest a concerted action in order to (1) estimate the prevalence of obstructive airway diseases in farmers across Europe, (2) identify the influence of inherent and occupation-related risk factors for the development of obstructive airway diseases in farmers across Europe, and (3) provide a European rationale for the development of control measurements to reduce the risk of obstructive airway diseases in farmers in the European community.

The study will comprise two steps: In the first, we will determine the prevalence of respiratory symptoms in cross-sectional samples of farmers by means of a standardised questionnaire part of which has been validated in the EC Respiratory Health Survey in 100,000 (short version) and 15,000 (long version) randomly selected subjects from the general population. Work exposure will he validated by qualitative methods.

The second step will focus on subpopulations of farmers with an increased risk for the development of obstructive airway disease.

The work-up of methods for quantitative exposure assessment is an important goal of the concerted action prior to measurement of a limited number of components by central laboratories. Four of them will care for the followinq tasks:
1 Dust measurements;
2 Measurement of airborne allergen, especially storage mite allergen;
3 Measurement of airborne micro-organisms and endotoxin, and
4 Analysis of serial peak flow records in farmers with symptoms suggestive of occupational asthma or bronchitis and asymptomatic farmers.

By the end of the study, we will have identified exposure-response relationships necessary for future European strategies on risk reduction.

Project leader:
Dr. Dennis NOWAK
Zentralinstitut/Ordinariat für Arbeitsmedizin
Adolph-Schönfelder-Strasse 5
DE 22083 Hamburg
Phone: +49 40 29 188 27 90
Fax: +49 40 29 188 27 85
Contract number: CT941554

Participants:

B. DANUSER, MD
Eidgenössische Technische Hochschule
Institut für Hygiene und Arbeitsphysiologie
Clausiusstr. 21
CH 8092 Zürich
Phone: +41 1 256 3986/2211
Fax: +41 1 262 4178

Ch. LUCZYNSKSA, PhD
Div. of Community Health,
Guy's and St. Thomas's Medical
and Dental Schools, Univ of London
Lambeth Palace Road
UK London SE1 7EH
Phone: +44 71 9289292
Fax: +44 71 9281468

E. MONSO, MD
Servei de Pneumologia, Hospital Germans Trias
i Pujol Institut Catala de la Salut
Ap. correus 72
ES 08916 Badalona, Catalonia
Phone: +34 3 3932556
Fax: +34 3 3954206

H. BRETERNITZ, PhD
Institut für Arbeitsmedizin, Medizinische
Hochschule Erfurt Zentrum für Hygiene,
Präventiv- und Umweltmedizin
Gustav-Freytag-Str. 1
DE 99096 Erfurt
Phone: +49 361 387 311
Fax: +49 361 387 314

M. IVERSEN, MD
Kommunehospital Lungeklinikken,
Universitet Aarhus
DK 8000 Aarhus C
Phone: +45 8612 5555/2233
Fax: +45 8613 8614

Prof. P. VERMEIRE, MD
Universiteit Antwerpen Dienst Longziekten
Universiteitsplein 1
BE 2610 Antwerpen
Phone: +32 3 820 2589
Fax: +32 3 820 2590

P. SHERWOOD BURGE, MD
Occupational Long Disease Unit
Birmingham Haertlands
UK East Birmingham B9 5ST
Phone: +44 21 7666611
Fax: +44 21 7736897

U. PALMGREN, PhD, & G. STRÖM
Pegasus Lab
Kunsgatan 113 - Box 97
SE 75103 Uppsala
Phone: +46 18 104700
Fax: +46 18 104500

U. RABE, MD
Fachkrankenhaus für Lungenkrankheiten und
Tuberkulose Abteilung Allergologie und Asthma
DE 14547 Beelitz
Phone: +49 33204 380
Fax: +49 33204 38 309

THE ROLE OF NEURAL AND EPITHELIAL MEDIATORS IN THE PULMONARY RESPONSE TO AIR POLLUTION

Key words
Atmospheric pollution, pulmonary disease, chronic inhalation.

Brief description
Atmospheric pollution is a major factor causing or exacerbating pulmonary disease, and the link between pollution and airway hyperactivity is well established. We have previously demonstrated that inhaled toxic and irritant compounds have a marked effect on the factors that control lung function, which we are produced by nerves, endocrine cells, vascular endothelium and airway epithelium. All of these factors are known to be involved in disease processes, including hyperactivity.

We therefore hypothesise that they are altered in hyperactive airways to a degree related to the severity of the disease, and plan to undertake long-term study of two major pollutants, nitrogen dioxide (no2) and ozone, to test this hypothesis. Tissues obtained by biopsy using a fibreoptic broncho-scope from subjects exposed to airway pollutants will be compared with that from age-matched controls with no respiratory disease to determine changes in their regulatory factors using immunocytochemistry and radio-immunoassay to determine storage of the factors, in-situ hybridisation to determine their rate of synthesis and in-vitro autoradiography to show changes in their sites of action (receptors). Surgically obtained lung tissue will be studied by pharmacological techniques with and without exposure to no2, ozone,or both.

The techniques employing morphology will all be quantified using appropriate forms of computerised analysis.

Results will be compared between the two subject groups and related to the severity of the pollution, the results of lung function tests including bronchial challenge to assess hyperactivity and the effects of experimentally inhaled no2 and ozone. To confirm mechanisms and to dissect the effects of individual pollutants and their timecourse, inhalation experiments will be performed in animals and lung tissues assessed morphologically and pharmacologically as for humans.

The findings of the study will be of benefit in disclosing the mechanism of disease caused by chronic inhalation of air pollutants. This will hopefully lead to better understanding of the pathogenesis, to allow the detection of individuals at greater risk and also to devise therapies to reverse or reduce the disease in sufferers.

Project leader:
Professor Julia M. POLAK
Royal Postgraduate Medical School
Du Cane Road 150
UK London W12 0NN
Phone: +44 81 740 32 31
Fax: +44 81 743 53 62
Contract number: CT941281

Participants:
Dr. C.E. MAPP
Inst. of Occupational Medicine, Univ of Padova
Via J. Facciolati 71
IT 35127 Padova

Prof. R.A. PAUWELS
Univ Hospital, Dept. of Respiratory Diseases
7 K12 IE
De Pintelaan 185
BE 9000 Ghent

Prof. S.T. HOLGATE
The Univ of Southampton, Faculty of Medicine,
Medicine 1 Level D, Centre Block,
Southampton General Hospital
Tremona Road
UK Southampton SO9 4XY

EARLY DETECTION, RISK ASSESSMENT AND PREVENTION OF OCCUPATIONAL ALLERGY CAUSED BY ORGANIC ACID ANHYDRIDES: AN INTERNATIONAL MULTIDISCIPLINARY APPROACH

Key words
Organic Acid Anhydrides, inhalation exposure, exposure limits, exposure-measement.

Brief description
Organic Acid Anhydrides (OAA) are widely used in industry. The compounds are volatile and there is thus risk of inhalation exposure. Studies in the present laboratories have shown high prevalence of sensitization to OAA and of symptoms from the airways, in spite of very low exposure levels. However, the relationship between exposure and risks is nearly unknown.

Such information is i.e. necessary for establishing of permissible exposure limits. The pathomechanism is in some cases an allergy type I reaction, but in other cases the mechanism is not known.

In the first step of the study, exposure-measurement are performed (air and biologic monitoring) and prevalence of symptoms from airways and specific antibodies are studied. The meaning of background factors, such as smoking and atopy is considered.

In the next step, nonspecific bronchial reactivity in a subgroup of exposed subjects and controls are studied. In subjects complaining of work-related asthmatic symptoms and in matched exposed controls lung function at work will be assessed. In exposed symptomatic (sensitized and nonsensitized) subjects and exposed controls, specific nasal challenge tests are performed. Symptoms and nasal inspiratory peak-flow are registred and nasal lavage fluid obtained for studies of mediators and cells.

Subjects with workrelated asthmatic symptoms are challenged bronchially, using a mobile challenge equipment, developed for challenge with low doses of OAA.

Before and after, sputum is collected for study of cells. Later, cells from sputum of the same subjects and from exposed and nonexposed controls will be obtained in the workplace, using the same technique. In one subgroup, bronchial lavage will be performed and cells and mediators studied.

Through the proposed concerted action, larger populations in varying exposures can be studied. The cooperation between laboratories already active in the field, but with different competences, will increase the scientific output, i.e. information is crucial for preventive action in important industries. furthermore, there will be an exchange of knowledge between the laboratories.

Project leader:
Professor Staffan SKERFVING
Department of Occupational and Environmental Medicine,
Lund University
SE 221 85 Lund
Phone: +46 46 173171
Fax: +46 46 173180
Contract number: CT941521

Participants:

Dr. H. DREXLER
Institut für Arbeits- und Sozialmedizin,
Universität Erlangen-Nürnberg
Schillerstrasse 25 und 29
DE 8520 Erlangen
Phone: +49 9131 85 61 12
Fax: +49 9131 85 23 17

Dr. G. MOSCATO
Fondazione Clinica del Lavoro
Via Boezio 26
IT 27100 Pavia
Phone: +39 382 59 22 56
Fax: +39 382 201 14

Dr. P. MAESTRELLI
Instituto di medicina del Lavoro
Via Facciolati 71
IT 35127 Padova
Phone: +39 49 821 66 27
Fax: +39 49 821 66 31

Dr. H. NORDMAN
Institute of Occupational Health
Haartmanskatu 1
FI 00290 Helsinki
Phone: +358 0 474 73 02
Fax: +358 0 41 24 14

Dr. K.M. VENABLES
Royal Brompton National Heart & Lung Hospital
Sydney Street
UK London SW3 6NP
Phone: +44 71 351 83 28
Fax: +44 71 351 83 36

I.3 BIOMEDICAL TECHNOLOGY

Introduction

Biomedical engineering has been an integral part of the EC biomedical and health research programmes since their quite modest beginnings in 1978, when only three collaborative research projects - 'Concerted Actions' - were supported by the EC. Collaboration is not natural and spontaneous within the scientific community, which rather believes in competition to ensure scientific progress. In fact, biomedical engineering, in the early period of the EC programme, may be said to have served as the driving force in the process of fostering some collaboration spirit in the European biomedical research community. It was so successful that in 1987, biomedical engineering consumed nearly 45 percent of the total programme's budget within the 16 projects running!

The ultimate goal of the biomedical engineering sub-area is to contribute to the improvement of the quality of health care, as well as to the containment of costs. Health technology assessment has gained further importance in view of the realization of the internal market within the EC. Such assessment may provide essential information for decision making at all levels (i.e., political, health services, medical). Because of the extremely rapid development of technology, results of assessment studies should become available quickly. Besides, evaluation of biomedical devices is expensive in financial and manpower terms, mainly because of the qualified personnel involved and the need to recruit patients. Inappropriate use of technology, not technology in itself, adds to the increase in health costs. Accordingly, health technology assessment, in particular assessment of technical and clinical efficacy comes under the biomedical technology heading of BIOMED.

Multi- and inter-disciplinary has always characterized the projects supported in the biomedical engineering part of the EC programme, and such an approach still is strongly encouraged. In biomedical engineering, the necessity for a closer collaboration between engineers and clinicians has always been felt, although it is not easy to promote such collaboration in concrete situations, which is exactly what the EC programme has tried to do. Against such a background, the submission of proposals is encouraged on the following topics:
- comparison of new technologies with existing ones in diagnosis, therapy, and rehabilitation;
- development and application of imaging techniques;
- biomedical applications of information science and technology;
- research on biomaterials for artificial organs;
- research on micro- and biosensors and stimulators.

Dr. Viviane Thévenin
Dr. Olivier Le Dour

ELECTRICAL IMPEDANCE TOMOGRAPHY

Key words
Electrical Impedance Tomography.

Brief description
Electrical Impedance Tomography (EIT) is a new medical imaging modality which can produce images of the distribution of the specific electrical impedance within the human body. Data for image reconstruction is relatively inexpensive to collect, although the design of data collection equipment is not trivial, but difficult to reconstruct into images. Nevertheless significant progress has been made in Europe and there is now a substantial body of expertise in this area within the European Community.

This concerted action will draw together this expertise in order to promote the development of EIT and encourage its introduction into appropriate clinical areas. The general aims are to encourage exploration of the scientific and technical limits of EIF, stimulate collaboration in research and development of EIT, covering theoretical, technical and clinical aspects and to disseminate technology and expertise to appropriate scientific and clinical groups.

Since EIT is currently a developing technique, with several important scientific questions still to be answered, the concerted action will concentrate principally on facilitating information transfer between participants, mainly through the mechanism of conferences, workshops and worker and data exchanges. In addition the Concerted Action will promote standardised methods of quantifying system performance, including standard phantoms.

Project leader:
Dr. David C. BARBER
Medical Physics and Clinical Engineering,
Royal Hallamshire Hospital
Glossop Road
UK Sheffield SI0 2JF
Phone: +44 742 766 222
Fax: +44 742 729 981
Contract number: CT920037

Participants:

Dr. B. BLOTT
Dept. Physics,
niv of Southampton
UK Southampton SO9 5NH
Phone: +44 703 592113
Fax: +44 703 585813

Dr. D. EVANS
GI Science Res Unit, London
Hosp Med College
26 Ashfield Street
UK London E1 2AJ,
Whitechapel
Phone: +44 71 377 0977
Fax: +44 71 375 2103

Dr. D. HOLDER
Dept. of Physiology,
Univ Coll London
Gower Street
UK London WC1E 6BT
Phone: +44 71 387 7050
Fax: +44 71 383 7005

Dr. E. GERSING
Zentrum Physiologie und
Pathophysiologie der Univ
Humboldt Allee 23
DE 3400 Gottingen
Phone: +49 551 395 891
Fax: +49 551 395 923

Dr. E.T. McADAMS
Northern Ireland
Bioengineering Centre,
Univ of Ulster
UK Co Antrim BT37 0BQ
Northern Ireland
Phone: +44 232 365131
Fax: +44 232 362804

Dr. F. BAISCH
DLR - Institut fur
Flumedizin, Linder Hohe
P.O. Box 906058
DE 5000 Koln 90
Phone: +49 2203 601
Fax: +49 2203 67310

Dr. G. VANTRAPPEN
Dept. Med and Div
Gastroenterology,
U Z Gasthiusberg
Herestrant
BE 3000 Leuven
Phone: +32 16 214 218

Dr. H. GRIFFITHS
Dept. Med Physics & Bio
engineering,
Univ Hosp of Wales
Heath Park
UK Cardiff CF4 4XW
Phone: +44 222 742033
Fax: +44 222 742012

Dr. H. STODKILDE-
JORGENSEN
Inst. of Exp Clin Res,
Univ of Aarhus,
Municipal Hosp
DK 8000 Aarhus C
Phone: +45 86 125 555

Dr. J. JOSSINET
INSERM U281
151 Cours Albert Thomas
FR 69424 Lyon Cedex 03
Phone: +33 72 33 10 03
Fax: +33 72 35 05 09

Dr. J. ROSELL
Dept. Eng Electronica,
Univ Polytechnic Catalunya
Campus Nord-Modul C4
ES 08071 Barcelona
Phone: +34 3 401 67 69
Fax: +34 3 401 67 56

Dr. M. EYUBOGLU
Dept. of Electrical and
Electronic Engineering,
Hacettpe Univ
TR Ankara

Dr. M. PIDCOCK
Dept. Computing &
Math Sciences,
Oxford Polytechnic
Gipsey Lane
UK Oxford OX3 0BP
Headington
Phone: +44 865 483 668
Fax: +44 865 483 666

Dr. P. RECORD
Dept. Biomedical
Engineering & Med Physics,
Univ of Keele
Thornburrow Drive
UK Stoke on Trent ST4 7QB
Phone: +44 782 717079
Fax: +44 782 747319

Dr. S.P. DEVANE
Dept. Child Health,
Fred Still Ward,
King's Coll Sch of Med
Bessemer Road
UK London SE5 9PJ
Phone: +44 71 274 6222
Fax: +44 71 326 3564

Dr. Z. IDER
Dept. Electronic & Electrical
Eng, Middle East
Techn Univ
TR Ankara
Phone: +90 4 210 1000
Fax: +90 4 210 1261

Prof. B. PERSSON
Dept. Radiation Physics,
Univ of Lund
SE 221 85 Lund
Phone: +46 46 173 110
Fax: +46 46 127 163

Prof. B.H. BROWN &
Dr. D.C. BARBER
Med Physics & Clin
Engineering, Floor 1,
Royal Hallamshire Hosp
Glossop Road
UK Sheffield S10 2JF
Phone: +44 742 827041
Fax: +44 742 827036

Prof. L.M.A. AKKERMANS
Dept. of Surgery,
Univ Hosp Utrecht
P.O. Box 85500
NL 3508 GA Utrecht
Phone: +31 30 508 065
Fax: +31 30 541 944

Prof. J.N. SAHALOS
School of Sciences, Dept.
Physics, Aristotle Univ of
Thessaloniki
GR TK 540 06 Thessaloniki
Phone: +30 31 991 422
Fax: +30 31 206 138

Prof. J.P. MORUCCI
INSERM U305, Centre
Hospitalier Hotel Dieu
FR 31052 Toulouse Cedex
Phone: +33 61 77 82 76
Fax: +33 61 59 46 36

Prof. U. FAUST
Inst. fur Biomedizinische
Technik, Univ of Stuttgart
Seidenstrasse 36
DE 7000 Stuttgart 1
Phone: +49 711 1212 370
Fax: +49 711 1212 371

Prof. W. SANSEN
Dept. Elektrotechniek, Kath
Univ Leuven, Afd. ESAT
Kardinaal Mercierlaan 94
BE 3030 Leuven
Phone: +32 16 220 931
Fax: +32 16 221 855

POSITRON EMISSION TOMOGRAPHY (PET) OF CELLULAR REGENERATION AND DEGENERATION

Key words
Positron Emission Tomography (PET), functional imaging, cellular regeneration and degeneration, pharmacology, clinical research.

Brief description
Most of the 30 European PET Centres will participate in the Concerted Action on PET investigation of cellular regeneration and degeneration. The programme will cover basic and methodological research in instrumentation, functional imaging, pharmacology and radiochemistry, as well as clinical research in neurology, psychiatry, cardiology, and oncology.

The main activities in these various fields will concern 3D acquisition and reconstruction of PET data (instrumentation), data normalization of PET brain activation maps (functional brain imaging), the creation of interaction between PET groups and pharmaceutical companies, the preclinical assessment of new radiopharmaceuticals for receptor imaging, the dosimetry reconsideration of specific radiopharmaceuticals (pharmacology), the evaluation of Alzheimer's disease in a collaborative study which will open the unique possibility to obtain a positive diagnosis (neurology), the establishment of guidelines for optimal clinical neuroleptic treatment by receptor occupancy measurement with PET (psychiatry), the assessment of myocardial blood flow/metabolism mismatch in patients suffering from dysfunctioning of the myocardium (cardiology), the comparison of in vivo PET measurement of glucose in tumours to in vitro assays of neoplastic function in biopsy samples and the evaluation of amino acids brain tumour uptake as a diagnostic imaging test (oncology).

It is hoped that this Concerted Action will contribute to provide answers to important clinical questions, will increase the technical quality of PET within European Community and will contribute to create plasticity and sense of collaboration between European scientists.

Project leader:
Dr. D. COMAR
Centre de Recherches du
Cyclotron, Univ de Liège
Bâtiment 30 Sart-Tilmant
BE 4000 Liège
Phone: +32 41 56 23 60
Fax: +32 41 56 29 45
Contract number: CT920160

Participants:
BTZ/ZYKLKOTRON
Universität Hamburg
DE 22761 Hamburg

Dr. A. DONATH
Div de Medecine nucléare,
Hopital cantonal univ
CH 1200 Geneve

Dr. A. LUXEN
Centre de recherches du
Cyclotron, Univ de Liège
BE 4000 Liege

Dr. B. LANGSTROM
Univ of Uppsala, Chemistry
SE 751 21 Uppsala

Dr. B. NEBELING
Krankenhausbetriebsgesell-
schaft Bad Oeynhausen
P.O. Box 100361
DE 32545 Bad Oeynhausen

Dr. Desmond CROFT
Clin Pet Centre,
St Thomas' Hospital
UK London SE1

Dr. GOLDMAN
Serv de Cyclotron, Univ
Libre de Bruxelles
BE 1070 Bruxelles

Dr. Gernot BIELKE
Stiftung Deutsche Klinik fur
Diagnostik GmbH
DE 65191 Wiesbaden

Dr. Gian Luigi BURAGGI
Div di Med Nucl, Inst. dei
Tumori di Milano
IT 20133 Milano

Dr. J. MELIN
Centre de Med Nucl, Univ de
Louvain, UCI 5430
BE 1200 Bruxelles

Dr. K. LEENDERS
Paul Scherrer Institut
CH 5234 Villigen

Dr. L. TRON
Hungarian Pet Center, c/o
Biomed Cycl Lab,
HU 4012 Debrecen

Dr. N. EVANS
Dept. of Biomed Physics
and Bioengeneerings,
Univ of Aberdeen
UK Aberdeen AB9 2ZD

Dr. R.J. OTT
Physics dept., The Inst. of
Cancer Research, Royal
Marsden Hosp
UK Sutton SM2 SPT

Dr. T. JONES
MRC Cyclotron Unit,
Hammersmith Hosp
UK London W12 OHS

Dr. W. VAALBURG
Dep of Nucl Med,
Univ Hosp
NL 9713 Groningen

Prof. A. SYROTA
Serv Hosp Frederic Joliot,
CEDA/DB Hopital d'Orsay
FR 91406 Orsay

Prof. DE ROO
Dept. of Nuclear Med,
Univ Hosp Gasthuisberg
BE 3000 Leuven

Prof. Dr. B. JOHANSSEN
Bioanorganische und Radio-
pharmazeutische Chemie
DE 01324 Dresden

Prof. Dr. FELIX
Radiologische Klinik,
DE 10117 Berlin

Prof. Dr. Gustav HOR
Zentrum der Radiologie,
Klin der J W Goethe Univ
DE 60596 Frankfurt/Main

Prof. Dr. G. STOCKLIN
Inst. fur Nuklearchemie,
DE 52428 Julich

Prof. H. HUNDESHAGEN
& Prof. Dr. G.J. MEYER
Medizinische Hochschule
Hannover
DE 30625 Hannover

Prof. Dr. H.H. COENEN,
Prof. Dr. Chr. REINERS
Arbeitsgruppe fur Nuklear-
chemie und Radiopharmazie,
Univ Klin Essen
DE 45122 Essen

Prof. Dr. H.J. MACHULLA
Radiologische Universitats-
klinik
DE 72076 Tubingen

H.W. MULLER-GARTNER
Nuklearmedizinische Klinik,
Heinrich Heine Univ
Dusseldorf
DE 40225 Dusseldorf

Prof. Dr. M. SCHWAIGER
Nuklearmed Klin u Poliklinik
rechts der Isar
DE 81675 Munchen

Prof. Dr. STRANGFELD
Humboldt Univ Berlin
DE 10117 Berlin

Prof. Dr. S.N. RESKE
Radiologische KLilik und
Poliklinik, Univ Ulm
DE 89081 ULM

Prof. Dr. U. BULL
Klin fur Nuklearmedizin,
Med Fak der RWTH Aachen
DE 52057 Aachen

Prof. Dr. Walter J. LORENZ
Ab Biophysik u Med
Strahlenphysik, Deutsches
Krebsforschungszentrum
DE 69120 Heidelberg

Prof. Dr. W.D. HEISS
Max Planck Inst. fur
neurologische Forschung
DE 50931 Koln

Prof. F. FAZIO
Dip di Scienze e Technologic
Biomediche, Univ di Milano
IT 20132 Milano

Prof. F. KNUTSSON
Karolinska Inst.,
Dep of Clin Neurophysiology
SE 10401 Stockholm

Prof. G.L. LENZI
Dip di Scienze Neurologiche,
Univ di Roma La Sapienza
IT 00185 Roma

Prof. J. De REUCK
Dept. of Neurology,
Univ Hosp
BE 9000 Gent

Prof. J.D. PICKARD
Neurosurgery Unit, Univ of
Cambridge Clin Sch, Level 4
A Block Addenbrooke's
Hospital
UK Cambridge CB2 2QQ

Prof. J.M. DERLON,
Dr.` J.C. BARON
CYCERON
FR 14021 Caen

Prof. L. DONATO
CNR, Inst. di Fisiologia
Clinica
IT 56100 Pisa

Prof. Marco SALVATORE
Ist di Neurochirurgia,
Ospedale C T O
IT 80131 Napoli

Prof. Mike MAISEY
Div of Radiol Sciences,
Guy's Hospital
UK London SE1 9RT

Prof. M. DEFRISE
Exp Med Imaging NUGE,
Vrije Univ Brussel
BE 1090 Brussel

Prof. O.B. PAULSON
Dept. of Neurology, Rigshos-
pitalet, Univ Hospital
DK 2100 Copenhagen

Prof. U. WEGELIUS
Dept. of Radiotherapy, Turku
Med Cyclotron Project
FI 20520 Turku

EUROPEAN STANDARDIZED COMPUTERIZED ASSESSMENT PROCEDURE FOR THE EVALUATION AND REHABILITATION OF BRAIN-DAMAGED PATIENTS (ESCAPE)

Key words
Neuropsychology, Memory, Aphasia, Perception, Attention, Problem Solving, Evaluation, Rehabilitation, Artificial Intelligence, Diagnostic Imaging.

Objectives
1 Develop a coherent system for assessment and rehabilitation of brain-damaged patients with impaired memory, language, problem solving, perception or attention.
2 Define and promote harmonized methodology, compatibility, common standards and guidelines, and evaluate the efficacy of biomedical technology and artificial intelligence resources applied to Clinical Neuropsychology.

Due to the diversity and intricacy of cognitive functions, the concerted action research is performed on a multidisciplinary basis in six sub-areas and one integration sub-project as follows.

Brief description
The project is structured into a network of experts from several fields involved in sub-projects covering different cognitive domains and one sub-project concerned with their interactions and daily-life dimensions. Methodological issues of concern are also considered and results are evaluated in large samples of patients engaged in multicentred studies.

Memory: It determines the functional locus of memory disorders within the theoretical framework of Working Memory, and compares the effects of rehabilitation techniques differing in their underlying principles and contents.

Language: It develops cross-linguistically adapted batteries for the evaluation of lexical disturbances according to the information processing approach, with expert systems for diagnosis and computerized rehabilitation.

Problem solving: It documents number processing, calculation and problem solving disorders, for planning the rehabilitation of patients with focal brain lesions or, in patients of Alzheimer type, as possible early cognitive markers of degenerative disease.

Perception: It develops a standardized test for the assessment of non-visual neglect, analyses the role of attention deficits and examines the typical sequence of recovery of several abilities on a cohort of acute stroke patients with unilateral visual neglect.

Attention: It evaluates the efficiency of computerized rehabilitation exercises with reference to the battery of test designed, adapted and standardized by this workgroup.

Children: In complement to the research on adult patients, it develops batteries for the assessment of cognitive functions in children with learning disabilities or with acquired disorders.

Integration: It evaluates the patient in broader terms than the usual syndrome analysis, considering emotional, personality and social dimensions with the ultimate goal to combine the specific types of assessment and rehabilitation tools developed by the specialized sub-projects into a holistic view.

The 3-year project will be managed by a Project Leader, assisted by a Committee. The sub-projects will be carried out by exchange of personnel and mobility facilities, and coordinated by the Project leader.

Project leader:
Dr. G. DELOCHE
Hôpital de la Salpetriere
47, Bd de l'Hôpital
FR 75651 Paris Cedex 13
Phone: +33 1 45 70 32 26
Fax: +33 1 45 70 20 45
Contract number: CT920218

Participants:
Dr. P. KITZING (SE)

Dr. H. KREMIN (FR)

Dr. R. LAAKSONEN (FI)

Dr. I. LE BOHEC (FR)

Dr. M. LECLERCQ (BE)

Dr. L. LORENZI (IT)

Dr. C. LUZZATTI (IT)

Dr. E. MAYER (CH)

Dr. C. MELJAC (FR)

Dr. METZ-LUTZ (FR)

Dr. M.U. NEUMANN (AT)

Dr. J. NIMATOUDIS (GR)

Prof. P. NORTH (FR)

Dr. O. ÖKTEM-TANÖR (TR)

Dr. H. OLSEN (DK)

Prof. P. PAQUIER (BE)

Dr. A. PASSADORI (FR)

Dr. I. PAVAO-MARTINS (PT)

Prof. L. PIZZAMIGLIO (IT)

Dr. R. QUINIOU (FR)

Dr. A. REIS (PT)

Dr. M. RENOM (ES)

Dr. D. RIVA (IT)

Dr. I. ROBERTSON (UK)

Dr. V. ROSENTHAL (FR)

Prof. M. ROUSSEAUX (FR)

Dr. A. SALLA (ES)

Dr. U. SCHURI (DE)

Prof. C. SEMENZA (IT)

Dr. A. SHIEL (UK)

Dr. L. SPINAZZOLA (IT)

Prof. F.J. STACHOWIAK (DE)

Prof. W. STURM (DE)

Dr. I. TAUSSIK (AR)

Dr. T. TEASDALE (DK)

Dr. R. TEGNER (SE)

Dr. C. TESSIER (FR)

Dr. V. TRETNJAK (SI)

Prof. A. TZAVARAS (GR)

Dr. S. UNVERHAU (DE)

Dr. M. Van de SANDT-
KOENDERMAN (NL)

Dr. M. VON ASTER (CH)

Dr. S. WALKER (UK)

Dr. J. WALSH (IE)

Dr. D. WEBER (NL)

Dr. H.R. VAN DONGEN (NL)

Dr. A. VAN HOUT (BE)

Dr. F. VARGHA KHADEM (UK)

Prof. J.M. VENDRELL (ES)

Dr. P. VENDRELL (ES)

Dr. E. VISCH-BRINK (NL)

Dr. E. WEBER (DE)

Dr. D. WENIGER (CH)

Dr. K. WILLMES (DE)

Prof. B. WILSON (UK)

Dr. W.H. ZANGEMEISTER (DE)

Dr. P. ZIMMERMAN (DE)

Dr. P. ZOCCOLOTTI (IT)

Dr. A. AGNIEUL (FR)

Dr. J.M. ANNONI (CH)

Prof. A. BADDELEY (UK)

Dr. A. BASSO (IT)

Dr. D. BEAUCHAMP (FR)

Dr. N. BESCHIN (IT)

Dr. L. BRAGA (BR)

Dr. O. BRUNA (ES)

Dr. T. CANAVAN (DE)

Dr. A. CANTAGALLO (IT)

Dr. S. CARLOMAGNO (IT)

Dr. M. CASANOVAS (ES)

Prof. A. CASTRO-CALDAS (PT)

Dr. A.L. CHRISTENSEN (DK)

Dr. D. CLAROS-SALINAS (DE)

Dr. N. CREMEL (FR)

Dr. J. DAVIDOFF (UK)

Dr. M. DE AGOSTINI (FR)

Dr. R. DE BLESER (DE)

Dr. DEELMAN (NL)

Dr. S. DELLA SALA (UK)

Dr. G. DELLATOLAS (FR)

Prof. F. DENES (IT)

Dr. M.A. DESI (FR)

Prof. M. TOURNILHAC (FR)

Dr. J. EVANS (UK)

Dr. A. FAHLBÖCK (AT)

Dr. B. FIMM (DE)

Dr. J. FONSECA (PT)

Dr. S. FRANKLIN (UK)

Prof. F. GAILLARD (CH)

Prof. J. GIOT (BE)

Prof. G. GOLDENBERG (AT)

Dr. G. GREITEMANN (DE)

Dr. W. GRIEßl (DE)

Prof. M. GROSS (DE)

Prof. H. GUYARD (FR)

Dr. P. HALLIGAN (UK)

Dr. K. HIRSH (UK)

Prof. V. HÖMBERG (DE)

Dr. D. HOWARD (UK)

Dr. A. IAVARONE (IT)

Dr. D. IONESCU (RO)

Dr. I. JAMBAQUÉ (FR)

Dr. M. JEHKONEN (FI)

Dr. R. KASCHEL (DE)

ASSESSMENT OF QUALITY OF BONE IN OSTEOPOROSIS

Key words
Osteoporosis, bone density, bone quality, NMR, MRI, QCT, photonabsorptiometry, fracture.

Objectives
The first objective is to explore the relationship between bone composition, micromacrostructure and bone physical properties (material and whole bone), leading to techniques for measurement of physical properties *in vivo*. The ultimate aim is to find, with a multimodality approach, new determinations of bone strength and fracture resistance.
The second objective is to assess the role of ultrasound to Serve as a primary Screening tool for osteoporosis, complementary to established ionising techniques.
The third objective is to standardize the present commercially available ultrasound systems by creating European reference and calibration phantoms along the lines done in the previous COMAC-BME Concerted Action 'Quantitative Assessment of Osteoporosis Study' (contract no. MR4*-CT900308).

Brief description
Although osteoporosis is the most common bone disease in the Western world, the diagnosis of osteoporosis or risk for osteoporosis remains problematic despite major advances in technology to measure bone mass in recent years. There is a need to perform more fundamental Studies on bone in normal and pathological conditions, in order to make progress in our knowledge and to detect patients at risk for osteoporotic fracture in time.
Twenty-three centres with recognized expertise in the assessment of bone micro-macrostructure, biochemistry, geochemistry and biomechanics will concert their findings on ex vivo bone tissue samples, with the aim to discover a new assessment or combination of assessments for the appreciation of bone quality in vivo. The following modalities for assessment of bone in addition to the established techniques such as radiogrammetry, photonabsorptiometry, DEXA, QCT and single photonabsorptiometry, will be incorporated: mechanical testing and fracture mechanics, ultrasound, bone biochemistry, three dimensional imaging, magnetic resonance spectroscopy and imaging.
Special attention will be given to the standardisation of ultrasound velocity and attenuation measurements in a working group bringing together the experience of 10 centres.

Project leader:
Professor Dr. Jan DEQUEKER
Arthritis and Metabolic Bone Disease Research Unit,
K.U.Leuven - U.Z. Pellenberg
Weligerveld I
BE 3212 Pellenberg
Phone: +32 16 333720
Fax: +32 16 335724
Contract number: CT920296

Participants:

Dr. Christian LANGTON
Dept. of Medical Physics,
University of Hull,
Princess Royal Hospital
Sutton
UK Hull HU8 9HE
Phone: +44 482 676 698
Fax: +44 482 702 147

Prof. RUEGSEGGER
Inst. for Biomedical Engin.
and Medical Informatic,
University of Zurich
Moussonstrasse 18
CH 8044 Zurich
Phone: +41 1 632 4598
Fax: +41 1 261 5187

Prof. Dr. W.B. STERN
University of Basel,
Geochemical Laboratory
Bernoullistrasse 30
CH 4056 Basel
Phone: +41 61 267 36 22
Fax: +41 61 267 36 13

Prof. Dr. P. LIPS
Free University Hospital,
Dept. of Endocrinology
P.O. Box 7057
1007 MB Amsterdam
Phone: +31 20 444 0614
Fax: +31 20 444 0502

Prof. Dr. Paolo BIANCO
Univ. of Rome La Sapienza,
Dept. Human Biopathol.,
Policlinico Umberto I
Viale Regina Elena 324
IT 00161 Rome
Phone: +39 6 490 526
Fax: +39 6 494 0896

Dr. Andrzej SAWICKI
National Food and Nutrition
Institute (NFNI), Mineral
Metabolism and Bone Disease
Dept.
ul. Powsinska 61/63
PL 02-903 Warsaw
Phone: +48 22 49 29 41
Fax: +48 22 23 44 51

Dr. Jacek GALAS
Institute of Applied Optics
(IAO)
ul. Kamionkowska 18
PL 03-805 Warsaw
Phone: +48 22 18 44 97
Fax: +48 22 13 32 65

Prof. Dr. Yuri DEKHTYAR
Riga Technical University,
Dept. of Microelectronics
1 Kalku Str.
LV-1658 Riga
Phone: +469 88 28034

Prof. Dr. M. RAKOVIC
Institute of Biophysics,
1st Medical Faculty,
Charles University
Salmovska 3
CZ 120 00 Prague 2
Phone: +42 2 295 603
Fax: +42 2 296 792

Prof. Dr. Alan BOYDE
University College London,
Dept. of Anatomy and
Developmental Biology
Gower Street
UK London WC1E 6BT
Phone: +44 71 387 7050
Fax: +44 71 391 1302

Dr. Pascal LAUGIER
Laboratoire d'Imagerie
Parametrique, Universite
Paris VI - URA CNRS 1458
15 rue de l'Ecole de
Medecine
FR 75006 Paris
Phone: +33 1 44 41 49 72
Fax: +33 1 46 33 56 73

Prof. Dieter FELSENBERG
Universitatsklinikum
Benjamin Franklin,
Abt. Roentgendiagnostik,
Minerallabor
Hindenburgdamm 30
DE 12200 Berlin
Phone: +49 30 798 3040
Fax: +49 30 793 59 18

Prof. Dr. Willi KALENDER
Siemens Medical Systems,
CTMP
Henkestrasse 127
DE 91050 Erlangen
Phone: +49 9131 84 77 36
Fax: +49 9131 84 63 65

Prof. LAVAL-JEANTET
Universite Paris VII,
C.N.R.S.
10 avenue de Verdun
FR 75010 Paris
Phone: +33 1 44 89 77 70
Fax: +33 1 44 89 78 00

Dr. Marie-Ch. HOBATHO
INSERM U305, Centre
Hospitalier Hotel Dieu
FR 31052 Toulouse
Phone: +33 61 77 82 84
Fax: +33 61 59 46 36

PHARMACOLOGIC STRESS ECHOCARDIOGRAPHY: A NEW, EFFECTIVE AND INEXPENSIVE METHOD FOR NON-INVASIVE DIAGNOSIS OF CORONARY DISEASE IN CLINICAL CARDIOLOGY

Key words
Cardiology, Coronary Artery Disease, Ultrasound, Stress Echocardiography, Myocardial Ischemia, Stress Testing, Noninvasive Imaging, Diagnosis, Prognosis.

Objectives
The ultimate goal is to set up a cost-effective clinical algorithm for the diagnosis and prognosis of coronary artery disease with a noninvasive and widely available imaging tool. A stepwise approach has been planned through the Concerted Action aiming at:
a Mutual quality control in ongoing and future studies of stress echocardiography;
b Comparison of efficacy of different diagnostic methodologies with regard to diagnostic yield, practicability and cost effectiveness;
c Pooling of results acquired in the different centres on the same issue, but with different tools or on different clinical models;
d Attempt to develop a standardized cost-effective approach to the diagnosis of coronary artery disease, generating a pooled data bank also for prognostic assessment.

Brief description
The first part of the project will strengthen the network of the cardiological community in Europe, leading to a standardization of echocardiography techniques and stress testing methodology. In an area lacking standardization, which is a tremendous limitation to progress, this will establish a true supranational *European Stress Echo Laboratory (ESEL)* in which the very same methodology is applied to the same patients and identical criteria are adopted for transmitting the information. A sizeable number of European centres, indeed, already perform stress echocardiographic tests with various methodologies, different protocols and non-uniform criteria. The number of centres interested in stress echocardiography is, however, skyrocketing on the scientific evidence that the rationale of this approach is generally sound.

Harmonized methods of collection and analysis will lead to the building up of a central data bank with a single scientific 'currency'. In addition, sub-projects will emphasize the specific contibution and expertise of each of the participating centres, which, on one side, will bring patient data to the central bank and, on the other side, will receive organization support and facilities to carry on their own specific projects. The algorithm generated from the pooled data will hopefully lead to standardized criteria for patient treatment, reducing costs to an absolute minimum.

Thus, it is highly desirable - with a standardized and clinically feasible protocol to collect sufficient numbers and expertise to develop an authoritative result which could be substituted to the presently redundant, cost-ineffective, subjective approach to the diagnosis of coronary artery disease. This proposal eventually, will obtain much more accuracy in diagnosis and prognosis in much less time, at less cost, with simpler non invasive instrumentation and, therefore, without significant risks for the patients.

The time schedule of this Concerted Action comprises 36 months of research.

Project leader:
Professor A. DISTANTE
C.N.R., Clinical Physiology Institute,
University of Pisa Medical School
Via P. Savi 8
IT 56100 Pisa
Phone: +39 50 58 32 86
Fax: +39 50 55 34 61
Contract number: CT921318

Participants:
Alan FRASER
Div of Cardiology
UK Cardiff
Phone: +44 22 742338
Fax: +44 22 761442

Bengt WRANNE
Univ Hosp of Linkoping, Clin Physiology
SE Linkoping
Phone: +46 13 223351
Fax: +46 13 145949

Jos R.T.C. ROELANDT
Div of Cardiology, Thoraxcentre, Erasmus Univ
NL 3000 DR Rotterdam
Phone: +31 10 4635312
Fax: +31 10 4363096

Liv HATLE
Univ of Trondheim, Regional Hospital
NO Trondheim
Phone: +47 7 997327
Fax: +47 7 997546

Luc A. PIERARD
Div of Cardiology, Univ Hosp Sart Tilman
BE Liege
Phone: +32 41 667111
Fax: +32 41 667195

Pascal GUERET
Hopital Henry Mondor
FR Creteil
Phone: +33 1 42075141
Fax: +33 1 43959241

Peter HANRATH
RWTH Aachen, II Medical Clinic
DE Aachen
Phone: +49 241 8089705
Fax: +49 241 8088360

OTOACOUSTIC EMISSIONS

Key words
Hearing function, hearing impairment, auditory biophysics. early diagnosis.

Brief description
Research in hearing has advanced dramatically over the past decade. The advances began with the startling realization that existing knowledge and accepted concepts could not explain the response of the cochlea to sound and in particular otoacoustic emissions. The very understanding of both the physical basis for hearing and the nature of hearing impairment was challenged.

Otoacoustic emissions (OAE) of several different kinds were discovered. The action of the cochlear *efferent* system was at last demonstrated objectively in the human ear.

Until the beginning of the 1980's, the cochlea was being modelled as a linear, passive, broadly tuned mechanical structure, as detailed by von Békésy forty years earlier. By the mid 1980's the term *active mechanism*s had come to represent the process by which the whole mechanical response of the cochlea to sound comes to be actually under the control of physiological processes, thus linking together haircell motility, cochlear non-linearity, frequency selectivity, otoacoustic emissions, sensory hearing loss and the influence of higher cerebral functions on the auditory periphery.

However, despite these major changes in thinking, several basic aspects still remain to be explored further. For example, haircell motility, as presently observed, has not yet been proven as the basis of the mechanical amplifier although this is now widely accepted as being essential to normal cochlear function.

Theoreticians are only beginning to explore the implications of the *nonlinear and active processes* and have not yet been able to synthesize the new experimental data and concepts into a workable model.

On more practical ground, otoacoustic emissions can be measured with several different recording techniques (spontaneous emissions; transient evoked emissions; emissions produced by simultaneous continuous tones). All these techniques are in use in auditory research and are playing an increasingly important role in the audiological test battery to assess and monitor hearing function in neonates, children, adults as well as in the elderly.

Operationally, the Concerted Action is performed in four major sub-projects as follows:

1 Development of recording methods (probes, for all kinds of Otoacoustic Emissions [OAE]; response characterisation of OAE; new recording techniques).
2 Biophysics and physiological aspects (development of models for the overall behaviour and dynamics of OAE, relation to auditory performance in normal ears; effects of suppression and masking; maturation in neonates and children; noise exposure, contralateral stimulation).
3 Clinical applications (correspondence of OAE characteristics with psychoacoustic performance; relation to cochlear and retrocochlear pathologies; effects of drugs; functional exploration of the medial olivocochlear bundle efferent activity).
4 Screening trials (practical implementation of OAEs in neonatal screening tests; computation of sensitivity and specificity for screening normal full-term and NICU babies; comparison between OAE and Auditory Evoked Brainstem Responses).

Project leader:
Dr. Ferdinando GRANDORI
Centro Teoria dei Sistemi
CNR, Politecnico di Milano
Via Ponzio 34/ 5
IT 20133 Milano
Phone: +39 2 239 93 561
Fax: +39 2 239 93 412
Contract number: CT920270

Participants:
Dr. Alexandru PASCU
RO 76231 Bucharest

Dr. Ann M. BROWN
UK Brighton BN1 9QG

Dr. A. DAVIS
UK Nottingham NG7 2RD

Dr. A. SAMIVALLI,
Dr. R. JOHANSSON
FI 20520 Turku

Dr. A.R.D. THORNTON
UK Southampton SO9 5NH

Dr. Brenda
LONSBURY-MARTIN
US Miami Florida 33101

Dr. E. PANOSETTI
LU 1210 Luxembourg

Dr. P. RAVAZZANI,
Dr. G. TOGNOLA
IT 20133 Milano

Dr. G. SMOORENBURG
NL 3769 Soesterberg

Dr. G.A. van ZANTEN
NL 3000 Rotterdam

Dr. I.W.S. MAIR,
Dr. B. ENGDAHL,
Dr. A.R. ARNESEN
NO 0407 Oslo 4

Dr. Johnatan W.P. HAZELL
UK London W1P 5FD

Dr J.J. BARAJAS DE PRAT
ES 39004 Santa Cruz de
Tenerife, Islas Canarias

Dr. J. Marco ALGARRA
Dr. Sequi CANET
ES 46010 Valencia

Dr. J.C. STEVENS
UK Sheffield S10 2JF

Dr. MADEIRA DA SILVA, ·
Dr. J.L. REIS
PT 1300 Lisboa

Dr. J.M. ARAN,
Dr. R. DAUMAN
FR 33076 Bordeaux Cedex

Dr. L. COLLET,
Dr. J. WABLE,
Dr. M. GIARD
FR 69437 Lyon Cedex 03

Dr. Martine FRANCOIS
FR 775935 Paris Cedex 19

Dr. M.D. TSAKANIKOS
GR Athens

Dr. M.E. LUTMAN
UK Nottingham NG1 6HA

Dr. N. PEREZ
ES 31080 Pamplona

Dr. N.J. JOHNSEN
DK 3400 Hillerod

Dr. O. LIND,
Dr. J.S. RANDA
NO 5021 Bergen

Dr. P. AVAN
FR 63001 Clermont Ferrand

Dr. P. BONFILS
FR 75730 Paris Cedex 15

Dr. P. DOLHEN,
Prof. D. HENNEBERT
BE 1000 Bruxelles

Dr. P.G. ZOROWKA
DE 55101 Mainz

Dr. R.G. MATSCHKE
DE 45659 Recklinghausen

Dr. W.F. DECRAEMER
BE Antwerpen

Ozcan OZDAMAR
US Florida

Prof. Dr. K.SCHORN
DE 8000 Munchen 40

Prof. Dr. W. FRITZE
AT 1090 Wien

Prof. D.T. KEMP,
Dr. S. RYAN
UK London WC1X 8EE

Prof. F. AKDAS
TR 81190 Istanbul

Prof. G. CIANFRONEA,
Dr. G.M. MATTIA-
IT 00161 Roma

Prof. G. SALOMON
DK 2900 Hellerup

Prof. H. SKARZINSKI
PL 02 021 Warszawa

Prof. H.P. WIT
NL 9713 EZ Groningen

Prof. H.P. ZENNER,
Dr. P.K. PLINKERT
DE 7400 Tubingen

Prof. J. POCH-BROTO
ES 28046 Madrid

Prof. J. PYTEL
HU 7621 Pecs

Prof. J.M. NUNES-LEITAO
PT 1096 Lisboa Cedex

K. CIESLAK-BLINOWSKA
PL 00 681 Warszawa

Prof. P. OSTERHAMMEL,
Dr. A. RASMUSSEN
DK 2100 Copenhagen

Prof. R. PROBST,
Dr. F.P. HARRIS
CH 4031 Basel

Prof. R. PUJOL,
Dr. G. REBILLARD,
Dr. A. UZIEL
FR 34059 Montpellier

Prof. Y. ULGEN,
Prof. O. OZDAMAR
TR 80815 Bebek-Istanbul

Susan NORTON
US Seattle WA 98105-0371

OCULAR FLUOROMETRY: NEW METHODS AND INSTRUMENTATION FOR NON-INVASIVE DIAGNOSIS BY OCULAR FLUORESCENCE MEASUREMENT (EUROEYE)

Key words
Diabetes, eye, fluorescence, instrumentation, diagnosis.

Objectives
The main goal of the Concerted Action is the development of new methodologies for non-invasive diagnosis by ocular fluorescence measurement focusing on the development of novel instrumentation and its clinical evaluation. The development of new instrumentation will follow two main directions:
1 instrumentation with improved axial resolution for better definition of the permeabilities of the boundaries separating ocular compartments, using exogenous fluorophores.
2 instrumentation capable of spectral analysis by rapidly changing excitation and emission wavelengths for non-invasive quantitative analysis of endogenous fluorophores.

Brief description
Ocular Fluorometry may also be used for monitoring changes in naturally occurring fluorophores in the ocular structure. The information gaps in this area include the characterization of new exogenous and endogenous fluorophores, cost-benefit analysis and technical limitations of improved axial resolution, characterization of specific wavelengths to be used in the mapping and measurement of natural fluorophores and their correlation with local and systemic diseases.
An Atlas of Fluorophores is another important goal in this area and will be published at the end of this Concerted Action.
Instrumentation Centralized Facilities where new instrumentation prototypes are to be assembled and tested will be located in Coimbra, Copenhagen and London. Exchanges and visits will be encouraged.
The Clinical Component will include a multicenter trial designed to test ocular florometry as a screening test to select patients at risk of developing diabetic retinopathy. This Multicenter Trial will create the necessary data pool to validate future studies to test new drugs to stabilize or prevent diabetic retinopathy-one of the major causes of blindness in Europe. It will serve as a reference for testing new developments in instrumentation.

Project leader:
Dr. E. LEITE
Dept. of Ophthalmology,
Coimbra University Hospital
PT 3049 Coimbra Codex
Phone: +351 39 71 71 82
Fax: +351 39 266 65
Contract number: CT920477

Participants:
Albert ALM
Dept. of Ophthalmology,
Univ Hosp
SE 75185 Uppsala

Andrea PERDICCHI
Clinica Oculistica II,
Univ La Sapienza
IT 00185 Roma

Carlos CORREIA
Dept. of Physics,
Univ of Coimbra
PT 3000 Coimbra

Dr. A. PERDICCHI
Clinica Oculista II,
Università 'La Sapienza'
IT 00185 Roma

Dr. J. BENITEZ DEL
CASTILLO
Dept. of Ophthalmology,
Univ Hospital San Carlos
ES 28040 Madrid

Dr. J. VAN BEST &
dr J.P. BOETS &
dr W. SWARTZ
Dept. of Ophtalmology,
Univ Hospital
NL 2333 leiden

Dr. M. DIESTELHORST
Universtats Augenklink
DE 5000 Koln

Dr. R. SCHALNUS
Zentrum der Augenheilkunde,
J.W. Goethe Universitat
DE 6000 Frankfurt am Main

Dr. S. FANTAGUZZI
Clinica Oculistica,
Università di Milano
IT 20132 Milano

Dr. V. ROSAS
Dept. of Ophthalmology,
S. Joao Hospital
PT 4200 Porto

Elmer MESSMER
Dept. of Ophtalmology,
Univ Hosp
CH 8091 Zurich

Franco DOCCHIO
Departimento di Elettronica
per l'Automazione,
Univ di Brescia
IT 25123 Brescia

Gabriel COSCAS
Clinique Ophtalmologique
Univ, Hopital de Creteill
FR 94010 Creteil cedex

Hendrik LUND-ANDERSEN
Dept. of Ophthalmology,
Gentofte Univ Hosp
DK 2900 0404 Hellerup

Jaap van BEST
Dept. of Ophthalmology,
Univ Hosp
Rijnsburgerweg 10
NL 2333 Leiden

Jean-Jacques de LAEY
Dept. of Ophthalmology,
Univ Hosp
BE 9000 Ghent

John MARSHALL
Dept. of Ophthalmology,
Block 8, UMDS,
St Thomas Hosp
UK London SE1 7EH

Jose Benitez del CASTILLO
Dept. of Ophtalmology,
Univ Hosp San Carlos
ES 28040 Madrid

Jose CUNHA-VAZ
Dept. of Ophthalmology,
Coibra Univ Hosp
PT 3049 Coimbra

Jose Paulo DOMINGUES
Dept. of Physics,
Univ of Coimbra
PT 3000 Coimbra

Maria Carolina MOTA
Dept. of Ophtalmology,
Coimbra Univ Hosp
PT 3049 Coimbra

Michael DIESTELHORST
Universitats-Augenklinik
DE 5000 Koln

Peter DALGAARD
Statistical Research Unit,
Univ of Copenhagen
DK 2200 Copenhagen N

Prof. A. ALM
Dept. of Ophthalmology,
Univ Hospital
SE 75185 Uppsala

Prof. E. MESSMER
Dept. of Ophthalmology,
Univ Hospital
CH 8091 Zürich

Prof. F. DOCCHIO
Dipt. di electtronica per
l'Automazione,
Università di Brescia
IT 25123 Brescia

Prof. G. COSCAS
Clinique Ophthalmologique
Universitaire,
Hôpital de Créteil
FR 94010 Créteil

Prof. H. LUND-ANDERSEN
& Dr. C.ENGLER &
Dr. B.SANDER
Dept. of Ophthalmology,
Gentofte Univ Hospital
DK 2900 0404 Hellerup

Prof. J. CUNHA-VAZ
Dept. of Ophthalmology,
Coimbre Univ Hospital
PT 3000 Coimbra

Prof. J. MARSHALL
Dept. of Ophthalmology,
Block 8, St. Thomas hospital
UK London SE1 7EH

Prof. J.J. DE LAEY
Dept. of Ophthalmology,
Univ Hospital
BE 9000 Ghent

Prof. W. LOHMANN
Institut für Biophysic,
Just Liebig Universitat
DE 6300 Giessen

Rainer SCHALNUS
Zentrum der Augenheilkunde,
Johann-Wolfgang-Goethe
DE 6000 Frankfurt am Main

Robert van VELZE
Dept. of Ophthalmology,
Coimbra Univ Hosp
PT 3049 Coimbra

Sergio FANTAGUZZI
Clinica Oculistica,
Univ di Milano,
IT 20132 Milano

Victor ROSAS
Dept. of Ophthalmology,
S. Joao Hosp
PT 4200 Porto

Wolfgang LOHMANN
Inst. fur Biophysic der
Justus-Liebig-Univ,
Strahlenzentrum
DE 6300 Giessen

HEART ASSIST AND REPLACEMENT

Key words
MCSS, TAH, VAD, artificial organs, pumps.

Brief description
The topic of the Concerted Action is the technology and application of totally or partially implantable Mechanical Circulatory Support Systems (MCSS).

The objectives are grouped in the following homogeneous sub-areas:
- Development of MCSS covering the technological development and in-vitro testing of MCSS with reference to R & D guide-lines and regulations.
- Biomaterials for MCSS covering MCSS biomaterial selection criteria and use.
- In-vivo (animal) testing of MCSS covering inventories of in-vivo testing laboratories, and experimental protocols (pre-, intra-, and post-operative).
- Clinical Application of MCSS covering common clinical protocols guiding application of existing MCSS, and identification of clinical needs for the development of new MCSS.
- Skeletal Muscle Assist focusing on mechanical circulatory support by means of endogenous energy source (i.e. skeletal muscle).

Project leader:
Dr. B. MAMBRITO
Tecnobiomedica SpA
Via Vaccareccia 41
IT 00040 Pomezia
Phone: +39 6 912 43 11
Fax: +39 6 912 16 81
Contract number: CT920152

Participants:
Dr. D.J. DUARTE
Cirurgia Cardiovascular,
Hospital de la Princesa
ES 28006 Madrid

Dr. E. HENNING
Deutsches Herzzentrum
Berlin
DE 1000 Berlin 65

Dr. E. QUAINI
Div di Cardiochirurgia A
De Gasperis, Ospedale
Niguarda Ca 'Grande
IT 20162

Dr. F. WALDENBERGER
Kath Univ Leuven
BE 3000 Leuven

Dr. F.H. van der VEEN
Academic Hospital Maastricht
NL 6202 AZ Maastricht

Dr. G. RAKHORST
Univ of Groningen
BMTC - 25
NL 9713 EZ Groningen

Dr. G. TRIVELLA
Istituto di Fisiologia
Clinica del CNR
IT Pisa

Dr. G. WIESELTHALER
II depart of Surgery,
Univ of Vienna
AT 1090 Wien

Dr. H. SCHIMA
Bioengineering Lab
2nd Dept. of Surgery
AT 1090 Vienna

Dr. H.O. VETTER
Ludwig Maximilians
Univ Munchen
DE 8000 Munchen 70

Dr. Ing. Z. KRATOCHVIL
Tech Univ Brno
CS 61669 Brno

Dr. J. JARVIS
Human Anatomy and Cell
Biology,
Univ of Liverpool
UK Liverpool L69 3BX

Dr. J. NEVES
Centro de Cirurgia Exp,
Inst. do Caracao
PT Carnaxide 2795
Linda a Velha

Dr. J. del CANIZO LOPEZ
Hospital general Gregorio
Maranon
ES 28007 Madrid

Dr. L.H. KOOLE
Biochemie, Biomaterialen en
Polymeren Res Inst.,
Rijks Univ Limburg
NL 6200 MD Maastricht

Dr. M. MELI
Hesperia Hospital
IT 41100 Modena

Dr. P. FERRAZZI,
Dr. M. GLAUBER
Ospedali Riuniti di Bergamo
IT Bergamo

Dr. P. VAUDAUX
Hopital Cantonal
Universitaire de Geneve
CH 1211 Geneve 4

Dr. R. ELOAKLEY
Wythenshawe Hospital
UK Manchester M23 9LT

Dr. R. LO RUSSO
Ospedale Civile
IT 25025 Brescia

Dr. S. CHIECO
Tecnobiomedica S p A
IT 00040 Pomezia

Dr. T. POCHET
Univ de Liege, LHCN
BE 4000 Liege

Dr. T.L. HOOPER
Wythenshawe Hospital,
Dept. Cardiothoracic Surgery
UK Manchester M23 9LT

Dr. YIANNI
Biocompatibles Ltd,
Brunel Science Park
UK Uxbridge Middlesex
UB8 3PQ

Prof. A. PAVIE
Groupe Hospitalier La Pitie
Salpetriere
FR 75651 Paris Cedex 13

Prof. C.T. LEWIS
The London Hospital
(Whitechapel)
UK London E1 1BB

Prof. Dr. R. HETZER,
Dr. R. SCHIESSLER
Deutsches Herzzentrum
Berlin
DE 1000 Berlin 65

Prof. D. DUVEAU
Thoracic and Cardiovascular
Surgery Clinic,
Hop Guillaume et Rene
Laennec
FR 44035 Nantes Cedex 01

Prof. D. LOISANCE
Ctr. d'Exp Animale et de
Rech Chirugicales- Henri
Mondor, Univ Paris XII
FR 94010 Creteil Cedex

Prof. D.T. ARTS
State Univ of Limburg
NL 6200 MD Maastricht

Prof. H. REUL,
Dipl.-Ing. R. KAUFMANN
Helmholz Inst. for BME
DE 5100 Aachen

Prof. H. THOMA
Inst. fur Biomed Technik und
Physik,
Allgemeines Krankenhaus
AT Wien

Prof. J. DANKERT
Universiteit van Amsterdam
NL 1105 ZA Amsterdam

Prof. J. FEIJEN
Univ of Twente
NL 7500 AE Enschede

Prof. J.R. MONTIES
CHU Timone
FR 13385 Marseille Cedex 5

Prof. K. AFFELD
Free Univ of Berlin
DE 1000 Berlin 19

Prof. O. LARM
Medicarb AB
SE Bromma

Prof. S. SALMONS
• Human Anatomy and
Cell Biology,
Univ of Liverpool
UK Liverpool L69 3BX

Prof. S.D. MOULOPOULOS
Clin Therapeutics,
Univ of Athens,
Sch of Medicine
GR 115 28 Athens

Prof. U. CARRARO
Centro Fisiopatologia
Muscolare,
Univ degli Studi di Padova
IT 35121 Padova

Prof. W. FLAMENG
Ctr voor Exp Heelkunde en
Anesthesiologie,
Kath Univ Leuven
BE 3000 Leuven

LASER-DOPPLER FLOWMETRY FOR MICROCIRCULATION MONITORING

Key words
LD-flowmetry, LD-signal processing, LD-data bank, LD-perfusion imaging, Microcirculation monitoring.

Objectives
This Concerted Action shall improve the efficiency of medical and health research by facilitating development of the great potential of Laser-Doppler (LD) Flowmetry in the Member states. Groups from individual clinical fields shall develop internationally standardized protocols for acquisition of medical and, in conjunction with technical groups, LD-data, including a consensus on points and conditions of measurement for respective diseases.

Brief description
A pool of medical, LD-signal, and LD-imaging data will be established, and correlated to specific diseases and their courses. Technical/signal processing groups shall concurrently be engaged in standardization of the LD-devices and the measuring method, including development and testing of basic and advanced signal processing procedures, and use of computer simulation and new microprobes for the control of measuring depth to promote further quantitative microcirculatory assessment.

A central LD-data bank, of pivotal importance in pooling of data and information exchange between the clinical and technical/signal processing groups, will create an efficient basis for communication and coordinating the activities of the individual participants.

Improvement and standardization of the LD-technique in conjunction with the development of a unified system of medical data collection, exchange, and advanced signal processing shall lead to harmonization of methods and optimal interpretation of clinical data, resulting in an enhancement of the state-of-the-art as well as being conducive to substantial original work.

Project leader:
Dr. K.O. MÖLLER
Medizinische Universität
Lübeck,
Chirurgische Forschung
Ratzeburger Allee 160
DE 23562 Lübeck
Phone: +49 451 500 20 18
Fax: +49 451 500 21 61
Contract number: CT920006

Participants:
Dr. Andrew OBEID
Oxford Optronix Ltd,
Standangford House
UK Oxford OX4 1BA

Dr. Aneta STEFANOVSKA
Fac of Electrical and
Computer Engineering
SI 61000 Ljubljana

Dr Constantinos PATTICHIS
The Cyprus Inst. of
Neurology and Genetics
CY Nicosia

Dr. David POPIVANOV
Bulgarian Academy of
Sciences,
Inst. of Physiology
BG 1113 Sofia

Dr. Eric WAHLBERG
Dept. of Surgery,
Karolinska Hosp,
Div of Vasc Surg
SE 104 01 Stockholm

Dr. Folke SJOBERG
Dept. of Anesthesiology,
Univ Hosp
SE 581 85 Linkoping

Dr. Frits F.M. de MUL
Dept. of Applied Physics,
Univ of Twente
NL 7500 AE Enschede

Dr. Gerhard LITSCHER
Univ Klin Anasthesiologie,
Univ Graz
AT 8036 Graz

Dr. Jean CIUREA
Cl Hosp Dr. D Bagdasar,
Sos Berceni 10, Sector 4
RO Bucharest

Dr. Kjell BAKKEN
Perimed AB
SE 175 26 Järfälla

Dr L.N.A. van ADRICHEM
Streekziekenhuis Walcheren
NL 4380 DD Vlissingen

Dr. Luca A. RAMENGHI
Servizio di Patologia
Neonatale
IT 66100 Chieti

Dr. Nick J. BARNETT
Moor Instruments
UK Devon EX13 5DT

Dr. Vladimir KRAJCA
Dept. Neurology,
Fac Hosp Bulovka
CZ 180 81 Praha 8

Prof.Dr. A.N. NICOLAIDES
Ac Surg Unit, Irvine Lab,
St Mary's Hosp
UK London W2 1NY

Prof. A. COLANTUONI
CNR Inst. of Clin Physiolo-
gy, Univ di Pisa
IT 56100 Pisa

Prof. Dr. Bengt FAGRELL
Dept. of Med,
Karolinska Hosp
SE 104 01 Stockholm

Prof. Dr. Bo LILJA
Dept. of Clin Physiology,
Malmo General Hosp
SE 21401 Malmo

Prof. Dr. Gert E. NILSSON
Dept. of Biomedical
Engineering,
Linkoping Univ Hosp
SE 581 85 Linkoping

Prof. Dr. Gunnar WALLIN
Dept. Clin Neurophysiology,
Sahlgrenska Hosp
SE 413 45 Gothenburg

Prof. Dr. Gyula SZEGEDI
3rd Dept. of Med,
Univ Med Sch of Debrecen
HU 4004 Debrecen

Prof. Dr. Henri BOCCALON
Hopitaux de Toulouse, CHU
Rangueil, Angiologie
FR 31054 Toulouse Cedex

Prof. Dr. Henry SVENSSON
Dept. of Plastic Surgery,
Malmo Allmanna Sjukhuset
SE 214 01 Malmo

Prof. Dr. Herbert WITTE
Friedrich Schiller Univ Jena,
Inst. fur Med Stat,
Informatik und
Dokumentation
DE 07740 Jena

Prof. Dr. I. TAIVANS
Dept. fo Pulmonal
Physiology,
Latvian Academy of Med
LV 1007 Riga

Prof. Dr. Jens KASTRUP
Dept. of Cardiology,
Gentofte Hosp
DK 2900 Hellerup

Prof.Dr. L. JAZUKEVICIUS
Surgery Dept.,
Lithuanian Oncological
Centre
LT Vilnius 232600

Prof. Dr. P. Ake OBERG
Dept. of Biomedical
Engineering,
Linkoping Univ Hosp
SE 581 85 Linkoping

Prof. Dr. R. MANIEWSKI
Inst. of Biocybernetics &
Biomedical Engineering,
Polis Academy of Sciences
PL 02109 Warshaw

Prof. Silvia BERTUGLIA
CNR Inst. of Clin
Physiology,
Univ di Pisa
IT 56100 Pisa

Prof. Ivars BILINSKIS
Inst. of Electronics and
Computer Science
LV 1006 Riga

Prof. Stefanos KOLLIAS
Dept. of Electrical
Engineering,
Nat Tech Univ of Athens
GR 15773 Zographou

STUDY OF VARIABLE TRANSITION ZONES IN AN ATTEMPT TO USE EXCIMER LASERS IN PHOTO-REFRACTIVE KERATECTOMY FOR ADDRESSING HIGH MYOPIA

Key words
Myopia, excimer laser, photorefractive keratectomy, transition zones.

Brief description
Myopia and refractive errors involve 35% of the European Community population.
Photorefractive Keratectomy (PRK) is a new and promising technique for correction of such errors. Currently, the main factor that seems to be correlated with regression in the size of the operated zone.

The aim of the present study is to investigate the possibility of reducing postoperative regression in high myopic corrections by either utilizing aspheric corrections or using optical zones of several different sizes.

The main stages of the project include:
- modification of the mathematical model for aspheric lens surfaces, to achieve an aspheric corneal ablation;
- using excimer laser supplied with the modified computer-driven delivery system, a series of experiments will be conducted on human cadaver eyes, with different sizes of the final ablation zones;
- optical measurements, scanning and transmission electron microscopy will be used to assess the results of these experiments;
- on the basis of these preliminary studies a series of postoperative refractive status will be checked at varying times using streak retinoscopy;
- preliminary clinical studies will be undertaken on a series of blind eyes;
- at the final stage of the programme corrections will be carried out between -7.00D and -15.00D on a sighted eye series; both blind and sighted eye series will be studied using all current resources developed within the participating laboratories.

Project leader:
Professor I. PALLIKARIS
Dept. of Ophthalmology,
Eye Institute Vardinoyiannon,
University of Crete Medical School
P.O. Box 1352
GR 71110 Heraklion, Crete
Phone: +30 81 26 93 51 or 26 28 18
Fax: +30 81 26 18 50 or 26 19 78
Contract number: CT921185

Participants:

John MARSHALL
UMDS, Dept. of
Ophtalmology,
Block 8, South wind,
St Thomas Hosp
UK London SE1 7EH
Phone: +44 71 928 9292
Fax: +44 71 401 9082

Prof. T. SEILER
Universitatsklinikum
Carl Gustav Carus,
Augenklinik
Fetscherstr. 74
DE 01307 Dresden
Phone: +49 351 458 2388
Fax: +49 351 458 4335

Dr. E. LENS
Groupe d'Etucde Pluridiscipl-
inaire Stéthacoustique,
Clinique Reine Fabiola
BE-Courcelles
Phone: +32 71 462 068

RESTORATION OF MUSCLE ACTIVITY THROUGH FUNCTIONAL ELECTRICAL STIMULATION (FES) AND ASSOCIATED TECHNOLOGY (RAFT)

Key words
Neuroprostheses, rehabilitation engineering, paraplegia, functional electrical stimulation (FES).

Brief description
The objective of the proposed Concerted Action is to stimulate research and European cooperation in the field of reactivating paralysed or poorly controlled muscle function in order to permit patients with a wide range of disabling conditions to perform activities of daily living more effectively. This will in turn lead to an increase in their independence and reduce the financial burden of the support which such patients require from the various European national social security arrangements.

Three main objectives have been identified as major research topics:

Technical aspects: the nerves going to the muscles are made with a mixed population of fibres, including motor and sensitive pathways. Given this organization, the stimulation of a nerve trunk does not allow to get a good selectivity in terms of reaching the right muscle and obtaining a reliable modulation of force by recruiting the different motor units. Special investigations on animals and stimulation modality are required for that. In order to obtain an acceptable movement, it is also important to adapt the control strategies to the individual patient. This goal can be obtained a priori by considering the type and level of the lesion, the anthropometric, physiological and anatomical characteristics of each patient in conjunction with the results of specific tests (spasticity, paresis, etc.). From the dynamic point of view the optimal adaptation can be reached by quantitative analysis of the performance and by using simulation techniques in order to choose the best rules for muscle recruitment.

Clinical aspects: the selection of patients and the definition of a proper training before and after the implantation is the key point in order to reach valuable results. The spinal cord injury patient cannot feel the sensation of muscular fatigue like normal subjects and the composition of fibres (fast and slow) is very often modified in these patients. It is important to detect the fatigue in order to avoid the muscle damage by FES.

Evaluation: according to the great impact not only on health technology development but also on economical aspects, it is important to provide a multidisciplinary evaluation during the Concerted Action of all the clinical and research achievements.

This will be made mostly by means of clinical trials organized within the European clinical network established among the different spinal cord injury participating centres.

Project leader:
Professor A. PEDOTTI
Centro di Bioingegneria,
Politecnico di Milano,
Fondazione Pro.
Juventute IRCCS
Via Gozzadini 7
IT 20148 Milano
Phone: +39 2 400 92 260
Fax: +39 2 268 61 144
Contract number: CT921350

Participants:
Prof. J.P. DELWAIDE
Hopital de la Cittadelle,
Service de Neurologie
BE 4000 Liege

Prof. T. SINKJAER
University of Aalborg,
Dept. for Med. Inf. and
Image Analysis
DK 9220 Aalborg

Dr. F. BIERING-
SOERENSEN
Centre for Spinal Cord
Injured Righospitalet,
Rehabilitation Department
DK 31100 Hornbaek

Prof. J. HAASE
Aalborg Hospital S.,
Department of Neurosurgery
DK Aalborg

Prof. P. RABISCHONG
I.N.S.E.R.M. Unité 103,
Appareil Moteuret Handicap
FR 34090 Montpellier

Dr. M. HERLANT
Centre l'Espoir de
Teeducation Specialisé pour
Adultes
FR 59260 Lille Hellemes

Dr. F. OHANNA
Centre Propara
FR 34195 Montpellier

Prof. J. MASSION
Laboratoire de Neurosciences
Fonctionelles, C.N.R.S.
FR 13402 Marseille Cedex 2
Phone: +33 91 16 40 00
Fax: +33 91 77 50 84

Prof. T. BRANDT
Universitat Munchen
Klinikum Grosshardern
Ludwig-Maximili
DE 8000 München

Prof. K.H. MAURITZ
Klinik Berlin
DE 1000 Berlin 22

Prof. G. VOSSIUS
Universitat Karlsruhe,
Institut fur Biokybernetik und
Biomedizinische Techniku
DE 75 Karlsruhe 1

Prof. J. EDWARDS
University of Salford,
Dept. of Orthopaedics
Mechanics
UK Salford M5 4WT

Dr. K.R. KISHNAN
Mersey Regional Spinal
Injury Centre,
District General Hospital
UK Southport, Merseyside

Prof. J.P. PAUL
Wolsson Centre,
Bioengineering Unit,
University of Strathclyde
UK Glasgow G4 ONW

Prof. D. RUSHTON
Institute of Psychiatry,
Dept. of Rehabilitation,
Royal London Hospital
UK London SE1

Dr. J. STALLARD
Robert Jones & Agnes Hunt
Orthopaedic Hospital,
O.R.L.A.U.
UK SY10 7AG Oswestry

Prof. S. SALMONS
University of Liverpool,
Dept. of Human Anatomy
and Cell Biology
UK Liverpool L69 3BX

Dr. G. ANOGIANAKIS
Faculty of Medicine,
Dept. of Physiology,
University of Thessaloniki
GR 54006 Thessaloniki

Prof. G. FOROGLOU
Faculty of Medicine,
Dept. of Neurosurgery
GR 54006 Thessaloniki

Dr. X. MICHAEL
National Institute for
Rehabilitaiton
GR Nea Liosa, Athens

Dr. L. TESIO
Istituto Scientifico S.
Raffaele,
Servizio di Riabilitazione
Clinica Ortopedica
IT 20132 Milano

Prof. M. MARCHETTI
Istituto di Fisiologia Umana,
Universita' La Sapienza
IT 00185 Roma

Dr. S. SORBI
Ospedale di Careggi,
Dip. Scienze Neurologiche e
Psichiatriche,
Universit di Firenze
IT 50134 Firenze

Prof. G. BRUNELLI
Clinica Ortopedica,
Universita' di Brescia
IT 25124 Brescia

Prof. M.A. VANNINI
Ospedale di Montecatone,
Divisione di Recupero e
Rieducazione Funzionale
IT 40026 Imola

Prof. M. GARRETT
University College Dublin,
School of Physiotherapy,
Mater Hospital
IE Dublin 7

Dr. ALFONSO
Centro de Reabilitacao do
Alcoitao
PT 2765 Alcoitao

Dr. E. PORTELL
Institut Guttman
ES Barcelona

Prof. H. BOOM
Univ. of Twente, Biomedical
Engineering Division
NL 7500 AE Enschede

Dr. T. MULDER
St. Maartensklinick,
Research and Development
Nijmegen

Prof. G. ZILVOLD
Roessing Research &
Development BV
NL 7500 AE Enschede

CANCER AND BRAIN DISEASE CHARACTERIZATION AND THERAPY ASSESSMENT BY QUANTITATIVE MAGNETIC RESONANCE SPECTROSCOPY

Key words
Magnetic resonance spectroscopy (MRS), cancer, brain, biofluids, standardized methodologies.

Objectives
1 to identify MRS parameters for non-invasively monitoring metabolic status and effects of therapy in tumours, in relation to vascularity and cell proliferation;
2 to investigate antineoplastic drug pharmacokinetics and metabolism, including the effects of (multi-)drug resistance (MDR);
3 to characterize metabolic alterations induced in human brain by normal ageing processes, degenerative disorders; multiple sclerosis; vascular disorders; AIDS
4 to identify pathophysiological factors for prognosis and for monitoring the effect of treatment schemes in cancer and brain diseases;
5 multi-centre evaluation of high resolution MRS, in view of their possible transfer from experimental to clinical level, for analysis of biofluids, and bioptical specimens.

Brief description
The project will employ recent developments in Magnetic Resonance Spectroscopy (MRS) to non-invasively measure tissue metabolism and physiology, in order to improve the effectiveness of this biomedical technology in European countries.

The general purpose of the project is to provide new methodologies to increase understanding improve diagnosis and evaluate new therapies in cancer and brain diseases.

Investigation and evaluation of the new metabolic and physiological parameters provided by MRS, as *in-vivo* markers of diagnosis, prognosis and therapeutic response, require multicentre development of standardized methodologies for quantitative and reproducible measurements and their validation in well controlled clinical and experimental trials. By continuing previous efforts under the EEC COMAC-BME Concerted Action *Tissue Characterization by Magnetic Resonance Spectroscopy and Imaging* (1988-1992), the project develops quantitative MRS methodologies:
a to determine in-vivo metabolite and drug concentrations (in cells, model systems and clinical measurements);
b to elucidate metabolic mechanisms underlying clinical and laboratory observations and identify markers of diagnosis, prognosis and response to therapy;
c to define standard methodologies in MRS of biofluids, tumour biopsies and tissue extracts;
d to establish the bases for multi-centre pre-clinical and clinical pilot trials in tumour pathologies and brain diseases.

The time schedule of the concerted action comprises 36 months.

Project leader:
Dr. Franca PODO
Istituto Superiore di Sanità
Viale Regina Elena 299
IT 00161 Roma
Phone: +39 6 4990
Fax: +39 6 4440018
Contract number: CT920432

Participants:

Dr. Constance MOORE
UK Liverpool L69 3BX

Dr. A.E. BAERT
BE 1049 Brussels

Dr. C. SEGEBARTH
BE 1070 Bruxelles

Dr. D.H. MILLER
UK London WC1N 3BG

Dr. E. MARTIN
CH 8032 Zurich

Dr. E. MOSER
AT 1090 Wien

Dr. E.B. CADY
UK London WC1E 6AV

Dr. I. WILKINSON
UK London WIN 8AA

Dr. J.C. LINDON
UK Beckenham (Kent)

Dr. J.D. BELL
UK London W12 OHS

Dr. J.D. De CERTAINES
FR 35043 Rennes Cedex

Dr. J.T. ENNIS
IE Dublin 7

Dr. L. Le MOYEC
FR 75010 Paris

Dr. M. DECORPS
FR 38043 Grenoble Cedex

Dr. M. EUGENE
FR 75010 Paris Cedex 10

Dr. M. GYNGELL
DE 50931 Koln

Dr. M.C. MALET-
MARTINO
FR 31062 Toulouse Cedex

Dr. M.O. LEACH
UK Sutton SM2 5PT

Dr. P. CARLIER
FR 91401 Orsay Cedex

Dr. P. KOEHL
FR 67084 Strasbourg

Dr. R. SAUTER
DE 8520 Erlangen

Dr. R. de BEER
NL 2600 GA Delft

Dr. S. AKOKA
FR 37032 Tours Cede

Dr. S. CERDAN
ES 28029 Madrid

Dr. S. KEEVIL
UK London SE1 9RT

Dr. W.M.M.J. BOVEE
NL 2600 GA Delft

Prof. A. BRIGUET,
Dr D. GREVERON-DE
MILLY
FR 69622 Villeurbanne

Prof. B. BARBIROLI
IT 40138 Bologna

Prof. C. ARUS
ES 08193 Bellaterra
Barcelona

Prof. Dr. O. LUTZ
DE 72076 Tubingen

Prof. D. GADIAN
UK London WC1N 1EH

Prof. D. LEIBFRITZ
DE 28359 Bremen 33

Prof. D.J. GILI
ES 08035 Barcelona

Prof. G. RADDA
UK Oxford OX1 3QU

Prof. H. HENNING
DE 79106 Freiburg

Prof. J. CHAMBRON
FR 67085 Strasbourg Cedex

Prof. J.K. NICHOLSON
UK London WC1H 0PP

Prof. J.R. GRIFFITHS
UK London SW17 0RE

Prof. J.S. ORR
UK Glasgow G62 8HX

Prof. O. HENRIKSEN
DK 2650 Hvidovre
Copenhagen

Prof. P.J. COZZONE
FR 13005 Marseille

Prof. S. AIME
IT 10125 Torino

Prof. W. HEINDEL
DE 50924 Koln 41

AUTOMATED MOLECULAR CYTOGENETIC ANALYSIS

Key words
Automation, microscopy, opto-electronics, cameras, digital imaging, image analysis, pattern recognition, molecular cytogenetics, DNA analysis, in situ hybridisation.

Objectives
Molecular cytogenetic information is contained in the number of in situ hybridisation signals per cell, their colour, their positions and their intensities.

The main objective is to stimulate the scientific and technological basis for automated systems for molecular cytogenetic analyses by performing research into and development of the instrumentation and software for the rapid and automated detection of in situ hybridisation signals in metaphase and interphase cells: the analysis of these signals with respect to number, colour information and spatial relationship: size and intensity measurements of in situ hybridisation signals and correlation of signal locations with chromosome and cell morphology.

Additional objectives are: the proper definition of the speed and resolution requirements for each different cytogenetic application and establishment of system evaluation protocols.

Brief description
Cytogenetics has made major contributions to the understanding of the chromosomal basis of constitutional and acquired diseases. Its techniques are widely applied in clinical practice and significant contributions have been made to the prevention, diagnosis and treatment of severe conditions such as cancer and genetic diseases. They are also applied in environmental and occupational studies in order to monitor the biological effects of mutagenic and carcinogenic agents such as chemicals and radiation. In recent years a new technology, in situ hybridisation, has developed that extends the capabilities of cytogenetics to the molecular level. the field of molecular cytogenetics. Using specially designed molecules, called probes, it is possible to specifically mark multiple DNA targets with colours in metaphase and interphase cell nuclei, such that the marked regions can be visualized with the aid of fluorescence or bright-field microscopy. Deviations from the normal patterns of marked regions permit the highly specific identification of genetically aberrant cells. The new ability to analyze interphase cells greatly expands the diagnostic and prognostic potential of cytogenetics. This has a major impact in fields such as prenatal diagnosis, oncology. haematology, pathology and genetic toxicology. The number of cells that must be examined to achieve a reliable decision on the molecular cytogenetic make-up of a cell sample, the complexity of the images and the amount of analysis time available indicate clearly that instrumentation for the (semi)automated examination of microscope images is crucial to achieve the required objectivity and speed. Microscope systems capable of doing so do not yet exist.

The goal of the Concerted Action Automated Molecular Cytogenetic Analysis is, therefore, to stimulate the development of the scientific and technological basis for automated systems for molecular cytogenetic analyses. This involves the integration of a variety of technologies - in situ hybridisation, microscopy, opto-electronics, electro-mechanics, digital processors, image processing methodologies and pattern recognition techniques.

The Concerted Action is managed by a Project Management Group consisting of the co-ordinator and 6 members: 3 from the engineering and 3 from the molecular cytogenetic field. This coordination and information exchange is effectuated by organization of topical and plenary workshops, promotion of interlab exchanges of personnel and material and by dissemination of information via publications of the Concerted Action.

Project leader:
Dr. A.K. RAAP
Dept. of Cytochemistry
and Cytometry,
Leiden University
Wassenaarseweg 72
NL 2333 AL Leiden
Phone: +31 71 27 61 87
Fax: +31 71 27 61 80
Contract number: CT921307

Participants:

Dr. D. ARNDT-JOVIN
DE 3400 Goettingen

Dr. P.A. BENEDETTI
IT 56100 Pisa

Dr. C. CREMER
DE 6900 Heidelberg

Dr. H. VAN DEKKEN
NL 3000 DR Rotterdam

Dr. J. GARCIA-SAGREDO
ES 28034 Madrid

Prof. E. GRANUM
DK 9220 Aalborg East

Dr. J.A. ATEN
NL 1105 AZ

Prof. G. BRUGAL
FR 38041 Grenoble

Prof. T. CREMER
DE 6900 Heidelberg

Dr. A. FORABOSCO
IT 41100 Modena

Dr. J. GRAHAM
UK Manchester M13 9PT

Dr. A.G.J.M. HANSELAAR
NL 6500 HB Nijmegen

Dr. J.M.N. HOOVERS
NL 1105 AZ Amsterdam

Dr. A.H.N. HOPMAN
NL 6200 MD Maastricht

Prof. J.A. HOUGHTON
IE Galway

Dr. O.P. KALLIONIEME
FI 33521 Tampere

Prof. P. KLEINSCHMIDT
DE 94030 Passau

Dr. S. KNUUTILA
FI 00014 Helsinki

Dr. L. KOULISCHER
BE 4000 Sart Tilman

Dr. P. LICHTER
DE 6900 Heidelberg

Dr. D. LLOYD
UK Didcot, Oxon ORQ

Dr. C. LUNDSTEEN
DK 2100 Copenhagen O

Prof. P. MALET
FR 63001 Clermont Ferrand

Dr. J. PIPER
UK Edinburgh EH4 2XU

Dr. P. POPESCU
FR 78352 Jouy en Josas

Dr. F. POZO
ES 28040 Madrid

Prof. J.P. RIGAUT
FR 75251 Paris Cedex 05

Dr. M. ROCCHI
IT 70126 Bari

Dr. E. SOINI
FI 20521 Turku

Dr. F. SPELEMAN
9000 Gent

Prof. H.J. TANKE
NL 2333 AL Leiden

Dr. D. TARUSCIO
IT 00161 Rome

Dr. E.J. TAWN
UK Cumbria CA20 1PG

Dr. M. TSO
UK Manchester M60 1QD

Dr. D. WHITE
UK Cardiff CF4 4XN

Dr. J. WIENBERG
DE 8000 Munich 2

Prof. I.T. YOUNG
NL 2628 CJ Delft

CONCEPTION, ELABORATION AND DEVELOPMENT OF AN ORIGINAL OSTEOINDUCTIVE BIOCOMPOSITE MATERIAL FOR BONE SUBSTITUTION

Key words
Composite biomaterial, Apatitic phosphates, Elastin Peptides-Collagens matrix, Bone substitute.

Brief description
A new artificial connective matrix has been recently described and developed. This matrix results from the association between elastin peptides and collagens which association could markedly be improved by addition of fibronectin, laminin, type IV collagen and glycosaminoglycans. With a view to elaborating a bioactive bone substitute, the possible association of such a matrix with calcium phosphates (CaPh) was investigated. The main original idea was based on the property of CaPh, especially of Hydroxyapatite (HAP), to adsorb and retain proteins. Preliminary investigations have been performed which clearly showed that:
1 some elastin peptides (ESP) were irreversibly bound to several HAP samples,
2 these products kept the capacity to react with I + III collagens,
3 the yielded composite, made of mineral and organic moieties, was not toxic and allowed the osteoblast to grow. From these first results and within the scope of our project, several investigations have to be performed.

Selection of the most suitable CaPh material
The first criterium of CaPh selection will be the capacity of ESP adsorption. Therefore, the experimental conditions of CaPh synthesis will be optimized in order to determine the main parameters of mineral moiety which are responsible for ESP adsorption.

Physical and chemical characterization of the mineral/organic interface
This study implies the research of the nature of binding between organic and mineral moieties, and also the evaluation of the quantity and the quality of crystal growth sites.

Improvement of the composite elaboration
The bonds between CaPh, ESP and collagens can be reinforced by synergistic effects of connective proteins and glycosaminoglycans. To the yielded composite material, specific proteins of osseous tissue could be trapped, conferring to it the capacity to monitor hard tissue restoration.

Mechanical properties and biocompatibility testing of the new developed composite materials
The mechanical properties of the material will be studied by means of tension, compression, bending and fatigue tests performed in saline solutions. In vitro preliminary studies will be carried out with L 929 cell cultures for cytotoxicity tests, and human osteoblast cultures for basal and specific cytocompatibility. Short and long term implantations, in rats, rabbits or dogs, both in ectopic and osseous sites, will allow the determination of osteoblast biointegration on the material.

Project leader:
Dr. M. RABAUD
INSERM, Unité 306,
Université de Bordeaux II
146, rue Léo-Saignat
FR 33076 Bordeaux Cedex
Phone: +33 57 57 17 30
Fax: +33 56 90 05 17
Contract number: CT920254

Participants:
Dra. Isabel LOPEZ VALERO
Osteosynth
Carrer Major 65
ES 08629 Torrelles de Llobregat,
Barcelona
Phone: +34 3 689 10 46
Fax: +34 3 689 04 95

Dra. Antonetta GATTI
Centro di Stud dei Biomateriali,
Univ di Modena
Via del Pozzo 71
IT 41100 Modena
Phone: +39 59 37 26 42
Fax: +39 59 37 34 28

Dra. Nuria BASI
Centro de Investigacion y Desarrollo Aplicado
Argenters 6
ES Barcelona
Phone: +34 3 719 03 61
Fax: +34 3 718 96 67

Dr. Christian REY
Ecole de Chemie, Lab des PO4,
Univ de Toulouse
Rue des 36 Ponts 38
FR 31400 Toulouse
Phone: +33 61 55 65 32
Fax: +33 61 55 60 85

Dr. Josep PLANELL
Univ Politec de Catalunya,
Dept. di Ciencia de los Materiales
Diagonal 647
ES 08028 Barcelona
Phone: +34 3 401 67 08
Fax: +34 3 401 66 00

Dr. William BONFIELD
Queen Mary and Westfiels College
Mile End Road
UK London E1 NS
Phone: +44 71 975 51 51
Fax: +44 81 983 17 99

NEAR INFRARED SPECTROSCOPY AND IMAGING FOR NON INVASIVE MONITORING OF THE OXYGENATION AND HAEMODYNAMIC STATUS IN TISSUES

Key words
Near Infrared Spectroscopy, Optical Tomography, Oxygenation, Photon Propagation.

Objectives
1 To quantitate Near Infrared Spectroscopy (NIRS) measurements, by increasing the knowledge of absorption and scattering phenomena in tissues.
2 To aplly the quantitative measurements to basic research on tumours, the heart and cerebral tissues.
3 To use the refined NIRS methodology for clinical investigations such as oxygenation in neonatal brain, tumours, the heart, adult anaesthesia and CNS disorders.
4 To study photon propagation in blood perfused tissue, investigate the 'Forward Problem' and devise methods to solve the 'Inverse Problem' to reconstruct images of tissue.
5 Apply NIR imaging for breast cancer screening and neonatal cerebral studies.

Brief description
NIRS has been developed for non invasive assessment into the pohysiological and pathophysiological processes. There is now great potential to extend this methodology for clinical imaging (or biochemical imaging). However, a numer of clinical and biomedical tasks have been identified which need to be solved before NIRS and Imaging can be successfully aplied. These are outlined below:

Task 1 Quantitation: A major problem is to produce quantitative measurements. This problem will be solved by determining the optical path length in different biological tissues, the scattering and absorption coefficients of all relevant tissues and developing algorithms for the calculation of tissue chromophore concentrations. This work will be carried out using pico/femto second lasers and streak camera, and other optical instrumentation based on phase modulation techniques (PMS).

Task 2 Movements artefacts: This will be approached firstly by developing improved means (suction etc) with which to attach probes, especially for fetal apllication. In parallel with these attemps to make practical improvements theoretical analyses will be carried out to investigate the influences of movement artefacts. Direct measurement of pathlength using PMS techniques will also allow movements to be monitored and employ corrections.

Task 3 Development of NIRS Imaging: This will require instrumentation development and theoretical/mathematical research.

Instrumentation Imaging with NIRS has been demonstrated in limited laboratory studies. Basic research can be performed with the complex laser/streak systems, but these are expensive and not directly suited to clinical application. The instrumentation will therefore include pico second diode lasers and dedicated detectors as well as intruments based on PMS technique.

Image Reconstruction Photon propagation through biological tissue is complex and requires a special approach in order to derive equations for the 'Forward Problem'. The analysis then will be extended to the 'Inverse Problem' for developing reconstruction techniques.

Task 4 Development of test materials for NIRS spectroscopy/imaging phantoms: A design for a phantom material which matches the optical properties of tissue has been suggested. Both non-biological (Polystyrene) and biological (mitochondria, cells) suspensions will be used for this work.

Task 5 Tumour perfusion and oxygenation The radiosensitivity of tumours depends upon the cellular oxygenation which is difficult to assess. NIRS offers the possibility of monitoring oxygenation non invasively. There is a need to investigate possible correlations between cell proliferation, energy metabolism and oxygen levels in tumours. Assessment of normal and abnormal hepatic oxygenation will also be carried out using NIRS. There is a high incidence of primary and secondary carcinoma of the liver, and NIRS will provide useful information for basic research and surgical interventions.

Task 6 NIRS Investigation of myocardial oxygenation The basic optical properties of myoglobin will be determined as part of Task 1. The work will then be extended in order to allow application of NIRS to the exposed animal heart, exposed human heart, and in the longer term non-invasive interrogation of the human myocardium.

Task 7.1 Normal ranges of NIRS variables; Clinical Investigations NIRS has already shown that it can be used to measure cerebral blood volume and flow in infants, and can show abnormalities of oxygenation and haemodynamics during labour or following asphyxia. Studies in several clinical areas will establish normal ranges and variations for NIRS measured variables, and identify the differences observable in pathological or diseased states. It is essential to perform clinical validations and to determine the reliability in a variety of clinical situations. Multi centre trials with the Concerted Action would increase statistical strength of NIR monitoring techniques, especially CBF and CBV.

Task 7.2 Brain metabolic imaging with NIRS Work on imaging of the brain in neonates is already under way at several centres and NIR images of brain in the rat have been demonstrated. However, solutions to Tasks 3 and 4, need to be found before clinical functional imaging (or biochemical imaging) can be started.

Project leader:
Professor P. ROLFE
Department of Biomedical
Engineering &
Medical Physics,
Keele University
Thornburrow Drive
UK Stoke on Tent, Staffs
ST4 7QB
Phone: +44 782 71 66 00
Fax: +44 782 74 73 19
Contract number: CT921234

Participants:
Dr. D. ROSENTHAL
DE 6000 Frankfurt am Main

Dr. Gorm GREISEN
DK 2100 Copenhagen 0

Dr. Joanna DOBROGOWSK-
A-KUNICKA
PL 04 628 Warshaw

Dr. M. KASCHE
DE 7082 Oberkochen

Albert & Renate HUCH
CH 8091 Zurich

Prof. Berend OESEBURG
NL 6500 HB Nijmegen

Prof. C. CHOPIN
FR 59037 Lille Cedex

Prof. C. STREFFER,
Dr. F. STEINBERG
DE 4300 Essen 1

Prof. David DELPY
UK London WC1E 6JA

Prof. David EDWARDS
UK London W12 ONN

Prof. Dawood PARKER
UK Swansea SA6 6NL

Prof. Dr. M. KESSLER
DE 8520 Erlangen

Prof. Nils SVENNINGSEN
SE 221 85 Lund

Prof. G.DUC
CH 8091 Zurich

Prof. Marco FERRARI
IT 67100 L'Aquila

Prof. Paul CASAER
BE 3000 Leuven

Prof. Stephan SCHMIDT
DE 5300 Bonn 1

CHEMICAL SENSORS FOR IN VIVO MONITORING

Key words
Chemical sensor, *in vivo*, glucose, biomaterials, biosensor.

Objectives
The Concerted Action will target reliable, continuous, short-term *in vivo* monitoring of glucose as its principal goal. It will also target a significant advance in *in vivo* monitoring of at least one other analyte.

Brief description
Recent advances in sensor technology have brought the ambitious goal of reliable continuous in vivo sensing closer to clinical reality. The Concerted Action on chemical sensors for in vivo monitoring acts as a core research base in pursuit of more stable, biocompatible and specific sensors for *in vivo* monitoring. The biological interface is a major area where problems must be resolved for the future success of such sensors. The information gaps which will receive attention include:
Biomaterials: membrane/packaging; biophysics of cell surface interactions, tissue polymer interactions; sensor/surface characterization prior to and after implantation: physical, chemical, biochemical; novel materials: modified electrodes, modified membranes and newer conducting materials and feasibility of their biological use. Continuous monitoring versus discrete monitoring: tissue biochemistry and physiology and physiopathology, analyses subject to tissue modification; sensor reliability versus accuracy in relation to significance of physiological data; physiology/pathophysiology of *in vivo* sensing site.
In vivo calibration, requirements, possibilities, reference methods; *in vitro* evaluation of sensors: procedure, duplication of matrix. enzyme and/or mediator leaching toxicology; *in vivo* evaluation of implanted sensors: animal model, implantation mode, calibration procedure, drift assessment, inflammatory assessment, clinical evaluation. Scale-up of production of microsensors; reference electrodes: fabrication, failings and interfacing signal processing: molecular engineering, to include natural sensors; quality assurance.
The programme will be based on a series of workshops, which will provide convenient assessment points for evaluation of progress and cues for the preparation of reports; exchanges of personnel; and a centralised information facility including an established database and a quarterly Newsletter. The key stages of the Concerted Action correspond to subjects covered in the workshop programme.

Workshop Programme
Year 1: (i) 'Biomaterials & Biointeractions'.
   (ii)'Chronobiology In Relation to *In Vivo* Monitoring'.
Year 2: (i) 'Technology Evaluation'.
   (ii)'Design & Fabrication of Sensing Systems'.

The Concerted Action on Chemical Sensors for *In Vivo* Monitoring is funded under BIOMED for 24 months.

Project leader:
Professor A. TURNER
Biotechnology Centre,
Cranfield University
Cranfield
UK Bedford MK43 0AL
Phone: +44 234 75 43 39
Fax: +44 234 75 09 07
Contract number: CT920015

Participants:

Prof. P. BERGVELD
NL 7500 AE

Dr. B. DANIELSSON
SE 22100 Lund

Dr. D. de ROSSI
IT 56100 Pisa

Dr. F.J. SCHMIDT &
Dr. A.J.M. SCHOONEN
NL Groningen

Dr. G. REACH
FR 75004 Paris

Dr. H. BAUSER
DE 7000 Stuttgart 80

Dr. Ir. C. INCE
NL Rotterdam

Dr. J. LEKKALA
FR 33101 Tampere

Dr. J.C. PICKUP
UK London SE1 9RT

Dr. J.M. TELLADO
ES 28007 Madrid

Dr. P. JACOBS
BE 3030 Heverlee

Mrs. S. KOCH
DE 80920 Munchen

Prof. A. BASZKIN
FR 92296 Chatenay Malabry

Prof. A. MACHADO
PT 4000 Porto

Dr. S.J. ALCOCK
UK Bedford MK43 0AL

Prof. B. MATTIASSON
SE 22100 Lund

Prof. B. OESEBURG
NL 6500 HB Nijmegen

Prof. D.R. THEVENOT
FR 94010 Creteil Cedex

Prof. G. PALLESCHI
IT 00173 Rome

Prof. J. FEIJEN
NL 7500 AE Enschede

Prof. J.M. KAUFFMAN
BE 1050 Bruxelles

Prof. K. SCHUGERL
DE 3000 Hannover 1

Prof. L. CAMPANELLA
IT 00185 Rome

Prof. M. KARAYANNIS
GR Ioannina

Prof. M. MASCINI
IT 50121 Firenze

Prof. M.P. COUGHLAN
IE Galway

Prof. M.R. SMYTH
IE Dublin 9

Prof. N. de ROOIJ &
Dr. M. KOUDELKA
CH 2000 Neuchatel 7

Prof. O. BESKARDES
TR Ankara

Prof. O.
SIGGAARD-ANDERSEN
DK 2730 Herlev

Prof. O. WOLFBEIS
AT 8010 Graz

Prof. P. ROLFE
UK Stoke on Trent ST4 7BQ
Hartshill

Prof. P.M. VADGAMA
UK Salford M6 8HD

Prof. BIOMATECH
FR 38670 Chasse sur Rhone

Prof. R. PICKARD
UK Cardiff CF1 1XL

Prof. S. ALEGRET
ES 08193 Bellaterra

Prof. T. SCHEPER

DE 4400 Munster

Prof. U. FISCHER
NL Rotterdam

Prof. W. KERNER
DE 23538 Lubeck

DEVELOPMENT AND HARMONISATION OF THE NORMS AND PARAMETERS IN BIOLOGICAL TESTING PROTOCOLS DESIGNED FOR ROOT CANAL SEALERS IN THE EUROPEAN COMMUNITY

Key words
Biological testing, dental materials, harmonisation, in vitro (non animal) testing, in use testing.

Objectives
1 To provide a starting point for the implementation of new European Standards (ENs) setting out the biological testing methods to be used for all dental materials.
2 Standardisation of test methods between different centres by use of defined protocols.
3 Comparison of results obtained in various modes of testing to determine the relevance of individual test and the relationship between data obtained from different tests.
4 To develop new methods of biological testing.
5 To develop simple biological testing protocols which do not inhibit the development of new materials and involve minimal use of animals, while protecting humans.

Brief description
A coordinated series of studies will be carried out in 8 European centres in which the results of in vitro (non animal) testing will be compared with results obtained in vivo in animals models. Obtaining data from different centres will expedite the harmonisation of the individual testing protocols and hence improve the reproducibility of the results. The multi-centre approach will allow data obtained by subjecting the same material to the wide range of methods of biological testing to be compared.

Tests described in the ISO protocols will be carried out. These comprise:
1 Initial testing using cell culture methods. The cells used are fibroblasts.
2 Secondary testing involving implantation of materials contained in biocompatible tubes into living tissues.
3 Usage tests in the root canals of selected animal models.

Three new initial tests will be carried. These will seek to:
A Develop and evaluate the use of osteoblasts in culture. Root canal sealing materials may come into contact with bone.
B Develop the use of immune competence testing as a means of screening the toxicity of root canal sealing materials.
C Investigate the use of the chorioallantoic membrane of the chick egg as a non mammalian tissue culture system.

Four commonly used root canal sealing materials will be subjected to initial secondary and usage testing. Each individual test will be carried out in at least 2 centres. A series of workshops, expert meetings and exchanges of personnel and data will facilitate the project.

Project leader:

Dr. A. WATTS
Glasgow Dental Hospital and School
378 Sauchiehall Street
UK Glasgow Scotland G2 3JZ
Phone: +44 41 332 70 20
Fax: +44 41 331 27 98
Contract number: CT920419

Participants:

Dr. HENSTEN-PETTERSEN
Dept. of Biological and
Clinical Testing, NIOM
Kirkeveien 71B
NO 1344 Haslum
Phone: +47 67 580100
Fax: +46 67 591530

Prof. R.C. PATERSON &
D.G. MacDonald
Dept. of Adult Dental Care,
Dental Hospital and School
378, Sauchiehall Street
UK Glasgow G2 3JZ
Phone: +44 41 3327020
Fax: +44 41 3312798

Dr. A. WENNBERG
Dept. of Endodontics, School
of Dentistry
Carl Gustavs Vag 34
SE 21421 Malmo
Phone: +46 40 323000
Fax: +46 40 925359

Dr. E.C. MUNKSGAARD
Dept. of Dental Materials
Science,
Univ School of Dentistry
Norre alle 20
DK 2200 Copenhagen
Phone: +45 353 71700
Fax: +45 353 71743

Dr. F.M. ANDREASEN
Dept. of Paediatric Dentistry,
Univ School of dentistry
Norre Alle 20
DK 2200 Copenhagen
Phone: +45 353 71700
Fax: +45 353 71743

Dr. J.O. ANDREASEN
Dept. of Oral Medicine and
Oral Surgery, Univ Hospital
18, Tagensvej
DK 2200 Copenhagen
Phone: +45 354 57565
Fax: +45 354 57506

Dr. T. LAMBRIANIDIS
Dept. of Dental Pathology
and Therapeutics,
Aristole Dental School
GR 54006 Thessaloniki
Phone: +30 32 991017/023
Fax: +30 32 266321

Prof. G. SCHMALZ
Policlinic für Zahnerhaltung
und Parodontologie
Franz Josef Strauss Allee 11
DE 93042 Regensburg
Phone: +49 941 9446024
Fax: +49 941 9446025

Prof. J. SZABO
Difchka U 5,
School of Dentistry,
Univ of Pecs
HU 7621 Pecs
Phone: +36 72 315130
Fax: +36 72 315130

Prof. M. CERVINKA
Facultas Medica,
Universitas Carolina
SK 87050038 Hradec Kralove
Phone: +42 49 23048
Fax: +42 49 23048

Prof. BERGENHOLTZ &
Dr. M.G. JONTELL
Dept. of Endodontology/
Oral diagnosis,
Faculty of Odontology
Medicinaregatan 12
SE Goteburg
Phone: +46 31 853250
Fax: +46 31 826416

Prof. R.M. BROWNE
Dept. of Oral Pathology,
The Dental School
St Chad's Queensway
UK Birmingham B4 6NN
Phone: +44 21
2368611/5866
Fax: +44 21 6258815

SKELETAL IMPLANTS

Key words
Biocompatibility, biomaterials, bioactive materials, implant retrieval analysis, skeletal implants.

Brief description
To establish a major grouping of 41 laboratories across Europe, with the two objectives of:
1 Implant retrieval analysis.
2 Innovation of second generation skeletal implants.

A project of this scale is essential if Europe is to establish the conceptuel medical technology required to deal with the escalating percentage of repeal operations.

Project leader:
Professor W. BONFIELD
IRC in Biomedical Materials
Mile End Road
UK London E1 4NS
Phone: +44 71 975 51 51
Fax: +44 81 983 17 99
Contract number: CT931275

Participants:
Dr. A. RAVAGLIOLI &
Dr. A. KRAJEWSKI
National Research Council,
Research Inst. for Ceramics
Technology
Via Granarolo 64
IT 48018 Faenza

Dr. B. McCORMACK,
Dr. A. CARR
Dept. of Mechanical
Engineering,
School of Engineering
Univ College Dublin
IE Dublin 4

Dr. D. JONES
Dept. of Cell Biology,
Universitity of Munster
Domaghstrasse 3
DE 4400 Munster

Dr. D. MUSTER
L.E.E.D. Biomateriaux,
Lab de Recherche de
la Chaire de Stomatologieet
Chirurgie Maxillofaciale
P.O. Box 426
FR 67091 Strasbourg

Dr. E. GABRIEL
Chir Universtat Klinik
Josef Schneider Strasse 2
DE 8700 Wurzburg

Dr. E. SCHNEIDER
Arbeitsbereich Biomechanik,
Technische Universitat
Hamburg-Harburg
Denickenstrasse 15
DE 2100 Hamburg 90

Dr. J. CORDEY
AO Research Inst.
Clavadelerstrasse
CH 7270 Davos-Platz

Dr. J.J. FICAT
Clinique Saint Jean
20 Route de Revel
FR 31077 Toulouse Cedex

Dr. J.T. TRIFFITT
MRC Bone Laboratory,
Nuffield Orthopaedic Centre
Windmill Road
UK Headington OX3 7LD

Dr. L. AMBROSIO,
Prof. G. NICOLAIS
Dept. of Materials and
Production Engineering,
Univ of Naples
Piazzala Tecchio
IT 80125 Napoli

Dr. M.F HARMAND LEMI
Technopole Montesquieu
FR 33650 Martillac

Dr. P. THOMSEN
Dept. of Anatomy,
Univ of Gotenberg
P.O. Box 33031
SE 400 33 Gothenberg

Prof. A. BEZERIANOS
Dept. of Medical Physics,
School of Medicine,
Univ of Patras
GR 26500 Patras

Prof. C. BAQUEY
Universite de Bordeaux II
146 Rue Leo Saignat
FR 33076 Bordeau Cedex

Prof. C. LACABANNE
Laboratoire de Physique
des Solides,
Paul Sabatier Universite
118 Route de Narbonne
FR 31062 Toulouse Cedex

Prof. C. MIGLIARESI
Dept. of Materials
Engineering,
Univ of Trento
IT 38050 Mesiano-Trento

Prof. C. REY
Labatoire de Physico-Chemie
des Solides, Ecole Nationale
Superieure de Chemie,
38 Rue de 36 Ponts
FR 31400 Toulouse

Prof. E. BONUCCI
Departimento di Biopatologia
Umana, Universita Degli
Studi di Roma La Sapienza
Viale Regina Elena 324
IT 00161 Roma

Prof. G. DELLING,
Dr. M. HAHN
Institut für Pathologie,
Universität-Krankenhaus
Eppendorf
Universität Hamburg
Martin Strasse 52
DE 200 Hamburg 20

Prof. G. MAROTTI
Instituto di Anatomia
Umana Normale,
Unversita di Modena
Via del Pozzo 71
IT 41100 Modena

Prof. G. PAPANICOLAOU
Applied Mechanics
Laboratory,
Dept. of Mechanical
Engineering
University of Patras
GR 26110 Patras

Prof. AUDEKERCKE,
Prof. G. van der PERRE
Dept. Werktuigkunde,
Katholieke Universiteit
Leuven
Celestijnenlaan 200 A
BE 3001 Haverlee

Prof. G.W. HASTINGS,
Dr. K.E. TANNER
Queen Mary and Westfield
College
Mile End Road
UK London E1 4NS

Prof. I. HVID
The Orthopaedic Hospital,
Univ of Aarhus
DK 8000 Aarhus C

Prof. Jack van RECK
Institut de Stomatologie,
Hopital Univ. St Pierre
322 Rue Haute
BE 1000 Brussels

Prof. J. HELSEN
Dept. MTMK.U.
Leuven de Croylaan 2
BE 3001 Haverlee

Prof. J. PLANELL,
Prof. F. DRIESSENS
Dept. Cienia de los Materials
e Ingenieria Metalurgica
Universidad Politecnica
de Cataluna
Diagonal 647
ES 08028 Barcelona

Prof. K. de GROOT,
Dr. C.P.A.T. KLEIN
Dept. of Biomaterials,
Univ of Leiden
Rijnburgerweg 10
NL 2333 AA Leiden

Prof. L. SEDEL,
Prof. A. MEUNIER
Faculte de Medecine
Lariboisiere St Louis
10 Avenue de Verdun
FR 75010 Paris

Prof. M. BARBOSA
Rue D Manuel II
PT 4003 Porto Codex

Prof. N. AKKAS
Technical Univ
TR Ankara

Prof. P. REVELL
Rowland Hill Street
UK London NW3 2PF

Prof. P. TORMALA
P.O. Box 527
FI 33101 Tampere

Prof. TRANQUILLI
LEALI,
Dr. A.MEROLLI
IT 00168 Roma

Prof. P.N. VRYZAKIS
GR 14565 Athens

Prof. R. BOURGOIS
Dept. of Civil Engineering,
Royal Military Academy
Renaissancelaan 30
BE 1040 Brussels

Prof. R. HUISKES
Inst. for Orthopaedics,
Univ of Nijmegen
De Craanenlaan 7
NL 6500 Nijmegen

Prof. R. THULL
Universitatsklinik und
Polikliniken fur Zahn-,
Mund-, und
Kieferkrankheiten
Pleicherwall 2
DE 8700 Wurzburg

Prof. U. GROSS
Universitatsklinikum Steglitz,
Freie Universitat Berlin
Hindenburgdamm 30
DE 1000 Berlin 45

Prof. Y. MISSIRLIS
Biomedical Engineering
Laboratory, Dept. of Physics,
Univof Patras
GR Patras

COMPUTER AIDED ORTHODONTICS

Key words
Orthodontics, biomechanics, FEM, CAD, bone remodelling, laser scanning.

Brief description
The aim of orthodontic treatment is the correction of malpositions of the teeth. This is achieved by the application of forces that are generated by orthodontic appliances. To prevent damage of the teeth and the supporting biological structures, orthodontic forces have to be of correct magnitude, direction, and duration.
The objective of the proposed project is to gain a thorough knowledge about the behavior of the biological structures of the jaws when loaded with orthodontic force systems. To assess the treatment effects of an appliance, the induced morphological changes, i.e., movements of the teeth and reorganisation of adjacent structures, have to be measured. Using this data in combination with experimentally determined force systems generated by an orthodontic appliance allows the elaboration of a theoretical model of tissue behavior. This model forms the basis of a specialised design system that is used to develop improved appliances with a higher degree of effectiveness and reliability.
Matching clinical observations with theoretical and experimental results requires four major research tasks: CAA (computer aided analysis).
Development of a measuring device to obtain the spatial information of orthodontically induced tooth movements, FEM (finite element methods).
Development of 3D-FEM models of the teeth, periodontal and bony structures. Elasto-static analysis of structural reorganisation induced by orthodontic forces (bone remodelling), CAD (computer aided design).
Development of a specialised CAD-system for the design of orthodontic appliances utilising FEM calculations and 3D-data input obtained by CAA, CAT (computer aided testing).
Testing and validation of the newly designed appliances using a 3D-force-measurement system.

Project leader:
Dr. D. DRESCHER
Poliklinik für Kieferorthopaedie der
Universität Bonn
Welschonnenstrasse 17
DE 53111 Bonn
Phone: +49 228 287 24 49
Fax: +49 228 287 24 44
Contract number: CT931712

Participants:

Prof. A. KANARACHOS
National Technical
Univ of Athens
Mechanical Design and
Control
P.O. Box 64078
GR 15710 Athens
Phone: +30 1 771 6016
Fax: +30 1 973 4180

Dr. David BROOME
Univ College London,
Dept. of Mechanical
Engineering
Torrington Place
UK London WC1E 7JE
Phone: +44 71 387 7050
Fax: +44 71 380 0180

Dr. Christoph BOURAUEL
Poliklinik für
Kieferorthopädie der
Universität Bonn
Welschonnenstr 17
DE 53111 Bonn
Phone: +49 228 287 2332
Fax: +49 228 287 2444

APPLICATION OF STABLE ISOTOPES IN CLINICAL MEDICINE

Key words
Nitrogen isotopes, isotope labeling, spectrum analysis, mass, breath tests, diagnosis, digestive system, carbon isotopes.

Brief description
This Concerted Action is concerned with the development and applications of non-radioactive (i.e. stable isotope) techniques for diagnostic use in clinical and epidemiological studies.
The aim is to coordinate research in eight different nations to ensure that:
- Adequate European references are established so that all centres provide the same results.
- Standardized test protocols are developed to enable trans-European comparisons of results that can be interpreted with well-understood levels of specificity and sensitivity.

Because there is some disparity as to the extent to which progress in these areas has already been made, there is diversity in the proposed clinical applications:
1 Standard procedures now exist for the diagnosis of Helicobacter Pylori infection in children and adults.

We propose their use in an epidemiological study of the frequency of the infection in children in less-privileged areas of Europe in relation to diarrhoeal disease and growth faltering.
2 In a clinical context there is rather too much diversity in the way in which tests are carried out and results presented.

Existing tests will be developed, standardized and organized so that data gathered across Europe on problems of malassimilation of carbohydrates, lipids and proteins can be integrated in a meaningful way.
Particular attention will be given to digestive function in children with cystic fibrosis.
The measurement of gastric emptying will provide additional insights in these main digestive functions:
3 Current applications for investigation of metabolism are mainly with respect to liver microsomal capacity as applied in studies on alcoholic liver disease, hepatitis, liver transplantation, drug treatment, xeno-biotic substances.
4 The curious interactions that bring together mass-spectrometry and clinical medicine means that neither medical or mass-spectrometric bibliography adequately cover the field of the proposed concerted action.
We intend to initiate a bibliography for users of stable isotopes in clinical medicine.

Project leader:
Professor Dr. Y. GHOOS
University Hospital Gasthuisberg,
Lab.Digestie & Absorptie,
Catholic University of Leuven
Herestraat 49
BE 3000 Leuven
Phone: +32 16 34 43 97
Fax: +32 16 34 43 99
Contract number: CT931239

Participants:

A. ANDIULLI
Ospedale Casa Solievo della
Sofferenza
Viale dei Cappuccini
IT 71013 San Giovanni
Rotondo
Phone: +39 882 410263
Fax: +39 882 411879

Br. DRUMM
Univ College Dublin
Belfield
IE Dublin 4
Phone: +353 1 556901
Fax: +353 1 555307

C. JACOBS
Acad. Hospitaal
Vrije Universiteit
De Boelelaan 1117
NL 1081 HV Amsterdam
Phone: +31 20 5389111
Fax: +31 20 5484898

D. HALLIDAY
Clinical Research Centre,
Watford Road
UK Harrow,
Middlesex HA1 3UJ
Phone: +44 81 8693203
Fax: +44 81 4231275

D. RATING
Ruprecht-Karls-Universität
Kinderklinik
Im neuenheimer Feld 150
DE 6900 Heidelberg 1
Phone: +49 6221 562311
Fax: +49 6221 564388

G. ODERDA
Pediatrics-Gastroenterology,
University of Turin
Piazza Polonia 94
IT 10126 Torino
Phone: +39 11 6927304
Fax: +39 11 6631925

J.P. GALMICHE
Hopital G et R Laennec,
Hepato-Gastro-Enterologie
P.O. Box 1005
FR 44035 Nantes Cedex 01
Phone: +33 40 165742
Fax: +33 78 775743

J.P. RIOU
Faculte de Medecine
A. Carrell
Rue G. Paradin
FR 69372 Lyon Cedex 08
Phone: +33 78 009898
Fax: +33 78 778612

L. WEAVER, J. THOMAS,
A. COWARD
Dunn Nutrition Centre
Downhamslane, Milton Road
UK Cambridge CB4 1XJ
Phone: +44 223 426356
Fax: +44 223 426617

M. QUINA
Hospital de Pulido Valente,
Medicina III
Alameda das Linhas de
Torres 117
PT 1799 Lisboa Codex
Phone: +351 1 7586603
Fax: +351 1 7586603

Ph. JOHNSON
Bureau of Stable Isotope
Analysis
Brook Lane North
Brentford,
Middlesex TW8 0PP
Phone: +44 81 847 3955
Fax: +44 81 847 5053

P. KRUMBIEGEL
UFZ-Umweltforschungs-
zentrum
Promosorstrasse 16
DE 7050 Leipzig
Phone: +49 341 23922246
Fax: +49 341 2352288

R. VONK
Universiteit - Research Lab
Bloemsingel 10
NL 9712 KZ Groningen
Phone: +31 50 632772
Fax: +31 50 632606

RAPID DIAGNOSIS OF MYOCARDIAL INFARCTION
WITH A NEW MARKER AND BIOSENSOR

Key words
Myocardial infarction, instable angina, biosensor, immunosensor, fatty acid-binding protein, myoglobin, bed-side diagnosis.

Brief description
The Concerted Action aims at coordinating individual research activities on the development and evaluation of new, highly specific and rapid methods and novel instrumentation for the diagnosis of acute myocardial infarction and of minor myocardial damage (instable angina) in man. The methods are based on the newly established infarction marker fatty acid-binding protein (FABP) and modern immunosensor technology which allows rapid (within 10 minutes) bed-side analysis of specific proteins in plasma. By monitoring FABP in plasma the assessment or exclusion of an infarction is possible as early as 1.5- 3 hours after onset of first symptoms of acute myocardial infarction, which time is important for starting successful treatment.

The Concerted Action should accelerate the multi-center evaluation and final technical improvement of the FABP-immunosensor, necessary for its introduction into European medical practice. It is expected that the FABP-immunosensor dévice will improve quality and reduce laboratory costs of infarction diagnostics. The accurate discrimination between patients with and without myocardial infarction at an earlier point in time will markedly reduce costs of clinical treatment of patients initially suspected of having an acute myocardial infarction.

Project leader:
Dr. J. GLATZ
Dept of Physiology, Cardiovascular
Research Institute, Maastricht (CARIM)
P.O. Box 616
NL 6200 MD Maastricht
Phone: +31 43 88 12 08
Fax: +31 43 67 10 28
Contract number: CT931692

Participants:
Dr. A.P.M. GORGELS
Dept. of Cardiology,
Academic Hospital
Maastricht
P.O. Box 5800
NL 6202 AZ Maastricht

Dr. C.J. McNEIL
Dept. of Clinical
Biochemistry/Biosensors
Research Group,
The Medical School,
Univ of Newcastle-upon-Tyne
Framlington Place
UK Newcastle-upon-Tyne NE2 4HH

Dr. R. RENNEBERG
Institut für Chemo- und Biosensorik e.V.
Nottulner Landweg 90
DE 48161 Münster-Roxel

Prof. Dr. K. THYGESEN
Dept. of Cardiology, Arhus Univ Hospital
Tage-Hansens Gade 2
DK 8000 Arhus-C

Prof.Dr. M. HORDER
Dept. of Clinical Chemistry,
Odense Univ Hospital
DK 5000 Odense-C

ASSESSMENT OF ADEQUACY OF ANAESTHESIA BY SPONTANEOUS AND EVOKED BRAIN ELECTRICAL ACTIVITY

Key words
Monitoring, electroencephalogramm, evoked response, somatosensory, auditory, depth of anaesthesia, neutral network, knowledge based system.

Brief description
The aim of the study is to assess simultaneously EEG, SEP, AEP and tcM-MEP (see sect. 3) during general anaesthesia in addition to systemic variables which are related to CNS function, arterial and/or end-expiratory carbon dioxide concentrations, arterial oxygen saturation, heart rate, and blood pressure. The degree of muscle paralysis will be assessed by a standard train-of-four test of peripheral muscles.

1 In a first step all variables will be analyzed and correlated in order to identify those parameters which will give the best information on depth of anaesthesia and specific conditions such as intraoperative arousal and movement in response to surgical incision.

2 In a second step all data will be subjected to further analysis such as bispectral EEG analysis, neural network based classification of EEG, SEP, AEP, tcM-EEP patterns, and knowledge based self-learning algorithms in order to identify variables which best predict depth of anaesthesia. These will be very innovative approaches for analyzing the complex and heterogeneous brain electrical activity. No studies have been reported so far using these very promising computerized techniques.

3 The ultimate goal is the development and characterization of monitoring variables for the assessment of depth of anaesthesia which is as yet an unsolved problem. A standard procedure for brain monitoring will be defined which can be used for the development of a commercial unified monitor of depth of anaesthesia.

Project leader:
Dr. E. KOCHS
Dept of Anaesthesia, University
Hospital Eppendorf
Martinistrasse 52
DE 20246 Hamburg
Phone: +49 40 4717 2415
Fax: +49 40 4717 4963
Contract number: CT931506

Participants:
Christine THORNTON
Anaestetic Dept., St. Mary's Hospital
Medical School Northwick Park Hospital
Watford Road
UK Harrow HAI 3UJ

Dr. Cor J. KALKMAN
Dept. of Anaestesia, Academic Hospital,
Univ of Amsterdam
Meibergdreef 9
NL 1105 AZ Amsterdam

Prof. Dr. Ewal KONECNY
Professur für Medizintechnik,
Medical Univ of Lübeck
Ratzeburger Allee 160
DE 223538 Lübeck

Prof. Dr. Hermann KUPPE
Dept. of Anaesthesia,
Medical Univ of Lübeck
Ratzeburger Allee 160
DE 23538 Lübeck

OBJECTIVE COMPETITIVE ASSESSMENT OF THE TECHNOLOGIES USED IN THE DIAGNOSIS OF JAUNDICE (IC-TEC)

Key words
Jaundice, health technology assessment, diagnosis of jaundice, computed diagnosis.

Brief description
It assesses the technologies used in the diagnosis of jaundice by comparing them to one another objectively against the standard provided by the clinical data. An objective base-line of clinical data is available from 9000 cases observed in the Euricterus project. From it a patient's clinical data can provide a computed diagnosis.

The efficacy of a technology is the percentage increment by which its results raises the computed diagnosis above the level provided by the clinical data. The clinical data and the results of the technologies wil be recorded on proforma in the 17 major diseases involved. The protocol is devised by the 75 participating hospitals in 24 countries. Each hospital will gather 5 cases of each disease, total 300. The cases will be entered on a floppy disk and mailed monthly to the data centre. After validation, they are entered in a relational database and analysed by Bayesian techniques which display the increment provided by each technology, over the clinical data. The performance of his data is fed back to the assessing doctor, in comparison with that of the database as a whole, to monitor quality. The heart of the assessment is a Bayesian diagnostic program. It returns a percentage as the clinical data is entered and again as the result of each technology is entered The increment given by a technology is a measure of its contribution to diagnosis by comparing the average costs of the tests to the average diagnostic increment the cost benefit and opportunity-cost are obtained for each disease group.

The diagnostic probabilities for the technologies are obtained from a database compiled in the course of the project, which will include about 100 clinical and 60 technological and cost data only the technologies needed for the management of the individual are used and recorded. They include ultrasound, Ercp, PTCG etc. Where test results are numeric (ALT =256) the results are divided into 5 equinumeric bands from 'low' to 'high'. Where the results are text, they are divided into significant statements such as 'common bile duct 'dilated'. The occurrence of the statements is counted in each disease The frequencies are expressed as centimas with confidence intervals. The efficacy of each test is correlated with its cost. A rank order of test by cost benefit is made for each disease, providing an optimum path of investigation.

Project leader:
Professor B.E. LEONARD
Dept of Experimental
Medicine,
Clinical Science Institute
University College,
IE Galway 90
Phone: +353 91 250 46
Fax: +353 91 265 05
Contract number: CT931036

Participants:

Dr. A. GONZALEZ
ES Barcelona

Dr. MALCHOW MOELLER
DK Svendborg

Dr. A. SANTOS
PT Lisboa

Dr. A. TANNER
UK Cleveland

Dr. A. THEODOSSI
UK Croydon, Surrey

Dr. A.VIEIRA
PT Aveiro

Dr. B. Van HOEK
NL Leiden

Dr. D. O'BRIEN
IE Galway

Dr. E. ELIAS
UK Birmingham

Dr. E. LISSEN
ES Sevilla

Dr. F. GONZALEZ
ES Salamanca

Dr. F.CUNNINGHAM
IE Co Meath

Dr. G. MACEDO
PT Porto

Dr. G. ROHR
DE Mannheim

Dr. J. CROWE
IE Dublin 7

Dr. J. MORRIS
UK Brigend Wales

Dr. J.E. MILLAN
ES Cadiz

Dr. L. TOME
PT Coimbra

Dr. M. KLOPPENBURG
NL Drachten

Dr. M. SALVAGNINI
IT Sandrigo

Dr. M. SARTORI
IT Novara

Dr. M. SERRA
ES Valencia

Dr. P. ALMASIO
IT Palermo

Dr. P. HENRIQUES
PT Viseu

Dr. P. LEDERER
DE Forchheim

Dr. R. COZZOLONGO
IT Bari

Dr. R. SAINZ
ES Zaragoza

Dr. R.M. dos SANTOS
PT Combria

Dr. S. DAWIDS
DK Copenhagen

Dr. S. MATERN
DE Aachen

Dr. T. O'GORMAN
IE Galway

Dr. U. TAGE-JENSEN
DK Aalborg

Prof. EFSTRATOPOULOS
GR Athens

Prof. A. GAUTHIER
FR Marseille

Prof. C. MERKEL
IT Padova

Prof. C. TIRIBELLI
IT Trieste

Prof. C.GIPS
NL Groningen

Prof. D. TSANTOULAS
GR Athens

Prof. D. TSIFTSIS
GR Herakleion Crete

Prof. G. BUDILLON
IT Napoli

Prof. G. MAGGI
IT Erba

Prof. G. MOLINO
IT Torino

Prof. J. RODRIGO
ES Valencia

Prof. J.H.F. WILSON
NL Rotterdam

Prof. K. KEHAGIOGLOU
GR Athens

Prof. N. McINTYRE
UK Hampstead

Prof. Ph.JANNE
BE Brussels

Prof. P. AVAGNINA
IT Orbassano

Prof. R. CARRATU
IT Naples

Prof. V. CUERVAS-MONS
ES Madrid

ULTRASONIC SCANNER: QUANTITATIVE DYNAMIC IMAGING

Key words
Echography, tomography, ultrasounds, quantitative imaging.

Brief description
This action aims to establish the feasability of a dynamic control of organs on the basis of a multi-parametric cartography (impedance, attenuation, velocity) evolving With time and adapted to tissue characterization. The real-time high definition image offered to the practitioner, can be frozen as required, enabling the reading of acoustic, spatial and kinematic characteristics.

The mode of investigation envisaged consists of measuring transmitted and reflected ultrasonic waves, the doppler information of which is used for the reconstruction of a tomographic (or simply echographic) image. The quantitative measurements delivered are necessary for an efficient prevention evaluation.

The major innovations aimed for during the next two years are:
- Control of activation to improve the measurement of information (high quality imaging)
- Resolution of the diffraction inverse problem in a multi-parametric tomographic frame - quantitative data estimation, physical modelisation and parameter synthesis, (e.g. density).
- Tridimensional visualisation by stereoscopic representation, imaging of superimposed parameters.

The social benefits expected from such a coherent system of diagnosis are cost reduction and quality improvement of the systematic screening of pathologies (cardiology, cancerology). Ultrasound imaging system development should give Europe a relative autonomy in this growing market.

Thus the scope of the information delivered, the small amount of space required (portable apparatus) and the relatively low cost of the system appear as true medical, practical and economic prescriptions.

Project leader:
Dr. S. MENSAH
Digilog Scientific Department
B.P. 16000
FR 13791 Aix-en-Provence Cedex 3
Phone: +33 42 39 93 19
Fax: +33 42 24 38 06
Contract number: CT931292

Participants:
Isabelle MAGNIN
Laboratoire Traitement du
Signal et Ultrasons, URA 1216
Avenue Albert Einstein
FR 69621 Villeurbanne Cedex

S.J. SAROUFAKIS
Institut of Informatique & Telecommunications
NRCPS Demokritos
P.O. Box 60228
GR 153 10 Paraskevi/Attiki

Prof. Uwe FAUST
Institut für Biomedizinische Technik
Seidenstrasse 36
DE 70174

DEVELOPMENT OF VIDEOREFRACTION TECHNIQUES FOR PAEDIATRIC VISION SCREENING

Key words
Videorefraction, vision, screening, paediatric, refractive errors.

Brief description
The project will combine expertise from four European centres on videorefractive instrumentation, used for measuring the refractive state of the eyes in children who are too young to communicate verbally with examiner. These methods are rapid, non-invasive, and require no restraint or contact with the patient. They are of particular value in large-scale screening programmes for detecting visual problems in young children.

The goal is to develop a new instrument which will be the first effective autorefractor for infants and pre-school children.

The instrument will:

a use up-to-date digital technology to create a compact and portable device;

b incorporate automatic image analysis to compute quantitative refractive error from the optical distribution of light returning from the eyes, without the need for interaction with the operator;

c allow direct and natural interaction between the operator and an infant patient;

d optimise the user interface for effective and trouble-free use by clinical personnel;

e Provide hard copy of the images, for inclusion in medical records.

The project will exploit experience with current instruments to select and combine the optimal features of different designs and to add a number of novel but essential design features. It will use optical computations and empirical data to determine the light distributions from different source/lens configurations to provide the basis for designing sensitive and robust algorithms for image analysis. It will attempt to minimize instrument costs, to encourage wide usage and distribution within and outside the EC.

Designs will be evaluated in laboratory testing, with adults and children with known refractive errors, and in field trials in infant refractive screening programmes at a number of European centres in conjunction with a Concerted Action on infant vision screening (co-ordinator Dr J Atkinson).

Successful development of such an instrument would be expected to have a great impact on the cost-effectiveness of paediatric vision screening and assessment.

Project leader:
Dr. J. WATTAM-BELL
Visual Development Unit,
Department of Psychology,
University College London
Gower Street
UK London WC1E 6BT
Phone: +44 71 387 7050 Ext. 5358
Fax: +44 71 436 4276
Contract number: CT931409

Participants:

Dr. B. RASSOW
Univ of Hamburg,
Medical Optics Laboratory,
Unversity Eye Clinic
Martinistrasse 52
DE 2000 Hamburg 20
Phone: +49 40 4717 2313
Fax: +49 40 4717 4906

Dr. Frank SCHAEFFEL
Univ of Tübingen,
Experimental Opthalmology,
Univ Eye Hospital
Rontgenweg 11
DE 72076 Tübingen
Phone: +49 7071 295926
Fax: +49 7071 295038

Dr. Mario ANGI
Università di Padova,
Clinica Oculistica, Servizio di
Oftalmologia Preventiva
Via Giustiniani
IT 35121 Padova
Phone: +39 49 875 2350
Fax: +39 49 875 2384

Ing. Aldo COCCHIGLIA
FORTUNE OPTICAL srl
Via Giorgione 50
IT 35020 Albignasego (Padova)
Phone: +39 49 880 3696
Fax: +39 49 880 4933

COORDINATION AND DEVELOPMENT OF HEALTH CARE TECHNOLOGY ASSESSMENT IN EUROPE (EUR-ASSESS)

Key words
Health care technology assessment, effectiveness, costeffectiveness of health care, standards.

Brief description
The proposal has the basic aim of stimulating and coordinating developments in the field of health care technology assessment (HCTA) in Europe. Beginning in the mid-1980s, European countries have begun to develop national and regional bodies to carry out health care technology assessment as a way of improving the effectiveness and costeffectiveness of health care. Thus far, there has been little coordination of these national efforts.

The project will organize sub-groups around topics important for every agency involved in such work: priority-setting, methods of assessment, and dissemination and evaluation of impact. In addition, the subject of relations between payment decisions and technology assessment will be investigated.

The goal in these sub-projects is to improve and harmonize methods between different agencies so that information may be more useful and can be shared between agencies more effectively.

There will also be one international study organized concerning the effectiveness and appropriate use of radiotherapy in cancer in selected countries. This study will use standards of appropriate use being developed by the Swedish Council on Technology Assessment in Health Care (SBU). A successful European effort in health care technology assessment will help assure improving the health of European populations and contributing to a stable climate for industrial innovation.

Project leader:
Professor David BANTA
Centre for Medical Technology,
Netherlands Organization for Applied Scientific Research
P.O. Box 430
NL 2300 AK Leiden
Phone: +31 71 181483
Fax: +31 71 181901
Contract number: CT941250

Participants:
Dr. A. GRANADOS
Dep. de Sanitat i Seg.Soc.
Traverssera de les Corts 131-159
ES 08028 Barcelona
Phone: +34 3 3391111
Fax: +34 3 4111114

Dr. E. BORST-EILERS
Health Coucil
P.O. Box 90517
NL 2509 LM The Hague
Phone: +31 70 3441800
Fax: +31 70 3837109

Dr. L. LIAROPOULOS
Inst. for Health Systems Management (IMOSY)
9D Pirou Stret
GR 1527 Athens
Phone: +30 1 7795225
Fax: +30 1 7795225

Dr. P. LAZARO
Sanitaria Ministerio de Sanidad y Consumo
Antonio Grilop 10
ES 28015 Madrid
Phone: +34 1 5421800
Fax: +34 1 5413280

Dr. S. van der KOOIJ
Ziekenfondsraad
P.O. Box 396
NL 1180 BD Amstelveen
Phone: +31 20 5478911
Fax: +31 20 6473494

Dr. T. SHELDON
Centre for Health Economics, Univ of York
UK York YO1 5DD
Phone: +44 904 433718
Fax: +44 904 433644

Dr. P.B. ANDREASEN
Danish Medical Research Council, Dept. of
Clinical Medicine, Gentofte Hospital
Niels Andersensvej 65
DK 2900 Hellerup
Phone: +45 31 651200
Fax: +45 31 681698

Mr T. JORGENSEN
Danish Hospital Inst.
Landemaerket 10
DK 1119 Copenhagen K
Phone: +45 33 115777
Fax: +45 33 931019

Prof. Dr. F. BESKE
Inst. for Health Systems Research, WHO Collaborating Centre for Public Health Research
Weimarer Strasse 8
DE 2300 Kiel-Wik
Phone: +49 431 389520
Fax: +49 431 389555

Prof. E. JONSSON & Prof. L. WERKO
Swedish Council for Health Care Technology
Assessment (SBU), The Karolinska Inst.,
Dept. of Medicine
P.O. Box 16158
SE 10324 Stockholm
Phone: +46 8 6111913
Fax: +46 8 6117973

Prof. M. PECKMAN & Dr. C HENSHALL
Research and Development Dept. of Health
Richmond House,
79 Whitehall
UK London SW1 2NS
Phone: +44 71 210 5556
Fax: +44 71 210 5868

Prof. S. GARATTINI & Dr. A. LIBERATI
Istituto M. Negri
Via Eritrea 62
IT 20157 Milan
Phone: +39 2 29014 540
Fax: +39 2 33200 231

Prof. Y. MATILLON
Agence Nationale pour le Developpement
de l'Evaluatio Medicale (ANDEM)
5 bis, rue Perignon
FR 75015 Paris
Phone: +33 1 4438 5000
Fax: +33 1 4734 9146

ENHANCEMENT OF BIOMEDICAL TECHNOLOGY USAGE IN THE DIAGNOSIS OF ACUTE ABDOMINAL PAIN

Key words
Acute abdominal pain, diagnostic biomedical technology.

Brief description
1 Each year between two and three million people in the EC attend hospital with acute abdominal pain. Minimum estimates place a value of over 1.5 billion ECU's per annum on the cost of treating such patients. Around 10% of this is spent on diagnostic biomedical technology.
2 Previous detailed studies have shown that such technology is potentially highly effective - adding approximately 15% to initial unaided diagnostic accuracy. However, there is wide variation in usage of biomedical technology (particularly as regards newer imaging technology). As a result, technology is failing to achieve its full potential.
3 The present project aims to assist existing technology to achieve its full potential, by collecting (from across EC countries) information concerning the use and value of biomedical technology in diagnosing acute abdominal pain patients - information so comprehensive, so authoritative, and so meticulously collected that it will allow authoritative guidance to be given on objective evidence to young inexperienced clinicians throughout the Community.
4 The project will therefore collect and analyse a database of clinical information concerning not less than 10,000 patients representative of EC practise. The project will (i) document existing practise in varying institutions and countries, (ii) evaluate the intrinsic value and added diagnostic benefit of each form of technology, (iii) develop guidelines, circulate these, and (iv) analyse feedback to produce a final report.
5 The proposed study network involves many of the most relevant experienced scientific workers and clinicians throughout the Community. The study will employ proved methodology, and a wide network of contacts involving national and European Societies for dissemination of results.
6 Successful prosecution of this work will result in enhanced value of the biomedical technology used, a better service for (potentially) 2.3 million ECU's.

Project leader:
Prof. F. T. DE DOMBAL
University of Leeds,
Clinical Information Science Unit
22 Hyde Terrace
UK Leeds L3 9LN
Phone: +44 532 334 961
Fax: +44 532 429 078
Contract number: CT941597

Participants:
Dr. J. IKONEN (FI)

Dr. B. BJERREGAARD (DK)

Dr. B. SCOLLA &
Dr. C. CAMMA &
Dr. P. PARISI (IT)

C. IONESCU-TRIGOVISTE (RO)

Dr. C. VICOL (RO)

Dr. D. ANTONELLIS (IT)

Dr. D. PRUNA (RO)

Dr. E. OSCH (LU)

Dr. E. STANCIU (RO)

Dr. E. STICKLEY (UK)

Dr. F. IORDACHE &
Dr. V. NITESCU (RO)

Dr. F. TURCU (RO)

Dr. F. TINE' (IT)

Dr. G. DUNCAN (UK)

Dr. G. FENYO (SE)

Dr. G. MALIZIA (IT)

Dr. H. KLOTTER &
Dr. A. ZIELKE (DE)

Dr. H. de BAERE (BE)

Dr. I. ASCHIE (RO)

Dr. J. HENRIQUES (PT)

Dr. J. HOFFMAN (DK)

Dr. J. PETIT (NL)

Dr. K. ROWSELL (UK)

Dr. K. SIMPKINS (UK)

Dr. M. ESKELINEN (FI)

Dr. M. IMHOF (DE)

Dr. M. JORGENSEN (DK)

Dr. M. SAVU (RO)

Dr. O. HOSTMALINGEN (NO)

Dr. P. van ELK (NL)

Dr. R. DOWIE (UK)

Dr. R. PISA (IT)

Dr. S. BARNES (UK)

Dr. S. GAVRILESCU (RO)

Dr. M. GEORGESCU (RO)

Dr. V. ULMEANU &
Dr. I. ORSANU (RO)

Dr. V. SALVADORI &
Dr. P. GIGANTE &
Dr. D. ISCARO (IT)

Dr. W. SWOBODNIK (DE)

Dr. W. ZMYSLOWSKI &
Dr. A. JOZWIK (PL)

Dr. A. BUCCALLATO (IT)

Dr. A. FINGERHUT (FR)

Dr. E. PEPE &
Dr. G. ROSONE (IT)

Dr. H. SITTER (DE)

Dr. L. GRANDE (ES)

Dr. V. DALLOS (UK)

Mr A.D. JOHNSON (UK)

Mrs. S.E. CLAMP (UK)

Mr. A.A. GUNN (UK)

Mr. I.J.W. WALLACE (UK)

Mr. L.R. JENKINSON (UK)

Mr. N. ZOLTIE (UK)

Mr. W.A.F. McADAM (UK)

Prof. C. OHMANNN (DE)

Prof. C. PERA & Dr. J.C.
GARCIA-VALDECASAS (ES)

Prof. E. CASTANAS (GR)

Prof. E. ERKOCAK (TR)

Prof. E. NEUGEBAUER &
Dr. R. LEFERING (DE)

Prof. F. LARGIADER (CH)

Prof. G. FEIFEL (DE)

Prof. H. BLUM &
Prof. W. VETTER (CH)

Prof. H. TROIDL (DE)

Prof. H. WULFF (DK)

Prof. I.A.D. BOUCHIER (UK)

Prof. L. CAPURSO & Dr. M.
KOCH & Dr. G. BAZURO &
Dr. C.PAPI (IT)

Prof. M. CLASSEN (DE)

Prof. M. ROTHMUND (DE)

Prof. N. GOURTSOYIANNIS
(GR)

Prof. O. WINDING (DK)

Prof. S. LAVELLE (IE)

Prof. VONDERSCHMITT (CH)

Prof. W. FUCHS (CH)

Prof. W.U. WAYAND (AT)

Prof. Y. FLAMANT &
Prof. J.M. HAY (FR)

ENHANCEMENT OF EEG-BASED DIAGNOSIS OF NEUROLOGICAL AND PSYCHIATRIC DISORDERS BY ARTIFICIAL NEURAL NETWORKS

Key words
EEG, neurological and psychiatric disorders, artificial neural networks, diagnosis, neurological and psychiatric diseases or disorders, schizophrenia.

Brief description
The objective of this project is to enhance the diagnosis of neurological and psychiatric diseases or disorders based on EEG, by further developing the method of artificial neural networks for automatic classification and interpretation of the EEG data. Artificial neural networks have proven many times to be a suitable method for processing complex non-linear and possibly noisy data.

In first prototypes - many of them developed by the partners in this project - they have also shown their potential in classifying and mapping spatiotemporal or stationary EEG input. This project aims at Concerting European efforts to develop the method based on these prototypes, into practically useful tools for daily clinical routine.

Research on artificial neural networks and their application to EEG data will be carried out by all the partners in close cooperation with clinics, hospitals or clinical university departments. The main expertise of the consortium is three-fold.

One group consists of computer scientists with a strong background on neural networks who will do most of the necessary research and development on, and implementation of different neural network systems.

The second group are engineers with a large background in preprocessing the raw EEG data and in signal processing in general.

The third group are clinical partners with the necessary medical expertise providing the main applications.

The project is expected to fulfil the objectives of the Biomed 1 program in two ways: First, the results will be advanced devices for diagnosis, in this case for neurological and psychiatric disorders but with some potential to be expandable to other domains as well. Since better diagnosis often means earlier treatment, the project can contribute to public health in europe.

Secondly, the research to be conducted promises to also advance the knowledge about neurological and psychiatric diseases, for instance through providing novel ways of classification of types into sub-types in schizophrenia.

Project leader:
Dr. Georg DORFFNER
Austrian Research Institute
for Artificial Intelligence
Schottengasse 3
AT 1010 Vienna
Phone: +43 15 35 32 81
Fax: +43 15 32 06 52
Contract number: CT941129

Participants:

Dr. K. THAU
Universitätsklinik für Psychiatrie,
Elektrophysiologisches Labor
Währinger Gürtel 18-20
AT 1090 Wien
Phone: +43 1 40 400 35 84
Fax: +43 1 40 400 36 05

Dr. H. WERNER
FGNN, Universität Gesamthochschule Kassel
Heinrich-Plett-Strasse 40
DE 3500 Kassel
Phone: +49 561 804 4618
Fax: +49 561 804 4244

M.S. PEKKA ELO
Tampere Univ of Technology,
Institut of Electronics
Korkeakoulunkato 1, P.O. Box 692
FI 33101 Tampere
Phone: +358 31 316 2064
Fax: +358 31 316 2620

Prof. B. GALLHOFER
Independent Clinical Psychopathology Unit,
Dept. of Psychiatry Justus-Liebig-Univ,
School of Medicine
AM Steg 24
DE 6300 Giessen
Phone: +49 641 70 23 829
Fax: +49 641 70 23 858

Prof. G. PFURTSCHELLER
Medizinische Informatik und Neuroinformatik
(LBMI)
Brockmanngasse 41
AT 8010 Graz
Phone: +43 316 821 694
Fax: +43 316 81 29 64

Prof. H. WITTE
IMSID, Medical Faculty of the
Friedrich Schiller Univ of Jena
Jahnstrasse 3
DE 6900 Jena
Phone: +49 36 41 822 31 33
Fax: +49 36 41 254 47

Prof. P. RAPPELSBERGER
Inst. of Neurophysiology
Waehringerstrasse 17
AT 1090 Wien
Phone: +43 14 04 80 622
Fax: +43 14 02 85 25

NON-INVASIVE METHODS FOR ASSESSING CARDIOVASCULAR HYDRODYNAMICS (INVADYN)

Key words
Non-invasive methods, cardiovascular hydrodynamics, hemodynamic evaluation, medical imaging, cardiovascular diseases, diagnostics, cardiovascular hemodynamic assessment.

Brief description
Assessing the cardiac function and vascular status, in terms of hemodynamic evaluation and medical imaging, is a multidiciplinary scientific area.

Its importance is underscored by the very high incidence of cardiovascular diseases in the European countries. Consequently diagnostics and treatment of patients suffering from these diseases has a major social and economical impact on all industrialized countries.

In order to optimize the reliability and efficiency of various methods for cardiovascular hemodynamic assessment it is essential to evaluate the methods used scientifically and clinically today. It is also of paramount importance to evaluate sensitive, reliable and practically obtainable hemodynamic parameters in order to exchange clinical and biomedical knowledge across the borders. This proposal also gives an input to a European standardization on recommended measures for experimental and clinical hemodynamic evaluation. This will provide an improved diagnostic basis for optimal medical or surgical treatment of patients.

Project leader:
Dr. J. Michael HASENKAM
Dept. of Cardio-Thoracic Surgery,
Skejby Sygehus
Brendstrupgaards vej
DK 8200 Aarhus
Phone: +45 86 78 45 11
Fax: +45 86 78 32 34
Contract number: CT941761

Participants:
Prof. Per ASK
Dept. of Biomedical
Engineering, Linköping Univ
SE 581 85 Linköping

Dr. F. FLASCHKAMPF
II Medical Clinic,
RWTH Aachen
DE Aachen

Dr. F. PINTO
Univ Hospital of Santa
Maria, Clinico Médica-Piso
Av Prof. Egas Moinz
PT 1699 Lisabona Codex

Dr. F. RECUSANI
IRCCS Policlinoco San
Matteo, Div.e di Cardiologia
Piazzale Golgi 2
IT 27100 Pravia

Dr. H. BAUMGARTNER
2nd Dept. of Internal Medi-
cine/Cardiology Krankenhaus
der Barmherzigen Schwestern
Seilerstätte 4
AT 4020 Linz

Dr. J. HARTIALA
Dept. of Clinical Physiology
Kiinamyllumkato 4-8 (TYKS)
FI 20520 Turku

Prof. B. ANGELSEN
Dept. of Biomedical Engin-
eering, Univ of Trondheim
NO 7006 Trondheim

HARMONIZATION OF THE IN VITRO ASSESSMENT OF THE BIOLOGICAL BEHAVIOUR OF METALLIC BIOMATERIALS

Key words
In vitro corrosion, biocompatibility, metallic biomaterials, dental alloys, corrosion tests, biological tests of biomaterials.

Brief description
The principal points of the present research project are the harmonization of methodology of existing *in vitro* corrosion and biocompatibility tests and the assessment of corrosion resistance of metallic biomaterials (in particular dental alloys) in the biological environment.

The main point is the combination of conventional electrochemical corrosion tests and current biological tests of biomaterials.

The first part of the CA concerns the selection and determination of reference materials and of the experimental conditions.

The principal corrosion tests considered are impedance spectroscopy, anodic polarization, crevice corrosion, and other electrochemical corrosion tests such as open circuit, galvanic and pitting.

After evaluation in inorganic media, the selected and improved methods will be applied to corrosion tests in the biological environment in a specific bioreactor.

These tests will be performed in the presence of relevant bacterial strains for human pathology in monocultures and mixed populations.

As to mammalian cell types, the program has foreseen relevant immune cells (lymphocytes and monocytes) in suspension cultures. Target cells in monolayer cell cultures, such as gingival epithelial cells, osteoblasts, osteoclasts, etc. will finally be aplied.

The biological test methods must be relevant and lead to quantitative assessments of cell viability and cell differentiation, of inflammatory and cytotoxic effects.

The last part in the elaboration of a proposal for a harmonized test-concept including (i) the evaluation of tests and methods with respect to their clinical relevance and to their significance for the biocompatibility of metallic biomaterials, (ii) the establishment of a methodological test spectrum for a classification of metallic biomaterials with respect to corrosion resistance in the biological environment, and (iii) the evaluation of the possibility to generalize the use of the biological test methods to other non-metallic biomaterials.

In European Countries exist a general trend for the reduction of costs in public health-care service and subsequently for the use, whenever possible, of alternatives involving lower costs, as long as no risks arise to the patients.

It is therefore very important to evaluate this risk, and above all, to combine test methods associating two aspects traditionally seen apart and which may have synergistic effects when biomaterials are placed in the human organism.

With this in mind, the present program has also foreseen to adapt a bioreactor for standardized corrosion tests in biological environments.

Project leader:
Dr. H. HILDEBRAND
Groupe de Recherches sur les Biomatériaux
Place de Verdun 1
FR 59045 Lille Cédex
Phone: +33 20 626964
Fax: +33 20 883664
Contract number: CT941539

Participants:
Dr. Ing K. LIEFEITH
I.B.A.
Rosenhof
DE 37308 Heiligenstadt
Phone: +49 3606 671170
Fax: +49 3606 671200

Prof. dr E. LENZ
Poliklinik für Stomatologie
Nordhäuser Strass 74
DE 99089 Erfurt
Phone: +49 361 792033
Fax: +49 361 792033

Prof. dr. J. BREME
Werkstoffwissenschaften
Gebäude 22
DE 66041 Saarbrücken
Phone: +49 681 3022908
Fax: +49 681 3024385

Prof. dr. J. HELSEN
Dept. M.T.M., Kath. Universiteit Leuven
De Croylaan 2
BE 3001 Leuven
Phone: +32 16220931 ext. 1263
Fax: +32 16207995

Prof. dr J. WIRZ
Zahnärzliches Institut, Abteilung
Zahnärtzliche Technologie
Petersplatz 14
CH 4051 Basel
Phone: +41 612618040
Fax: +41 612619713

QUANTITATIVE METHODS AND TEXTURE ANALYSIS IN MAGNETIC RESONANCE IMAGING (MRI) - TISSUE CHARACTERISATION THROUGH MORPHOLOGICAL, STRUCTURAL AND FUNCTIONAL MEASUREMENT

Key words
Magnetisation transfer, magnetic resonance imaging, texture analysis, tissue structure, relaxation times, diffusion imaging.

Brief description
The project is designed to progress the quantitative application of magnetic resonance imaging (MRI) as a clinical diagnostic tool by means of a concerted European research and testing programme. This will maximise the value of this expensive technology and help to spread expertise from specialist centres throughout the community. The impact on the overall diagnostic power of the method in brain diseases is expected to be very significant.

Three areas of collaborative investigation are planned - texture analysis of the MRI image data to extract the maximum information on tissue structure and characteristics measurement of the relaxation times Tl and T2 in as accurate and reproducible a manner as possible and study of the possibility of diffusion imaging (which may allow tissue blood perfusion and microcirculation to be investigated.) Much of this work progresses naturally from the MRI part of a previous Concerted Action COMAC-BME II.2.3. *Tissue Characterization by MRS and MRI* and largely involves the same research teams whose successful collaboration was a key feature of this programme.

The project will progress by means of plenary meetings, topical workshops, exchange fellowships and central software development and data collection.

The term is three years and, at present 12 groups of researchers form the basic core of the programme but it is expected that invited corresponding experts will augment the research base. Industrial collaboration will be encouraged.

Project leader:
Dr. R.A. LERSKI
Medical Physics Dept.,
Ninewells Hospital and Medical School
UK Dundee DD1 9SY
Phone: +44 382 632700
Fax: +44 382 632970
Contract number: CT941274

Participants:
Ass. Prof. Dr. E. MOSER
Arbeitsgruppe NMR,
Inst. of Medical Physics Univ of Vienna
Waringerstrasse 13
AT 1090 Vienna
Phone: +43 222 40480379
Fax: +43 1 4024030

Dr. A. BRUNO
Laboratoire Traitement du Signal et de l'Image
Université de Rennes 1
Campus de Beaulieu
FR 35042 Rennes Cedex
Phone: +33 99 286220
Fax: +33 99 286917

Dr. A. RYS
Center for Medical Technology,
School of Public Health Univ of Cracow
ul. Grzegorzecka 20
PL 31531 Cracow
Phone: +48 12 188857
Fax: +48 12 12217447

Dr. K. STRAUGHAN
Dept. of Electric Engineering,
Imperial College
Exhibition Road
UK London SW7 2BT
Phone: +44 71 225 8528
Fax: +44 71 225 1099

Dr. L. MASCARO
Servizio di Fisica Sanitaria,
Spedali Civili di Brescia
IT 25100 Brescia
Phone: +39 30 3995284
Fax: +39 30 3995927

Dr. L. SCHAD
German Cancer Research Centre
Institut of Nuclear Medicine
Im Neuenheimer Feld 280
DE 6900 Heidelberg
Phone: +49 6221 422569
Fax: +49 6221 411307

Dr. P. RING
MR Afdeling-Afsnit,
Hvidovre Hospital
Kettgard Alle 30
DK 2650 Copenhagen
Phone: +45 36 32 2884
Fax: +45 31 47 0302

Dr. L. GULACSI
Hungarian Inst. for Quality of Health Care,
Coordinating Officefor Health Technology
Assessment
Bem ter 8
HU 4026 Debrecen
Phone: +36 52 323264

Dr. R. CHRZANOWSKI
Swiss Public Health Institute, ISH
rue Bugnon 21 A
CH 1005 Lausanne
Phone: +41 21 3132424
Fax: +41 21 3132423

Prof. A. SPISNI
Istituto di Chimica Biologica,
niversita di Parma Ospedale Maggiore
Viale Gramsi 14
IT 43100 Parma
Phone: +39 521 290360
Fax: +39 521 988952

Prof. Dr. P.A. RINCK
MR Center
NO 7006 Trondheim
Phone: +47 73 99 7681
Fax: +47 73 94 2133

Prof. D. ENACHESCU
Director National Inst. for Health
Services and Management
Str. Dr. Leonte nr. 1-3
RO 76256 Bucaresti

Prof. I. ISHERWOOD
Univ of Manchester, Dept. of Dianostic
Radiology, Stopford Building
Oxford Road
UK Manchester M13 9PT
Phone: +44 61 275 5114
Fax: +44 61 275 5594

Prof. J. CHAMBRON
Institut de Physique Biologique
4 rue Kirshleger
FR 67085 Strasbourg Cedex
Phone: +33 88361144
Fax: +33 88371497

Prof. R. LUYPAERT
MR Centre, Academie Hospital
Vrije Universiteit Brussel
Laarbeeklaan 101
BE 1090 Brussels
Phone: +32 2 4775295
Fax: +32 2 4775800

Prof. R.N. MULLER
Dept. of Organic Chemistry NMR
Faculté de Medecine
Université de Mons
BE 7000 Mons
Phone: +32 65 373520
Fax: +32 65 373520

A NOVEL ULTRA-SENSITIVE BIOASSAY TECHNIQUE BASED ON SCANNING PROBE TECHNOLOGIES

Key words
Immunoassays, microscopic immunoassay, scanned probe technologies, antibody, antigen binding, immunosensors.

Brief description
The main aim of this proposal is to assess the practical feasibility of new method of measurement which has the potential to lead to novel instrumentation of benefit within the field of immunoassays and related applications. Presently used immunoassays have sensitivities in the nanomole per litre to picomole per litre range and involve several procedural steps. The proposed scanned force microscopic immunoassay (SFMIA) system uses scanned probe technologies to detect antibody/antigen binding by physical imaging of the binding event.

In its simplest form this novel approach is likely to deliver sensitivities comparable to existing immunoassay methodologies but with less procedural steps, thereby leading to significant economies in assay time and materials consumption. Furthermore, parallel imaging SFMIA instruments based on emerging technologies are likely to lead to significant improvements in sensitivity into the femtomole per litre to attomole per litre sensitivity range. SFMIA is suitable for the development of on-line and in-situ immunosensors for clinical and industrial use.

When compared to established and emerging techniques, SFMIA has three main advantages:
1. SFMIA directly images the capture event and therefore does not require the antibody (or antigen) to be labelled;
2. SFMIA's theoretical sensitivity is higher as, in principle, one single antibody/antigen capture event can be detected;
3. SFMIA instruments are self-validating.

Project leader:
Dr. L. McDONNELL
Dept. of Applied Physics,
Cork Regional Technical College
IE Cork 30
Phone: +353 21 54 52 22
Fax: +353 21 54 53 43
Contract number: CT941745

Participants:
Dr. L. HELLEMANS
Dept. of Chemistry, Katholieke Universiteit Leuven
Celestijnenlaan 200 D
BE 3001 Heverlee
Phone: +32 16 201015
Fax: +32 26 201368

Dr. A. THERETZ
UM103, Biomerieux Ecole
Normale Superieure de Lyon
Allee d'Italie 46
FR 69364 Lyon Cedex 07
Phone: +33 72 72 83 63
Fax: +33 72 72 85 33

Dr. F. GRUNDFELD
NIMA Technology Ltd.
The Science Park
UK Coventry CV4 7EZ
Phone: +44 203 419457
Fax: +44 203 692511

Dr. O. WOLTER
Dr. Olaf Wolter GmbH,
IMO Building
Im Amtmann 6
DE 6330 Wetzlar-Blankenfeld
Phone: +49 6441 77155
Fax: +49 6441 77181

EUROPEAN TASK FORCE ON IMPLANTABLE DEVICES FOR INSULIN DELIVERY

Key words
Diabetes, clinical trial, intraperitoneal insulin treatment, implantable pump, subcutaneous, insulin treatment.

Brief description
This project is designed to create a European network for planning and implementing a clinical trial on the efficacy of intraperitoneal insulin treatment in reducing incidence of severe hypoglycaemias in type 1 diabetic patients.

The project will be extended over a three year period.

The first part comprises the creation of the European network, with arrangement of local pre-existing resources and establishment and implementation of a project management system.

The second part of the project comprises the organization of the clinical protocol with detailed attention to the standardization of procedures and definition of quality indicators. The implementation of the clinical protocol will include recruitment of patients, treatment with intraperitoneal insulin using an implantable pump or with subcutaneous intensive insulin treatment, and a two-year patient follow-up with monthly visit to the centres.

Project leader:
Professor Dr. Piero MICOSSI
Dept. of Medicine and
Dept. of Epidemiology and Statistics,
C/O Hospital San Raffaele
Via Olgettina 60
IT 20132 Milano
Phone: +39 226432759
Fax: +39 226434704
Contract number: CT941689

Participants:
Dr. E. BALLEGOOIE
Dept. of Internal Medicine,
Ziekenhuis De Weezenlanden
Groot Weezenland 20
NL 8011 JW Zwolle
Phone: +31 38 299911
Fax: +31 38 299125

Dr. J.L. SELAM
Hotel Dieu, dept. of Diabetology
1 Place du Paris Notre Dame
FR 75181 Paris cedex 04
Phone: +33 1 42348376
Fax: +33 1 43541564

Dr. N. JEANDIDIER
Pavillon Leriche,
Hospitaux Universitaires
FR 67091 Strasbourg
Phone: +33 88 161149
Fax: +33 88 161262

Prof. K.D. HEPP
Diabetes Center,
Hospital Bogenhousen
Englschalkinger Strass 77
DE W8000 München
Phone: +49 89 92702111
Fax: +49 89 92702116

NON-INVASIVE EVALUATION OF THE MYOCARDIUM (NEMY)

Key words
Myocardium, non-invasive examination of the heart, cardiac electrical sources, non-invasive examination, electromagnetic sensing, electrocardiographic techniques.

Brief description
The overall objective of the NEMY proposal is to improve the diagnostic information content of electromagnetic data by developing standardized systems for non-invasive examination of the heart. This proposal promotes harmonization of techniques and measurement systems, leading to the definition of European standards for the accurate recovery and visualization of cardiac electrical sources from remote (i.e. body surface) measurements. The NEMY Concerted Action brings together leading European experts in this field to reach this objective.

The project features a supervisory workpackage called Harmonization and Evaluation during which all partners combine to collaborate and define standards for collection and interchange of information. Subsequent modelling and clinical measurement workpackages are closely coordinated by the Technical Coordinator of the Project to ensure a consistent approach to evaluation of the results.

The method used for non-invasive examination is to compute the myocardial potential distribution from body surface measurements using thoracic models derived from a library of actual MRI scans. Expertise in 'forward modelling' is well established and the consortium includes the world's leading experts in the effort to develop and refine the 'inverse solution' which is the objective of this project.

By the conclusion of the project, coherent trans-European methodology will have been developed whereby the condition of the myocardium can be derived and visualized from non-invasive measurements and the diagnostic efficiency of this methodology assessed in those classes of cardiac disease where electromagnetic sensing can be expected to enhance the performance of existing electrocardiographic techniques.

Project leader:
Professor D.M. MONRO
University of Bath,
School of Electrical
Engineering
Claverton Down
UK Bath BA2 7AY
Phone: +44 225 826833
Fax: +44 225 826073
Contract number: CT941025

Participants:
Dr. F. KORNREICH
Vrije Universiteit Brussel
(VUB), Unit for Cardio-
vascular Research and
Engineering
BE 1090 Brussels
Phone: +32 2 5554050
Fax: +32 2 5554049

Dr. R. EASTON-ORR
Beaufort European Ltd (BEL)
12 Gloxinia Walk
UK Hampton, Middlesex
Phone: +44 81 783 1218
Fax: +44 81 783 1218

Prof. A. van OOSTEROM
Katholieke Universiteit van
Nijmegen (NIM), Laboratory
of Medical Physics
NL 6525 EZ Nijmegen
Phone: +31 80 614248
Fax: +31 80 541435

Dr. S.W. EDWARDS
Univ of Bath, School of Elec-
tronic Electrical Engineering
UK Bath BA2 7AY
Phone: +44 225 826833
Fax: +44 225 826073

Prof. E. MUSSO &
E. MACCHI
Universita Degli Studi di
Parma (PAR), Dept. di Bio-
logia e Fisiologia Generali
IT 43100 Parma
Phone: +39 521 905624
Fax: +39 521 905673

Prof. J. WILLEMS
UZL, Div. of Medical
Informatics
BE 3000 Leuven
Phone: +32 16 343801
Fax: +32 16 343796

Prof. T. KATILA
HUT, Laboratory of
Biomedical Engineering
FI 02150 Espoo
Phone: +358 0 4513173

DEVELOPMENT AND STANDARDIZATION OF NEW DYNAMIC RADIOTHERAPY TECHNICS 'DYNARAD'

Key words
Dynamic radiotherapy, radiation therapy, radiation surgery, treatment planning procedure, dose distribution, stereotactic radiation surgery.

Brief description
This Concerted Action (CA) concerns dynamic Radiation Therapy and Radiation Surgery, using high energy (MeV) photon beams shaped in transverse cross section and modulated in spatial distributions.

The majority of cancer patients are treated by Radiation Therapy using external photon beams.

The clinical results of the treatment depends on the dose distribution in the patient for small and medium size tumours, which are usually more curable and controlable than large ones, the dose distributions obtained by dynamic technics are usually superior to those obtained by ordinary stationary fields.

Up to now, the application fo dynamic technics (Conformation Radiotherapy) is very limited because of the complicated set ups, the lack of algorithms for computing the dose distribution and the lack of adequate diagnostic knowledge concerning the location size and shape of the tumour and of the vital organs.

This project aims to face and solve these problems for both Radiation Therapy and Radiation Surgery.

European Institutions are involved. Each Institution is particulary interested in and belongs to one or more of the six subject areas of the project. Each of the six groups is coordinated by a topical expert who acts as the Group Magager (GM). The six GMs and the Project Coordinator (PC) constitute the Project Managing Group (PMG).

It is planned to:

a compare the existing diagnostic technics on the basis of their accuracy, simplicity and availability in defining the tumour and the surrounding healthy structure.

b select the most promising diagnostic technics for Radiation Therapy and Radiation Surgery and incorporate them in the treatment planning procedure by developing the necessary software.

c compare the existing technics of dynamic therapy on the basis of their simplicity and effectiveness in controling the dose distribution.

d select the best of these technics for small and medium size tumours.

e simplify, further develop and standardize these dynamic technics and devices for specific kinds of tumours.

f develop the corresponding algorithms and software to compute the dose distribution for the selected as standard technics.

g apply these technics in clinical practice.

A similar procedure will be followed for Stereotactic Radiation Surgery with emphasis in the geometric accuracy for the positioning of the patient and the definition of the narrow photom beam. The products of this (procedure, technics, software and devices) will be made available to all participating Institutions.

The resulting information and data will be offered through scientific publications to all interested.

This way, Radiation Therapy and Surgery by photon beams will offer superior physical results (dose distributions) through simpler and more easily applicable technics in every day practice. This physical and technological advancement will have a corresponding improvement to the clinical results. The social scientific and technological impact for Europe is obvious.

Project leader:
Professor Basil S. PROIMOS
School of Medicine,
Dept. of Medical Physics,
University of Patras
GR 265 00 Patras
Phone: +30 61997620
Fax: +30 61992496
Contract number: CT941783

Participants:
Prof. Dr. R. SPELLER
Univ College Hospital,
UK London WC1E 6 JA
Phone: +44 71 38 09 700
Fax: +44 71 38 09 577

Dr. D. EMRE
Cerrahpasa Tip Fakultesi
Radyasyon Onkolojisi
Anabilim Dali
TR 34 303 Instanbul
Phone: +90 1 58 84 800
Fax: +90 1 58 61 528

Dr. D. LEFKOPOULOS
Hospital Tenon, Dept. de
Radiotherapie
Rue de la Chine 4
FR 75970 Paris Cedex 20
Phone: +33 140 30 7000
Fax: +33 140 30 7933

Dr. E. DEAN
St. Bartholomews Hospital,
Dept. of Medical Physics
UK London EC1A 7BE
Phone: +44 71 601 8376
Fax: +44 71 601 8356

Dr. G. CHIEREGO
U.L.SS.N8. Vicenza
Presidio, Ospedaliero
IT 00158 Roma
Phone: +39 444 993474

Dr. J.C. ROSENWALD
Service de Physique
Medicale, Institut Curie
FR 75231 Paris Cedex 05
Phone: +33 14 4324004

Dr. K. OLSEN
Dept. Medical Physics,
Rigshospitalet
Blegsdamvej 9
DK Copenhagen
Phone: +45 35 453994
Fax: +45 35 453990

Dr. M. BENASSI
CRS, Instituto Regina Elena
Via delle Messi d'Oro 156
IT 00158 Roma
Phone: +39 649 85535
Fax: +39 641 80473

Dr. N. THROUVALAS
Piraeus Anti Cancer Hospital
Radiation Therapy Dept.
GR Piraeus
Phone: +30 1 451 6233

Dr. P. BEY
Dept. Radiotherapy,
Centre Alexis Vautrin
Av. de Bourgogne
FR 54511 Vandoevre-Les
Nancy
Phone: +33 83 598400
Fax: +33 83 446071

Dr. L. PEDRO
Centro de Oncologia de
Coimbra, Radiotherapy Dept.
PT 3003 Coimbra Codex
Phone: +351 3 940 1717

Prof. B. LIND & BRAHME
Karolinska Instituet
P.O. Box 60 211
SE 104 01 Stockholm
Phone: +46 872 94718
Fax: +46 8 34 3 525

PROF. J. DEMOPOULOS &
N. PAPADAKIS
Univ of Patras, Medical
School Radiotherapy Dept.
GR 26110 Patras
Phone: +30 61 999 216
Fax: +30 61 993 987

Prof. Dr. F. NUSSLIN
Radiologische Univ. klinik
Hoppe-Seyler-Str. 3
DE 72076 Tubingen
Phone: +49 70 71 292176
Fax: +49 70 71 295920

Prof. Dr. T. KATILA
Helsinki Univ,
Dept. of Technical Physics
FI Helsinki
Phone: +35 80 451 3172
Fax: +35 80 451 3182

Prof. F. S. DOBLADO
Facultad de Medicina, Dept.
Fisiologia y Biofisica
Avda Sanchez Pizijuan 4
ES 41009 Sevilla
Phone: +34 54 3715 46
Fax: +34 54 9000 67

Prof. J. van DIJK
AMC
Meibergdreef 9
NL 1105 AZ Amsterdam
Phone: +31 20 566 4231
Fax: +31 20 566 4440

Prof. O. DAHL
Haukeland Hospital, Dept. of
Radiation Oncology
NO 5021 Bergen
Phone: +47 059 72010
Fax: +47 059 72046

Prof. R. van LOON
Dept. ELEC, V.U.
Pleinlaan 2
BE 1050 Brussel
Phone: +32 2 6412953
Fax: +32 2 6412850

Prof. SEITZ
Universitätskliniken Strahlen-
therapie und Strahlenbiologie
Alser str. 4
AT 1090 Wien
Phone: +43 14 400 3382
Fax: +43 222 46400

IMPROVING CONTROL OF PATIENT STATUS
IN CRITICAL CARE (IMPROVE)

Key words
Critical care, intensive care, monitoring physiological signals, control of patient status, physiological variables, physiological models, interpretative analysis, multi signal fusion, digital signal processing, monitoring systems, vector median hybrid filtering.

Brief description
The vital functions of the patient can be monitored continuously in critical care i.e. in the Operating Theatre or the Intensive Care Unit (ICU) to avoid complications and to correct them when they appear. During the last decades commercial equipment for monitoring physiological signals, variables and trends have been developed technically enormously. However, monitoring systems only rarely are designed taking patient outcome into consideration being far away from intelligent systems. There are obvious needs and opportunities to improve the control of patient status in critical care. Increasingly complex and demanding operations during anaesthesia or ICU require an even more sophisticated interpretation of physiological variables. The diagnosis of the state of patient must be based on real evaluated I physiological models and knowledge. The provided alarms and diagnosis need to be more reliable and to avoid unnecessary interventions. Using systems able to predict and establish the status of patient properly, the treatment of a patient can be enhanced. Such next generation monitoring systems for cardiovascular and respiratory functions, brain function, blood chemistry, temperature, fluid balance, etc. can be produced utilizing techniques capable of combining algorithmic, interpretative analysis and multi-signal fusion in real-time environments.
The development of Digital Signal Processing (DSP) techniques for detecting significant patterns has been tremendous in the past decade. The DSP-techniques are divided into linear and nonlinear algorithms. Linear DSP-methods have been extensively applied to various areas including critical care. However, the physiological processes that are monitored and treated are not linear requiring exploration of more advanced methods. In many cases outside medicine nonlinear methods have been proven to be superior compared to typically used linear methods (e.g. colour image-, image sequence and audio signal processing). Examples of nonlinear methods are FIR-median hybrid-, polynomical-, statistic-, and morphological filters and neural network techniques.
The current monitoring systems there is also an evident shortage of the use of spatial and temporal interpretation for making higher level diagnosis and providing decision support based on for example models of the functions of the nervous system. Multivariate modelling methods and knowledge based techniques are appropriate tools for analyzing correlations between different physiological variables and the transfer functions between the variables. In this proposed Concerted Action (CA) multivariate autoregressive modelling supported by the use knowledge based tools for the interpretation of results and nonlinear multivariate tools, such as vector median hybrid filtering, will be applied in critical care. These methods may be used in critical care to improve the quality of interpretation of the signals and thus to avoid for example false alarms and even false diagnosis.
The overall goal is to apply novel nonlinear, linear, multivariate and/or knowledge based algorithms to improve the on-line assessment and management of the patient state in ICU and Operating Theatre environments. The operational goal is to enhance the research

efforts of the participating groups in the area of nonlinear and multivariate modelling techniques through concertation of efforts.

The basic objective of the CA is to create a consortium with appropriate clinical and technical experience within critical care, which is capable of harmonized development, application and evaluation of existing and new DSP-methodologies. This includes the definition and collection of a library of well documented patient cases including raw data. The project can be divided into subgoals as follows:

Goal 1:   To increase the knowledge for analyzing real-time physiological signals and improve care in critical environments by organization of workshops, meetings and exchange of persons forI short-term periods.

Goal 2:   To enlarge the methodological knowledge for the development of enhanced monitoring systems for the ICU and Operating Theatre.

Goal 3:   To increase the algorithmical knowledge in the areas of nonlinear and multi-variate techniques.

Project leader:
Prof. Niilo SARANUMMI
Technical Research Centre
of Finland,
Information Technology
P.O. Box 1206
FI 33101 Tampere
Phone: +358 31 316 33 00
Fax: +358 31 317 41 02
Contract number: CT941768

Participants:
Dr. A. KARI
Kuopio University Hospital,
Department of Intensive Care
FI 70210 Kuopio
Phone: +358 71 173 428

Prof. A. ROSENFALCK
Department of Medical
Informatics and Image
Analysis, Aalborg University
DK 9220 Aalborg SO
Phone: +45 98 158 522

Dr. P.J.M. CLUIGMANS
Eindhoven University
of Technology,
Division of Medical
Electrical Engineering
NL 5600 MB Eindhoven
Phone: +31 40 473 335

Prof F. DEL POZO
Universidad Politecnica
Madrid, Bioengineering
Department, Cuidad
Universitaria
ES 28040 Madrid

Dr. I. PITAS
University of Thessaloniki,
Dept. of Electrical
Engineering
P.O. Box 463
GR 54006 Thessaloniki
Phone: +30 31 996 317
Fax: +30 31 274 868

Dr. W. FRIESDORF
Universität Ulm/Klinikum,
Sektion Anästhesiologische
Technologie und
Verfahrensentwicklung
Steinhövelstrasse 9
DE 89075 Ulm
Phone: +49 731 502 79 18
Fax: +49 731 502 66 99

Prof. A. D'HOLLANDER
Hopital Erasme, Department
of Aneasthesiology
Route de lemmik 808
BE 1070 Brussels
Fax: +32 2 2 555 4363

Prof. J.H. VAN BEMMEL
Erasmus University,
Dept. of Medical Informatics,
Faculty of Medicine and
Health Sciences
P.O. Box 1738
NL 3000 DR Rotterdam
Phone: +31 10 408 70 50
Fax: +31 10 436 28 82

Prof. E. CARSON
City University,
Centre for Measurement and
Information in Medicine
Northhampton Square
UK London EC1V 0HB
Phone: +44 71 477 83 70
Fax: +44 71 477 85 79

Prof. J.L. COATRIEUX
Universitaire de Rennes I,
Laboratorie Traitement du
Signal et de l'Image,
Campus de Beaulieu
Batiment 22
FR 35042 Rennes Cedex
Phone: +33 99 286 220
Fax: +33 99 286 917

Prof. S. CERUTTI
Polytechnic University of
Milan, Department of
Biomedical Engineering
Piazza Leonardo da Vinci 32
IT 20133 Milan
Phone: +39 2 239 935 57
Fax: +39 2 239 935 87

Prof. M. BRACALE
Universita di Napoli,
Dipartimento di Ingegneria
Elettronica
Via Claudio 21
IT 80125 Naples
Phone: +39 81 593 85 22

METHODOLOGY FOR IT: THE ASSESSMENT OF IT-BASED DECISION SUPPORT IN DIABETES CARE (MFIT)

Key words
Diabetes care, diabetes, information technology, expert systems, decision support systems.

Brief description
Diabetes is a lifelong condition that affects around 1.5% of the population of Europe, with an estimated further 1.5% undiagnosed. Diabetes affects all sections of society, regardless of sex, age or race. Its complications are severe and include blindness, amputation and renal failure. Fortunately, the onset of these complications can be delayed or avoided entirely by good control of blood sugar levels using insulin and regular screening and appropriate education.

The key to good health for people with diabetes is well organised delivery of care over long periods of time. The expertise necessary to deliver the required care is generally only found in expensive, and hence scarce, specialist centres. Community physicians often do not possess the skills, or lack the confidence, to care for people with diabetes without support. One way to make the necessary knowledge more accessible is to disseminate it through the use of Information Technology. Expert Systems and Decision Support Systems will bring to the desktop of the community physician the expertise of the hospital specialist.

Much work has been done towards representing the skills of specialist diabetologists in computerised form. Although the technology largely exists in prototype form, the process of introducing it to the medical community at large has proved to be problematic. The project we are proposing will address this problem by developing and testing methodologies for integrating a number of technical solutions and for allowing multi-national evaluative studies of the technology in a way that is clinically relevant.

The proposed consortium will consist of six participants from Hungary, Italy, Denmark and the United Kingdom. Between us we will bring a wide range of skills and disciplines to bear on the problems addressed by the project. The pan-European dimension of the work will enable the experiences of representatives of different countries to be pooled to address this shared problem. The funds available through the Biomed programme will help sponsor this much needed consensus activity and thus lead to an improvement in the delivery of care to diabetics in Europe.

Project leader:
Professor Peter SOENKSEN
Dept of Endocrinology and
Chemical Pathology,
St Thomas Hospital
Lambeth Palace Road
UK London SE17EH
Phone: +44 71 8289292
Fax: +44 71 9284226
Contract number: CT941629

Participants:
Dr. L. FLETCHER
Newton Building, Room S36a
UK Salford M5 4WT

Dr. S. ANDREASSEN
Inst. of Electronic Systems,
Strandvejen 19
DK 9000 Aalborg

Dr. Tibor DEUTSCH
Computing Inst. Semmelweis,
Univ of Medicine
Kalvaria ter 5
HU 1089 Budapest

Prof. E. CARSON
Dept. of Systems Science,
City Univ
Northampton Square
UK London EC1V OHB

Prof M. MASS-BENEDETTI
Instituto di Patologia Speciale
Medica et Metodologica
Clinica
Via del Pozza
IT 6100 Perugia

EXPERIMENTAL TOMOGRAPHY BY ELECTRON SPIN RESONANCE IMAGING (EPRI) AND PROTON ELECTRON DOUBLE RESONANCE IMAGING (PEDRI)

Key words

Electron Spin Resonance Imaging (EPRI), Proton Electron Double Resonance Imaging (PEDRI), paramagnetic contrast agent, relaxation times.

Brief description

Electron Spin Resonance Imaging (EPRI) and proton Electron Double Resonance Imaging (PEDRI) produce images representing the distribution of exogenous paramagnetic probes. They are being developed to obtain at very low magnetic field the same sensitivity of high field MRI and to determine more physiological and functional parameters. The data obtained by PEDRI and EPRI are strictly complementary and this makes important a close connection for their development. In PEDRI the NMR resonance of the sample is observed while an ESR resonance of a paramagnetic contrast agent is excited. Saturation of the ESR transition causes a strong reduction of the relaxation times of the protons interacting With the unpaired electrons of the contrast agent. The NMR signal from these protons being relaxed is enhanced and these regions will exhibit a greater intensity in the final image. EPRI permits the direct localization of endogenous and/or exogenous paramagnetic molecules in living species. Using nitroxide free radicals as paramagnetic probes the technique has reached micromolar sensitivity. EPRI and PEDRI on large samples are performed at field values of the order of 5-10 mT. The ESR transitions are then betwenn 140 and 280 Mhz and the NMR frequencies between 200 and 500 khz. The concerted action will address the the following aspects:

a Development of instrumentation that can be used in EPRI and/or PEDRI experiment and verifications of the results of different experimental approaches;

b Experimental aspects of magnets and gradient coils design;

c Experimental techniques for the reduction of power deposition on the sample;

d Use and effect: paramagnetic probes of different linewidths;

e Resolution and sensitivitv of PEDRI and EPRI in phantoms, small animals and microscopic samples;

f Probe distribution through EPRI and PEDRI and its relation to NMR signal enhancement;

g Mathematical techniques to improve the resolution of PEDRI and EPRI images.

Project leader:
Professor Antonello SOTGIU
Consorzio INFM-Unità L'Aquila,
Tecnologie Biomediche e di Biometria,
Presso Dipartimento di Scienze B
Università dell'Aquila
Collemaggio
IT 67100 L'Aquila
Phone: +39 862 439862
Fax: +39 862 433433
Contract number: CT941352

Participants:

Dr. R. DEMEURE
Université Catholique de Louvain,
Dept. of Radioloqy
Cliniques Universitaires Saint-Luc
BE Louvain
Phone: +33 2 764 7340
Fax: +33 2 764 7363

Dr. D.J. LURIE
Dept. of Bio-Medical Physics and
Bio-Engineering Univ of Aberdeen
and Grampian Health Board
Foresthill
UK AB9 2ZD Aberdeen
Phone: +44 224 681818
Fax: +44 224 685645

Dr. K. GOLMAN
Hafslund Nycomed
P.A. Hanssons vag 41
SE 20512 Malmo
Phone: +46 40 32 1300
Fax: +46 40 32 1313

Dr. M. SYMONS
Dept. of Chemistry, Univ of Leicester
Univ Road
UK LEI 7HR Leicester
Phone: +44 533 522522
Fax: +44 533 522200

Dr. D. GRUCKER
Inst. de Physique Biologique Université
Louis Pasteur de Strasbourg
4 rue Kirschleger
FR 67085 Strasbourg Cedex
Phone: +33 8836 1144
Fax: +33 8837 1497

Prof. A. RASSAT
Ecole Normale Superieure
Laboratoire de Chimie
24 Rue Lhomond
FR 75231 Paris Cedex 05
Phone: +33 1 4707 1973
Fax: +33 1 4707 6856

Prof. F. MOMO
Dipartimento di Chimico-Fisica
Università di Venezia
Calle Larga Santa Marta
IT 30100 Venezia
Phone: +39 41 5298599
Fax: +39 41 5298594

Prof. L.H. SUTCLIFFE
Dept. of Chemistry and Physics
Univ of Surrey
UK Guilford Surrey GU2 5XH
Phone: +44 483 300800
Fax: +44 483 300803

Prof. T. MEHLKOPF
Delft Univ of Technology Faculty of
Appleid Physics, Section SSt-SI Imaging
Lorentzweg 1
NL 2628 CJ Delft
Phone: +31 15 785394
Fax: +31 15 624978

COMPUTERIZED RESPIRATORY SOUND ANALYSIS TECHNIQUES, STANDARDIZATION AND CLINICAL EVALUATION (CORSA)

Key words
Computerized respiratory sound analysis, clinical evaluation, pulmonary diseases, asthma, chronic bronchitis, lung sounds, auscultation, respiratory sounds, noninvasive techniques.

Objectives
The main objectives of the Concerted Action are the following:
1 To assess the need for general harmonization of the instrumentation and analysis techniques. This includes standardization of the way signals are captured, recorded, processed, analyzed, and interpreted (WP 1).
2 To coordinate basic research for the development of computerise stethoscope (WP 2).
3 To assess the advantages of home monitoring, monitoring during sleep an telecommunication of sound signals (WP 3).
4 To compare signal processing methods and automatic feature recognition for diagnostic purposes (WP 4).
5 To validate the methods in physiological and clinical terms and to assess the fitness of these methods in diagnosing and monitoring pulmonary diseases.(WP 5).
These objectives can be grouped into the various workpackages (WP) indicated above.

Brief description
Pulmonary diseases in many European countries are very common. The prevalence of asthma has increased to 3-6 per cent of the population and that of chronic obstructive pulmonary disease (COPD) is between 15-20% of the smoking population. A great deal of patients with asthma or chronic bronchitis produces pathological lung sounds by ordinary auscultation. Also, most other lung diseases and some cardiac diseases cause abnormal respiratory sounds.
These abnormal sounds contain clinically relevant information, and have features typical for the disease, correlate with its severeness, pulmonary function and the underlying structural changes.
Since the discovery by Laennec in 1816, the stethoscope has been commonly used for lung sound auscultation. However, by ordinary auscultation, only subjective evaluation of the sound can be carried out with no facility for recording, measurement, analysis or documentation. In 1955, the first lung sound spectrograms were published by McKusic and the first results analyzed with a computer were reported in the late 1970's. Modern digital signal processing methods offer powerful means for analyzing respiratory sound data. The results may be used for diagnosis, for follow-up of the disease, for assessing of the effect of treatment and physical rehabilitation and for the monitoring of patients. Recent results of comparative clinical studies indicate that adventitious lung sounds such as crackles which occur in various diseases contain features with a high discriminating power and that changes in bronchial obstruction reflect systematic alternations in lung sound spectra. Furthermore computerized analysis increases the sensitivity to detect abnormal features of respiratory sounds.
The sound signal is easily accessible with noninvasive techniques and an objective record can be obtained. The newest digital signal processing equipment and techniques facilitate

a fast and versatile respiratory sound analysis. Automated pattern recognition methods could be used to assist the diagnosis. The size of the equipment needed for lung sound analysis has decreased. Thus prerequisites for a computerized stethoscope and bed-side monitoring have become a reality.

Research groups in the United States, Canada, Japan, Israel and in several European countries are presently quite independently developing systems and methods for respiratory sound analysis. An International Lung Sound Association has been active for 17 years. In Europe alone, there are about 15 active groups in the field with different research profiles. last year the Respiratory Sounds European Club was founded to promote and disseminate the European science in the field. However, comparison of the data at different laboratories in Europe as well as in other continents is difficult due to the lack of accepted standards. These and the lack of sufficient clinical data also hamper the industrial development of computerized lung sound analyzers.

Project leader:
Dr. Anssi SOVIJÄRVI
Lung Function Laboratory,
Helsinki University
Central Hospital
SF 00290 Helsinki
Phone: +358 0 417 25 53
Fax: +358 0 471 40 18
Contract number: CT940928

Participants:
Dr. J. EARIS
Fazakerley Hospital,
Aintree Chest Centre
UK Liverpool
Phone: +44 51 794 45 09
Fax: +44 51 794 45 40

Dr. S.A.T. STONEMAN
University College of
Swansea, Dept. of
Mechanical Engineering
UK Swansea
Phone: +44 792 295 701

Prof. J. VANDERSCHOOT
Leiden University,
Medical Informatics
NL Leiden
Phone: +31 71 276 793
Fax: +31 71 276 782

Dr. H.W.J. SCHREUR
University Hospital
of Leiden,
Dept. of Pulmonology
NL Leiden
Phone: +31 71 210 714
Fax: +31 71 263 261

Prof. T. KATILA
Helsinki University of
Technology, Institute of
Biomedical Engineering
FI Espoo
Phone: +358 0 451 31 73
Fax: +358 0 451 31 82

Prof. G. CHARBONNEAU
Universite Paris-Sud, Institut
d'Electronique Fondamentale
FR Orsay Cedex
Phone: +33 1 6941 79 39
Fax: +33 1 6019 25 93

Dr. J.L. RACINEUX
Centre Hospitalier Regional,
Clinique de Pneumologie
FR Angers Cedex

Dr. J.W. SCHÄFER
ENT Clinic University of
Ulm, Section Rhinology
and Rhonocopatheis
DE Ulm
Phone: +49 731 179 42 54
Fax: +49 731 179 24 23

Dr. F. DALMASSO
Ospedale Mauriziano
Umberto I di Torino,
Divisone di Pneumologia
IT Torino
Phone: +39 11 5080 444
Fax: +39 11 616 394

Prof. G. RIGHINI
Instituto Elettrotecnico
Nazionale Galileo Ferraris
IT Torino
Phone: +39 11 650 76 11

Dr. M. ROSSI
Ospedale Sclavo,
Fisiopatologia Respiratoria
IT Siena
Phone: +39 577 299 761
Fax: +39 577 270 678

Dr. C.F. DONNER
Clinica del Laboro
Foundation, Divisione
di Pneumologia
IT Veruno
Phone: +39 322 830 101
Fax: +39 322 830 294

Prof. W. SANSEN
Katholieke Universiteit
Leuven,
Dept. Elektrotechniek
Kardinaal Mercierlaan 94
BE 3030 Heverlee
Phone: +32 16 22 09 31
Fax: +32 16 22 18 55

I.4 HEALTH SERVICES RESEARCH

Introduction

Most European Health Care Systems are facing similar problems.The important demographic changes,the new social attitudes and the increasing pressure of the scientific and technical progress are factors that are raising the health care expenses to unbearable limits and that have motivated fundamental health care reforms.

The increasing longevity leads to the growing rate of chronic diseases and consequently to the increase of health services consumption which is funded by a decreasing active population. The economic and social development leads to a higher health care demand,and in addition to a better quality in health care delivered. The technological progress, which cannot be ignored, increases the health costs. And all Health Systems, whatever their organisation and financing mechanisms are, must answer to the rising health care demand and at the same time contain the health care expenditure. These seem to be, at first glance, opposite objectives which jeopardize some basic ideas strongly deeprooted in a democratic Europe such as the equity, the solidarity and the quality of care, and which promote the search for the equilibrium between efficiency and quality in an optimum, equal and universal health care system.

The Biomedical and Health Research Programme, BIOMED I, through the Health Services Research specific programme, has participated in the search of this relationship between efficiency and quality, financing research projects to go towards the harmonisation of methodologies and protocols in health care services, financing mechanisms, workforce gestion, information systems and the best and most efficient way to prevent and to treat diseases. From 1991 to 1994, the activity period of this programme, financial support for the coordination of more than 300 research teams, who have worked on different projects, has been given. Now, thanks to their valuable collaboration, they are published in this chapter.

Maria Cruz Razquin

COMPARATIVE STUDY ON TASK PROFILES OF GENERAL PRACTITIONERS IN EUROPE

Key words

Research, Family Practice, Health Care Systems, Cross Cultural Comparisons, Job Description, Task Performance, Consultation and Referral, Workload, Europe, World Health Organization.

Objectives

The aim of the study is, firstly to describe the differences within and between health care systems in the WHO European Region with regard to the tasks performed by general practitioners and, secondly, to explain these differences from a number of possible determinants. In this survey services provided by general practitioners will be related to those provided by medical specialists.

Brief description

Research variables:

GP activities and their variation are described along a number of dimensions:

1 The range of performed tasks, i.e: (a) the degree involvement in rather specialised medical techniques; (b) involvement in diagnosis and treatment of non-medical problems; (c) involvement in anticipatory and preventive procedures; (d) provision of supplementary tasks (e.g. in public health etc.).

2 The population served; the general population or are certain categories excluded and allocated to the care of other physicians.

3 Working hours and workload, i.e. numbers consultations and visits; involvement in emergency service; administration; continuous education etc.

Variation of these dimensions will be related to a number of possible characteristics. These can be divided in two categories: determinants of variation of GP task performance between health care systems and determinants of variation of profiles within health care systems. Characteristics used in this study are specified below.

A Health care system determinants ('between variation'):

- health care system features as expressed in a country's health legislation and regulation (e.g. the system of remuneration)
- the level of professional education and training; e.g. the (period of) special training to become a GP; postgraduate training

B Practice dependent determinants ('within variation'):

- the level of practice equipment
- practice location factors; low health care supply in rural areas and a high level of facilities in cities may be related to different ranges of services provided by GPs.

Methodology:

A cross-sectional survey with a multi level design has been chosen, with data collection both on individual GP level and on the level of health care systems.

The method of data collection is threefold:

1 a questionnaire (in 25 languages) containing sections relevant to task performance and developed in co-operation with the participants in the study;

2 a simple one-week activities diary (in combination with the questionnaire) developed in a similar procedure as the questionnaire;

3 desk research to obtain information on health systems in the countries.

Currently the study has been implemented in 32 countries.

The sampling procedure facilitates intra-country analyses of subgroups of GPs practising in different conditions of urbanisation. GPs working in inner cities, in towns and in rural areas will be compared as regards services provided. The total sample size per country is dependent on the expected response rate. The number of completed questionnaires required per country has been fixed at 250 GPs (less in small countries). In due course, data regarding separate countries will be at the disposal of the national coordinators for their own purposes.

Interpretation of results will, again, be a joint activity of NIVEL and the national coordinators. After the reports of the international comparison have been drawn up, the complete database will be at each participants disposal for specific comparisons.

Project leader:
Dr. W.G.W. BOERMA
Netherlands Institute of
Primary Health Care
P.O. Box 1568
NL 3500 BN Utrecht
Phone: +31 30 319946
Fax: +31 30 319290
Contract number: CT921636

Participants:
Dr. Bonaventura BOLIBAR
Catalan Inst. of Health ICS
ES 08227 Terrassa

Dr. Brendan O'SHEA
Irish College of General
Practitioners
IE Naas Co.Kildare

Dr. Claude DIAZ
National Inst. of Health and
Mecical Research INSERM
FR 75251 Paris Cedex 05

Dr. Daniel BERGER
Interdisciplinary Research
Centre IFZ
CH 9007 St. Gallen

Dr. D. PRADOS TORRES
Andalusian Inst. of Health
ES Malaga

Dr. Derek BARFORD,
Dr. Douglas FLEMING
Royal College of General
Practitioners
UK Birmingham B17 9DB

Dr. D.J. BOUILLIEZ
Walloon Scientific Society
of General Medicine
BE 6120 Nalinnes

Dr. Elise KOSUNEN
Univ of Tampere, Dept. of
Public Health Sciences
FI 33101 Tampere

Dr. Frede OLESEN,
Dr. Lone BAK
Univ of Aarhus,
Inst. of Family Medicine
DE 8000 Aarhus C

Dr. Gianluigi PASSERINI,
Dr. Davide LAURI
Inst. of Farmacological
Research 'M Negri'
IT 20157 Milano

Dr. Guy MEISCH,
Dr. Romain STEIN
Association of Physicians
and Dentists
LU 2680 Luxemburg

Dr. Ingbert WEBER
Zentralinstitut fur die
Kassenarztlliche Versorgung
DE 5000 Cologne 41
Dr. Kaj KOGEUS,
Dr. Christina NERBRAND
Swedish Ass for Gen Med
SE 10726 Stockholm

Dr. Knut HOLTEDAHL
Univ of Tromso, Inst. of
Community Medicine
NO 9001 Tromso

Dr. Leo PAS
Flemish Inst. of General
Practice
BE 1970 Weezenbeek-Oppem

Gerhard HOLLER,
Dr. Michaela MORITZ
Austrian Federal Inst.
of Health Care
AT 1010 Vienna

Prof. John KYRIOPOULOS
Athens School of Public
Health, Dept. of
Health Economics
GR 11521 Athens

Prof. Dr. Zaida AZEREDO
Univ of Porto, Dept. of
Community Medicine
PT 4000 Porto

Prof. P. GROENEWEGEN,
Prof. J. van der ZEE
Netherlands Inst. of
Primary Health Care NIVEL
NL 3500 BN Utrecht

HOSPITAL USE, CASE MIX AND SEVERITY: ANALYSIS OF DIFFERENCES IN EUROPE

Key words
Hospital Information Systems (N$_4$.452.515.360), Case Mix (N$_2$.421.589.473.100), Europe (Z$_1$.542.49).

Objectives
1 To describe differences in the pattern of care provided for patients with particular diseases and at various levels of severity within and among European countries. This will include the threshold for admission to hospital, length of stay and, to a limited extent, outcome.
2 To analyze factors contributing to the differences found, including differences of individual health care systems, and treatment patterns by doctors.
3 To estimate implications for hospital costs of the differences found and analyze the contribution of factors other than case-mix and severity to these differences.

Brief description
The project has been organized in two phases. The first phase is devoted to statistical analysis of hospital Minimum Basic Data Sets (MBDS) of European countries to derive empirical results on variability in hospital use by patients, adjusted by case-mix and severity. At the same time, different tools for measuring case-mix and severity will be tested in European databases. Some high volume or high cost pathologies will be selected for more detailed analysis of the components of care, severity, and to a limited extent, outcomes. The potential impact on cost will be estimated for these high volume-high cost conditions by differences in length of stay after controlling by case mix and severity. The second phase will be oriented to apply geographical information systems to population-based databases to describe differences in hospital admission rates, and to obtain information on doctor's opinions and perceptions of patterns of care for well-defined types of patients where empirical differences have been found , by means of a *soft* methodology.

Two central data handling facilities have been established, one in Barcelona and one in London. The facility in Barcelona provides secretarial assistance and coordination as well as computing facilities for collecting, processing and grouping the data, and performing the first phase analysis. The facility in London will apply geographic information systems to the population-based databases.

MBDS databases from different European countries have been pooled together in the best possible comparable way, following the preliminary experience and network of collaborating teams in EURODRG Concerted Action. The response to the project from European teams has been very large, including Eastern and Central European teams. A database of around 4,000,000 discharges has been collected from 12 countries. Four of them are declared population-based. These data have been processed and grouped with three case-mix and severity tools (Diagnosis Related Groups; All Patient Refined Diagnosis Related Groups, and Disease Staging), this being the first time such a large European database has been used with all these measurement systems. Currently the data analysis of the first phase is being performed, and its results are going to be presented in the first Workshop in June 1994.

The existing network and preliminary experience constitutes a unique opportunity for a large European study on profiles of resource use for high volume/ high cost hospital conditions. It is recognized that important differences exist among health care systems in European countries, and that these differences influence medical practices. The more widespread use of case mix and severity measures in Europe will enable research in different areas to move beyond the current level of health systems comparisons, based on descriptions of structures and processes, to a situation where the effects of different systems and types of care provided and resulting outcome for particular conditions, can be compared.

Project leader:
Dr. M. CASAS
IASIST S.A.
Ronda Universidad 23
ES 08007 Barcelona
Phone: +34 3 301 40 61
Fax: +34 3 317 25 97
Contract number: CT920231

Participants:
Francis Roger FRANCE
Univ Cath de Louvain,
Clin Univ Saint-Luc
Av. Hippocrate 10
BE 1200 Brussels
Phone: +32 2 764 47 11
Fax: +32 2 764 45 00

Gemma VOSS
Academisch Ziekenhuis
Maastricht, Stafbureau
P.O. Box 1918
NL 6201 BX Maastricht
Phone: +31 43 876543
Fax: +31 43 877878

Hugh SANDERSON
National Case Mix Office
Stoney Lane 5
UK Winchester-Hampshire
+44 962 864 698

Anita ALBAN
Danish Hospital Inst.
Niaopostipa 18
DK 1602 Copenhagen
Phone: +45 33 11 5777
Fax: +45 33 93 1019

Eve BERLICZA
Medical Univ of Debrecen
HU 4012 Debrecen
Phone: +36 52 17 524
Fax: +36 52 17 524

Francesco TARONI
Instituto Superiore di Sanita
Viale Regina Elena 299
IT 00161 Roma Nomentano
Phone: +39 6 49 90 572
Fax: +39 6 44 69 938

Jacob HOFDIJK
Hofbrouckerlaan 8
NL 2341 LN Oegstgeest
Phone: +31 712 56708
Fax: +31 711 55682

Jean Marie RODRIGUES
U. de Saint Etienne,
Dept. Sante Publique
FR St. Jean Bonnefonds
Phone: +33 77 421425
Fax: +33 77 427970

Linda JENKINS
CASPE Research
14 Palace Court
UK London W2 4HT
Phone: +44 1 229 87 39
Fax: +44 1 737 27 33

Margarita BENTES
Ministerio da Saude,
Gabinete do Secretario
de Estado Adjunto
Av. da Republica 34
PT Lisboa
Phone: +351 1 793 19 19
Fax: +351 1 76 30 47

Martin McKEE
London School of Hygiene
and Tropical Medicine
Keppel Street
UK London WC1E 7HT
Phone: +44 71 636 86 36
Fax: +44 71 436 36 11

Miriam M. WILEY
Economic and Social
Research Inst.
Burlington Road 4
IE Dublin 4
Phone: +353 1 760 115
Fax: +353 1 686 231

Rosa TOMAS
IASIST
Ronda Universidad 23
ES 09007 Barcelona
Phone: +34 3 3014061
Fax: +34 3 3172597

Tim SCOTT
Barnes Hospital,
Health Strategies
Kingsway, Cheadle
UK Cheshire SK8 2NY
Phone: +44 61 491 55 51
Fax: +44 61 491 42 54

Veronique KOEHN
Service Cantnale de
Recherche E d'Information
Statistiques
Rue Sant Martin 7
CH 1014 Lausanne

HARMONISED APPROACHES TO AMBULATORY CARE OUTCOME MEASUREMENT IN EUROPE

Key words
Health outcome, primary care, hospital care, quality of life, health status measurement.

Objectives
1 To develop strategies and tools to promote harmonised European ambulatory care outcome measurement;
2 To evaluate the utility of health outcome measurement appropriate to European ambulatory health care;
3 To clarify a conceptual framework supporting harmonisation of health outcome measurement;
4 To create a standardised bibliography as a shared resource for the Action;
5 To create a framework of compatible data structures to facilitate the sharing and comparison of research results;
6 To compile a directory of selected multi-language health measurement instruments;
7 To share human resources and train research staff;
8 To raise awareness of health outcome measurement.

Brief description
The assessment of the outcome of ambulatory health care provision is a complex process. Comparison between health systems or individual units has traditionally used relatively finite but insensitive outcome measures such as death or serious disability. But these measures, although still used to compare between health systems, are now being supplanted by instruments which are more responsive. Developmental work is now going on internationally to construct and refine measures of health status and quality of life as measures of outcome. Since not every health status or quality of life measure is, or can be, used as an outcome measure, the selection, validations and utility of outcome measures has become a priority for many national health services.

Aim: The aim of this Concerted Action is to use current research on outcome measurement within the research group as a basis for understanding the concepts, methodologies and utility of outcome measurement. A utility evaluation will encompass the practical as well as the methodological issues. Between the 9 participants there are currently 15 ambulatory care outcome research studies being undertaken in both hospital ambulatory care and in general practice. As these projects are completed they will be drawn together as a series of monographs. Principally, however, they will provide the vehicle for an evaluation of the health outcome measures in use in the studies.

Progress: During the first year of the Action substantive progress has been made on all of the objectives. The work has been to clarify a conceptual framework for outcome measures and to use this to classify measures in two ways. First, to identify which health status measures are suitable for use as health outcome measures, which has resulted in a first stage consensus of the choice of measures.

The second major step has been to identify health status measures for which multi-language translations exist whilst at the same time developing with the help of external colleagues a set of criteria against which to measure the validity of the translated instruments. Already substantial interest is being shown by researchers across Europe in this element of the work and it will form an interim deliverable in 1994 as a directory of multi language measures.

The Action also set out to create a standardised bibliography which the participants and associated research teams could access. However, copyright held by the major data bases limits the use of a data base to a customer organisation thus preventing shared access between participants. This problem provided the stimulus to assess the various taxonomies available on health outcome, resulting in a common set of keywords which is now in use across the Action.

Ethical issues in the exchange of data between member states who have very different data projection rules proved a further constraint. As a result each participant is now providing data sets which is integrated by the owner institution to a standard format. The first feasibility study of this work is now completed.

Overall, and in each of the goal areas, substantial progress has been made. Health outcome measures scientific criteria have been developed and the translation work has proceeded ahead of schedule. The Action is now refocussing the goals towards published products and has expanded the work to include a feasibility study of multi-national, multi-cultural outcome measurement in 1994. This will provide an enhanced final product from the research programme.

Project leader:
Professor A. HUTCHINSON
Centre for Health Services
Research, University of
Newcastle Upon Tyne
Claremont Place 21
UK Newcastle Upon Tyne
NE2 4AA
Phone: +44 91 222 62 60
Fax: +44 91 222 60 43
Contract number: CT920204

Participants:
Ms. E. MCOLL
Univ of Newcastle u. Tyne,
Centre for Health Serv Res
21 Claremont Place
UK Newcastle upon Tyne
NE4 2AA
Phone: +44 91 2227047
Fax: +44 91 2226043

Berit R. HANESTAD
Dept. of Public Health &
Primary Health Care
Ulriksdal 8C
NO 5009 Bergen
Phone: +47 5 206162
Fax: +47 5 206130

Dr. C. KONIG
Dept. of General Practice and
Social Medicine
Verlengde Groenestraat 75
NL 6525 EJ Nijmegen
Phone: +31 80 613137
Fax: +31 80 541862

Dr. H. Van WEERT &
Dr. Nico Van DUIJN
Dept. of General Practice
Meibergdreef 15
NL 1105 AZ Amsterdam
Phone: +31 20 5664744
Fax: +31 20 6918806

Dr. K. Van HOECK &
Prof. J. HEYERMAN
Katholic Univ of Leuven,
Dept. of General
Minderbroederstraat 17
BE 3000 Leuven
Phone: +32 16 337468
Fax: +32 16 220920

Dr. P.L. FERREIRA
Universidade de Coimbra,
Fac de Economia
Av Dias da Silva 165
PT 3000 Coimbra
Phone: +351 39 715897
Fax: +351 39 403511

Dr. S.H. SCHUG
Abt Allgemeinmedizin MHH
DE 30623 Hannover 61
Phone: +49 511 5324927
Fax: +49 511 5324176

Mr. K. MEADOWS
Univ of Hull, Dept. of Public
Health Medicine
UK Hull HU6 7RX
Phone: +44 482 466021

Prof. B. MEYBOOM-
DE JONG
Dept. of Family Medicine
Ant. Deusinglaan 4
NL 9713 AW Groningen
Phone: +31 50 632963
Fax: +31 50 632964

Prof. F. TOUW-OTTEN
Univ of Utrecht, Dept.
of General Practice
Bijlhowerstraat 6
NL 3511 ZC Utrecht
Phone: +31 30 538188
Fax: +31 30 538105

Prof. J. De MAESENEER
Dept. General Practice
De Pintelaan 185
BE 9000 Gent
Phone: +32 92 403542
Fax: +32 92 404967

Prof. N.BENTZEN
Inst. of Community Health,
Dept. of General Practice
J.W. Winslowsparken 17
DK 5000 Odense C
Phone: +45 66 158600
Fax: +45 65 918296

Prof. V. GRABAUSKAS
Kaunas Medical Academy
Mickeviciaus Str. 9
LT 3000 Kaunas
Phone: +3707 226110

HEALTH CARE FINANCING AND THE SINGLE EUROPEAN MARKET

Key words
Health care financing, efficiency, cross-border care, impact research, convergence.

Objectives
1 To identify aspects in health care financing which are of relevance in a single market, including differences in health care and its financing in EC member states which set incentives for interaction between systems;
2 To analyze cross-border health care with respect to its legal regulation, empirical extent, financing, and to investigate possibilities for alternative organization;
3 To explore and analyze current and future impacts of the single market on health care financing, including impacts on organization and performance of health care.

Brief description
The project aims at the analysis of financing issues of different national health care systems that interact in the single market and with the single market. It comprises three working areas, the topics of which are briefly sketched below:
Current EC health care financing systems: Differences of national health care financing in organization and in performance set incentives for interaction: e.g. patients may react to differentials in availability or insurance coverage of services; provides of medical technology to differentials in reimbursement, regulation and quality control; authorities contracting out for health care services to differentials in price and quality.
Cross-border care: This refers to patients insured in one member state, but receiving care in another one. This is subject to a number of current EC rules. The quantity of cross-border care is partly linked to the general mobility within the single market, partly to the cross-border accessibility of health care.
Impacts of the single market and future developments: Effects on economic integration may affect financing by various ways (e.g. through prices for health care goods and services such as medical technology, pharmaceutical products.) Furthermore, the question of convergence of EC health care and financing systems emerges.
The first and the third area will be analyzed by one working group, the second by another working group. These working groups will first explore their research issues, then specify their research protocols, collect data, and then process the protocols. This involves, among others, base-line descriptions of selected health care financing issues, the identification of major interactions between the single market and health care financing, the analysis of trends towards a possible convergence, and the analysis of current cross-border care and its alternative regulations.

Project leader:
Professor Dr. R. LEIDL
Scientific Administration, Grant Rhodes MSc,
Department of Health Economics,
University of Limburg
P.O. Box 616
NL 6200 MD Maastricht
Phone: +31 43 881727
Fax: +31 43 670960
Contract number: CT920740

Participants:

Dr. Bert HERMANS
Health Care Policy and Management
P.O. Box 1738
NL 3000 Dr. Rotterdam
Phone: +31 10 408 80 03
Fax: +31 10 436 07 17

Dr. George FRANCE
Instituto di Studi Sulle Regioni
Lungotevere delle Armi 22
IT 00195 Roma
Phone: +39 6 321 6061/3/9
Fax: +39 6 321 6071

Dr. John ROBERTS
European Office of the World
Health Organization
8 Scherfigsvej
DK 2100 Copenhagen
Phone: +45 39 171717
Fax: +45 31 181120

Dr. Markus SCHNEIDER
BASYS GmbH Beratungsgesellschaft für
angewandte Systemforschung mbH
Reidingerstrasse 25
DE 8900 Augsburg 1
Phone: +49 821 257 940
Fax: +49 821 57 93 41

Dr. Michael CALNAN
The Univ of Canterbury, Centre for
Health Serv Studies George Allen Wing
UK Canterbury CT2 7NF Kent
Phone: +44 227 76 40 00
Fax: +44 227 45 90 25

Mrs. SANDIER CREDES
Rue Paul Cezanne 1
FR 75008 Paris
Phone: +33 1 40 768215
Fax: +33 1 45 635742

Mr. Ray ROBINSON
King's Fund Inst.
126 Albert Street
UK London NW1 7NF
Phone: +44 71 485 9589
Fax: +44 71 482 3584

Prof. Dr. Hans MAARSE
Univ of Limburg, Dept. of Health
Policy and Administration
P.O. Box 616
NL 6200 MD Maastricht
Phone: +31 43 881560

Prof. Dr. John KYRIOPOULOS
Athens School of Public Health,
Dept. of Health Economics
Alexandras Av. 196
GR 11521 Athens
Phone: +30 1 64 35 328
Fax: +30 1 64 49 571

Prof. Dr. Juan ROVIRA
SOIKOS Centre d'Estudis en Economia de la
Salut i de la Politica Secial SL
Carrer Arizala 1-3 Entl. 1a
ES 08028 Barcelona
Phone: +34 3 449 80 70
Fax: +34 3 33 44 935

Prof. Dr. Peter OBERENDER
Univ Bayreuth, Lehrstuhl fur
Volkswirtschaftslehre
P.O. Box 10 12 51
DE 8580 Bayreuth
Phone: +49 921 55 28 80
Fax: +49 921 55 28 86

Prof. Peter ZWEIFEL, Mr. Luca CRIVELLI
Institut für empirische Wirtschaftsforschung
Kleinstr. 15
CH 8008 Zürich
Phone: +41 1 251 63 23
Fax: +41 1 261 91 66

Prof. Dr. Reiner LEIDL
Univ of Limburg, Dept. of Health Economics
P.O. Box 616
NL 6200 MD Maastricht
Phone: +31 43 881727
Fax: +31 43 670960

Prof. Dr. W. van EIMEREN, Dr. Jürgen JOHN
GSF Medis Inst.
Ingolstädter Landstrasse 1
DE 8042 Neuherberg
Phone: +49 89 3187 4032
Fax: +49 89 3187 3017

Prof. Jean HERMESSE
Alliance Nationale des Mutualites Chretiennes
Rue de la Loi 121
BE 1040 Bruxelles
Phone: +32 2 237 41 11
Fax: +32 2 237 33 00

SOCIO-ECONOMIC INEQUALITIES IN MORBIDITY AND MORTALITY IN EUROPE: A COMPARATIVE STUDY

Key words
Socio-economic status, mortality, health surveys, physical disability, epidemiologic factors, social class, cause of death, health status indicators, chronic diseases.

Objectives
1 To measure the size of socio-economic inequalities in morbidity and mortality in different European countries, and to compare the size of these inequalities between countries;
2 To measure the size of socio-economic inequalities in *determinants of* morbidity and mortality in different European countries, to compare the size of these inequalities with those in morbidity and mortality, and to make inferences on the causes of international variation in inequality in morbidity and mortality.

Brief description
This project aims at increasing the understanding of socio-economic inequalities in health by studying international variation in the size of inequalities in health and in specific determinants of health.

The following indicators of health are included: prevalence of chronic conditions; prevalence of short-term and long-term disability; perceived general health; mortality by cause of death. The following determinants of health are included: cigarette smoking; alcohol consumption; physical exercise; obesity and dietary habits; housing and working conditions; use of preventive, curative and rehabilitative health care services.

Data on mortality come from longitudinal studies or cross-sectional studies, whereas data on morbidity and determinants come from health interview (and similar) surveys. Most data sources are nationally representative. Much attention is given cross-country comparability of these data, and to the development of summary indices on the extent of health inequalities.

Project leader:
Prof. J.P. MACKENBACH
Department of Public Health,
Faculty of Medicine and
Health Sciences,
Erasmus University
P.O. Box 1738
NL 3000 DR Rotterdam
Phone: +31 10 4087714
Fax: +31 10 4366831
Contract number: CT921068

Participants:
Dr. U. HELMERT
Bremer Institut für Präven-
tionsforschung und
Sozialmedizin (BIPS)
DE 2800 Bremen 1
Phone: +49 421 59 59 6 0
Fax: +49 421 59 59 665

Dr. A. LECLERC
INSERM Unité 88
FR 75634 Paris Cedex 13
Phone: +33 1 45 846374
Fax: +33 1 45 838302

Dr. A. MIELCK
GSF-Medis
DE 8042 Neuherberg
Phone: +49 89 31 87 53 00
Fax: +49 89 31 87 33 75

Dr. A. MIZRAHI and
Dr. M. SOURTY
Credes
Rue Paul Cézanne
FR 75008 Paris
Phone: +33 1 42 894573
Fax: +33 1 42 894582

Dr. A. RITSAKAKIS
World Health Organisation
DK 2100 Copenhagen
Phone: +45 39 171717
Fax: +45 31 181120

Dr. A.S. ANDERSEN
Statistics Norway, Div for
Analysis of Demography and
living conditions
NO 0033 Oslo 1
Phone: +47 2 864500
Fax: +47 2 864973

Dr. B. NOLAN
The Economic and Social
Research Inst.
IE Dublin 4
Phone: +353 1 760 115

Dr. C.E. MINDER
Inst. Sozial- und
Präventivmedizin
CH 3012 Bern
Phone: +41 31 648631
Fax: +41 31 237956

Dr. D. VAGERÖ
Stockholm Univ, Swedish
Inst. for Social Research
SE 10691 Stockholm
Phone: +46 816 20 00
Fax: +46 815 46 70

Dr. E. LAHELMA
Univ Helsinki,
Dept. Sociology
FI 00550 Helsinki
Phone: +358 0 70 84 614
Fax: +358 0 70 84 619

Dr. E. REGIDOR
Min de Sanidad y Consumo
Pasio del Prado 18-20
ES 28071 Madrid

Dr. E. van DOORSLAER
IMTA/Erasmus Univ
NL 3000 Dr. Rotterdam
Phone: +31 10 4 087317
Fax: +31 10 4 087738

Dr. F. PAGNANELLI
Inst. Nazionale di Statistica
Via C. Balbo 16
IT 00100 Roma
Phone: +39 6 46 73 1
Fax: +39 6 46 73 41 73

Dr. G. DESPLANQUES
INSEE
Bd. Adolphe Pinard 18,
Room no. 647
FR 75675 Paris Cedex 14
Phone: +33 1 41 175050
Fax: +33 1 41 176666

Dr. J.T.P. BONTE,
Dr. J. van den BERG
Centraal Bureau voor de
Statistiek
NL 2270 AZ Voorburg
Phone: +31 70 3 37 38 00
Fax: +31 70 3 87 74 29

Dr. L. GRÖTVEDT,
Dr. J.-K. BORGAN
Div. for Health,
Statistics Norway
NO 0033 Oslo 1
Phone: +47 2 864500
Fax: +47 2 864973

Dr. L. ROVERI
Instituto Nazionale
di Statistica
IT 00142 Roma
Phone: +39 6 59 43 100
Fax: +39 6 59 43 257

Dr. N. RASMUSSEN
Danish Inst. for Clinical
Epidemiology
DK 2100 Copenhagen
Phone: +45 31 20 77 77
Fax: +45 31 20 80 10

Dr. O. ANDERSEN
Danmarks Statistik
DK 2100 Copenhagen O
Phone: +45 31 298222
Fax: +45 31 184801

Dr. O. LUNDBERG
Stockholm Univ, Swedish
Inst. for Social Research
SE 10691 Stockholm
Phone: +46 816 20 00
Fax: +46 815 46 70

Dr. R. LAGASSE
Université Libre de Bruxel-
les, Ecole de Santé Public
Campus Erasme CP 590
BE 1070 Brussels
Phone: +32 2 555 40 84
Fax: +32 2 555 40 49

Dr. R.J. BUTCHER
OPCS, Social Survey Div
UK London WC2B 6JP
Phone: +44 71 242 02 62
Fax: +44 71 405 30 20

Dr. Th. SPUHLER
Bundesamt für Statistik
CH 3003 Bern
Phone: +41 31 618772
Fax: +41 31 617856

Prof. A SISSOURAS
Univ of Patras, Sch of Engin-
eering, Dept. of Management
and Operational Res
GR Patras
Phone: +30 61 991684
Fax: +30 61 997260

Prof. A.E. PHILALITHIS
Univ Crete-School of
Health Sciences
GR Iraklion
Phone: +30 81 262675
Fax: +30 81 262674

Prof. Dr. W. LINKE
Bundesinstitut für Bevölke-
rungsforschung
DE 6200 Wiesbaden 1
Phone: +49 611 46 11 65
Fax: +49 611 72 40 00

Prof. J. FOX
OPCS, Medical Statistics
UK London WC2B 6JP
Phone: +44 71 242 02 62
Fax: +44 71 405 21 67

Prof. J.P. MACKENBACH
Erasmus Univ, Dept. of
Public Health and
Social Medicine
NL 3000 Dr. Rotterdam
Phone: +31 10 408 77 14
Fax: +31 10 436 68 31

Prof. M. do ROSARIO
GIRALDEZ
Escola Nacional de
Saude Publica
PT 1699 Lisboa Codex
Phone: +351 1 758 55 99
Fax: +351 1 758 27 54

Prof. T. VALKONEN
Dept. of Sociology
(Univ Helsinki)
Hämeentie 68 B
FI 00550 Helsinki
Phone: +358 0 70 84 624
Fax: +358 0 70 84 619

THE MANAGEMENT OF END STAGE RENAL DISEASE IN EUROPE: APPROACHING A CONSENSUS

Key words
End Stage Renal Disease, Comorbidity, Clinical Guidelines.

Objectives
1 To determine the survival of patients commencing Renal Replacement Therapy over a seven year period in major centres in five European countries, taking into account age and comorbidity.
2 To develop and evaluate protocols for the treatment of anaemia and bone disease in patients undergoing Renal Replacement Therapy and in addition to develop guidelines to manage patients with positive cytomegalovirus status as well as those with active infection.

Brief description
The survival of patients on Renal Replacement Therapy (dialysis or transplantation) is the ultimate outcome measure. Over the years this has become more difficult to analyze and compare between areas because more elderly patients now receive RRT in developed countries as do patients with diseases of organs other than the kidney (eg heart disease, peripheral vascular disease). Such diseases are known as comorbid conditions. Using a risk stratification protocol we are determining the effect of age and comorbidity on survival on Renal Replacement Therapy. The data will further be analyzed using Cox's proportional hazard model also taking into account age and the different comorbid illnesses.

To improve the patient care of those undergoing RRT we are developing and monitoring protocols on three aspects of the management of such patients - anaemia, bone disease and the patient's CMV status and CMV infection. This new approach will not only allow more rational patient management but ultimately permit us to cost each aspect of the Renal Service. We now wish to study such Health Care interventions in our different Renal Units in five countries. Protocols will be compared in an attempt to reach a consensus on the best and most effective forms of management.

Project Leader:
Dr. A.M. MacLEOD
Department of Medicine and
Therapeutics, Medical
School, Univ of Aberdeen
Polwarth Building,
Foresterhill
UK Aberdeen AB9 2ZD
Phone: +44 224 681818
Fax: +44 224 699884
Contract number: CT920932

Participants:
Dr. I. HENDERSON
Ninewells Hospital,
Renal Unit
UK Dundee DD1 9SY
Phone: +44 382 60111

Dr. M. PAPADIMITRIOU
Aristotelian Univ of
Thessaloniki,
Hippokration Gen Hosp
GR Thessaloniki
Phone: +30 31 828595
Fax: +30 31 835955

Dr. R.A.P. KOENE
Academisch Ziekenhuis
Nijmegen, Afd. Nierziekten
Geert Grooteplein 8
NL 6500 Nijmegen
Phone: +31 80 614 761
Fax: +31 80 540 788

Prof. E. RITZ
Klinikum der Universitat
Heidelberg
Bergheimer Strasse 56a
DE 6900 Heidelberg
Phone: +49 6221 91120
Fax: +49 6221 162476

Prof. J.P. SOULILLOU &
Dr. D. CANTAROVICH
Centre Hospitalier Regional
et Univ de Nantes
P.O. Box 1005
FR 44035 Nantes
Phone: +33 40 083284
Fax: +33 40 356697

THE ESTABLISHMENT OF A EUROPEAN ORTHODONTIC QUALITY ASSURANCE SYSTEM (EUROQUAL)

Key words
Quality, quality-assurance, effectiveness, efficiency, objectivities standards, indices, criteria, evaluation, orthodontics, dentistry.

Objectives
1 The formulation of a patient entered evaluation system.
2 The formulation of a practitioner entered evaluation system.
3 Methods to maximise effectiveness and efficiency in orthodontic care.

Brief description
Orthodontics is a branch of dentistry that deals with the treatment of irregularities of the teeth and abnormalities of their relation to the surrounding facial structures.

With the removal of national barriers in Europe, an appraisal of the provision of orthodontic care throughout Europe and the establishment of guidelines for quality regarding orthodontic care becomes an issue of importance.

In a Concerted Action of orthodontic Quality Assurance System.

The goal of the Concerted Action will be to reach consensus regarding the development of systematic measures to assure and improve the appropriateness and effectiveness in orthodontic care throughout Europe.

Three tasks have been defined:
1 Formulation of a patient centred evaluation system.

  The criteria that patients apply in their evaluation of treatment may differ from that of practitioners.

  In order to develop a patient centred evaluation system, criteria and norms will be developed to assess information from patients regarding their perception of treatment desires, the treatment process and treatment outcome.
2 Formulation of a practitioners centred evaluation system.

  Several objective measures have been developed to attempt to categorise malocclusion into groups according to the level of treatment need. At present there is no internationally agreed approach to assess need for treatment.

  In order to develop a practitioners centred evaluation system criteria and standards will be developed to assess treatment need and treatment outcome by means of peer- or self assessment.
3 Methods to maximise appropriateness and effectiveness of orthodontic care.

  Quality in orthodontic services depends on the degree to which technical and diagnostic skills match the complexity of treatment and the extent to which performance is influenced by the working environment, resource and financial constraints.

  In order to improve rationalisation and integration in orthodontic service, criteria and standards to maximise effectivity, efficiency and quality of orthodontic care will be developed.

The proposed methodology in the development of the Quality Assurance System comprises:
- research;
- workshops;
- consensus meetings;
- training of auditors;
- validation studies;
- field trials.

After development of the Quality Assurance System, an implementation phase has been planned.

Project leader:
Professor B. PRAHL-ANDERSEN
Orthodontic Department,
Academic Centre for Dentistry (ACTA)
Louwesweg 1
NL 1066 EA Amsterdam
Phone: +31 20 518 88 88
Fax: +31 20 518 85 66
Contract number: CT920145

Participants:
Dr. A. SANDHAM
Academic Centre for Dentistry (ACTA)
Louwesweg 1
NL 1066 EA Amsterdam
Phone: +31 20 5188330
Fax: +31 20 5188333

Dr. A. STENVIK
Univ of Oslo Dental Faculty
Geitmysveien 71
NO 0455 Oslo
Phone: +47 2 357080
Fax: +47 2 373146

Dr. I.P. ADAMIDIS
Univ of Athens, Faculty of Dentistry
Thivon Street 2
GR 115 27 Athens, Goudi
Phone: +30 1 3605460

Dr. S. RICHMOND
Univ of Manchester Dental School
Higher Cambridge Street
UK Manchester M15 6FH
Phone: +44 61 275 6661
Fax: +44 61 275 3438

Prof. F. MIOTTI
Univ of Padova, Faculty of Dentistry
Via A. Gabelli 14
IT 35121 Padova
Phone: +39 49 821 2041
Fax: +39 49 876 1210

Prof. G. REHAK
Heim Pal Hospital for Sick Children
Zoltan u. 18
HU 1954 Budapest
Phone: +36 1 1316529
Fax: +36 1 1335172

Prof. J. CANUT
Univ of Valencia, Faculty of Dentistry
Grabador Esteve 10
ES Valencia 46004

Prof. R. BERG
Universitat des Saarlandes,
Abt Kieferorthpadie
DE 6650 Homberg-Saar
Phone: +49 6841 164910
Fax: +49 6841 164950

EQUITY IN THE FINANCE AND DELIVERY
OF HEALTH CARE IN EUROPE

Key words
Equity, income distribution, health economics.

Objectives
1 Enlargement and update of cross-country comparison performed in Phase 1 of the project.
2 Analyses of equity consequences of changes to health care system in 14 European countries.
3 Refinement and further development of methods to assess equity.
4 Analysis of the sources of cross-country differences in equity

Brief description
This Concerted Action (CA) is a continuation of an earlier CA which investigated the equity characteristics of 10 health care systems. The present CA aims at filling some remaining gaps in the knowledge about equity in health care. The cross-section of countries has been enlarged with research teams from five new countries (Belgium, Finland, Germany, Norway and sweden) to investigate how their systems compare in terms of equity. Progressivity of health care finance is being assessed using standard progressivity indices, as in our earlier work. Inequalities in health are quantified by means of illness concentration indices. The issue of 'equal treatment for equal need' is examined by testing for differences in expenditure figures across income groups after standardizing for morbidity, age and gender. Simulation is used in 'what if' analyses of proposed reforms to health care finance and delivery. Finally, it is hoped that the enlarged datasets (both cross-sectionally and over time) and the extensions and refinements of the methodology will allow the exploration of possible sources of any inequities detected. Such information is deemed to be highly relevant for the current health policy debates in many European countries.

Project leader:
Professor E. VAN DOORSLAER
Department of Health Care Policy and Management,
Erasmus University
P.O. Box 1738
NL 3000 DR Rotterdam
Phone: +31 10 4087317
Fax: +31 10 4087738
Contract number: CT920608

Participants:

Dr. Adam WAGSTAFF
Univ of Sussex, School of
Social Sciences
UK Brighton BN1 9QN
Phone: +44 273 606755
Fax: +44 273 678466

Dr. Andreas MIELCK
GSF-Medis
Ingolstädter Landstr. 1
DE 8042 Neuherberg
Phone: +49 89 3187 5325
Fax: +49 89 3187 3375

Dr. Carol PROPPER
Univ of Bristol,
Dept. of Economics
8 Woodland Road
UK Bristol BS8 1TN
Phone: +44 272 303030
Fax: +44 272 737803

Dr. Claire LACHAUD
Univ Claude Bernard, Centre
National de la Recherche
Scientifique
43 Bd du 11 Nov. 1918
FR 69622 Villeurbanne
Phone: +33 72 448264
Fax: +33 72 440573

Dr. Guido CITONI
Istituto di Studi per la Pro-
grammazione Economica
Corso V. Emanuele 284
IT 00186 Roma
Phone: +39 6 3873503
Fax: +39 6 3872422

Dr. Jes SOGAARD
Odense Univ
Winslowparken 17, 1
DK Odense
Phone: +45 661 58600
Fax: +45 659 18296

Dr. Jozef PACOLET
Inst. of Labour Research
(HIVA)
E. van Evenstraat 2E
BE 3000 Leuven
Phone: +32 16 283335
Fax: +32 16 283344

Dr. Jurgen JOHN
GSF-Medis
Ingolstädter Landstr. 1
DE 8042 Neuherberg
Phone: +49 89 3187 5325
Fax: +49 89 3187 3375

Dr. Lise ROCHAIX
Ministère de l'Economie
et Finances
Rue de Bercy 139
FR 75572 Paris Cedex 12
Phone: +33 1 40 249718
Fax: +33 1 43 452283

Dr. Marisol Rodriguez
Univ of Barcelona,
Fac of Economics
Avds. Diagonal 690
ES 0834 Barcelona
Phone: +34 3 280 5161
Fax: +34 3 280 2378

Dr. Pierella PACI
City Univ, Dept. of
Social Sciences
Northampton Square
UK London EC1V 0HB
Phone: +44 71 477 8000
Fax: +44 71 477 8580

Dr. Richard JANSSEN
Limburg Univ, Dept.
of Health Economics
NL 6200 MD Maastricht
Phone: +31 43 883439
Fax: +31 43 219080

Dr. Terker CHRISTIANSEN
Odense Univ, Center for
Health & Social Policy
Winslowparken 17, 1
DK 5000 Odense C
Phone: +45 661 58600
Fax: +45 659 18296

Dr. Ulf GERDTHAM
Stockholm School of
Economics, Centre for
Health Economics
P.O. Box 6501
SE 11383 Stockholm
Phone: +46 8 7369283
Fax: +46 8 313207

Mr. Carlos Gouveia PINTO
Instituto Superior
de Economia
Lupi 20
PT 1200 Lisbon

Mr. Jean HERMESSE
Landbond Chr. Mutualiteiten
Wetstraat 121
BE 1040 Brussel
Phone: +32 2 237 4111
Fax: +32 2 237 3300

Mr. Joao PEREIRA
School of Public Health
Av. Padre Cruz
PT 1699 Losboa Codex
Phone: +351 1 7575599
Fax: +351 1 7582754

Mr. Owen O'DONNELL
Univ of York, Centre for
Health Economics
UK York YO1 5DD
Phone: +44 904 433668
Fax: +44 904 433644

Mr. Unto HÄKKINEN
National Agency for
Welfare & Health
P.O. Box 220
FI 00531 Helsinki
Phone: +358 0 3967 2327
Fax: +358 0 3967 2459

Prof. Barbara WOLFE
Russel Sage Foundation
112 East 64th Street
US New York 10021
Phone: +1 212 750 6022
Fax: +1 212 371 4761

Prof. Bengt JÖNSSON
Stockholm School of Eco-
nomic, Economics
P.O. Box 6501
SE 11383 Stockholm
Phone: +46 8 7369281
Fax: +46 8 302115

Prof. Brian NOLAN
Economic and Social Re-
search Inst.
4 Burlington Road
IE Dublin 4
Phone: +353 1 760 115
Fax: +353 1 686 231

Prof. Dr. F.F.H. RUTTEN
Erasmus Univ Rotterdam,
Inst. for Medical
Technology Assessment
P.O. Box 1738
NL 3000 Dr. Rotterdam
Phone: +31 408 7317
Fax: +31 408 7783

Prof. Dr. Robert LEU
Univ of Bern, Volkswirt-
schaftliches Institut
Vereinsweg 23
CH 3012 Bern
Phone: +41 31 654090
Fax: +41 31 653783

Prof. Peter GOTTSCHALK
Dept. of Economics,
Boston College
Chestnut Hill
US Massachusetts 02167
Phone: +1 617 5523670
Fax: +1 617 5528828

RESOURCE USE, COSTS AND OUTCOME OF DIFFERENT PACKAGES OF CARE FOR STROKE

Key words
Resource, Cost, Stroke.

Objectives
1 To maintain hospital, and community based stroke registers for recording the care and outcome of stroke patients in 9 centres in England, France, Italy, Germany and Portugal.
2 To measure the resources used by each centre treatment package for stroke patients e.g. home/hospital care, level of rehabilitation support.
3 To assess the costs of different packages of care and analyze the reasons for cost variations between centres eg. are they due to differences in the price, type, or volume of input?
4 To compare packages of care in the different centres in terms of resource use and outcome i.e. mortality, disability, handicap and quality of life.
5 To provide a framework which allows other European centres to assess the resource and cost implications of establishing desired treatment packages in their locality.

Brief description
During the first four months the project leader (CW) and the Senior Research Fellow in Operational Research visited all participating centres to assess the structure and process of care for stroke patients admitted to the hospital. The proposed methodologies were discussed for their feasibility and means of data collection for the resource use and cost elements established.

The first meeting of the Concerted Action was help in London in July 1993 to establish the protocol for hospital based registries. It was agreed that all stroke patients registered in the participating hospitals would be assessed on admission, at three months and one year after the stroke. Separate recording of recurrent strokes or deaths will also occur. A minimum data set to enable the objectives of the Concerted Action to be fulfilled was drawn up. In the following month amendments and standardisation of the terminology occurred. Data collection commenced in September 1993 and to data 200 stroke patients have been registered. It is proposed to meet in Florence in February to assess progress and problems of data collection as well as establish studies to assess inter centre agreement.

Project leader:
Dr. C.D.A. WOLFE
Division of Community Health,
United Medical and Dental Schools of
Guy's and St. Thomas's Hospitals
St. Thomas Campus
UK London SE1 7EH
Phone: +44 71 9289292
Fax: +44 71 9281468
Contract number: CT920272

Participants:

Dr. A. RUDD
St. Thomas's Hospital,
Care of the Elderly Unit
UK London SE1 7EH
Phone: +44 71 928 9292
Fax: +44 71 928 1468

Dr. B. Haussler
Inst. fur Gesundheits und
Sozialforschung GmbH (IGES)
Otto Suhr Allee 18
DE 1000 Berlin 10
Phone: +49 30 348 070
Fax: +49 30 348 0770

Dr. R. BEECH
St. Thomas's Campus,
Div. of Community Health UMDS
UK London SE1 7EH
Phone: +44 71 928 92 92
Fax: +44 71 928 14 68

Dr. D. BARER
Royal Liverpool Univ Hosp,
Univ Dept. of Geriatric Medicine
P.O. Box 147
UK Liverpool L69 3BX
Phone: +44 51 706 4062
Fax: +44 51 706 4064

Dr. J. BERGER
Univ of Hamburg, Inst. fur Mathematik
und Datenverarbeitung in der Medizin
Martini Strasse 52
DE Hamburg 20
Phone: +49 40 468 3652
Fax: +49 40 468 4882

Dr. J.A.A. DIAS, Prof. M. CARRAGETA
Divisao de Epidemiologia
Alameda D. Alfonso Henriques no 45
PT 1056 Lisboa Dodex
Phone: +351 793 3441
Fax: +351 176 7525

L. RICHARDSON
Kent and Sussex Hospital, Research Associate
Mount Ephrain, Tunbridge Wells
UK Kent TN4 8AT
Phone: +44 892 526111

Prof. L. AMADUCCI, Prof. D. INZITARI
Universita Degli Studi di Firenze,
Ospedale Careggi
V. le Morgagni
IT 85 50134 Firenze
Phone: +39 55 432224
Fax: +39 55 413603

Prof. M. GIROUD
Centre Hospitalier Regional Univ de Dijon,
Service de Neurologie
Rue du Faubourg-Raines 3
FR 21033 Dijon Cedex
Phone: +33 80418141
Fax: +33 80293683

Prof. SPITZER
Univ of Hamburg-Eppendorf,
Dept. of Neurology
Martinistr. 52
DE 2000 Hamburg 20
Phone: +49 40 468 3771
Fax: +49 40 468 5086

Prof. S. EBRAHIM
The Royal London Hospital,
Dept. of Health Care of the Elderly
Bancroft Road
UK London E1 4DG
Phone: +44 71 377 7894
Fax: +44 71 377 7862

FREQUENCY AND RISK FACTORS OF MATERNAL MORBIDITY AND MORTALITY 'AVOIDABLE' DEATHS AND EVALUATION OF CARE

Key words
Maternal morbidity, maternal mortality, pregnancy.

Brief description
Maternal mortality is not only a dramatic event. It is also an indicator of the quality of care. But important discrepancies in maternal mortality rates are recorded in Europe without knowing if these differences are related to the notification and the registration of deaths, or to the deficiency of health care systems.

The project has two objectives:

1 To compare the notification and the actual frequency of the maternal mortality between countries of the European Union.

2 To identify risk factors related to the patients or to the health care conditions.

Two different surveys should be carried out, both or separately:

- a study of validation of maternal mortality rates will bear on a representative sample (or the whole) of maternal deaths. The certifying doctors will be asked to provide complementary information on the gravid condition of the woman (aborted or pregnant or within 42 days of termination of pregnancy). All deaths concerning a woman in gravido-puerperal conditions, identified before and/or by the survey, will be examined by a committee of medical experts. This committee will have to classify maternal deaths into direct or indirect obstetrical causes and fortuitous causes.

- the second survey will refer to mortality and morbidity. It will be based on hospital statistics, on a geographical area and related to five pathologies: haemorrhage, eclampsia, infection, thrombo-embolism and cardiomyopathy.

The WHO definition will be used for maternal mortality. About severe morbidity, a complete and operational definition will have to be determined. Enquiries will be done with standardized questionnaires. In the frame of this European approach, the frequency of maternal mortality could be evaluated in each country and risk factors related to the health care system could be highlighted, taking account of the factors related to the patient.

Project leader:
Mrs. Marie-Hélène BOUVIER-COLLE
INSERM, Unité 149,
Recherches Epidemiologiques
sur la Santé des
Femmes et des Enfants
Avenue Paul Vaillant Couturier 16
FR 94807 Villejuif Cedex
Phone: +33 1 45 59 59 90
Fax: +33 1 45 59 50 89
Contract number: CT931064

Participants:

A. MacFARLANE
National Perinatal
Epidemiology Unit
Radcliffe Infirmary
UK Oxford OX2 6HE
Phone: +44 865 224 876
Fax: +44 865 726 360

C. WOLFE
UMDS, Div. of
Community Health,
Dept. of Public
Health Medicine
Lambeth Palace Road
UK London SE1 7EH
Phone: +44 71 928 9292
Fax: +44 71 928 1468

Dra. M. Da PURIFICAÇAO
ALAUJO
Direction Générale des soins
de santé, Div. de SM-PF
Al D. Afonso Henriques 45
PT 1000 Lisboa
Phone: +351 1 847 55 19
Fax: +351 1 847 66 39

Dr. A. TABOR
Herlev Hospital,
University of Copenhagen
Herlev Ringrej 75
DK 2730 Herlev
Phone: +45 44 53 53 00
Fax: +45 44 53 53 32

Dr. D. CHOPIN
O.N.E.
Av. de la Toison d'Or 64
BE 1060 Bruxelles
Phone: +32 2542 12 11

Dr. G.M. McILWAINE
Greater Glasgow Health
Board,
Glasgow Royal Maternity
Hospital
Rottenrow
UK Glasgow G4 ONO
Phone: +44 41 552 3400 218
Fax: +44 41 552 0737 280

Dr. Pr. Hermann WELSCH
Candid Str. 20/VII
DE W-8000 Munchen 90
Phone: +49 652456

Dr. P. JASZCZAK
Herlev Hospital,
Unversity of Copenhagen
Herlev Ringrej 75
DK 2730 Herlev
Phone: +45 44 53 53 00
Fax: +45 44 53 53 32

Dr. S. ALEXANDER
Ecole de Santé Publique,
Campus Erasme-ULB-CP
590/6
BE 1070 Bruxelles
Phone: +32 2 555 40 63
Fax: +32 2 555 40 49

F. HATTON
Institut National de la Santé
et de la Recherche Médicale,
U 149
Bd. de Port-Royal 123
FR 75014 Paris
Phone: +33 34 80 24 30
Fax: +33 34 80 24 48

G. BREART
Institut National de la Santé
et de la Recherche Médicale,
U 149
Bd. de Port-Royal`123
FR 75014 Paris
Phone: +33 43 26 00 46
Fax: +33 43 26 89 79

J.P. MACKENBACH
Faculteit der Geneeskunde en
Gezondheids-Wetenschappen
P.O. Box 1738
NL 3000 Dr. Rotterdam
Phone: +33 31 10 408 77 20
Fax: +33 31 10 436 68 31

Dr. J.BENNENBROEK
GRAVENHORST
Dept. of Obstetrics,
Univ Hospital
Rijnsburgerweg 10
NL 2333 AA Leiden
Phone: +31 71 269 111
Fax: +31 71 223 462

P.BUEKENS
Ecole de Santé Publique,
Campus Erasme-ULB-CP
590/6
BE 1070 Bruxelles
Phone: +32 3 555 40 18
Fax: +32 2 555 40 46

COORDINATED CASE-CONTROL STUDIES TO DETERMINE WAYS OF REDUCING SUDDEN INFANT DEATH SYNDROME, SIDS, RATES IN EUROPE

Key words
Sudden Infant Death Syndrome (SIDS), child health care, infant care practices.

Brief description
Sudden infant Death Syndrome, (SIDS) is a major cause of infant mortality but rates vary in different parts of Europe and very recently rates have fallen rapidly in some countries.

Concerted Action is therefore proposed to harmonize protocols and coordinate a network of case-control enquiries in 15 centres from 12 European countries. By combining data from these studies and meta analysis exploiting differences between countries, the project will obtain scientific data to improve the effectiveness of child health care. specifically the study will examine the extent to which pronation is currently used in Europe and possible risks associated with other current practices of putting infants to sleep, including clothing, bedding heating and co-sleeping.

Also in view of the changes in mortality, the study will re-assess previously known risk factors eg:- socio-economic status. maternal age parity and history of infection in pregnancy and infancy;parental smoking sex; low birth weight; multiple birth; bottle feeding; season of birth; history of apnoea; history of infection; etc.

CA will make it possible to evaluate the prevalence of high risk practices quickly, to examine a wider range of infant care practices than would otherwise be possible, and to study interactions between risks and how these vary in relation to the socio-cultural background.

The project is expected to lead to recommendations on measures to reduce the risk of SIDS.

Project leader:
Dr. Robert CARPENTER
London School of Hygiene and Tropical Medicine
Keppel Street
UK London WC1E 7HT
Phone: +44 71 927 22 61
Fax: +44 71 436 42 30
Contract number: CT931207

Participants:

Dr. E.M. TAYLOR
The Children's Hospital
Western Bank
UK Sheffield S10 2TH
Phone: +44 74 276 1111
Fax: +44 74 275 5364

Dr. K.W. TIETZE
Institut fur Sozialmedizin
und Epidemiologie des
Bundesgesundheitsamtes
Werner-Voss-Damm 62
DE 1000 Berlin 42
Phone: +49 30 185 4044
Fax: +49 30 786 1036

Dr. C. BACON
Yorkshire Health,
The Queen Building
Park Parade
UK Harrogate HG1 5AH
Phone: +44 423 500066
Fax: +44 423 568253

Dr. C. MORLEY
Dep of Paediatrics,
Addenbrooke's Hospital
Hills Road
UK Cambridge CB2 2QQ
Phone: +44 223 33 6886
Fax: +44 223 33 6996

Dr. G. WENNERGREN
Dept. of Pediatrica I,
Gothenburg Univ,
East Hospital
SE 416 85 Gothenberg
Phone: +46 31 37 4000
Fax: +46 31 84 3010

Dr. K. HELWEG LARSON
Inst. of Forensic Medicine,
Univ of Copenhagen
DK Copenhagen
Phone: +45 3 537 3222
Fax: +45 3 537 1651

Dr. STRAMBA-BADIALE
Univ of Milan,
Clinica Medica
Via Francesco Sforza 35
IT 20122 Milan
Phone: +39 2 551 3366
Fax: +39 2 545 1666

Dr. P. FLEMING
Dept. of Child Health,
St. Michael's Hospital
Southwell Street
UK Bristol BS2 8EG
Phone: +44 27228 5226
Fax: +44 27228 5751

D.C. EINSPIELER
Dept. of Physiology,
Univ of Graz
Harrach Gasse 21/5
AT 8010 Graz
Phone: +43 316 380 4276
Fax: +43 316 383 686

J.H. JOHANSSON
Patologisk Institut
IS 121 Reykjavik
Phone: +35 4160 1930
Fax: +35 4160 1904

Ms. B. KIBERD
Registrar &
Research Officier,
Carmichael House
North Brunswick Street 4
IE Dublin 7
Phone: +353 1872 6199
Fax: +353 1872 6056

Prof. A. KAHN
Univ Hosp for Children,
Queen Fabiola
Avenue J.J. Crocq 15
BE 1020 Bruxelles
Phone: +32 2 477 3280
Fax: +32 2 477 3289

Prof. E. MALLET
Pediatrie, Hospital du Nicolle
FR 76031 Rouen
Phone: +33 3 508 8187
Fax: +33 3 508 8188

Prof. G. JORCH
Univ Muster, Klinik und
Poli fur Kinderheilkunde
Albert Schweitzer Strasse 33
DE 4400 Muster
Phone: +49 2 51 831
Fax: +49 2 51 836 960

Prof. J. HUBER
Univ Hosp for
Children & Youth,
Wilhelmina Childrens
Hospital
P.O. Box 18009
NL 3501 CA Utrecht
Phone: +31 30 320 274
Fax: +31 30 334 825

Prof. L. IRGENS
Med Register of Norway,
Armauer Hansen Building,
Haukeland Hospital
NO 5021 Bergen
Phone: +47 55 298 060
Fax: +47 55 974 998

CONCERTED ACTION PROGRAMME ON QUALITY ASSURANCE IN HOSPITALS II

Key words
Quality assurance, hospitals, external QA programs.

Brief description
The concerted action programme on quality assurance in hospitals. It will be building on the network of 16 teams and 262 hospitals created during the first concerted action programme between 1990-1993.

This second programme will run from 1-7-93 to 1-12-95 and consist out of:

1 An action programme for hospitals, focusing on two multidisciplinary problem area's. After the preparatory phase hospitals can participate in an action phase during which they are asked to execute a quality assurance study and try to introduce change. During the evaluation phase results in terms of outcome of the studies and successfulness in implementing change Will be assessed by means of modified versions of previously used instruments.

2 Three Workshops will be held on discussing the effect on the implementation of quality assurance mechanisms of:

a the legal sytem;

b the financial system;

c external QA programs such as accreditation/certification.

Project leader:
Dr. Niek KLAZINGA
CBO, National Organization for
Quality Assurance in Hospitals
P.O. Box 20064
NL 3502 LB Utrecht
Phone: +31 30 96 06 47
Fax: +31 30 94 36 44
Contract number: CT931106

Participants:
A. GIRAUD
Centre National de L'Equipement Hospitalier
Rue Antoine Chautin 9
FR 75014 Paris
Phone: +33 1 40441515
Fax: +33 1 40448234

A. CASPARIE
Dept. of Health Policy and Management
P.O. Box 1738
NL 3000 Dr. Rotterdam
Phone: +31 10 4088003
Fax: +31 10 4360717

E. REERINK
CBO
P.O. Box 20064
NL 3502 LB Utrecht
Phone: +31 30 960647
Fax: +31 30 943644

R. SUNOL
Avedis Donabedian Foundation
Diagonal 341
ES 08037 Barcelona
Phone: +34 3 4592908
Fax: +34 3 2076608

COPING WITH PHYSICAL ILLNESS WITH A PARTICULAR FOCUS ON BLOOD DYSCRASIAS

Key words
Risk factors, protector factors, coping, resilience, haemophilia, thalassaemia.

Brief description
Most studies of families confronted with adversity focus on ill health.

In contrast, the theoretical foundations of this project are based on risk, protective factors and coping. The aim of the study is to explore the factors associated with coping and resilience in families and children in which one parent suffers from haemophilia, or a child from Thalassaemia. For these purposes, we intend to address a cohort of families with a blood dyscrasia with the model of dyscrasia being haemophilia and thalassaemia. A battery of inventories will be applied relating to family and individual psychological qualities with particular reference to coping and resilience. Surprisingly this is a very poorly explored area with major informational gaps.

Haemophilia and Thalassaemia are stresseul conditions for families in their own right. They are chronic conditions, for example, haemophilia as characterised by recurrent bleeding, at times precipitated by only very minor trauma. Family life is disrupted not only by the diseases and their symptomatology, but also by frequent visits to the hospital for treatment, and even home treatment. The stress level in families may be very high.

The design to be used follows that employed in major studies or coping with social and other forms of psychological adversity. The availability of well developed and rigorously validated instruments for the measurement of psychopathology and behavioural adjustment means that the proposed research is now feasible.

It should be able to develop a profile of characteristics associated with coping, which will enable a better understanding of the nature of resilience. This information may provide assistance to care workers and also other families facing similar adversities.

Project leader:
Professor Israel KOLVIN
The Tavistock Centre
Academic Unit of Child
and Family Mental Health
Belsize Lane 120
UK London NW3 5BA
Phone: +44 71 435 71 11
Fax: +44 71 431 53 82
Contract number: CT931517

Participants:
Dr. Christine A. LEE
Haemophilia Centre,
Royal Free Hospital
Pond Street
UK London NW3 2QG
Phone: +44 71 794 0500
Fax: +44 71 431 8276

Prof. Brent TAYLOR
The Royal Free
Hosp School of Med,
Dept. of Child Health
Rowland Hill Street
UK London NW3 2QG
Phone: +44 71 794 0500
Fax: +44 71 830 2003

Prof. John TSIANTIS
Aghia Sophia Children's
Hospital, Dept. of
Psychological Paediatrics
Thivon and Mikras Asias
GR 11527 Goudi-Athens
Phone: +30 1 779 8748
Fax: +30 1 779 7649

Prof. P. M. MANNUCCI
Inst. of Internal Medicine,
Univ of Milano
Via Pace 9
IT Milano 20122
Phone: +39 2 551 6093
Fax: +39 2 551 6093

Prof. Titika MANDALAKI
2nd Reg Blood
Tranfusion Centre,
Laikon Gen Hosp of Athens
Agiou Thoma Str. 17
GR 11527 Athens Goudi
Phone: +30 1 77 71 138
Fax: +30 1 77 79 774

APPROPRIATENESS OF HOSPITAL USE: AN EUROPEAN PROJECT ASSESSING THE MEDICAL APPROPRIATENESS OF HOSPITAL UTILIZATION AND ITS STRUCTURAL, FINANCIAL AND SOCIAL DETERMINANTS

Key words
Appropriateness of hospital use, structural, organizational, social determinants, organizational/financial incentives.

Brief description
The objectives proposed are: to improve methods for evaluating the appropriateness of use of hospitals within Europe to develop a common methodology to measure appropriateness of hospital use and to identify its structural, organizational and social determinants accross Europe to promote and coordinate national pilot studies to test the yield of the common methodologic set-up during the initial phase of the project to assure effective dissemination of the findings from these studies to policy makers hospital administrators, and national organisations responsible for quality assurance to design and promote a multicenter European study aimed at quantifying the amount of inappropriate hospital use, its determinants with reference to the role of general practice and of different local organizational/financial incentives to the use of hospital resource.

Project leader:
Dr. Alessandro LIBERATI
Istituto di Ricerche Farmacologiche 'Mario Negri'
Via Eritrea 62
IT 20157 Milano
Phone: +39 23 901 44 86
Fax: +39 23 54 62 77
Contract number: CT931053

Participants:

Dr. Christian KOECK
Vienna City Hospital
Administration,
Organizational Development
Zelinkagasse 9/2
AT 1010 Vienna
Phone: +43 1 531 14 87751
Fax: +43 1 531 14 7931

Dr. Giovanni APOLONE
Laboratorio di
Epidemiologia Clinica,
Istituto Mario Negri
Via Eritrea 62
IT 20157 Milano
Phone: +39 2 39014519
Fax: +39 2 3320031

Dr. Gyles R. GLOVER
Charing Cross &
Westminster Medical School,
Dep of Community Med
Horseferry Road 17
UK London SWIP 2AR
Phone: +44 81 746 8157
Fax: +44 81 746 8806

Dr. Margherita BENDES
Direcao General
dos Hospitais
Avenida Republica No 61/4
PT 1000 Lisboa
Phone: +351 1 763047
Fax: +351 1 7931919

Dr. R. SUNOL
Quality Assurance Dept. &
Pharmacy Service,
Hosp de la Santa Creu
i Sant Pau
St. Antoni M. Claret 167
ES 08025 Barcelona
Phone: +34 3 347 3133
Fax: +34 3 456 0190

Dr. Thierry LANG
Serv de Biostatistique et
Informatique Medicale,
CHU Pietiè
Bd de l'Hopital
FR 75013 Paris Cedex
Phone: +33 1 4586 1998
Fax: +33 1 4586 5685

EFFICIENCY IN ORAL HEALTH CARE: THE EVALUATION OF ORAL HEALTH SYSTEMS IN EUROPE

Key words

Effectiveness, cost containment, quality of care, oral health care systems, outcome indicators, oral health status.

Brief description

Health policy in member states is required to address difficulties in the financing and delivery of health care and recently reform strategies have extended to a restructuring of the organisation of health care systems.

Within the reform strategies, particular emphasis has been placed on the design of systems for provider payment. The effectiveness of alternative strategies in terms of cost containment are reasonably clearly established.

The impact of payment systems on the quality of care as well as on the effective utilisation of services is much more problematic. The measurement of final outcome as the ultimate test of quality is even more difficult both for the health system as a whole and for individual services.

Oral health care systems share many of the structural challenges faced by health care in general. They have also been subject to review and redesign in terms of funding and payment policies. However, outcome indicators are more accessible in the context of oral health care because of the existence of well-established measures of oral health status.

These measures represent potential indicators of the impact of programme design on the content and outcome of interventions. They, therefore, represent an important tool for proceeding beyond process and cost evaluation to the level of the effectiveness of system design. In this sense, oral health care represents a marker for policy development with regard to health care systems as a whole.

In this project, a comprehensive analysis of six third party funding systems currently in operation in member states will be undertaken.

Information currently available on inputs and outputs will be collated following which the partners will develop agreed methods for their objective measurement. These agreed methods will then be piloted in each of the six systems for six months. The Final Report will include recommendations for measuring inputs into oral health care systems in such a way that their influence on oral health levels over time can be measured. Using oral health care as a model, recommendations will be made also on how to proceed in other health care areas to adopt systems which will allow the effects of inputs on health status to be measured.

Project leader:
Professor Denis O'MULLANE
Oral Health Services Research Centre,
Cork Farm Centre
Dennehy's Cross
IE Cork
Phone: +353 21 27 68 71
Fax: +353 21 54 53 91
Contract number: CT931624

Participants:

Dr. Carolina MANAU
Faculty of Odontology, L'Hospital Llobregat,
Dep of Prev and Comm Dentistry
Feixa Llarca Sin
ES Llobregat
Phone: +34 3 4024200
Fax: +34 3 4179266

Dr. David BARMES
World Health Organisation
CH P1211 Geneva 27
Phone: +41 227 912111
Fax: +41 227 910746

Dr. David PARKIN
Dep of Epidemiology and Public Health,
Univ of Newcastle Upon Tyne
UK Newcastle Upon Tyne NE2 4HH
Phone: +44 323 417000
Fax: +44 323 433517

Dr. Klaus KONING
Univ of Nijmegen Dental School
P.O. Box 9101
NL 6500 HB Nijmegen
Phone: +31 80 614043
Fax: +31 80 541314

Dr. Paul PETERSEN
The Royal Dental College Copenhagen,
Univ of Copenhagen
Norre Alle 20
DK 2200 Copenhagen N
Phone: +45 35 32 6790
Fax: +45 35 37 65 05

Mr. Dermot McCARTHY
National Economic and Social Council
Dublin Castle
IE Dublin
Phone: +353 1 713155
Fax: +353 1 713589

Ms. Jean TODD
Dental Data Service, Dental Practice Board
UK Eastbourne
Phone: +44 71 8373646
Fax: +44 71 9151233

Prof. Denis O'MULLANE
Dr. Helen WHELTON
Oral Health Services, Res Centre,
Cork Farm Centre
Dennehy's Cross
IE Cork
Phone: +353 21 27 68 71
Fax: +353 21 54 53 91

Prof. Martin DOWNER
Eastman Dental Hospital
Grays Inn Road 256
UK London WC1 X SLD
Phone: +44 91 222 6000
Fax: +44 01 222 8211

Prof. Pierre CAHEN
Univ Louis Pasteur, Fac Chir Dentaire
Place L'Hopital 1
FR 6700 Strasbourg
Phone: +33 88 362526
Fax: +33 88 212620

EC COORDINATION OF THERAPEUTIC TRIALS
IN SYSTEMIC VASCULITIS

Key words
ANCA (anti-neutrophil cytoplasmic autoantibodies), systematic vasculitis, multi-centre clinical trials, epidemiology, harmonising and optimising treatment.

Brief description
Presence of ANCA (anti-neutrophil cytoplasmic autoantibodies) is closely correlated to systemic vasculitis. European researchers have been leading in the description of ANCA and the possible pathogenic importance of ANCA for systemic vasculitis. Due to the growing understanding of these mechanisms and new options for modulating the immune response, treatment of systemic vasculitis has become a promising field.

Through the succesful work performed by the EC/BCR Group for ANCA Assay Standardisation, established in 1989 and now including 9 EC countries, an urgent need for co-ordinated multi-centre clinical trials in systemic vasculitis has been revealed. Although the prevalence of systemic vasculitis of 1:5,000 Europeans and the frequently severe condition of these patients implies a substantial socio-economic impact on the national health care systems, the annual incidence of patients available for clinical trials at most European University Centres is usually only around 10. As 100 patients are frequently necessary for conducting clinical trials, multi-centre trials are imperative. Moreover, as there are great differences in the incidence and prevalence of the individual diseases within the group of systemic vasculitises in the various European countries and as treatment modalities available to the different University centres are not uniform, the presently proposed project can be instrumental for describing the epidemiology of systemic vasculitis within the EC as well as serving the purpose of harmonising and optimising treatment of the individual disorders within the EC.

It is expected that a concerted action building on the established network of the EC/BCR Group for ANCA Assay Standardisation will increase the scientific value and the cost-effectiveness of therapeutic trials. In addition it is expected that the extension and reinforcement of this network will facilitate the spreading of improved treatment modalities to all parts of the EC and thus be of importance for reducing the estimated annual cost of 150 - 200 million ECU for treatment of patients with systemic vasculitis in the EC.

Project leader:
Dr. Niels RASMUSEN
Othopathology Laboratory,
Department of Othopathology
Blegdamsvej 9
DK 2100 Copenhagen
Phone: +45 35 45 28 07
Fax: +45 35 45 26 90
Contract number: CT931078

Participants:

Dr. A. G. TZIOUFAS
Dep of Internal Med,
Univ of Ioannina Med School
GR 451 10 Ioannina
Phone: +30 651 92728
Fax: +30 651 92944

Dr. Charles PUSEY
Royal Postgrad. Med School,
Renal Unit, Dep of Med,
Hammersmith Hosp
Du Cane Road
UK London W12 ONN
Phone: +44 81 740 3152
Fax: +44 81 746 2410

Dr. Chris HAGEN
Dept. of Nephrology,
Academisch Ziekenhuis
Leiden
P.O. Box 9600
NL 2300 RC Leiden
Phone: +31 71 26 21 48
Fax: +31 71 21 07 14

Dr. Daniel ABRAMOWICZ
Lab of Immunology,
Hopital Erasme,
Free Univ of Brussels
Route de Lennik 808
BE 1070 Bruxelles
Phone: +32 2 555 3862
Fax: +32 2 555 4499

Dr. David R.W. JAYNE
Dep of Med,
School of Clin Med,
Univ of Cambridge
Hills Road
UK Cambridge CB1 2QQ
Phone: +44 223 33 67 44
Fax: +44 223 41 10 52

Dr. Eduardo MIRAPEIX
Servicio de Nefrologia,
Hospital Clinic I Provincial
ES 08036 Barcelona
Phone: +34 3 454 26 12
Fax: +34 3 454 08 07

Dr. K.W.A. WESTMAN
Dep of Nephrology,
Univ Hosp of Lund
SE 221 85 Lund
Phone: +46 46 17 12 48
Fax: +46 46 11 17 65

Prof. C. KALLENBERG
Univ of Groningen,
Lab for Clin Immunology
Oostersingel 59
NL 9713 EZ Groningen
Phone: +31 50 61 29 45
Fax: +31 50 61 34 74

Prof. Konrad ANDRASSY
Sektion Nephrologie,
Klinikum der Univ
Heidelberg
Bergheimer Strasse 56a
DE 69115 Heidelberg
Phone: +49 6221 91 120
Fax: +49 6221 16 24 76

Prof. Loic GUILLEVIN
Hopital Avicenne,
Univ de Paris
Rue de Stalingrad 125
FR 93009 Bobigny Cedex
Phone: +33 1 48 95 53 51
Fax: +33 1 48 95 54 50

Prof. Paul Anthony BACON
Dep of Rheumatology,
Medical School,
Univ of Birmingham
Vincent Drive
UK Birmingham B15 2TT
Phone: +44 21 414 6776
Fax: +44 21 414 6790

Prof. Philippe LESAVRE
Dep. de Nephrologie 8
Inserm U90,
Hopital Necker
Rue de Sèvres
FR 75743 Paris Cedex 15
Phone: +33 1 44 49 00 00
Fax: +33 1 45 66 51 33

Prof. Renato Alberto SINICO
Dep of Nephrology,
Ospedale San Carlo
Borromeo
Via Pio II 3
IT 20153 Milano
Phone: +39 2 40 22 24 89
Fax: +39 2 40 22 22 22

Prof. Wolfgang L. GROSS
Rheumaklinik Bad Bramstedt,
Med Univ zu Lübeck
Oskar Alexander Strasse 26
DE 24576 Bad Bramstedt
Phone: +49 4192 90 25 76
Fax: +49 4192 90 23 89

THE EFFECT OF ORGANISATION AND MANAGEMENT ON THE EFFECTIVENESS AND EFFICIENCY OF INTENSIVE CARE UNITS IN THE COUNTRIES OF THE EUROPEAN COMMUNITY

Key words
Organisation, management, intensive care units, performance of ICUs.

Objectives
a make an inter-disciplinary inventory of the relevant characteristics of ICUs in Europe from a Health Services Research perspective;
b define performance indicators for evaluating the effectiveness of organisation and management (O & M) of intensive care units (ICUs);
c determine the operational aspects of O & M which influence the performance, effectiveness and efficiency of ICUs;
d harmonise approaches to the O & M of ICUs in the countries of the European community.

Brief description
Prospective study. In each ICU, the O & M, patient care, and manpower systems are studied according with the general system theory (inputs/ throughputs/outputs). The ICUs are studied on four levels of aggregation:
a individual ICU;
b global European sample;
c national samples;
d requirements of care (ICU Levels of Care) in previous samples.

Setting: In 4 to 8 ICUs of one national region in each of 13 European countries, enrolling 100 ICUs, 18,000 patient admissions, 4,000 ICU staff members, and involving 25 research teams of different disciplines (medicine health services research, economics, O & M, psychology and statistics).

Interventions: At ICU level: daily collection of Patient Care System data, during four months; collection of O & M and Manpower Systems data, during six months (questionnaires, site visits and interviews).

Measurements: Quantification of the variables identifying the relevant characteristics of inputs/throughputs/outputs of each of the three systems at ICU level, using available instruments. using individual patient and/or individual ICU data, analysis will firstly focus upon the modeling of ICU performance indicators, also aggregated into standardized ratios of the European sample and, secondly, associate the various observed levels of O & M and the corresponding levels of performance.

Results expected: Besides those indicated in pected that the programme will strengthen and extend the existing network of research, providing the EC member states with objective instruments for the standardized evaluation of performance of ICUs.

Project leader:

Dr. Dinis REIS-MIRANDA
Intensive Care Unit,
Department of Surgery,
University Hospital
Groningen
P.O. Box 30001
NL 9700 RB Groningen
Phone: +31 50 61 43 79
Fax: +31 50 61 48 73
Contract number: CT931340

Participants:

Dr. A. FRUTIGER
Dir. Interdisciplinary ICU,
Kantonsspital
Loestrasse 120
CH 7000 Chur

Dr. GRANADOS I
NAVARRETE
Cap de l'Oficina
Técnica d'Avaluacio
de Tecnologia Médica
Pavello Ave Maria 131-159
ES 08028 Barcelona

Dr. A. KARI
Dept. of Intensive Care,
Kuopio Univ Hospital
FI 70210 Kuopio

Dr. C. NOWOROL
Jagiellonian Univ,
Dept. of Work Psychology
and Ergonomics
Pilsudskiego 13
PL 31 110 Krakow

Dr. D. EDBROOKE
Intensive Care Unit,
Royal Hallamshire Hospital
UK Sheffield

Dr. D.W. RYAN
General ITU,
Freeman Hospital
High Heaton
UK Newcastle Upon Tyne
NE7 7DN

Dr. G. IAPICHINO
Reparto di Rianimazione E.
Vecla, Ospedale Maggiore de
Milano
Via F. Sforza 35
IT 20122 Milano

Dr. G. SANDERS
Dept. of Organisation,
Technology and Innovation,
Univ of Groningen
P.O. Box 800
NL 9700 AV Groningen

Dr. G. VAZQUEZ MATA
Jefe del Servicio
de M Intensiva,
H.G.E. Virgen de las Nieves
Avda Coronel Munoz 2
ES 18014 Granada

Dr. J.P. ALEXANDER
Middelheim General Hospital
Lindendreef 1
BE 2020 Antwerpen

Dr. K. ROWAN
Dept. of Public Health and
Primary Care,
Univ of Oxford
Radcliffe Infirmary
UK Oxford OX2 6HE

Dr. M. HEMMER
Centre Hospitalier
Rue Barblé 4
LU Luxembourg

Dr. MOREIRA BRANDAO
Serviço de Cuidados
Intensivos,
Hospital Geral de
Santo Antonio,
Largo da Escola Médica
PT 4000 Porto

Dr. Ph. LOIRAT
Centre Médico-Chirurgical
Foch
Rue Worth 40
FR 92151 Suresnes

Dr. P.F. HULSTAERT
Dept. of Surgery,
Univ Hospital Utrecht
Heidelberglaan 100
NL 3584 CX Utrecht

Dr. R. ABIZANDA
Medicina Intensiva,
Hospital Son Dureta
ES Palma

Dr. W.B. SCHAUFELI
Dept. of Work and
Organisational Psychology,
Univ of Nijmegen
P.O. Box 9104
NL 6500 HE Nijmegen

Miss B.L. ATKINSON
Clinical Services Manager,
Intensive Care Services,
Southampton General Hosp.
Tremona Road
UK Southampton SO9 4XY

Prof. A. WILLIAMS
Inst. for Research in the
Social Sciences,
Univ of York
Heslington
UK York YO1 5DD

Prof. Dr. F.F.H. RUTTEN
Inst. for Medical Technology
Assessment,
Erasme Univ
P.O. Box 1738
NL 3000 Dr. Rotterdam

Prof. Dr. L. DRAGSTED
Herlev Hospital,
Dept. of Intensive Care,
Univ of Copenhagen
Herlev Ringvej
DK 2730 Herlev

Prof. Dr. S. LEMISHOW
School of Public Health,
Unversity of Massachusetts
US Amherst MA 01003

Prof. Dr. W. Van ROSSUM
Dept. of Organisation,
Technology and Innovation,
Univ of Groningen
P.O. Box 800
NL 9700 AV Groningen

Prof. H. BURCHARDI
Georg-August Universität
Robert Koch Strasse 40
DE 3400 Göttingen

Prof. J.R. LE GALL
Réanimation Médicale,
Hospital St Louis
Av. Cloude-Vellefaux 1
FR 75010 Paris

EURO-CRIS EUROPEAN CLINICAL RESEARCH INFORMATION SYSTEMS

Key words
Database, randomized clinical trials, HIV, AIDS.

Brief description
Euro-cris is a feasibility study and implementation of a database of all randomized clinical trials in HIV-infected persons, in Europe. The data-base which will form the core of this information system will be:

a exhaustive: all trials will be eligible, regardless of country, participant(s), sponsor, phase of study and investigational agent(s), so long as they are properly randomized;

b up-to-date: data on all trials, whether on-going or terminated, will be kept and regularly updated;

c clinically useful: the database will contain information of direct relevance to clinicians and biostatisticians;

d easy-to-use: at the computer level, the man-machine interface of the system will be highly sophisticated according to the state of the art in the domain.

The system will be designed so as to be applicable to all disease areas, but as a first step it is proposed to carry out a feasibility study with trials in AIDS patients and HIV-infected persons.

A European network of experts will collaborate in the project. 11 teams are planned. At this time, top level representatives of each major European countries are engaged in EURO-CRIS. INSERM in France, Heidelberg University in Germany, the MRC in the United Kingdom, among others. Close collaboration with the ENTA has also been secured. After approval of the project by C.E., the existing network will immediately be expanded to include other member states (the Netherlands, Denmark, Portugal and Greece) in which no representative has yet been identified.

Project leader:
Dr. Marc BUYSE
International Institute for
Drug Development (ID2)
Avenue Louise 430
BE 1050 Bruxelles
Phone: +32 2 6468918
Fax: +32 2 6468662
Contract number: CT941610

Participants:
B. LEDERBERGER
Swiss HIV Cohort Study,
Coordination Center
Zürichbergstrasse 29
CH 8032 Zürich
Phone: +41 1 2621662
Fax: +41 1 2621674

F. LIBEAU
Hendyplan S.A.
59 rue du Prince Royal
BE 1050 Brussels
Phone: +32 2 5131854
Fax: +32 2 5142877

J. DARBYSHIRE
MRC HIV Clinical Trials
Centre Royal Brompton
National Heart and
Lung Hospital
Sydney Street
UK London SW3 6NP
Phone: +44 49 71 3518043
Fax: +44 49 71 3518096

J.F. CHAMBON
ARCAT-SIDA
57 rue Saint-Louis en l'Ile
FR 75004 Paris
Phone: +33 1 43546715
Fax: +33 1 46331142

J.P. ABOULKER
INSERM SC10,
Hôpital Paul-Brousse
16 avenue Paul Vaillant
Couturier
FR 94807 Villejuif Cedex
Phone: +33 1 45595113
Fax: +33 1 45595180

THE HARMONIZATION BY CONSENSUS OF THE METHODOLOGY FOR ECONOMIC EVALUATION OF HEALTH TECHNOLOGIES IN THE EC

Key words
Economic evaluation, health technologies.

Brief description
The objective of the project is to develop and propose a unified methodology for the economic evaluation of health technologies to be adopted by EC regulatory agencies, national administrations and European multinational companies operating in the health care field with the eventual aim of harmonizing regulatory practices across EC countries. The main benefit form that harmonization will be its contribution to the achievement of an effective single market through the reduction of artificial barriers to free trade. This is expected to increase the competitiveness of European companies in world markets and also ensure that EC members states secure health technologies for their populations at a cost-effective level. Other benefits will be inceased transferability of the results of the studies from one setting to an other, improvement in the quality of the studies and the availability of a basic tool for carrying out multinational economic evaluation studies.

Project leader:
Dr. Joan Rovira FORNS
University of Barcelona
Gran via de les Corts catalanes 585
ES 08071 Barcelona
Phone: +34 3 3184266
Fax: +34 3 3025947
Contract number: CT941252

Participants:

Dr. A. AMENT
Dept. of Health Economics
Universiteitensingel 50
NL 6229 ER Maastricht
Phone: +31 4388 1727
Fax: +31 4367 0960

Dr. B. JÖNSSON
Centre for Health Economics,
School of Economics
P.O. Box 6501
SE 11383 Stockholm
Phone: +46 8 7369281
Fax: +46 8 3021156

Dr. C. HANAU
Dipartamento di Statistica
Universita degli Studi
di Bologna
Via Belle Arti, 41
IT 40126 Bologna
Phone: +39 51 258250
Fax: +39 51 227997

Dr. E. SOUETRE
Benefit
2 rue Louis Armanad
FR 92600 Asnieres

Dr. F. ANTOÑANZAS
Facultad de Derecho
Obispo Fidel Garcia, s/n
ES 26004 Logroño
Phone: +34 41 250811
Fax: +34 41 254636

Dr. F. RAMOS
Escola Nacional de Saúde
Pública
Avda. Padre Cruz
PT 1699 Lisboa Codex
Phone: +351 1 7585599
Fax: +351 1 7582754

Dr. J. ROVIRA
Soikos, S.L.
Arizala 1, entlo. 1a
ES 08034 Barcelona
Phone: +34 3 4498070
Fax: +34 3 3344935

Dr. J.C. SAILLY
Cresge
1, rue Norbert Ségard,
BP 109
FR 59016 Lille Cedex
Phone: +33 20 571177
Fax: +33 20 151903

Dr. M. BUXTON
Health Economics Research
Group, Brunel Univ
UK Uxbridge UB8 3PP
Phone: +44 895 203331
Fax: +44 895 203330

Dr. M. SCHNEIDER
BASYS GmbH
Reisingerstrasse 25
DE 8900 Augsburg 1
Phone: +49 821 571093-2579
Fax: +49 821 579341

Dr. P. KOCH
Federal Office of Social Insurances,
Medical Div.
Effingerstrasse 33
CH 3003 Berne
Phone: +41 31 619125

Dr. R. CHRZANOWSKI
Swiss Public Health Inst.
Pfrudweg 14
CH 5001 Aarau
Phone: +41 64 247161
Fax: +41 64 245138

Dr. R.J. LAUNOIS
Université de Paris Nord UFR de Bobigny
FR 75116 Paris
Phone: +33 1 45048271

Dr. A. ALBAN
Dansk Sygehus Institut
Landemaerket 10
DK 1119 Copenhagen K
Phone: +45 3311 5777
Fax: +45 3393 1019

Dr. A. BRANDT
I.M.I.B.
Bachtelenweg 3
CH 4125 Riehen
Phone: +41 61 673810
Fax: +41 61 673754

Dr. T. SEEGER
Reimbursement Officer, Cochlear AG
Clarastrasse 12
CH 4058 Basel
Phone: +41 61 6819300

Ms. M.R. van MÖLKEN
Dept. of Health Economics
Universiteitensingel 50 (Wijk 29)
NL 6229 ER Maastricht
Phone: +31 4388 1727
Fax: +31 4367 0960

M. Pierre-Jean LANCRY
Credes
1, rue Paul Cézanne
FR 75008 Paris
Phone: +33 1 40768215
Fax: +33 1 45635742

M.Ph. BOIRON
Credes
14, Passage Dubail
FR 75010 Paris
Phone: +33 1 42380040
Fax: +33 1 40050456

Prof. F. ROSSI
Instituto di Economia Sanitaria
Via Boccaccio, 14
IT 20123 Milano
Phone: +39 2 4693460
Fax: +39 2 48195851

Prof. F. RUTTEN
Inst. for Med. Technology Ass.,
Erasmus Univ, Medical Faculty
P.O. Box 1738
NL 3000 Dr. Rotterdam
Phone: +31 10408 7317
Fax: +31 10436 0717

Prof. M. DRUMMOND
Center for Health Economics, Univ of York
Heslington
UK York YO1 5DD
Phone: +44 904 433709
Fax: +44 904 433644

Prof. P. BONDONIO
CRESA
Corso Massimo d'Azegklio, 42
IT 19125 Torino
Phone: +39 11 687708
Fax: +39 11 6699500

EUROPEAN CLEARING HOUSE ON
HEALTH SYSTEMS REFORMS

Key words
Health care systems, health care reformers, policy-makers, Clearing House.

Brief description
Many European health care systems are undergoing major organisational and managerial change founded on principles which are far-reaching but, as yet, largely based upon limited testing and evaluation.
Health care reformers are 'learning by doing'. Given the far-reaching nature of the reforms, it is important to collect and collate information about similarities and variations in their nature and impact. There is immense scope for cross-national learning which would be of enormous assistance to policy-makers and practitioners across Europe as well as the research community.
It is proposed to establish a Clearing House containing a central repository for information about the introduction and development of health systems reforms, together with an assessment based on the findings from research investigating their impact.
The Clearing House will initially comprise 3 centres: the Nuffield Institute for Health Services Studies (University of Leeds, UK) which will act as project coordinator; Escuela Nacional de Sanidad (Ministerio de Sanidad y Consumo, Madrid) and the Department of Public Health (University of Helsinki, Finland).
The first year of the project will be devoted by the 3 participating centres to expanding the network and membership of the Clearing House within the EC to those research centres active in the monitoring and evaluation of health systems reforms in their respective countries.
The Clearing House will provide a forum for information exchange between researchers and practitioners.
This will take the form of international meetings, visits to participating centres and those which might become participants, a newsletter to bring important research findings to the attention of key policy-makers, practitioners and managers, and workshops at which policy-makers can interrogate and learn from cross-national research in dialogue with practitioners and researchers.

Project leader:
Professor David James HUNTER
Nuffield Institute of Health,
University of Leeds
Clarendon Road 71-75
UK Leeds L3 9PL
Phone: +44 53 2459034
Fax: +44 53 2460899
Contract number: CT941258

Participants:
Dr. J.R. REPULLO
Escuela Nationale de Sanidad Ministerio
de Sanidad y Consumo
ES Madrid
Phone: +34 (91) 314 79 89
Fax: +34 (91) 323 37 7.7

Prof. Dr. A. de ROO
Tilburgs Instituut voor Academische Studies
Katholieke Universiteit Brabant
NL Tilburg
Phone: +31 13 66 31 44
Fax: +31 13 66 30 62

Prof. M. BROMMELS
Dept. of Public Health,
Univ of Helsinki
FI Helsinki
Phone: +358 0 434 6611
Fax: +358 0 434 6456

SUPER: THE EUROPEAN FOOD AND SHOPPING RESEARCH

Key words
Nutrition, promotion of healthy diets, health promotion, nutrition behaviour.

Brief description
Nutrition related diseases are one of the main cause of premature death in Europe; the promotion of healthy diets forms a major part of the health promotion agenda. Until now nutrition education (based on knowledge) has not been very successful in changing dietary patterns. Nutrition behaviour is a complex process. A holistic approach seems to be essential for implementing nutrition behaviour.

This proposal describes a nutrition promoting action research, in which six European cities collaborate (Liverpool, Valencia, Amadora, Rennes, Horsens and Eindhoven, all Healthy Cities). The project is based on the idea that change has to occur at multiple stages in the change process, including awareness, motivation, initiation, main-tenance and support for change. A combination of existing and new health promotion techniques is used.

The essential strategy is one of community action and the central place for intervention is the supermarket.In each of the cities, a three year working plan is followed, containing three main steps:

1 a baseline study,
2 nutrition promotional activities in social, commercial and health settings and,
3 an evaluation study.

The activities are based on the same methodologies and principles of community involvement. Research is carried out on:

1 the individual level (knowledge, attitudes, behaviour);
2 at community level (social networking, including the quality of participation from the different participants and conditions for cooperation) and,
3 on the level of the project as a whole (incorporation in the structure).

The project can be seen as a comparative study, consisting of 6 case-studies. Comparisons of the achievements of each city has the potential to draw conclusion about processes in force in community based projects. This offers prospects to develop strategies which are useful in any other European city.

Since national funding agencies have very little money for international meetings this application is being made for EC-funding through BIOMED 1, so that exchange of experiences can be guaranteed.

Project leader:
Dr. Maria KOELEN
Agricultural University,
Dept. of Extension Science
Hollandseweg 1
NL 6706 KN Wageningen
Phone: +31 8370 84310
Fax: +31 8370 84791
Contract number: CT941327

Participants:

C. MASSON
INSFA
65 Rue de St. Brieuc
FR 35042 Rennes
Phone: +33 99 287577
Fax: +33 99 287510

Dr. S. le BRIS
DHS Ville de Rennes
BP 26 A
FR 35031 Rennes
Phone: +33 99 285708
Fax: +33 99 285862

Dr. C. COLOMER & G. BOONEKAMP MSc
& A. NUÑEZ MSc
Institut Valencia D'Estudis en
Salut Publica (IVESP)
Juan de Garay, 21
ES 46017 Valencia
Phone: +34 6 3869369
Fax: +34 6 3869370

E. CALJÉ
Public Health Service Centro de Saude Amadora
Largo Dario Gandra Nunes 1
PT 2700 Amadora
Phone: +351 1 4930113
Fax: +351 45 31 181120

E. CARREIRAS
Town Hall of Amadora
Av. Mov. Forças Armadas
PT 2700 Amadora
Phone: +351 1 4940188/4942930
Fax: +351 1 4922082

J. HOUMAN & O. BJORNHOLT MSc
Sund By Projektet
Raadhustorvet 2
DK 8700 Horsens
Phone: +45 75 614344
Fax: +45 75 628060

J. TAYLOR, MSc
Liverpool Healthy City Project Coordinator
P.O. Box 88, Municipal Buildings
Dale Street
UK Liverpool L69 2DH
Phone: +44 51 2252881
Fax: +44 51 2252900

L. VAANDRAGER MSc
Dept. of Extension Science, Agricultural
Univ of Wageningen
Hollandseweg 1
NL6706 KN Wageningen
Phone: +31 8370 84310
Fax: +31 8370 84791

Madame A. SABOURAUD
Hôtel de Ville
BP 26 A
28, Rue de Paris
FR 35031 Rennes
Phone: +33 99 285693
Fax: +33 99 635207

Mme M. OULC'HEN
APRAS
4 Cours des Alliés
FR 35043 Rennes cedex
Phone: +33 99 315244

Prof. Dr. J. ASHTON
Mersey Regional Health Authority
Hamilton House
24, Pall Mall
UK Liverpool L3 6AL
Phone: +44 51 2363974
Fax: +44 51 2581371

S. JUDD & M. JONES
Sir Alfred Jones Memorial Hospital
Churchstreet Garston
UK Liverpool L19 2LS
Phone: +44 51 4943058

T. GRIBLING & M. SPERMON & J. COSIJN
Municipal Public Health Services
P.O. Box 2357
NL 5600 RB Eindhoven
Phone: +31 40 384112
Fax: +31 40 116647

EUROPEAN CONTRIBUTION TO AN INTERNATIONAL REGISTER OF RANDOMIZED CONTROLLED TRIALS (RCTS) OF HEALTH CARE

Key words
Randomized controlled trials, International Register, Health Care.

Brief description
The proposal has two main objectives. The first is to ensure that information published in European general health care journals concerning completed, ongoing and planned randomized controlled trials in Europe is contributed to an International Register of Randomized Controlled Trials of Health Care.
The second is to ensure that this Register is made easily accessible:
a to those preparing systematic reviews to inform health care policy decisions, so that effective forms of care can be promoted and ineffective or dangerous forms of care discouraged, and;
b to those planning new research, so that unnecessary and costly duplication of research within the Community is minimized, whilst highlighting those areas which could benefit from further research.

In addition to the coordinating centre (The Cochrane Centre) the following main participating centres are proposers of this project:
Dr. Peter Gotzsche; Dept. of Infectious Diseases M 7431, Rigshospitalet, Tagensvej 20, DK 2200 Copenhagen, Denmark.
Professor Jean-pierre Boissel; Hopital Neuro-Cardiologique, Unite de pharmacologie Clinique, P.O. Box 3041, 69394 Lyon Cedex 03, France.
Dr. SÖren Schmidt/Dr. Gerd Antes. Tumor Biology Centre, Institute for Clinical pharmacology, P.O. Box 1120, 7800 Freiburg, Germany.
Dr. silvia Marsoni/Ms Monica Flann/Ms Vanna pistotti/Dr. Maurizio Bonati. Laboratory of Clinical Epidemiology, Mario Negri Institute for pharmacological Research, via Eritrea 62, 20157 Milan, Italy.
Dr. Jos Kleijnen/prof. Paul Knipschild. Dept. of Epidemiology, University.

Project leader:
Mrs. Carol LEFEBVRE
Cochrane Centre, National
Health Service
Research and Development
Programme
Summertown Pavilion
Middle Way
UK Oxford OX2 7LG
Phone: +44 865 516300
Fax: +44 865 516311
Contract number: CT941289

Participants:
Dr. Peter GOTZSCHE
DK Copenhagen
Phone: +45 3545 5571
Fax: +45 3545 6528

Prof. Jean-Pierre BOISSEL
FR Lyon
Fax: +33 22 95 53 65

Dr. Gerd ANTES &
Dr. Sören SCHMIDT
DE Freiburg
Phone: +49 7612 0605
Fax: +49 7612 062899

Dr. Silvia MARSONI
IT Milan
Phone: +39 2 3901 4540
Fax: +39 2 3320 0231

Dr. Jos KLEIJNEN &
Prof. Paul KNIPSCHILD
NL Amsterdam
Phone: +31 20 5663 273
Fax: +31 20 6912 683

Dr. Ian CHALMERS
UK Oxford
Phone: +44 865 516 300
Fax: +44 865 516 311

ESTABLISHMENT OF A EUROPEAN CLEARING HOUSE ON HEALTH OUTCOMES

Key words
Health Outcomes, European Clearing House, outcome measures.

Brief description
Based on the existing UK Clearing House on Health Outcomes (established at the Nuffield Institute in January 1992) the Concerted Action aims to develop a European Clearing House on Health Outcomes.

The initial task is to establish a European network of health outcome users.

The initial participating organisations to the Concerted Action are necessarily limited due to the innovative nature of the project. The UK Clearing House on Health Outcomes is unique in Europe as too is the role played by the National Organisation for Quality Assurance (CBO) in the Netherlands.

The intention is to extend the network to known service practitioners and researchers active in the outcomes area in Europe.

The network will thus provide forum for information exchange. This will take the form of international meetings, site visits and personnel exchange, newsletter production and distribution to key stakeholders at ministry and sub-national levels, and the identification of good practice and innovation approaches (measures, applications and methods).

Finally, in-country workshops will be held to raise awareness about outcome measures and assessment methods.

An important aspect will be to encourage the development of country-based infrastructures based on the model of the UK Clearing House with a view to establish a register of applications and users of outcome measure and assessment methods within and thus across European countries. This would emphasise the field of appropriate application of measures and ways for its use within routine practice.

This will form the core of the European Clearing House on Health Outcomes.

Project leader:
Mr. Andrew LONG
University of Leeds,
Nuffield Institute for Health
Clarendon Road 71-75
UK Leeds L3 9PL
Phone: +44 532459034
Fax: +44 532460899
Contract number: CT941486

Participant:
Dr. J.W.K. KISTEMAKER MD
CBO-National Organisation for
Quality Assurance
P.O. Box 20064
NL 3502 Utrecht
Phone: +31 30 943644
Fax: +31 30 960647

EURO-REVES: HARMONIZATION OF HEALTH EXPECTANCY CALCULATIONS IN EUROPE

Key words
Health expectancies, European data base, evolution of the health status, health expectancy calculations, data collection.

Objectives
The development of guidelines for the construction and calculation of health expectancies with a view to European harmonization of concepts; data collection, and calculation methods.

To provide a European data base on health expectancies which may be put at the disposition of individuals and organizations involved in health research and development programmes.

To edit a reference document describing concepts, questionnaires and calculation methods which may be used as a basis for the further promotion of calculations by other countries both within and ouside Europe.

Brief description
Scientific background: Dramatic increases in life-expectancy constitute perhaps one of the most remarkable advances of the twentieth century. As the year 2000 approaches a further challenge confronts us: Are the additional years gained in life-expectancy spent in good health or in prolonged state of illness and dependancy. The recent development of indicators of disability-free life expectancy have provided a means of addressing this important question, fundamental both for understanding of evolution of the health status of populations and for the formulation of government policies directed at the provision of services.

The action should recommend guidelines for the harmonization of health expectancy calculations in Europe, constitute a central data collection centre, and provide a forum for the discussion of the future use of such information. It is important to note that the proposed European network does not aim to subsidize or initiate new health surveys (this is the responsibility of the NIS and its subsidiary Eurostat). EURO-REVES is designed to promote the exploitation of data presently available and to provide European guidelines for future population studies.

The need to harmonize calculations in order to facilitate joint planning of health programmes and for the comparison of the health of different communities and socio-economic groups within the futur Europe is recognized by all participating teams. If the principal objective of social and health systems is not only to prolong life but also to maintain its quality in terms of autonomy and social functioning for as long as possible then health expectancy comes close in theory to an ideal indicator for monitoring the realisation of health objectives in Europe.

Project leader:
Dr. Jean-Marie ROBINE
INSERM Equipe Démographie et Santé, Lab.
d'Epidémiologie, Université de Montpellier I
route de Ganges 555
FR 34059 Montpellier Cédex

Phone: +33 67611082
Fax: +33 67042401
Contract number: CT941491

Participants:

A. van der BERG-JETHS
RIVM Bureau VTV
Postbus 1
NL 3720 BA Bilthoven
Phone: +31 30 74 91 11

C. JAGGER
Univ of Leicester, Dept. of
Community Health Leicester
Royal Infirmary
P.O. Box 65
UK Leicester LE2 7LX
Phone: +44 533 52 32 11

C.H.R.U. BELLEVUE
Dpt. Rééd. et Réd. Fonct.,
Pierre Minaire
Bd. Pasteur
FR 42023 St. Etienne 2
Phone: +33 77 42 77 57

D. KAY
New Castle General Hospital,
Neurochemical Pathology
Westgate Road
UK New Castle-upon-Tyne
NE4 6BE
Phone: +44 91 273 5251

F. PACCAUD
Inst. Universitaire de Méde-
cine Sociale et Préventive
17 rue du Bugnon
CH 1005 Lausanne
Phone: +41 21 313 20 20

G. DESPLANQUES
18 Bd Adolphe Pinard
FR 75675 Paris Cedex 14
Phone: +33 1 41 17 54 27

G.A.M. van den BOS
Inst. for Social Medecine,
Academic Medical Center
Universiteit van Amsterdam
Meibergdreef 15
NL 1105 AZ Amsterdam
Phone: +31 20 566 46 02

H. PETTERSSON
Statistics Sweden, I/MET,
Swedish NIS participant
SE 11581 Stockholm
Phone: +46 8 783 4885

H.J. van OYEN
Inst. of Hygiëne and
Epidemiology
J. Wytmanstraat 14
BE 1050 Brussel
Phone: +32 2 642 5025/5111

H.P.A. van de WATER
Nederlands Inst. of
Preventive Health Care/TNO
NL 2300 AC Leiden
Phone: +31 71 17 87 78

I. POPA
National Inst. for Health
Services and Management
(INSSC)
HU Bucarest
Phone: +36 0 37 32 10

Jean-Pierre MICHEL
Institutions Universitaires
de Gériatrie de Genève
Route Mon-Idée
CH 1226 Thonex
Phone: +41 22 48 74 11

J.T.P. Bonte
Dept. for Health Statistics,
Nederlands Central Bureau
of Statistics
P.O. Box 959
NL 2270 AZ Voorburg
Phone: +31 70 337 38 00

K. RITCHIE
INSERM/Equipe veillisse-
ment cognitif,
Centre Val d'Aurelle,
Parc Euromédecine
FR 34094 Montpellier 5
Phone: +33 67 61 30 26

M.N. MUTAFOVA
Dept. of Social Medicine,
Medical Academy
Belo More Street, 8
BG 1504 Sofia
Phone: +359 2 77 41 24

M.R. BONE
Office of pop. Census and
Survey, Social Survey Div.
10 Kingsway
UK London WC2B 6JP
Phone: +44 71 242 0262

M.V. ZUNZUNEGUI
Centro Universitario
de Salud Publica
General Oraa 39
ES 28006 Madrid
Phone: +34 341 564 24 99

N. BROUARD
INED
27 Rue du Commandeur
FR 75675 Paris cedex 14
Phone: +33 1 43 20 13 45

N.K.R. RASMUSSEN
The Danish Inst. for
Clinical Epidemiology
25 Svanemollevej
DK 2100 Copenhagen O
Phone: +45 31 20 77 77

P. BARBERGER-GATEAU
Université de Bordeaux II,
Pascale Barberger-Gateau
146 rue Léo-Saignat
FR 33076 Bordeaux cedex
Phone: +33 56 24 74 43

R. GISPERT
Dep. Sanitat Generalitat de
Catalunya, Gabinèt Tècnic
Trav. de les Corst, 131-159
ES 08028 Barcelona
Phone: +34 3 339 1111

S. EVERS
Univ of Lindburg,
Dept. of Epidemiology
Postbus 616
NL 6200 MD Maastricht
Phone: +31 43 88 17 27

Th. SPUHLER
Swiss Federal
Statistical Office
Hallwylstr. 15
CH 3003 Zurich
Phone: +41 31 61 87 72

V. EGIDI
Universita La Sapienza,
Dipartimento di Scienze
Demografiche
Via Nomentana, 41 00
IT 161 Rome
Phone: +39 40 54 884

INTERNATIONAL LABORATORY BASED SALMONELLA SURVEILLANCE (SALM-NET)

Key words
Salmonellosis, salmonella database, prevention, salmonella surveillance.

Brief description
International collaboration to enhance surveillance is essential to improve the effectiveness of primary and secondary prevention of foodborne salmonellosis. Established international networks provide a basis for exchanging information on existing problems, but do not facilitate rapid data exchange whereby new problems can be recognised swiftly. Therefore the creation of an online common salmonella database linking a network of national reference laboratories represents a new initiative.

The proposal aims to improve the prevention of human salmonellosis within the European community through strengthening international laboratory based salmonella surveillance and creating an online distributed network salmonella database (Salm-Net).

This will be achieved through:
1 extending phage typing for the most common salmonella serotypes more widely;
2 introducing an international quality assurance scheme for laboratory performance of salmonella phage typing;
3 establishing a core set of data items to accompany, where possible, each laboratory confirmed and typed human salmonella isolate;
4 creating an international distributed database of human salmonella infections;
5 developing statistical analysis programmes that will provide an automate mechanism for detecting clustering of cases so as to facilitate outbreak recognition, especially recognition of international outbreaks;
6 bringing such clusters rapidly to the attention of participants.

This harmonisation of public health methodologies and protocols for salmonella surveillance will improve the effectiveness of EC wide prevention of foodborne salmonellosis.

Project leader:
Dr. Burnett ROWE
Laboratory of Enteric Pathogens Central,
Public Health Laboratory
Colindale Avenue 61
UK London NW9 5HT
Phone: +44 81 2004400
Fax: +44 81 2007874
Contract number: CT941484

Participants:

Dr. A. ECHEITA (ES)
Dr. C. BARTLETT &
Mr. I. FISHER (UK)
Dr. D. GRECO (IT)
Dr. F. VAN LOOCK (BE)
Dr. G. RASCH (DE)
Dr. H. KÜHN (DE)
Dr. I. PIRES (PT)
Dr. J. COWDEN (UK)
Dr. J.C. DESENCLOS (FR)
Dr. K. GAARSLEV (DK)
Dr. M. FANTASIA (IT)
Dr. M. PAIXA (PT)
Dr. M. SPRENGER (NL)
Dr. P. ANDRE (BE)
Dr. R. CANO (ES)
Dr. R.W.A. GIRDWOOD (UK)
Mrs. L. WARD (UK)
Mrs. W.J. van LEEUWEN (NL)
Mr. B. REILLY (UK)
Prof. J. FLYNN (IE)
Prof. P. GRIMONT (FR)
Prof. Herbert BUDKA &
prof. F. SEITELBERGER (AT)
Prof. K. JELLINGER (AT)
Dr. R. KLEINERT (AT)
Dr. H. MAIER (AT)
Dr. Peter PILZ (AT)
Prof. J.M. BRUCHER (BE)
Prof. J.J. MARTIN &
dr. P. CRAS (BE)
Prof. C.J.M. SINDIC (BE)
Dr. Eva MITROVA (CZ)
Prof. Henning LAURSON (DK)
Dr. P. S. TEGLBJAERG (DK)
Prof. Matti HALTIA (FI)
Dr. Hannu KALIMO (FI)
Dr. Jussi KOVANEN (FI)
Dr. M. B. DELISLE (FR)
Mme. J. DOERR-SCHOTT (FR)

Dr. D. DORMONT (FR)
Prof. F. DUBAS (FR)
Prof. Francoise GRAY (FR)
Prof. J.J. HAUW (FR)
Dr. Nicole HELDT (FR)
Prof. Jacqueline MIKOL (FR)
Prof. Claude VITAL (FR)
Dr. Jan W. BOELLAARD (DE)
Prof J. CERVOS-NAVARRO &
dr. S. PATT (DE)
Prof. Erwin DAHME (DE)
Dr. H. DIRINGER (DE)
Prof. Hans H. GOEBEL &
dr. Jürgen BOHL (DE)
Prof. Filippo GULLOTTA (DE)
Prof. M. KIESSLING (DE)
Dr. Harold KLEIN (DE)
Prof. H.A KRETSCHMAR (DE)
Prof. P. MEHRAEIN (DE)
Prof. W. POEWE &
dr.K. JENDROSKA (DE)
Pr. W SCHACHENMAYR (DE)
Prof. Wolfgang SCHLOTE (DE)
Prof. J.M. SCHRODER (DE)
Prof. Roland SCHRODER (DE)
Prof. D. STAVROU &
dr. R. LAAS (DE)
Prof. Benedikt VOLK (DE)
Prof. G.F. WALTER &
dr. A. HORI (DE)
Prof. O.D. WIESTLER (DE)
Dr. Katherine MAJTENYI (HU)
Dr. G. GEORGSSON (IS)
Prof. S.J BALLOYANNIS (GR)
Prof. P. DAVAKI (GR)
Prof. E. PATSOURIS &
prof. C. KITTAS &
prof. E. AGAPITOS (GR)
Dr. Catherine KEOHANE (IE)
Dr. W. KAMPHORST (NL)

Prof. Davide SCHIFFER (IT)
Prof. Orso BUGIANI (IT)
Prof. Alfredo LECHI &
prof. G. R. TRABATTONI (IT)
Prof. Giorgio MACCHI &
prof. Carlo MASULLO (IT)
Dr. Maurizio POCCHIARI (IT)
Prof. Sverre J. MORK (NO)
Dr. Pawel P. LIBERSKI (PL)
Dr. C. COSTA &
J. PIMENTEL & C. LIMA (PT)
Dr. Arcadiu PETRESCU (RO)
Prof. Mara POPOVIC (SI)
Dr. F. CRUZ-SANCHEZ (ES)
Dr. Jose A. BERCIANO (ES)
Dr. Fco. Javier FIGOLS (ES)
M. GUTIERREZ-MOLINA &
C. MORALES BASTOS (ES)
Prof. Arne BRUN (SE)
Prof. K. KRISTENSSON (SE)
Prof. Yngve OLSSON (SE)
Dr. E.C. GESSAGA (CH)
Prof. R.C. JANZER (CH)
Prof. Paul KLEIHUES (CH)
Dr. Bruno OESCH (CH)
Dr. Gianpaolo PIZZOLATO &
dr. Antonio CAROTA (CH)
Prof. J. ULRICH (CH)
Prof. M. VANDEVELDE (CH)
Prof. Ch. WEISSMANN (CH)
Dr. P.V. BEST (UK)
Prof. L.W. DUCHEN &
dr. F. SCARAVILLI (UK)
Dr. Margaret M. ESIRI (UK)
Prof. Peter L. LANTOS (UK)
Prof. Roy O. WELLER (UK)
Prof. Slobodan DOZIC (YU)

COMPARISON AND HARMNIZATION OF DENOMINATOR DATA FOR PRIMARY HEALTH CARE RESEARCH IN COUNTRIES OF THE EUROPEAN UNION

Key words
Comparable data, primary care.

Brief description
In most European countries, sentinel practice networks have been established as an epidemiologic tool in the ambulatory care system. In such networks, office-based physicians are gathered on a (mostly) non-commercial base to monitor defined events among their patients. Spatial units covered by such networks are communities, counties, or - at best - countries. Though surveillance systems can be very useful in small regions, national differences or global trends in the frequency and distribution of health problems can only be demonstrated by joining together the results of single sentinel networks.

Comparability of national results is, however, limited; partly due to the different national health systems influencing the demand of medical care, mainly by the lack of comparable data on the population from which the cases arose. Such denominator data is a vital premise to compare data from primary care research between different regions or Countries. In this proposed project, a methodological working group consisting of scientists from five European countries Belgium, France, Germany, the Netherlands, United Kingdom) with different health care systems shall work on the denominator problem. The objectives of denominators and national approaches which have been realised in existing sentinel networks shall viewed and described in detail.

The ultimate goal of this small Concerted Action is to increase comparability of denominator concepts, as a first step especially between countries with and without patient registration. As a second step, comparable denominator concepts with more information on the residential population both for countries with and without patient registration shall be discussed and developed respectively.

This proposed methodologic project has central relevance for the harmonisation of methodologies and protocols in health services research and for the further development of coordinated networks providing for adequate collection and interpretation of data on health status and health systems.

Project leader:
Professor F.W. SCHWARTZ
Medizinische Hochschule
Hannover, Abt. Eipemiologie
und Sozialmedizin
Postfach 610180
DE 30625 Hannover 61
Phone: +49 511 532 44 22
Fax: +49 511 532 53 47
Contract number: CT941580

Participants:
Dr. A. BARTELDS
NIVEL, Postbus 1568
NL 3500 BN Utrecht
Phone: +31 30 31 99 46
Fax: +31 30 31 92 90

Dr. P. GAMERIN
Faculty of Medicine, B3E
27 rue Chaligny
FR 75571 Paris Cedex
Phone: +33 1 4473 84 30
Fax: +33 1 4307 39 57

Dr. V. VAN CASTEREN
Institut d'Hygiène
et d'Épidémiologie
Rue Juliette Wytsman 14
BE 1050 Brussels
Phone: +32 2 642 51 11
Fax: +32 2 642 50 01

Dr. D. FLEMING
The Royal College of General
Practitioners
Lordswood House
54 Lordswood Road
UK Harborne Birmingham
Phone: +44 21 426 11 25
Fax: +44 21 428 20 84

ESTABLISHMENT OF A META-ANALYSIS COORDINATION UNIT

Key words
Meta-analyses, EORTC Data Center, harmonization of treatment, cancer, common database.

Brief description
Meta-analyses should be coordinated on a European wide level in order to maximize the resources available within the EC.

The first aim of this project is to create a Meta-Analysis Coordination Unit (centralized facility) within the EORTC Data Center. The establishment of such a unit will allow the EORTC to:

1 provide the scientific means and expertise required to identify, process and analyze the data from trials to be included in meta-analyses conducted by the unit.
2 co-ordinate and provide data for patients entered in EORTC trials to be included in meta-analysis projects undertaken by other research groups.
3 further develop an increasing network of links with other European cancer research centers and meta-analysis units, thus leading to the coordination of common research efforts between these centers and the EORTC and a subsequent harmonization of treatment.
4 provide an optimal framework for the conduct of meta-analyses and for the dissemination of results as widely and as rapidly as possible within the European Community, thus further improving the treatment and management of cancer within Europe. In this way as many patients as possible will profit from state of the art treatment, even those treated outside of research oriented institutes.
5 provide the means to further increase the coordination of common research activities on cancer within Europe.

By establishing contacts and exchange of data and information with other centers in Europe already carrying out meta-analyses (for example with the Clinical Trial Service Unit, Oxford, England), the EORTC will prove itself to be a valuable partner in the co-ordination of meta-analysis activities on an European and worldwide basis.

The first task of the Meta-Analysis Coordination Unit will be to carry out meta-analyses studying the value of intravesical chemotherapy in superficial bladder cancer and the value of bone marrow transplantation in acute myelogenous leukemia (AML) in order to better define the optimal treatment in these diseases.

Objectives of the superficial bladder cancer meta-analysis are to determine the prognostic factors associated with the development of muscle invasion, define risk groups and ascertain the long term value of intravesical chemotherapy in preventing invasive disease and death. Objectives of the AML meta-analysis are to create and regularly update a common database at the EORTC Data Center in order to perform a prospective overview of the value of bone marrow transplantation in terms of disease free survival and survival, determine the prognostic factors and analyse the immediate and long term treatment side effects and quality of life data.

Project leader:
Dr. Richard SYLVESTER
EORTC Data Center
Avenue Mounier 83
P.O. Box 11
BE 1200 Bruxelles
Phone: +32 2 7741613
Fax: +32 2 7712004
Contract number: CT941433

Participants:
Dr. B. LOWENBERG
HOVON, Dr. Daniel den Hoed Cancer Center
Groene Hilledijk 315
NL 3075 EA Rotterdam
Phone: +31 10 439 15 98
Fax: +31 10 486 10 58

Dr. C. BOUFFIOUX
EORTC, Hôpital Universitaire
du Sart Tilman
Bte 35
BE 4000 Liège
Phone: +32 41 66 72 53
Fax: +32 41 66 72 58

Dr. F. MANDELLI
GIMEMA, Dept. of Hematology,
Univ La Sapienza
Via Benevento 6
IT 00161 Roma
Phone: +39 6 85 79 51
Fax: +39 6 44 24 19 84

Dr. F. MEUNIER
EORTC Data Center
83 Avenue E. Mounier, Bte 11
BE 1200 Brussels
Phone: +32 2 774 16 30
Fax: +32 2 771 20 04

Dr. M. PARMAR
MRC Cancer Trials Office
5 Shaftesbury Road
UK Cambridge CB2 2BW
Phone: +44 223 31 11 10
Fax: +44 223 31 18 44

Dr. P. SMITH
MRC, St. James Univ Hospital
Becket Street
UK Leeds LS9 7TF
Phone: +44 532 43 31 44
Fax: +44 532 83 69 75

Dr. R. ZITTOUN
EORTC, Hotel Dieu
1 Place du Parvis Notre Dame
FR 75181 Paris Cedex 04
Phone: +33 1 42 34 84 13
Fax: +33 1 42 34 84 06

Dr. S. SUCIU
EORTC Data Center
83 Avenue E. Mounier, Bte 11
BE 1200 Brussels
Phone: +32 2 774 16 05
Fax: +32 2 772 35 45

Mr. R. GRAY
MRC, Clinical Trial Service Unit,
Radcliff Infirmary Univ of Oxford
UK Oxford OX2 6HE
Phone: +44 865 57 241
Fax: +44 865 72 60 03

INFLUENCE OF NATIONAL CULTURE ON MEDICAL EDUCATION AND THE PROVISION OF HEALTH CARE

Key words
Quality, health care delivery, upgrading, medical training, national cultures, cost effectiveness, HCD approaches.

Brief description
The quality of health care delivery and its socio-economic impact is a matter of great concern to the western world. The EC includes a variety of health care delivery systems determined not only by each memberstates legal background but also by medical training and resource availability. The free movement of doctors within the EC provides a unique opportunity to assess these systems, their educational and cultural background. These grass root contacts might lead to suggestions on health care organization, medical training and clinical research with an attendant improvement in health care delivery throughout the EC and an optimization of health care expenditures.

Taking advantage of the 1977 directive on the free circulation of manpower (Van Ypersele, de Strihou C. *Clinical investigation and the free circulation of physicians within the European Economic Community: the future of European medicine.* In: Eur. J. Clin. Invest. 7: 323-324, 1977.), we established a network of leading European academic departments of medicine. Our intent was to evaluate the European potential for education and transfer of medical technology to clinical practice, to disseminate through experts, going from one country to another, the expertise developed in the expert's host country, and to stimulate a European spirit in academic clinical medicine among both younger trainees and heads of departments of medicine. These goals were to be achieved by the multilateral exchange of trainees in internal medicine.

The result of this endeavour was the demonstration of the feasibility of such a scheme despite language barriers (Van YPERSELE, de STRIHOU C. *Evaluation of clinical practice in Hospitals. Potential for postgraduate training in internal medicine.* In: "Health Services Research and Primary Health Care" G. Brenner & I. Weber, Eds. Congress Proceedings 2nd European Conference, Köln 1990, Deutscher Ärzte-Verlag GmBH, Köln 1991, pp. 218-220.) and its potential importance in the upgrading of medical training and practice throughout Europe (Van Ypersele C, Dickinson C.J. *The European exchange scheme for junior doctors in internal medicine.* In: Lancet II: 1446-1448, 1986).

The present project intends to pursue this initiative with an emphasis on the assessment of the influence of national cultures on medical training and organization and on the cost effectiveness of different HCD approaches.

Project leader:
Professor C. VAN YPERSELE
Université Catholique de Louvain,
Service de Néphrologie
Avenue Hippocrate 10
BE 1200 Bruxelles
Phone: +32 2 764 1857
Fax: +32 2 764 2836
Contract number: CT941054

Participants:

Prof. J.P. GRUNFELD
Hôpital Necker
FR 75743 Paris
Phone: +33 1 4449 5411
Fax: +33 1 4449 5450

Prof. E. COCHE
Cliniques Universitaires St-Luc
BE 1200 Bruxelles
Phone: +32 2 764 1055
Fax: +32 2 764 3697

Prof. W. STAUFFACHER
Kantonsspital Basel
CH 4031 Basel
Phone: +41 61 265 4294
Fax: +41 61 265 5353

Prof. H. GRETEN
Universitäts-Krankenhaus Eppendorf
DE 2000 Hamburg 20
Phone: +49 40 4717 3910
Fax: +49 40 4830 65

Prof. N. TYGSTRUP
Rigshospitalet
DK 2100 Copenhagen
Phone: +45 31 386633
Fax: +45 31 532913

Prof. G. MANCIA
Ospedale Maggiore di Milano
IT 20122 Milan
Phone: +39 2 573360

Prof. D. WEIR
University of Dublin
IE Dublin 8
Phone: +353 1 543922

Prof. J.H.P. WILSON
University Hospital Rotterdam
NL 3015 GD Rotterdam
Phone: +31 10 463 9222
Fax: +31 10 463 3268

Prof. J. DICKINSON
Wolson Institute of Preventive Medicine
UK London EC1M 6BQ
Phone: +44 71 982 6219
Fax: +44 71 982 6270

Prof. A. GUZ
Charing Cross Hospital
UK London W6 8RF
Phone: +44 81 846 7181
Fax: +44 81 846 7170

Prof. D. LOUKOPOULOS
Laikon General Hospital
GR 11527 Athens
Phone: +30 1 7771 161
Fax: +30 1 3607 089

Prof. Keith PETERS
University of Cambridge
UK Cambridge CB2 2QQ
Phone: +44 223 33 67 38
Fax: +44 223 33 67 09

Prof. K.M. KOCH
Medizinische Hochschule Hannover
DE 30625 Hannover
Phone: +49 511 532 23 94
Fax: +49 511 55 23 66

Dr. A. REES
Hammersmith Hospital
UK London W12
Phone: +44 81 740 31 52
Fax: +44 81 746 24 10

Prof. J. FEVERY
U.Z. Gasthuisberg
BE 3000 Leuven
Phone: +32 16 33 22 11
Fax: +32 16 34 44 19

Prof. Levi CUERRA
Hopital de Sao Joao
PT 5200 Porto
Phone: +351 2 49 38 25

Prof. A. CORREIA DE CAMPOS
Escola Nacional de Saude Publica
PT 1699 Lisboa
Phone: +351 758 55 99

Prof. W. ERKELENS
A.Z. Utrecht
NL 3584 CX Utrecht
Phone: +31 30 50 73 97
Fax: +31 30 51 83 28

Prof. A. JUNOD
Hôpital Cantonal Universitaire
CH 1211 Genève
Phone: +41 22 372 9052
Fax: +41 22 372 91161

Area II

**MAJOR HEALTH PROBLEMS AND DISEASES OF
GREAT SOCIO-ECONOMIC IMPACT**

II.1 AIDS RESEARCH

Introduction

The Acquired Immune Deficiency Syndrome (AIDS) poses a great challenge to the world as a whole and to scientists in particular. The virus continues to defy the know-how of scientists and to affect more and more extensive stratums of the population. Unfortunately, we do not yet have an effective treatment.

In spite of these negative aspects, it is stimulating to observe our Community's ability to react faced with a challenge of this kind. In fact, in 1983, only two years after the first case of Acquired Immune Deficiency Syndrome description, the Commission, of the then Economic European Community, started the fight against this disease together with other institutions. Both the speed of this response and its continuity have resulted in a better knowledge of the etiopathogeny, the incidence and the prevalence, as well as a whole series of factors that influence either directly or indirectly this disease.

In 1987, the European Commission integrated a series of research activities on AIDS in Europe, which were still dispersed and not coordinated, under one of the specific research programme activity areas called The Fourth Medical and Health Research Programme (M.H.R.4). There are a lot of successes to be accounted for within the quoted programme, whose activity period was extended until 1991, but there is a risk that some progress may be omitted. Nevertheless, it is worthwhile to emphasise the importance of the creation of reference centres on subjects such as: Epidemiological monitoring, animal models and laboratory reagents. However, there is no doubt that the most important elements have been to go beyond national borders, the integration of efforts and the diffusion of outputs. All these elements have made the basis for the creation of the Europe of the researchers.

The BIOMED-I programme replaced and continued with the activities started in the M.-H.R.-4. Now and in this chapter, a view of all the research projects carried out within this BIOMED-I programme is given. It is still early to judge its results, success and omittance. Nevertheless, one of the objectives of the European Union, the scientific cooperation in Europe, has been reached through the financing of more than 400 teams from 17 different countries.

The dissemination of content of these projects, as well as of the participating teams, will provide other scientists of with the means contacting and exchanging their knowledge and experience with teams who already take part in this European research network.

Maria Cruz Razquin
André-Emmanuel Baert

AIDS PREVENTION AND CONTROL PROGRAMME
OF THE EUROPEAN COMMUNITIES

Key words
AIDS, HIV infection, Epidemiological Monitoring.

Objectives
The objectives of the Concerted Action are mainly to maintain and to develop the European system of surveillance of AIDS and HIV infection, which are the primary functions of the European Centre for the Epidemiological Monitoring of AIDS, as it was requested by the Council and the Ministry of Health of the member states resolution of December 1989.
Apart from maintaining and updating existing data bases (see following points on methods) the Centre will focus its activities through BIOMED 1 on the methodological improvement of surveillance instruments and comparability of European data.

Brief description
1 *Management of data bases*
a E.N.A.A.D.S. (European Non-Aggregate AIDS Data Set): contains detailed information on all AIDS cases reported by 24 countries of the 31 which are part of the European Region (March 1992 data file contains 99/0 of the 71067 AIDS cases reported by the 31 countries. Files are updated quarterly. Countries send their data by mail (diskettes or by electronic mail (Euraids-EARN network using ASCII format, Dbase, Lotus or Epi Info. Data files are computed in ASCII format at the Centre, and analyzed using Dbase or Epi Info.
b E.T.A.A.D.S. (European Transfusion-Associated AIDS Data Set): contains detailed information on AIDS cases due to blood transfusion with more stringent criteria than those requested for national surveillance purposes.
Specific analyses are done on E.T.A.A.D.S. for estimation of the incubation period. Predictions of the number of transfusion-associated AIDS cases.
c E.V.A.A.D.S. (European Vertically-Acquired AIDS Data Set). This data set is being implemented during 1992. It will contain detailed information on paediatric cases, focusing on the mother's risk factor, incubation period and survival. Methods used for data management and analysis will be similar to those used with E.T.A.A.D.S.. Ten European countries out of the 13 which have reported Vertically-Acquired paediatric AIDS cases have accepted to participate.
d European HIV Data Base. This data base contains information on methods and results of HIV sero surveys organised in European countries. For each survey entered, information has to be available on study design, starting date, geographic coverage recruitment site, target population, testing policy and sampling procedure. Results can be broken down by geographic subareas, transmission group, age and sex.

2 *Assessment of indicators of recent HIV infection*
HIV-infected patients with known dates of infection will be recruited from European cohort studies. Threshold levels of biological markers (CD4 lymphocyte counts; B_2, microglobulin; serum, neopterin, immunoglobulin) will be determined analysing their sensitivity, specificity, positive predictive value, 'receiver operator characteristic curve' (RDC), and likelihood ratio for different levels of the variables against the duration of

infection of one and two years, respectively.

3 *Analysis of surveillance data on diseases that could be considered as indicator of risk behaviour*
Following an exploratory research undertaken in 1992 to make an in-depth analysis of surveillance methods used in European countries for the surveillance of sexually transmitted diseases, Hepatitis B and Tuberculosis, the Centre will explore the possibilities for further cooperation in developing criteria and guidelines to harmonise surveillance systems and centralising comparable data obtained in European countries.

Project leader:
Dr. J.B. BRUNET
European Centre for the Epidemiological
Monitoring of AIDS,
Hôpital National de Saint-Maurice
rue du Val d'Osne 14
FR 99410 Saint-Maurice
Phone: +33 1 43 96 65 45
Fax: +33 1 43 96 50 81
Contract number: CT921125

Participants:
Dr. A. STROOBANT
Conseil Supérieur/Coordination contre le SIDA,
Inst. d'Hygiene et d'Epidémiologie
14 Rue Juliette Wytsman
BE 1050 Bruxelles
Phone: +32 2 642 50 29
Fax: +32 2 642 50 01

Dr. J.K. van WIJNGAARDEN
Med Officer Health, Infectious Diseases, Staatstoezicht op de Volksgezondheid
P.O. Box 5406
NL 2280 HK Rijswijk
Phone: +31 70 34 79 11
Fax: +31 70 340 53 94

Dr. M. MELBYE
Dept. of Epidemiology,
The State Serum Inst.
Artillerivej 5
DK 2300 Copenhague S
Phone: +45 31 95 28 17
Fax: +45 31 95 58 22

Dr. M.T. PAIXAO
Inst. Nacional de Saude
Avenida Padre Cruz
PT 1699 Lisbon Codex
Phone: +351 1 759 70 70
Fax: +351 1 759 04 41

Dr. N. GILL
Div HIV, STD & Hepatitis Surveillance, PHLS,
Communicable Dis. Surveillance Centre
61 Colindale Avenue
UK London NW9 5EQ
Phone: +44 81 200 68 68
Fax: +44 81 200 78 68

Dr. O. HAIKALA
National Agency for Welfare and Health
FI 00531 Helsinki 53
Phone: +358 0 3967 2263
Fax: +358 0 3967 2227

Dr. P. Huberty KRAU
Inspection Sanitaire, Direction de la Santé
4 Rue August Lumière
LU 1950 Luxembourg
Phone: +352 4 0801
Fax: +352 48 1349

Dr. T. PAPADIMITRIOU
AIDS Section, Public Health Div,
Min of Health, Welfare
Aristoteles Street 17
GR 10187 Athens
Phone: +30 1 522 23 93
Fax: +30 1 523 17 07

Mrs. B. GOKYAY
Directorate General of External Relations,
Ministry of Health and Social Assistance
Saglik Bakanligi Sihhiye
TR Ankara
Phone: +990 4 131 38 20
Fax: +990 4 133 98 85

Prof. M.A. KOCH
Bundesgesundheitsamt, AIDS-Zentrum
Reichpietschufer 74-76
DE 1000 Berlin 30
Phone: +49 30 25 00 94 30/31
Fax: +49 30 25 00 94 66

DESIGN, SYNTHESIS, EVALUATION AND DEVELOPMENT OF NEW ANTIVIRAL COMPOUNDS AGAINST AIDS

Key words
AIDS, Antiviral compounds, HIV, Anti-HIV drugs.

Objectives
1 Concerted Action as Centralized Facility,
2 through the cooperative help of more than 100 collaborating centres worldwide,
3 detection of active 'lead' compounds for the treatment of AIDS,
4 based on evaluation of anti-HIV activity,
5 using a variety of assay systems, cell types and HIV strains,
6 envisaging all possible targets of the HIV replicative cycle,
7 elucidating the molecular target of action of the active 'lead' compounds,
8 acquiring insight in the structure-function relationship,
9 that should allow the design, through molecular modelling,
10 of the optimal anti-AIDS drug candidate to be used in the clinic.

Brief description
Using a number of assay methods, with various HIV strains and cell systems, a high input Facility for the evaluation of potential anti-HIV drugs has been developed that would allow to identify, from the vast number of compounds synthesized by the collaborating centres, new 'lead' compounds for the treatment of HIV infections (i.e. AIDS). These 'lead' compounds are then examined for their mechanism of action and molecular targets (within the HIV replicative cycle) with which they interact. Based on the structure-function relationship of the active compounds, as well as the molecular coordinates of the target site, the 'lead' compounds can be further refined, through molecular modelling followed by chemical synthesis, so as to optimize their interaction with their molecular target site, and, hence, to achieve optimal activity and selectivity against HIV. This 'lead optimization' must then permit the identification of the optimal anti-AIDS drug candidate(s) that, after the necessary pharmacokinetic and toxicological studies, should be further pursued in the clinic for their potential in the therapy and/or prophylaxis of AIDS.

Project leader:
Professor E. DE CLERCQ
Rega Institute for Medical Research
Minderbroedersstraat 10
BE 3000 Leuven
Phone: +32 16 33 21 60
Fax: +32 16 33 21 31
Contract number: CT920460

Participants:
Dr. A. HOLY (CZ)

Dr. A. KARLSSON (SE)

Dr. A. MATSUDA,
Prof. Dr. T. UEDA (JP)

Dr. A.A. KRAYEVSKY (RU)

Dr. A.G. HABEEB (EG)

Dr. B. MEUNIER (FR)

Dr. C. McGUIGAN (UK)

Dr. C.F. PERNO (IT)

Dr. E.M. NASHED (US)

Dr. G. HOLAN (AU)

Dr. G. PALU (IT)

Dr. G. PILJAC,
Dr. V. PILJAC (HR)

Dr. H. GIEHRING,
Dr. D. SCHWENGERS (DE)

Dr. H.G. GENIESER (DE)

Dr. J. BERES (HU)

Dr. J.C. MARTIN,
Dr. M.L. RIORDAN (US)

Dr. J.F.T. TRONCHET (CH)

Dr. J.S. TANDON (IN)

Dr. K. HARTMANN (DE)

Dr. K. ONO (JP)

Dr. K.L. KIRK,
Dr. L.A. COHEN (US)

Dr. L.J. TUSEK-BOZIC (HR)

Dr. M. LEWIS (IE)

Dr. M. MORR (DE)

Dr. M. UBASAWA (JP)

Dr. M.L. QUIJANO (ES)

Dr. M.J. CAMARASA,
Dr. M.J. PEREZ-PEREZ (ES)

Dr. P. GOYA (ES)

Dr. P.F. TORRENCE (US)

Dr. P.J. BARR (US)

Dr. R. GOTTLIEB,
Dr. G. KLEIN (DE)

Dr. R. GRAYSHAN (UK)

Dr. R. HERRANZ,
Dr. M.T. GARCIA-LOPEZ
(ES)

Dr. R. HERSHLINE (US)

Dr. R.T. WALKER (UK)

Dr. R.W. ADAMIAK (PL)

Dr. R.W. HUMBLE (UK)

Dr. S. MANFEDINI,
Prof. Dr. P. BARALDI,
Dr. S. MIERTUS (IT)

Dr. S. OZAKI (JP)

Dr. T. MARUYAMA,
Prof. Dr. M. HONJO (JP)

Dr. T. PATHAK (IN)

Dr. V.E. MARQUEZ,
Dr. J.S. DRISCOLL (US)

Dr. Y. MORIZAWA (JP)

Dr. Y.B. CHAE,
Dr. Z. NO, Dr. C.K. LEE (KR)

PAPADAKI-VALIRAKI (GR)

Prof. Dr. A.M. BROOM (US)

Prof B. GOLANKIEWICZ,
Dr. J. BORYSKI (PL)

Prof. Dr. B. JASTORFF (DE)

Prof. Dr. B. ÖBERG (SE)

Prof. Dr. C. PAOLETTI (FR)

Prof C.A. BRUGGEMAN,
Dr. F.S. STALS (NL)

Prof. Dr. D. BROWN,
Dr. D. LOAKES (UK)

Prof. D.E. BERGSTROM (US)

Prof. Dr. D.K.F. MEIJER,
Dr. R.W. JANSEN (NL)

Prof. Dr. E. LUKEVICS,
Prof. Dr. M. LIDAKS (LV)

Prof. Dr. E. MARINELLO (IT)

Prof. Dr. E. ZBIRAL,
Dr. F. HAMMERSMIDT (AT)

Prof F. ALDERWEIRELDT,
Dr. E. ESMANS (BE)

Prof. Dr. F. SEELA (DE)

Prof. Dr. G. SHAW (UK)

Prof. G.M. BLACKBURN (UK)

Prof. Dr. H. GEISE (BE)

Prof. Dr. H. GRIENGL,
Dr. H. BAUMGARTNER (AT)

Prof. Dr. H. THORMAR (IS)

Prof. Dr. H. TIMMERMAN,
Dr. Van der GOOT (NL)

Prof. Dr. H.B. LAZREK (MA)

Pr. I.A. MIKHAILOPULO (DE)

Prof. Dr. J. GANGEMI (US)

Prof. Dr. J. HUET,
Prof. Dr. A. SAULEAU (FR)

Prof. J.C. MILHAVET (FR)

Prof. Dr. J.R. DIMMOCK (CA)

Prof. Dr. J.S. PAGANO,
Dr. M.S. SMITH, J. LIN (US)

Prof. Dr. J.W. LOWN (CA)

Prof. Dr. J.L. IMBACH,
Dr. G. GOSSELIN (FR)

Prof. Dr. K. BERG (DK)

Prof. Dr. K. HARRAP,
Dr. P. SERAFINOWSKI (UK)

Prof. Dr. L. OTVOS,
Dr. J. SAGI, G. SAGI (HU)

Prof. Dr. L. SPARFEL (FR)

Prof. Dr. M. CUSHMAN (US)

Prof. Dr. M. GRIFANTINI (IT)

Prof. Dr. M. HORZINĔK,
Dr. M. KOOLEN (NL)

Prof. Dr. M. MONSIGNY (FR)

M. PREOBRAZHENSKAYA
(RU)

Prof. M.F.G. STEVENS (UK)

Prof. M.H. CARUTHERS (US)

Prof. Dr. M.J. ROBINS (US)

Prof. Dr. N. CLUMECK (BE)

Prof. Dr. N.J. LEONARD (US)

Prof. Dr. P. CHANDRA (DE)

Prof. Dr. P. MOHAN (US)

Prof. Dr. P. WUTZLER (DE)

Prof. Dr. P.A.J. JANSSEN,
Dr. K. ANDRIES (BE)

Prof. Dr. P.J. STANG (US)

Prof. Dr. R. GUEDJ (FR)

Prof. R. MECHOULAM (IL)

Prof. Dr. R.C. TAYLOR (US)

Prof. R.T. BORCHARDT (US)

Prof. Dr. S. GOROG (HU)

Prof. Dr. S. SHIGETA,
Dr. M. BABA,
Dr. T. YOKOTA (JP)

Prof. S.W. SCHNELLER (US)

Prof. Dr. T. MIYASAKA,
Dr. H. TANAKA (JP)

Prof. U. RAGNARSSON,
Dr. L. GREHN (SE)

Prof. Dr. V. LOPPINET (FR)

Prof. V. NAIR (US)

Prof. Dr. V.S. GUPTA (CA)

Prof. W. PFLEIDERER (DE)

Prof. W.G. BENTRUDE (US)

Prof. Dr. Y. BENSAID (MA)

COORDINATION OF A EUROPEAN STUDY GROUP ON HIV INFECTION AMONG HETEROSEXUALS

Key words
HIV, AIDS, heterosexual transmission, women, natural history.

Objectives
The general objectives of the present concerted action are:
- to develop and coordinate new projects on HIV infection among heterosexual populations inside the existing European network of centres for the study of heterosexual transmission of HIV. The first field of research chosen by the European participants was HIV infection in women.
- to maintain scientific communication inside the above mentioned network, through regular meetings and scientific workshops involving researchers from outside Europe.

Brief description
1 Meetings and workshops
Meetings are held twice a year in Paris with all participating centres. One of these meetings will be associated to a larger workshop, involving researchers not belonging to the EC group in order to exchange experiences.

2 Implementation of a study on the natural history of HIV infection in women
Most of the biomedical aspects of HIV/AIDS in women are still under debate. Incubation time and survival after AIDS diagnosis do not seem different between men and women infected with HIV, but few cohort studies have enroled enough women to be able to have observed any statistical differences or gender specific co-factors of progression. Another important outcome of interest is the potential impact of pregnancy on clinical progression. Furthermore, much remains to be learnt regarding the timing of onset of gynaecological disease in relation to the level of immunodeficiency due to HIV infection. Studies examining the clinical features of HIV-related disease in women have frequently identified fungal and viral infections, in particular of the genital tract, as the most prevalent clinical manifestations preceding the diagnosis of AIDS. Associations have been reported between HIV infection and CIN (Cervical Intra Neoplasia). The respective influences of the degree of immunodeficiency and sexual behaviour on the occurrence of these gynaecological disorders are not clear. However, these disorders seem frequent among women infected with HIV. More information is needed to define with precision the extent and frequency of check-ups to be recommended.

Specific Objectives
1 The description of the natural history of HIV infection in women.
- Incubation time between infection and full AIDS.
- Dynamic of disease progression using biological markers.
- Survival.
- Incidence of pathologies known to be HIV-related (pathologies listed in the CDC classification), according to the level of immunodeficiency.
- Incidence of gynaecological pathologies suspected to be HIV-related such as cervical dysplasia, genital herpes, yeasts, condylomas, according to the level of immunodeficiency.

2 The potential role of several factors on the natural history.
- Date of infection and mode of acquisition of HIV infection.
- Circumstances for HIV testing, delay between infection and testing, access to health care, and other socio-demographic and economic background.
- Sexual behaviour and history of sexually transmitted diseases.
- Pregnancies.
- History of drug use.
- Repeated contacts with HIV after infection (unprotected sexual contacts with HIV-infected partners, needle sharing during drug use).
- Antiviral, immunological and antibiotic treatments.

3 Description of contraceptive behaviour, attitudes toward pregnancies, and safer sex practices Contraception, obstetrical history and sexual behaviour (number of partners, condom use...) will be describe both before and after diagnosis of HIV infection.

Project leader:
Dr. I. DE VINCENZI
European Centre for the
Epidemiological Monitoring
of AIDS, Hôpital National de
Saint-Maurice
14, rue du Val d'Osne
FR 94410 Saint-Maurice
Phone: +33 1 43 96 65 45
Fax: +33 1 43 96 50 81
Contract number: CT921032

Participants:
Dr. Anne JOHNSON
Univ Coll and Middlesex Sch
The Middlesex Hospital
UK London WN 8NN
Phone: +44 71 380 91 45
Fax: +44 71 32 30 355

Dr. A. ROUMELIOTOU,
Prof. PAPAEVANGELOU
Dept. Epidemiol Med Statist
Centre AIDS,
Athens Sch of Hygiene
P.O. Box 14085
GR Athens 11521
Phone: +30 1 646 7473
Fax: +30 1 64 44 260

Dr. A. SARACCO
AIDS UNIT, IRCCS
San Raffaele
Via Stamira d'Ancona 20
IT 20100 Milan
Phone: +39 2 26 43 79 85
Fax: +39 2 26 43 79 89

Dr. A. SOBEL
Service Immunologie
Clinique, Hop. H. Mondor
51 Av. de Lattre de Tassigny
FR 94010 Creteil
Phone: +33 1 49 81 21 11
Fax: +33 1 49 81 24 69

Dr. D. BUCQUET
Inserm U292, Hopital Bicetre
78 Avenue General Leclerc
FR 94275 Kremlin Bicetre
Phone: +33 1 45 21 23 56

Dr. G. CARDOSO
Service de Dermatologia,
Hosp de Curry Cabral
R. da Beneficienca
PT Lisbonne 1000
Phone: +351 1 793 30 80
Fax: +351 1 769 515

Dr. G. REZZA
Centro Operativo AIDS, Inst.
Superiore di Sanita
Viale Regina Elena 299
IT 00161 Rome
Phone: +39 6 4957 742
Fax: +39 6 4456 741

Dr. R. ANCELLE
European Centre for the
Epidemiological Monitoring
of AIDS Hopital National de
Saint-Maurice
14 Rue du Val d'Osne
FR 94410 Saint-Maurice
Phone: +33 1 43 96 65 45
Fax: +33 1 43 96 50 81

Dr. J. CASABONA,
Dr. TOR
Programa per a la Prevecio i
el Control de la SIDA Pavel-
lo Ave Maria
ES 08028 Barcelona
Phone: +34 3 330 80 11

Dr M. VANDENBRUAENE,
Dr. J. GOEMAN
Inst. of Tropical Medicine
BE 2000 Anvers
Phone: +32 3 247 63 20/28
Fax: +32 3 232 16 14 31

Dr. P. COSTIGLIOLA,
Dr. E. RICCHI, F. CHIODO
Centro screening e preven-
zione AIDS, Inst. malatti
infettive
Via Massarenti 11
IT 40138 Bologna
Phone: +39 51 6363 355
Fax: +39 51 34 14 49

Dr. W. HECKMANN,
Dr. KRAUS
Soz. pedagogoisches Inst.
Schulenburgring 130
DE 1000 Berlin 61
Phone: +49 30 786 20 27/28
Fax: +49 30 785 30 99

H. v. HAASTRECHT,
Dr. A. v/d HOEK,
Dr. R. COUTINHO
Dept. of Infectious Diseases,
P.O. Box 20244
NL Amsterdam

FUNCTIONAL ANALYSIS OF MEMBRANE
INTERACTING HIV PROTEINS

Key words
Virus-Membrane interaction, Viral maturation (Budding), Membrane proteins, Fusion, Pathogenesis, Myristoylation, Ion channels.

Objectives
1 Analysis of the viral maturation process at the cell membrane (budding):
- Identification of the molecular mechanism by which the viral core proteins induce budding.
- Characterization of the membrane proteins (of viral or cellular origin) with which the viral core proteins interact during the budding process.
- Analysis of the mechanism of insertion of viral envelope proteins, from HIV or other retroviruses, into the cell membrane and of the resulting structure.
2 Analysis of the viral infection process at the cell membrane (fusion):
- Determination of the conformational changes and essential interactions between viral gp120 (SU) and the cellular CD4 receptor required for the liberation of the fusogenic peptide of gp41 (TM).
- Identification of other cellular membrane proteins involved in the liberation of the gp41 (TM) fusogenic peptide and characterization of their interaction with gp120 (SU) during this process.
- Analysis of structural and conformational requirements for the gp41 (TM) fusogenic peptide to induce membrane fusion.
3 Analysis of the pathogenic interaction between HIV proteins and the cell membrane:
- Influence of gp120 (SU) membrane protein interaction on the cytosolic $Ca2+$ concentration.
- Elucidation of the HIV nef protein's role as a possible 'G'-protein and examination of the involvement of nef myristoylation on this function.
- Identification of the conformation requirements for nef interaction with cellular ion channels.

Brief description
HIV and related viruses are dependent during their life cycle upon intimate interactions with cellular membranes. The virus particle is formed within the context of existing membranes in the infected cell and enters the new target host cell by membrane fusion. Membrane interactions also modulate viral growth and cell functions as well as directing the way in which the viral antigens are presented to the cellular immune system.
- HIV maturation at the cell membrane.
- HIV infection via the cell membrane (receptor interaction and fusion).
- Pathogenic interaction of HIV proteins with the cell membrane.

Project leader:
Professor V. ERFLE
Institut für Molekulare
Virologie, GSF,
Forschungszentrum für
Umwelt und Gesundheit
Ingolstädter Landstrasse 1
DE 85758 Neuherberg
Phone: +49 89 31 87 30 04
Fax: +49 89 31 87 33 29
Contract number: CT920324

Participants:
Dr. J. BRUNNER
Lab fur Biochemie
Universitätsstrasse 16
CH 8092 Zurich
Phone: +41 1 256 30 03
Fax: +41 1 252 87 44

Dr. Mark MARSH
MRC Lab for Molecular Cell
Biology, Univ Coll London
Gower Street
UK London WC1E 6BT
Phone: +44 71 380 78 07
Fax: +44 71 380 78 05

Dr. Paul CLAPHAM
Chester Beatty Lab,
Inst. of Cancer Research
Fullham Road
UK London SW3 6JB
Phone: +44 71 352 81 33
Fax: +44 71 352 32 99

Dr. Quentin SATTENTAU
Centre Nat de la Recherche
Scientifique
Parc Scientifique de Luninay
FR 13288 Marseille cedex 9
Phone: +33 91 26 94 94
Fax: +33 91 26 94 30

Dr. Toon STEGMANN
Univ Basel
Klingelbergstr. 70
CH 4056 Basel
Phone: +41 61 267 21 94
Fax: +41 61 267 21 89

Dr. Torben SAERMARK
Lab of Membrane Biology,
The Panum Inst. (Build 18.5)
Blegdamsvej 3c
DK 200 Kobenhavn N
Phone: +45 3135 79 00
Fax: +45 3135 95 77

Prof. Dr. Andreas SCHEID
Inst. fur Med
Mikrobiologie/Virologie,
Univ Dusseldorf
Universitatsstr. 1 / Geb 22/21
DE 4000 Dusseldorf
Phone: +49 211 311 22 25
Fax: +49 211 311 22 27

Prof. Dr. A.G. SICCARDI
Dept. di Ricerca Biologica e
Technologica, H.S. Raffaele
Via Olgettina 60
IT 20132 Milano
Phone: +39 2 2643 47 61

Prof. Dr. Arsene BURNY
Dept. de Biologie
Moleculaire,
Univ Libre de Bruxelles
BE 1640 Rhode St. Genese
Phone: +32 2 650 98 24
Fax: +32 2 650 51 13

Prof. Dr. Felix M. GONI
Dept. de Bioquimica,
Facultad de Ciencias,
Univ del Pais Vasco
P.O. Box 644
ES 48080 Bilbao
Phone: +34 4 464 77 00

Prof. Dr. Henrik GAROFF
Dept. of Molekular Biology,
Karolinska Inst.
Blickagangen 6
SE 14157 Huddinge
Phone: +46 8 608 91 00

Prof. Jacopo MELDOLESI
Dip di Ricerca Biologica e
Technologica, H S Raffaele
Via Olgettina 60
IT 20132 Milano
Phone: +39 2 2170 27 70
Fax: +39 2 2643 24 82

Prof. Dr. Jan WILSCHUT
Lab of Physiol Chemistry,
Univ of Groningen
Bloemsingel 10
NL 9712 KZ Groningen
Phone: +31 50 63 27 33
Fax: +31 50 63 26 06

Prof. Dr. GLUCKMAN
Lab de Biol et Genetique des
Pathologies Immunitaires
CNRS URA 1463 -
83 Boulevard de L'Hopital
FR 75651 Paris Cedex 13
Phone: +33 1 4570 38 34
Fax: +33 1 4570 38 32

Prof. J.M. RUYSSCHAERT
Laboratoire des Macromole-
cules,
Univ Libre de Bruxelles
CP 206/2
67 Rue des Chevaux
BE 1640 Rhode St. Genese
Phone: +32 2 650 53 77
Fax: +32 2 650 51 13

Prof. CHIECO-BIANCHI
Inst. di Oncologia,
Univ di Padova
Via Gattamelata 64
IT 35128 Padova
Phone: +39 49 807 18 63
Fax: +39 49 807 28 54

Prof. Dr. M. DIERICH
Inst. fur Hygiene,
Leopold Franzens Univ
Fritz PLregl Strasse 3
AT 6010 Innsbruck
Phone: +43 512 507 22 40
Fax: +43 512 507 35 99

Prof. M. PAPAMICHAIL
Dept. of Immunology, Hel-
lenic Anticancer Inst.
171 Alexandras Ave.
GR 11522 Athens
Phone: +30 1 643 00 83
Fax: +30 1 642 10 22

Prof O SANTOS-FERREIRA
Faculdade de Farmacia,
Univ de Lisboa
Ave das Forcas Armadas
PT 1699 Lisboa
+351 1 793 30 64
+351 1 793 42 12

EUROPEAN AIDS-VIRUS SEROSURVEILLANCE PROGRAMME (EASP): PROVISION OF SERUM TYPING INFORMATION FOR FUTURE ANTIGENIC CHARACTERIZATION

Key words

AIDS, HIV subtypes, molecular epidemiology, European HIV strains, vaccines, antigenic variation, serotyping.

Objectives

The Objective of the Concerted Action *European AIDS-virus Serosurveillance Programme (EASP)* is to characterize HIV RNA from sera of HIV infected individuals at different Stages of infection and from different riskgroups and geographic areas throughout Europe. Special attention will be paid to the genomic characterization of the HIV envelope. In the initial phase of the EASP Concerted Action typing of HIV RNA isolated from serum will be compared to typing of HIV RNA from virus supernatants.

Brief description

Currently it is known that HIV-1 subtype B was the predominant HIV strain in Europe in the eighties, except for Eastern Europe, where also other HIV-1 subtypes are prevalent.

The goal of EASP is firstly to map the current HIV envelope variation in Europe and Subsequently provide viruses and sera for further antigenic and biological characterization. Therefore, viruses and sera/plasma's are collected in almost all European countries. Stocks are being produced from all 100-150 viruses collected. A virus typing procedure is evaluated that complements the WHO efforts concerning HIV isolation and characterization. Viral RNA is isolated and cDNA are produced containing the gp120 coding region. Both the input RNA and the PCR amplified cDNA are characterized by the RNAse A mismatch analysis. Subsequently the RNAse A mismatch results are compared to results obtained by other genetic screening techniques like temperature gradient gel electrophoresis (TGGE) and the heteroduplex mobility assay (HMA). Sequence analysis and V3 peptide serology is used to confirm and extend the results obtained by the genetic screening techniques. Serotyping will be performed of the European viruses by using neutralization assays and gp120 binding assays, using natural sera in competition with well characterized antibody populations. Antibody specificities will be assessed by peptide binding assays and competitive binding assays with emphasis binding assays with emphasis on Vl/V2 antibodies, V3 antibodies, C4 and C7 antibodies. Variation in these particular epitopes, most likely crucial to vaccine efficacy, will be a special focus of attention. New sample sets will be collected from newly infected individuals in future European vaccine evaluation sites.

Project leader:
Professor Dr. J. GOUDSMIT
Human Retrovirus Laboratory,
University of Amsterdam
Meibergdreef 15
NL 1105 AZ Amsterdam
Phone: +31 20 566 38 53
Fax: +31 20 691 65 31
Contract number: CT920379

Participants:

Prof. Dr. H. RUBSAMEN-WAIGMANN,
Dr. M. GREZ
Georg Speyer Haus,
Chemotherapeutisches Forschungsinstitut
DE Frankfurt

Dr. F. de WOLF
Dept. Human Retrovirus Lab,
Univ of Amsterdam
Meibergdreef 15
NL 1105 AZ Amsterdam

Prof. Dr. J. WEBER,
Dr. C. CHEINGSONG-POPOV
G.U. Medicine and Communicable Diseases,
St Mary's Hosp Med Sch
UK London

Prof. Dr. J.P. LEVY,
Dr. S. SARAGOSTI
Dept. of Retrovirology,
Inst. Cochin de Genetique Moleculaire (ICGM)
FR Paris

Prof. Dr. P. PIOT,
Dr. G. van der GROEN
Dept. of Microbiology,
Inst. of Trop Med
BE Antwerpen

Prof. Dr. R. NAJERA,
Dr. C. LOPEZ GALINDEZ
Centro Nacional de Biologia Celular y Retrovi-
rus, Inst. de Salud Carlos III
ES Majadahonda (Madrid)

PATHOLOGY OF THE NERVOUS SYSTEM IN HIV INFECTION

Key words
AIDS, HIV, retrovirus, Nervous System, Central Nervous System, Peripheral Nervous System, Brain, Neuropathology.

Brief description
The purpose of this Concerted Action is to coordonate the pathological study of lesions of the nervous system in HIV infection.

Involvement of the nervous system (NS) is frequent in AIDS. 40-50% of the patients with AIDS have neurological symptoms which represent a major cause of disability and the principal cause of death in that population. Neuropathological studies have shown that 80-100% of AIDS patients have neuropathological abnormalities. Because of their very unusual aspect and multiplicity, the definition and classification of the neurological complications of this new disease, allowing a better diagnosis of the clinical and radiological symptoms, a better understanding of their pathogenetic mechanisms and assessement of any possible treatment, have to be settled on pathological data.

Among these neurological complications, lesions due to a direct infection of the NS by HIV have been observed with increasing frequency; they represents a frequent and increasing cause of dementia, peripheral neuropathies and death in AIDS patients. The characteristic neuropathological features of HIV-related encephalopathy, myelopathy and peripheral neuropathies are now roughly described. However the definition of lesions, their nomenclature and their diagnostic criteria vary which explains partly the variations of incidence of these lesions in the different series.

The pathogenetic mechanisms involved in the lesions of HIV-related encephalopathy, myelopathy and peripheral neuropathies are not yet understood. Understanding of the interactions of HIV and the NS requires collaborative studies of neuropathologists with virologists and molecular biologists.

The understanding of the neurologic manifestations is insufficiently precise to enable development of clinical diagnostic criteria at this time. Prospective studies with detailed and quantified correlation of stage of disease and clinical and radiological symptomatology with type, extent and distribution of cerebral changes are needed. Finally, since the onset of the AIDS epidemic new development have arisen mainly related to improvement in treatment. A pathological survey is necessary to assess the increase or decrease of some AIDS-related neurological complications and to precise the mechanism of complications of treatment such as zidovudine myopathy.

Project leader:
Professor F. GRAY
Département de Pathologie,
Hôpital Raymond Poincaré
FR 92380 Garches
Phone: +33 1 49 81 27 35
Fax: +33 1 49 81 27 26
Contract number: CT920118

Participants:
Dr. Bruno HURTREL
Dept. des Retrovirus,
Unité d'Oncologie Virale,
Inst. Pasteur
28 Rue du dr. Roux
FR 75724 Paris Cedex 15
Phone: +33 40 68 89 01
Fax: +33 1 45 68 88 85

Dr. Catherine KEOHANE
Dept. of Pathology,
Cork regional Hospital
IE Wilton-Cork
Phone: +353 21 546 400
Fax: +353 21 343 307

Dr. F. ENCHA-RAZAVI
Dept. de Pathologie,
Hop Henri Mondor
FR 94010 Creteil Cedex
Phone: +33 1 49 81 27 46
Fax: +33 1 49 81 27 35

Dr. Francesca CHIODI
Inst. for Virologi, c/o SBL,
Karolinska Hosp
SE 105 21 Stockholm
Phone: +46 8 735 1000

Dr. F. SCARA VILLI
Dept. of Path, Inst. of Neu-
rology, The Nat Hosp
Queen Square
UK London WC1 3BG
Phone: +44 71 837 36 11
Fax: +44 71 278 50 69

Dr. Frederic MORINET
Serv Central de
Microbiologie-Bacteriologie-
Virologie-Hygiene,
Hopital Saint Louis
FR 75475 Paris Cedex 10
Phone: +33 1 42 49 94 78

Dr. Irina ELOVAARA
Dept. of Clin sciences,
Univ of Tampere
P.O. Box 607
FI 33101 Tampere
Phone: +358 31 156 111
Fax: +358 31 156 164

Dr. J. Claudie LARROCHE
Unite INSERM 29,
Hopital Port Royal
123 Boulevard de Port Royal
FR 75674 Paris Cedex 14
Phone: +1 43 26 14 97

Dr. Jeanne E. BELL
Dept. of pathology, Neuro-
path Lab, Western General
Hospital
UK Edinburgh EH4 2XU
Phone: +44 31 332 2525
Fax: +44 31 332 4087

Dr. J. ARTIGAS
Inst. fur Pathologie am
Auguste Viktoria
Krankenhaus
DE 1000 Berlin 41
Phone: +49 79 03 23 82

M. GUTIERREZ MOLINA
Dept. Anatomia Patogica,
Hosp La Paz
Paseo dela Castellana 261
ES Madrid 28046
Phone: +34 1 372 08 11

Dr. Margaret ESIRI
Dept. of Neuropathology,
Radcliffe Infirmary
UK Oxford OX2 6HE
Phone: +44 865 249891
Fax: +44 865 790493

Dr. Pierre TROTOT
Serv de Radiologie,
Hôpital de l'Institut Pasteur
FR 75724 Paris Cedex 15
Phone: +33 1 40 61 38 00
Fax: +33 1 45 68 82 18

Prof. Dominique HENIN
Serv d'Anatomie et de Cyto-
logie Pathologiques, Hôpital
Beaujon
100 Bvd du General Leclerc
FR 92118 Clichy Cedex
Phone: +33 1 40 87 54 60
Fax: +33 1 47 30 48 63

Prof. Georg GOSZTONYI
Inst. fur Neuropathologie,
Klin Steglitz der
Freien Univ Berlin
Hindenburgdamm
DE 1000 Berlin 45
Phone: +49 30 798 2339
Fax: +49 30 798 4141

Prof. Dr. Hans GOEBEL
Path Inst., Neuropathologie
Johannes Gutenberg-Univ
Langenbeckstrasse 1
DE 6500 Mainz
Phone: +49 6131 1773 08
Fax: +49 6131 1766 06

Prof. Dr. Paul KLEIHUES
Inst. fur Neuropathologie,
Dept. Pathologie, Universi-
tatsspital
Schmelzbergstrasse 12
CH 8091 Zurich
Phone: +41 1 255 21 07
Fax: +41 1 255 44 02

Prof. H. BUDKA
Neurological Institute
of the Univ of Vienna
AT 1090 Vienna
Phone: +43 1 40480 254
Fax: +43 1 4034077

Prof. Jacqueline MIKOL
Serv Central d'Anatomie et
de Cytologie Pathologiques,
Hopital Lariboisiere
FR 75475 Paris Cedex 10
Phone: +33 1 49 95 84 94
Fax: +33 1 49 95 82 12

Prof. Maryse HURTREL
Serv d'Anatomie Pathologi-
que, Ecole Nat Veterinaire de
Nantes
FR 44087 Nantes Cedex 03
Phone: +33 40 68 76 57
Fax: +33 40 25 25 90

Prof. Matti HALTIA
Dept. of Pathology,
Univ of Helsinki
FI 00290 Helsinki
Phone: +358 0 43 461
Fax: +358 0 434 6700

Prof. Nicolo RIZZUTO
Istituto di Clinica Neurolgica,
Ospedale Policlino
Borgo Roma
IT 37134 Verona
Phone: +39 45 933285

Prof. Peter L. LANTOS
Dept. of Neuropathology,
Inst. of Psychiatry
Denmark Hill
UK London SE5 8AF
Phone: +44 71 703 8403
Fax: +44 71 708 3895

Prof. Romain GHERARDI
Dept. de Pathologie (Neuro-
pathologie), Hosp. Henri
Mondor
FR 92010 Creteil Cedex
Phone: +33 1 49 81 27 46

Prof. U. DE GIROLAMI
Neuropathology Div.,
Harvard Med Sch,
Brigham and Woman's Hosp
75 Francis Street
US Boston Massachusetts
Phone: +1 617 732 7532

IMPACT OF TOXOPLASMA GONDII STRAIN DIFFERENCES ON SEROLOGICAL DIAGNOSIS AND DISEASE IN AIDS PATIENTS WITH CEREBRAL TOXOPLASMOSIS AND IN OTHER GROUPS OF PATIENTS

Key words
Toxoplasma gondii, toxoplasmosis, strain, strain differences, serology, diagnosis, standardization, AIDS.

Objectives
1 To standardize diagnostical tests by defining and characterizing reference T. gondii strains for use in defined test systems.
2 To establish a classification system of T. gondii isolates and to identify antigens that are important for diagnosis and that might be specific for humanpathogenic T. gondii strains.
3 To analyze sporozoites, which might be the source for strain differences. Sporozoite antigens might be identified that will be useful as potential vaccine candidates for use in cats.
4 To determine the regional prevalence of toxoplasmic encephalitis in AIDS patients throughout Europe.

Brief description
The overall aim of this project is to achieve a deeper knowledge about epidemiology, diagnosis, treatment and prevention of toxoplasmosis especially in immunocompromised patients. An infection with T. gondii generally presents mild or asymptomatic diseases in healthy adults leading to the development of persisting cysts predominantly located in the brain of infected individuals. In immunocompromised patients, reactivation of cysts may result in cerebral toxoplasmosis, a disease that often has fatal outcome in AIDS patients. In addition to reactivated toxoplasmosis, an acute infection acquired in utero can cause serious or fatal illness in the infant. Diagnosis of T. gondii infection has mainly to rely on serological methods, which often are insufficient in diagnosing congenital infection or cerebral toxoplasmosis in AIDS patients. Since serological methods for detection of T. gondii-specific antibodies are not standardized throughout Europe, contrary results may occur. In addition, T. gondii strain-dependent human antibody response may also explain differences of test results. So far, no serological typing of T. gondii isolates is available, although it was demonstrated by several investigators that strain differences do exist. International scientific investigations on toxoplasmosis generally analyze the mouse-virulent laboratory reference strain RH, although it is known that most recent clinical isolates are non-mouse lethal. The RH strain is the one that is used in most serological tests as the antigenic source. Since it is not clear, whether all "RH-strains" are identical, this Concerted Action is planning to characterize reference T. gondii strains that were obtained from different diagnostical laboratories. Reference strains should be compared with clinical isolates in regards of differences in genotype and phenotype to establish a classification system upon which epidemiological studies could be possible. Representative isolates should be tested in diagnostical laboratories throughout Europe to determine parasitic factors/antigens that might be critical for standardized diagnosis. To perform such studies, this Concerted Action will cooperate with the Concerted Action "congenital Toxoplasmosis". Two identical European strain collections of T. gondii will be estab-

lished, that are available to the scientific community for further studies. Since sporozoites might be the source for strain differences, sporozoite antigens might be identified that could be useful as potential vaccine candidates for use in cats. Finally, in order to analyze the epidemiology of toxoplasmosis, the regional prevalence of reactivated toxoplasmosis (encephalitis/disseminated toxoplasmosis) shall be determined throughout Europe.

The meetings of all participants are organized every 6-10 months and are held in connection with international workshops *Toxoplasma gondii Research in Europe*. Past workshops have taken place in Würzburg (Germany) and Oxford (United Kingdom). The next workshop will take place in Vienna in April or May 1994. Further information is available from the project leader.

Project leader:
Dr. U. GROSS
Institute of Hygiene and Microbiology,
University of Würzburg
Josef-Schneider Strasse 2
DE 97080 Würzburg
Phone: +49 931 201 39 01
Fax: +49 931 201 34 45
Contract number: CT921535

Participants:
Dr. Andreas HASSL
Clin Inst. for Hygiene,
Univ of Vienna
Kinderspitalgasse 15
AT 1095 Vienna
Phone: +43 1 40490238
Fax: +43 1 40490242

Dr. Jean F. DUBREMETZ
INSERM U42
369 Rue Jules Guesde
FR 59651 Villeneuve d'lAscq Cedex
Phone: +33 20911462
Fax: +33 20059172

Dr. J.P. FERGUSON
Nuffield Dept. of Pathology and Bacteriology,
Univ of Oxford
UK Oxford OX3 9DU
Phone: +44 865 220524

Dr. J.P. OVERDULVE
Dept. Parasitology and Trop Vet Med,
State Univ of Utrecht
Yalelaan 1
NL 3508 TD Utrecht
Phone: +31 30 532559
Fax: +31 30 540784

Dr. Moni F. CESBRON-DELAUW
Centre d'Immunologie et de
Biologie Parasitaire,
Unite Mixte INSERM U167-CNRS 624,
Inst. Pasteur
1 Rue du Prof. A. Calmette
FR 59019 Lille Cedex
Phone: +33 20877965
Fax: +33 20877888

Dr. M. ROMMEL
Dept. of Vet Med, Inst. for Parasitology,
Univ of Hannover
Bunteweg 17
DE 3000 Hannover 71
Phone: +49 511 9538793
Fax: +49 511 9538870

PRECLINICAL STUDIES IN CHIMPANZEES AND RELEVANT PRIMATE MODELS: TOWARDS EFFECTIVE VACCINES AND THERAPEUTIC STRATEGIES FOR AIDS

Key words
Chimpanzees, nonhuman primates, preclinical, AIDS, vaccines, therapeutics, immunotherapy, biotechnology, clinical trials.

Objectives
1 To perform *efficacy testing of HIV-1* vaccines for prevention of HIV-1 infection. The ultimate goal is to identify a vaccine giving long lasting enduring immunity and heterologous cross protection from infected cells and viruses across mucosal barriers.
2 To elucidate mechanisms or *correlates of protective immunity to HIV-1 infection or disease* and to define prognostic parameters of protection for assessment of clinical trials; and
3 To investigate and *compare the pathogenesis of HIV-1 infection in man vs chimpanzees*: towards identifying new therapeutic strategies for the treatment of AIDS.

Brief description
The development of a safe effective vaccine or vaccines for the prevention of human immunodeficiency virus (HIV) infection is of international importance to halt or slow the current pandemic of AIDS. The principle cause of AIDS is HIV-1, a retrovirus with an enormous potential for variability both within the human host and within the population. In order to appropriately design, test and evaluate vaccines intended to protect humans from infection with this virus, an animal model must be available which responds to HIV-1 infection similar to man. Until recently HIV-1 had been proven only to infect man and his great ape relatives, while seemingly only able to cause AIDS in man. Of the great apes, only captive bred chimpanzees (man's closest relative) have been found to be practical models for HIV-1 vaccine or immunoprophylatic research. The near homologous nature of chimpanzees (>98% genomic DNA sequence homology) and man, means that the fine immunological and mechanistic events of HIV-1 infection can be studied comparatively in this species as in no other. The unique envelope (env) characteristics of HIV-1 necessitates the use of the chimpanzee model for final testing of HIV-1 vaccine efficacy. HIV-1 differs importantly from HIV-2 and the Simian Immunodeficiency Virus (SIV) in terms of envelope conformation and neutralization epitopes, proven to be important in protective immunity. Other common laboratory primates such as rhesus macaques are unfortunately only suitable for SIV/HIV-2 studies. Captive breeding facilities for chimpanzees with housing for HIV-1 infected chimpanzees are an uncommon and an invaluable resource in this regard. The search for other primate models of HIV-1 infection is ongoing and studies are planned to explore the possibility that Macaques may also be infected with a chaemeric SIV virus containing the HIV-1 envelope (SHIV) an hence a suitable model for HIV-1 infection.

This proposal aims to provide a European Centralized Facility for true centralized standardized efficacy testing of HIV-1 vaccines utilizing the chimpanzee model as the critical test and for establishing clinical trials guidelines, while HIV-1 efficacy studies of a more preliminary nature for testing new vaccine strategies are proposed to be first carried out using the SHIV macaque model.

Project leader:
Dr. J.L. HEENEY
Biomedical Primate Research Centre TNO, The laboratory of viral Pathopenesis
Lange Kleiweg 151
NL 2280 HV Rijswijk
Phone: +31 15 84 26 61
Fax: +31 15 84 39 99
Contract number: CT921203

Participants:
Dr. A. VENET, Dr. E. GOMARD,
J.P. LEVY
Immun et Oncologie des Maladies Retrovirales,
Inst. Cochin de Genetique Moleculaire,
INSERM U 152
Rue du Faubourg Saint Jacques 27
FR 75014 Paris
Phone: +33 1 46330293
Fax: +33 1 46339297

Dr. C. BRUCK
Virology, Smith Kline Beecham Biologicals
Rue de l'Inst. 89
BE 1330 Rixensaert
Phone: +32 2 6568111
Fax: +32 2 6568000

Dr. F. MIEDEMA, Dr. H. SCHUITEMAKER
Dept. of Clin Viral Immunology,
Central Lab for Blood Transfusion
Plesmanlaan 121
NL 1066 CX Amsterdam
Phone: +31 20 5123314
Fax: +31 20 5123310

Dr. G. van der GROEN
Dept. of Microbiology, Inst. of Tropical
Medicine, Prins Leopold
Nationalestraat 155
BE 2000 Antwerpen
Phone: +32 3 2476320
Fax: +32 3 2476333

Dr. H. HOLMES, Dr. G. SCHILD
AIDS Collaborating Center, Nat'l Inst.
of Biological Standards and Control
Blanche Lane South Kimms Potters bar
UK Herts EN6 3QG
Phone: +44 707 547 53
Fax: +44 707 467 30

Dr. M. GIRARD
Direction des Applications de la Recherche,
Inst. Pasteur
Rue de Docteur Roux 28
FR 75724 Paris Cedex 15
Phone: +33 1 45 688091
Fax: +33 1 43 069835

Prof. Dr. A. OSTERHAUS, Dr. C. van ELS
Dept. of Immunobiology, RIVM
P.O. Box 1
NL 3720 BA Bilthoven
Phone: +31 30 749111
Fax: +31 30 742971

Prof. Dr. B. WAHREN
Dept. of Virology,
The National Bacteriology Laboratory
SE 10521 Stockholm
Phone: +46 8 735 1000
Fax: +46 8 730 3248

Prof. Dr. J. GOUDSMIT, Dr. T. TERSMETTE
Section of Human Retrovirology, Dept. of
Med Virology Academic Med Center,
Univ of Amsterdam
Meibergdreef 9
NL 1105 AZ Amsterdam
Phone: +31 20 5664853
Fax: +31 20 6716531

Prof. Dr. K. KROHN
Dept. of Biomedical Sciences,
Univ of Tampere
P.O. Box 607
FI 33101 Tampere
Phone: +358 31 156111
Fax: +358 31 156170

Prof. Dr. L. MONTAGNIER
Viral Oncology, Inst. Pasteur
25 Rue de Dr. Roux
FR 75015 Paris
Phone: +33 1 45688000
Fax: +33 1 45688916

EUROPEAN VACCINE AGAINST AIDS (EVA)

Key words
Vaccine, AIDS, Immunodeficiency syndrome, Lentivirus, Prophylaxis, HIV, SIV.

Objectives
1 Selection and titration of candidate viruses for primate challenge experiments.
2 Support for international studies on virus epidemiology to define the viruses circulating in regions where efficacy trials of vaccines may take place.
3 Evaluation of candidate vaccines in the SIV model.
4 Supporting studies on new concepts in vaccine design such as the use of genetically modified viruses as vaccines, direct immunization with nucleic acids and improved adjuvants and delivery systems.
5 Development of reagents for use in and in support of vaccine trials.
6 Programme EVA Reagent Programme and Reference Centre.
7 Support for European pre and post-exposure clinical trials.

Brief description
Studies of candidate vaccines in chimpanzees are of central importance because they are the only primates that can be reliably infected with HIV-I. To date, there have been a small number of reports of vaccine-mediated protection and there is an urgent need to confirm and extend these studies. So far, all the challenge studies that have been reported were based on a laboratory strain of HIV-I (HTLV-IIIB). Programme EVA has decided to give priority to the preparation of a challenge stock based on a European field isolate. Several strains are urgently being evaluated with the intention of selecting one strain for *in vivo* titration.

The Programme is also working closely with the WHO in supporting studies on viral epidemiology so as to define the nature of the viruses circulating in regions where vaccine efficacy trials may take place. Information generated in these studies will help to ensure that vaccines are formulated to match the range of viruses that they may meet in the field.

Studies on new concepts of vaccine design are being supported. For example, EVA is funding a European Collaborative experiment in which an attenuated live nef-deleted SIV is being tested in macaques as a potential vaccine against a wide range of challenge viruses. Work on other deletion mutants, on the direct immunization with DNA and on improved adjuvants and delivery systems are also being actively supported by the Programme. Such studies are underpinned by the provision of key reagents needed for AIDS Research, a considerable number of which are now available from the Programme's Centralised Facility, and by occasional state-of-the-art Workshops, bringing together researchers actively pursuing common objectives.

Project leader:
Dr. H.C. HOLMES
National Institute for Biological Standards and Control (NIBSC)
Blanche Lane, South Mimms
UK Potters Bar (Herts) EN6 3QG
Phone: +44 707 65 47 53
Fax: +44 707 64 98 65
Contract number: CT921065

Participants:

Dr. G. HUNSMANN
Deutsches Primatenzentrum Gmbh
Kellnerweg 4
DE 3400 Gottingen
Phone: +49 551 38510
Fax: +49 551 3851 228

Dr. SCHILD NIBSC
Blanche Lane, South Mimms,
Potters Bar
UK Herts EN6 3QG
Phone: +44 707 54753
Fax: +44 707 46730

Dr. J. KARN
MRC Lab of Molecular Biology
Hills Road
UK Cambridge CB2 2QH
Phone: +44 223 248011
Fax: +44 223 412282

Dr. Marc GIRARD
Inst. Pasteur
Rue de Dr. Roux 28
FR 75724 Paris Cedex 15
Phone: +33 1 45 688740
Fax: +33 1 43 069835

Dr. R. NAJERA MORRONDO
Instituto de Salud Carlos III
ES 28220 Majadahonda, Madrid
Phone: +34 1 638 24 39
Fax: +34 1 638 06 13

Prof. A.BURNY
Fac des Sciences, Lab de Chimie Biol,
Univ de Bruxelles
67 Rue des Chevaux
BE 1640 Rhode Saint Genese, Brussels
Phone: +32 2 650 2111
Fax: +32 2 650 9999

Prof. Dr. J. GOUDSMIT
Human Retrovirus Lab, AMC,
Dept. of Virology, Room L1-157
Meibergdreef 15
NL 1105 AZ Amsterdam
Phone: +31 20 5664853
Fax: +31 20 916531

Prof. G.B. ROSSI
Dept. of Virology, Ist Superiore di Sanita
299 Viale Regina Elena
IT 00161 Rome
Phone: +39 6 4457116
Fax: +39 6 4453904

Prof. H. WIGZELL
Karolinska Inst., Dept. of Immunology
P.O. Box 60400
SE 10501 Stockholm
Phone: +46 8 286400
Fax: +46 8 328878

Prof. K. KROHN
Inst. of Biomedical Sciences,
Univ of Tampere
P.O. Box 607
FI 33101 Tampere
Phone: +358 31 156666
Fax: +358 31 156736

Prof. L. MONTAGNIER
Unite d'Oncologie Virale,
Institut Pasteur
Rue du Dr. Roux 28
FR 75724 Paris Cedex 15
Phone: +33 1 45 688740
Fax: +33 1 45 689816

Prof. M. PAPAMICHAIL
Helenic Anti-Cancer Inst.
Alexandria Avenue
GR 171 Athens 11522
Phone: +30 1 640 0462
Fax: +30 1 642 0146

Prof. V. ERFLE
GSF, Abteilung fur Moleculare Zellpathologie
Ingolstadter Landstrasse 1
DE 8042 Neuherberg
Phone: +49 89 31 874216
Fax: +49 89 31 873322

MONKEY MODELS FOR AIDS RESEARCH

Key words

AIDS research, vaccine trial, pathogenesis treatment, immune response, experimental infection, HIV, SIV, rhesus monkey.

Objectives

1 To design and perform concerted experiments in the area of AIDS pathogenicity, therapy, and vaccine development, using the experimental infection of macaques.
2 To mobilize, coordinate, and focus available European resources for these experiments.

Brief description

The objectives will be achieved through improved communication, standardization of experimental procedures, and coordination of concerted trials.

Results of common experiments as well as the know-how of the individual participants will freely be exchanged.

The mobility of researchers is encouraged by support of short-term visits to other participating laboratories.

Areas of scientific cooperation

As in the past, scientists from ten centres able to perform experiments with SIV- or HIV-infected macaques will cooperate in three major areas of AIDS research, namely (i) pathogenesis, (ii) experimental therapy, and (iii) vaccine development.

Moreover, the intended pooling of valuable and limited resources will ensure its effective use, speed-up the development, increase the international competitiveness of European AIDS research, improve the well-fare of experimental animals and reduce the overall number of monkeys required for this type of work.

Experimental approach

In the first phase we will concentrate on vaccine development by initiating experiments to:
- identify the protecting immunogen;
- develop resources for such immunogens (e.g. peptides, recombinant proteins, tissue culture grown virus);
- compare various challenge virus stocks (e.g. PBMC-grown virus);
- investigate different routes of inoculation (e.g. mucosal versus intravenous application of challenge, cell associated virus challenge);
- monitor the duration of protection in different experiments;
- elucidate the nature of the protecting immune mechanism
- examine the potentials of life recombinant vaccines and viral chimeras
- search for and implement new experimental systems, in particular, the infection of pigtailed macaques (Macaca nemestrina) with HIV-1 or rhesus and cynomolgous macaques with SIV recombinants carrying the HIV envelope.

First experimental protocol

Protection against PBMC-grown challenge virus with life recombinant SIV vaccines. Recently, a genetically attenuated SIV (SIVmac239 nef) was shown to replicate poorly in rhesus monkeys. Animals infected with these recombinant SIV were, however, protected against high doses of a complete pathogenic SIVmac.

We will examine attenuated recombinant SIV immunogens deleted in their nef or vpr or rev genes or in several of these non-structural genes. The purpose is to find out whether protection against monkey PBMC-grown challenge viruses or challenge stocks derived so ex vivo can be achieved. Moreover, we want to elucidate the mechanisms by which infection with the challenge virus is abrogated. Currently, we are concerned about the safety of potential recombinant life HIV-vaccines. However, the results of the planned experiment would help to define the protecting immune mechanisms which we then would try to induce with safer vaccines potentially applicable in humans.

In a first concerted experiment we will investigate the protective potential of an SIVmac239 nef recombinant against various titrated challenge viruses.

Project leader:
Professor G. HUNSMANN
Deutsches Primatenzentrum
Kellnerweg 4
DE 37077 Göttingen
Phone: +49 551 385 11 55
Fax: +49 551 385 12 28
Contract number: CT920634

Participants:
Dr. A. OSTERHAUS, Dr. P. de VRIES
National Inst. of Public Health (RIVM)
Antonie van Leeuwenhoeklaan 9
NL 3720 Bilthoven
Phone: +31 30 74 21 42
Fax: +31 30 74 29 71

Dr. D. DORMONT, Dr. R. LE GRAND
Centre de Recherches du Services
de Sante des Armees
60-68 Av de la Div. Leclerc
FR 92265 Fontenay aux Roses Cedex
Phone: +33 1 46 548122
Fax: +33 1 46 549180

Dr. J. HEENEY
Primate Center TNO
Lange Kleiweg 151
NL 2280 HV Rijswijk
Phone: +31 15 84 28 42
Fax: +31 15 84 39 98

Dr. Pete KITCHIN, Dr. Jim STOTT
National Inst. for Biol Standards and Control
Blanche Lane, South Minns, Potters Bar
UK Hertfordshire EN6 3QG
Phone: +44 707 5 47 53
Fax: +44 707 4 98 65

Dr. P. GREENAWAY, Dr. G. FARRAR
Div. of Pathology, PHLS, Centre for
Appl Microbioly and Research
Porton Down, Salisbury
UK Wiltshire SP4 0JG
Phone: +44 980 61 03 91
Fax: +44 980 61 10 96

Prof. Dr. G. BIBERFELD, Dr. P. PUTKONEN
The National Bacteriological Laboratory
Lundagatan 2
SE 105 21 Stockholm
Phone: +46 8 735 10 00
Fax: +46 8 735 41 36

Prof. Dr. G. ROSSI, Prof. Dr. P. VERANI
Dip di Virogia, Ist Superiore di Sanita Roma
299 Viale Regina Elena
IT 00161 Rome
Phone: +39 6 445 71 16
Fax: +39 6 445 39 04

Prof. Dr. R. KURTH, Dr. S. NORLEY
Paul Ehrlich Institut
Paul Ehrlich Strasse 51059
DE W-6070 Langen
Phone: +49 6103 755 0
Fax: +49 6103 755 123

Prof. Dr. V. ERFLE, Dr. A. KLEINSCHMIDT
Gesellschaft fur Strahlen- und Umweltforschung
Ingolstadter Landsstrasse 1
DE W-8042 Neuherberg
Phone: +49 89 31872416

DEVELOPMENT OF AIDS VACCINE STRATEGIES USING THE FELINE IMMUNODEFICIENCY VIRUS MODEL

Key words
AIDS, HIV, vaccination, FIV.

Objectives
The Concerted Action will use feline immunodeficiency virus (FIV) infection of cats to develop vaccines that are of relevance to vaccination against HIV. The major objectives are:
1 To produce the SU protein of FIV in several expression systems and to compare the efficacy of each as a vaccine in experimental challenge by live FIV.
2 To define the T and B cell epitopes of FIV SU which are involved in protective immunity.
3 To determine the influence of variation in the SU amino acid sequence among FIV isolates on vaccinal immunity.

Brief description
In the dynamics of infection, immune response, pathogenesis and immunological defects, FIV infection of the cat closely resembles HIV infection in man.
Consequently FIV is considered to be excellent model to study vaccination against HIV. The ready availability of experimental cats permits the rapid assessment of the efficacy of candidate vaccines.
A prototypic vaccine based on chemically inactivated virus protects cats against challenge by virus. This protection is virus-specific and appears to correlate with the level of virus neutralising antibodies induced in vaccinated cats. Research is now in progress to define the immunogens necessary for protection and to determine the immunological mechanisms by which the protection is achieved. Since virus neutralisation may be important in immunity, emphasis is placed initially on the surface glycoprotein of the virus, gp120 (SU) as an immunogen.
The SU immunogens to be tested are expressed in four systems in different laboratories: vaccinia recombinants in mammalian cells, adenovirus recombinant in mammalian cells, baculovirus recombinants in insect cells and recombinant proteins in *E. coli*.
The response of cats to these vaccines can be monitored by induction of antibodies, particularly virus neutralising antibodies, by the induction of cytotoxic T cells, and ultimately by challenge against live virus.
The extent of heterologous protection against different FIV isolates will be assessed. Challenge viruses are available that are either antigenically related or unrelated to vaccinal viruses by virus neutralisation. How these antigenic differences are reflected in amino acid sequence variation within the variable regions of the SU protein of the appropriate viruses will be examined.

Project leader:
Professor O. JARRETT
Dept. of Veterinary Pathology,
Veterinary School,
University of Glasgow,
Bearsden
UK Glasgow G61 1QH
Phone: +44 41 330 57 73
Fax: +44 41 330 56 02
Contract number: CT920879

Participants:
Dr. Anne MORAILLON
Ecole Nationale Veterinaire d'Alfort
Avenue du General de Gaulle 7
FR 94704 Maisons-Alfort Cedex
Phone: +33 1 43 96 71 32
Fax: +33 1 43 96 71 31

Dr. Anthony de RONDE
Fac der Diergeneeskunde, Rijksuniv te Utrecht
P.O. Box 80 165
NL 3508 TD Utrecht
Phone: +31 30 534195
Fax: +31 30 536723

Dr. Hans LUTZ
Veterinar Med Klin, Univ Zurich
Winterthur Strasse 260
CH 8057 Zurich
Phone: +41 1 365 1219
Fax: +41 1 313 0046

Dr. Pierro SONIGO
Inst. Cochin de Genetique Moleculaire,
Lab de Genetique des Virus
22 Rue Mechain
FR 75014 Paris
Phone: +33 1 40 51 75 59
Fax: +33 1 40 51 72 10

Prof. Dr. Albert DME OSTERHAUS
Rijksinstituut voor Volksgezondheid
en Milieuhygiene
Antonie van Leeuwenhoeklaan 9
NL 3720 BA Bilthoven
Phone: +31 30 742142
Fax: +31 30 250493

Prof. Mauro BENDINELLI
Univ di Pisa, Dip di Biomedicina
Via S Zeno 35-39
IT Pisa
Phone: +49 50 553 562
Fax: +49 50 555 477

DEVELOPMENT AND EVALUATION OF IMMUNOLOGICAL AND VIROLOGICAL PROGRESSION MARKERS TO BE USED FOR MONITORING OF THERAPY IN HIV INFECTION

Key words
AIDS, immunology, prognosis, therapy.

Objectives
Development, implementation, standardization and evaluation, in ongoing European cohort studies, of new immunological and virological markers that are suitable for staging of HIV infection and are surrogate markers for clinical end-points in evaluation of therapy in HIV infection.

Brief description
Evaluation of selected immunological and virological markers in therapy trials
The core activity of the CA will be to implement and evaluate selected markers simultaneously and in a coordinated fashion in several European treated and untreated cohorts of HIV infected people. First T cell functional assays and HIV phenotype will be studied.
T cell functional tests This will include:
1 PWM-driven culture systems in whole blood and on purified leucocytes;
2 Anti-CD3 (several Mabs) and PHA driven systems employing purified cells;
3 An anti-CD3 driven system performed in whole blood cultures using an IgE anti-CD3 Mab available through the CLB, Amsterdam.

HIV phenotyping. Phenotyping of HIV variants to detect SI variants that are predictive for rapid CD4 decline based on selective growth and CPE induction of syncytium-inducing variants in MT2 cells.
Flow chart. In the first year, to make these markers operational in the different laboratories, standard reagents and cell lines will be produced and distributed, including anti-CD3 Mab, reference virus strains and the MT2 cell line. Criteria and requirements for these assays, i.e. quality control of reagents, standardization and user-friendliness, will be established. In bilateral collaborations personnel will be trained in laboratories that have developed specific assays but short wet-workshops for on-the-site training of researchers from several participating laboratories will also be organised.
In the second year and the first part of the third year, these prognostic tests will be used to prospectively monitor ongoing trials with anti-viral drugs and to retrospectively analyze treated groups for these novel variables.
In the third year the project will be finalized, pooling and comparing results obtained in cohort studies of the participating groups in terms of reliability, predictive value for progression, relation to CD4 counts and other variables that may be in use (antigenemia) using standard statistical methods. By evaluating these markers simultaneously in several cohorts in a short time great statistical power can be generated.
Identification of Novel Immunological Progression Markers
To identify new predictive markers that are pathogenetically involved in the natural history of HIV infection knowledge on immune abnormalities and mechanisms of immune deficiency, which is being accumulated in rather independent disciplines of immunomorphology/pathology, cellular immunology and viro-immunology, will be inte-

grated by directed communication during 2 plenary CA meetings to be held in the first and the third year. In these larger format meetings, in addition to the participants to the core-project described above, relevant researchers will be invited to take part. These groups are designated as non-core participants to the CA.

Project leader:
Dr. F. MIEDEMA
Dept. of Clinical Viro-Immunology, CBL,
University of Amsterdam
Plesmanlaan 125
NL 1066 CX Amsterdam
Phone: +31 20 512 33 17
Fax: +31 20 512 33 10
Contract number: CT921451

Participants:
Dr. B. AUTRAN
Lab d'Immunol Cell Tiss,
Hop Pitie-Salpetriere C.E.R.V.I.
83 Boulevard de l'Hopital
FR 75013 Paris
Phone: +33 1 45703819
Fax: +33 1 45702045

Dr. E. DICKMEISS
Dept. Clin Immunol, Sec 2032/
Blood Bank, Rigshospitalet
9 Blegdamsvej
DK 2100 Copenhagen
Phone: +45 35352032
Fax: +45 35452053

Prof. F. AIUTI
Univ La Sapienza,
Cattedra Allergologia Immun Clin
IT 00161 Roma
Phone: +39 6 4454941
Fax: +39 6 4463328

Prof. G. JANOSSY
Dept. of Clin Immunol, Royal Free Hosp
Pond Street
UK London NW3 2QG
Phone: +44 71 4310879
Fax: +44 71 4310879

Prof. J. ECONOMIDOU
Dept. Immunol Histocomp,
Evangelismos Hosp Athens
45-47 Ipsilantou Street
GR 10676 Athens
Phone: +30 1 7220101
Fax: +30 1 7291808

Prof. M. SELIGMANN
Serv D'Immunohematologie, Hopital Saint Louis
Avenue Claude Vellefaux 1
FR 75475 Paris Cedex 10
Phone: +33 1 42499690
Fax: +33 1 42494040

Prof. V. GEORGOULIAS
Dept. of Clin Oncology, Univ General Hosp
P.O. Box 1352
GR 711 10 Heraklion Crete
Phone: +30 81 269747
Fax: +30 81 261433

MECHANISMS OF CD4+ CELL DEPLETION
IN AIDS PATHOGENESIS

Key words
HIV, SIV, AIDS, T lymphocytes, Apoptosis, Receptors, superantigen.

Objectives
The aim of the Concerted Action is to analyze the mechanism of CD4 cell depletion in
the course of HIV infection, which is central to the immunopathogenesis of AIDS. First
a standardization of experimental procedures was planned in order to study spontaneous
and activation-induced apoptosis in patients' lymphocytes, to study the Vß T cell repertoire and to analyze the influence of cytokines on the growth of specific T cell subpopulations. Then the contributions of several mechanisms contributing to CD4 cell depletion
will be studied: induction of apoptosis in non infected cells, influence of superantigens
(bacterial and viral) on CD4 cell depletion, rol of autoantibodies, influence of $\tau\delta$ T cell
subpopulations in AIDS. A model that would account for the progressive depletion of
CD4+ T cells in vivo and the possible clinical implications will be derived.

Brief description
Despite a low rate of HIV infection in peripheral CD4 T cells, a decline of the immune
system occurs including dysfunction of monocytes and of CD4 helper T cells, polyclonal
activation of B cells and a progressive CD4 T cell depletion leading to AIDS. Since
these effects are unlikely to be only due to small amounts of HIV-infected lymphocytes,
indirect immunological mechanisms have to be envisaged. Recent developments in our
laboratory have suggested that the loss of CD4 T cells is associate with lymphocyte
activation: antigenic or mitogenic stimulation of T lymphocytes from patients results,
instead of proliferation and cytokine secretion, in death of a fraction of activated cells
through a mechanism known as programmed cell death or apoptosis (Gougeon et al.).
This phenomenon is enhanced by superantigens, which are known to interact with the Vß
domain of the T cell Receptor (TCR). Deletions of TCR Vß expressing T cell subsets
has been found in the early stages of the disease (Dalgleish et al.) and at the AIDS stage
(Primi et al.). Vß specific anergy was also observed in a large fraction of asymptomatic
HIV-infected individuals (Gougeon et al.). These findings indicate that superantigens are
involved in AIDS pathogenesis and the participation of HIV has to be considered.
Several models have been proposed and are currently testes for the mechanism of CD4+
T cell activation and subsequent deletion of non-infected cells in AIDS:
- the delivery of wrong co-signals to T cells by HIV-infected monocytes (this aspect is
  studied by J. Heeney in the chimpanzee model);
- the delivery to T cells through the HIV envelope gp 120-CD4 interaction of inhibitory
  signals which would program CD4 cells for apoptosis or induce it (Piacentini et al.);
- the allogenic stimulation of T cells consequently to the mimicry of MHC by gp120
  (Dalgleish et al.);
- a superantigenic activity associated to HIV (Gougeon et al.).

Another related question concerns the renewal of these depleted CD4 T cells: Is there
any defect in the maturation of precursor T cells into mature T cells in patients? This
aspect is analyzed through the identification of T cell subsets that express the $\tau\delta$ TCR,
which are significantly enhanced during HIV-infection and which seem to inhibit in vitro

the maturation of bone marrow T cell precursors into mature T cells (Rossol et al.). Characterization of the repertoire and the function of these $\tau\delta$ subsets is in progress (Gougeon et al.) and the mechanisms responsible for their inhibitory effect (cytokines vs cytotoxic activity) are currently under investigation (Rossol et al.).

Project leader:
Professor L. MONTAGNIER
Unité d'Oncologie Virale,
Département SIDA et Rétrovirus,
Institut Pasteur
28 Rue du Dr. Roux
FR 75724 Paris Cedex 15
Phone: +33 1 45 688740
Fax: +33 1 45 688916
Contract number: CT921571

Participants:
Drs. M. PIACENTINI, V. COLIZZI
Dip Di Biologia, II Univ Degli Studi Di Roma
Via E. Carnevale
IT 00173 Roma
Phone: +39 6 72594370
Fax: +39 6 2023500

Dr. Daniele PRIMI
Conbiotec - Consorzio per le Biotecnologie,
Lab di Biotecnologie
Piazzale Spedale Civili no 1
IT 25123 Brescia
Phone: +39 30 383 439
Fax: +39 30 397 045

Dr. G. BIRD
HIV Immunol Lab,
Blood Transfusion Service
41 Lauriston Place
UK Edinburgh EH3 9HB Scotland
Phone: +44 31 2292585
Fax: +44 31 2285238

Dr. Jonathan HEENEY
Div of Health Res, TNO, Inst. of
Applied Radiobiology and Immunology
P.O. Box 5815
NL 2280 HV Rijswijk
Phone: +31 1584 2660
Fax: +31 1584 3999

Dr. Rita ROSSOL
Bio Pharm GMBH
Justinianstrasse 22
DE 6000 Frankfurt am Main
Phone: +49 69 245 53 253
Fax: +49 69 55 16 21

Prof. Angus DALGLEISH
Div of Oncology, St. George's Hospital
Cranmar Terrace
UK London SW17 ORE
Phone: +44 81 672 9944
Fax: +44 81 784 2649

Prof. D. HOELZER
Dep Hematologie, Univ Klin Frankfurt,
Zentrum Innere Medizin
Theodoor Stern Kai 7
DE 6000 Frankfurt am Main 70
Phone: +49 69 6301 5194
Fax: +49 69 6301 7326

CENTRALIZED FACILITY FOR HIV GENOME ANALYSIS

Key words
HIV, base sequence, variation.

Objectives
The CF for HIV Genome Analysis helps European AIDS researchers to manage the large amount of sequencing work required to understand the different phenotypic properties of HIV resulting from the extreme variability of its genome. An automated laser fluorescence (A.L.F.) machine and a set of premade primers allows rapid sequencing of full length HIV-1 genomes and the *env* region of HIV-2. Additional primers will be synthesized for other regions of the HIV-2 genome or for the simian viruses, if required. Sequencing projects include the fields of vaccine development, molecular epidemiology, pathogenesis, tropism or drug resistance.

Brief description
Concentration of the sequencing efforts at the CF allows to perform this work in a more time- and cost efficient way: the strategy of premade primers derived from consensus sequences is especially useful in cases where many similar sequences have to be determined. The CF works with primers originally designed from an HIV-1 consensus sequence which included European/US and prototypic African strains. This primer set was then extended by primers synthesized for the individual projects sequenced in the past at the CF. These projects included strains from different subtypes of HIV-1 and parts of the HIV-2 genome. Today, 135 fluorescent labelled primers are available for HIV-I, 25 for HIV-2 and 13 for various cloning vectors. These primers can be used in future sequencing projects at the CF. Further HIV-2 or SIV primers will be synthesized if required.

Sequencing is performed by an automated laser fluorescence machine (A.L.F.), where fluorescent labelled sequencing products are detected by a fixed laser during the gel run. Data are transferred to a computer and evaluated with the corresponding software.

Several technical improvements during the last years of the CF's activity resulted in longer reading lengths per gel lane, up to 650 basepairs. Also, direct sequencing of PCR products on a solid phase was established. Indepently of the primers, the label of the sequencing products can now also be introduced via a labelled nucleotide (fluoro-dATP). Thus, depending on the kind of the project, several approaches can be used.

Applications from the different fields of HIV research are sent to the CF and proofed by a steering committee consisting of 8 members from 7 European countries. This steering committee decides on relevance and priority of the projects. So far, more than 100 kb of evaluated sequence data have been generated for 9 different projects.

Project leader:
Professor H. RÜBSAMEN-WAIGMANN
Georg-Speyer-Haus
Paul-Ehrlich-Strasse 42-44
DE 60596 Frankfurt am Main 70
Phone: +49 69 63 39 50
Fax: +49 69 63 39 52 97
Contract number: CT921667

Participants:
Dr. A. BURNY
Université Libre de Bruxelles
Laboratoire de Chimie Biologique
rue des Chevaux 67
BE 1640 Rhode-St-Genèse
Phone: +32 2 650 99 99

Dr. P. GREENAWAY
PHLS Center for Applied Microbiology
and Research, Division of Pathology
Porton Down
UK Salisbury Wiltshire SP4 0JG
Fax: +44 980 61 10 96

Dr. K. KROHN
Institute of Biomedical Sciences
University of Tampere
P.O. Box 607
FI 33101 Tampere
Fax: +358 31 15 61 70

Dr. R. NAJERA-MORRONDO
Instituto de Salud Carlos III
Ctra. Majadahonda
ES Madrid
Fax: +34 1 323 42 96

Prof. A. SICCARDI
DIBIT, Instituto H.S. Raffaele
Via Olgettina 60
IT 20132 Milano
Fax: +39 2 2643 47 67

Dr. P. SONIGO
Institut Cochin de Génétique Moléculaire
CNRS UPR-0415
22 rue Méchain
FR 75014 Paris
Fax: +33 1 4051 72 10

Dr. S. WAIN-HOBSON
Institut Pasteur, Unité de Biologie
et Immunologie Moleculaire
25/28 Rue de Dr. Roux
FR 75724 Paris Cedex 15
Fax: +33 1 4568 88 74

DEVELOPMENT OF NOVEL TSAO DERIVATIVES AS A TOOL FOR DELINEATING THE MOLECULAR MECHANISMS OF HUMAN IMMUNODEFICIENCY VIRUS RESISTANCE AND CIRCUMVENTING THE EMERGENCE OF RESISTANT VIRUS STRAINS

Key words
HIV-1, HIV-2, SIV, TSAO compounds.

Brief description
TSAO nucleoside analogues represent a structural class of compounds that inhibit the replication of human immunodeficiency virus type 1 (HIV-l), but not HIV-2, simian immunodeficiency virus (SIV) or other DNA or RNA viruses.

Their mechanism of action and biological properties are similar to the previously discovered HIV-l-specific TIBO, HEPT, nevirapine, pyridinone and BHAP derivatives.

However, TSAO derivatives represent the first molecules for which the active pharmacophore (i.e. the 4 moiety) could be identified. Indeed, the 4 of glutamic acid (Glu) at position 138 of the reverse transcriptase.

Mutant HIV-l strains that are selected for resistance against TSAO are characterized by an RT, that invariably contains Lysine (Lys) at position 138 instead of Glu.

These findings open interesting perspectives to design a of TSAO molecules instead of Glu-138 and thus can inhibit TSAO-resistant viruses.

Moreover, since positions 137 and 136 of the RT contain asparagine (Asn) residues that are highly conserved in all HIV-1, HIV-2 and SIV strains, it is our intention to synthesize a series of molecules currently available TSAO molecules.

Thus, synthesis of rationally designed 2nd and 3rd generation-TSAO molecules will be performed and the novel TSAO derivatives will be evaluated on their antiretroviral action against HIV-l, HIV-2 and SIV strains, including HIV-l strains that are resistant to the currently available TSAO molecules.

In addition, mutant virus strains resistant against the novel TSAO compounds will be selected in lymphocytes and macrophages, isolated and characterized at the molecular level (reverse transcriptase).

Introduction of different amino acids at positions 138, 137 and 136 of the RT by site-directed mutagenesis will provide us with valuable information on the mechanism of resistance development, and the nature of interaction of the TSAO molecules with their target enzyme.

The pathogenicity of several TSAO-resistant HIV-l strains will be studied in SCID mice constituted with human PBL.

In addition, emergence of TSAO-resistant HIV-l strains in mice under TSAO therapy will be investigated and molecularly characterized.

These TSAO-resistant HIV-l strains - if they emerge - will be evaluated on their sensitivity to other HIV-l-specific compounds.

Eventually, the susceptibility of these mutant HIV-l strains to be inhibited by other HIV-l-specific compounds will be examined.

Project leader:
Dr. Jan BALZARINI
Laboratory of Experimental Chemotherapy,
Rega Institute for Medical Research
Minderbroedersstraat 10
BE 3000 Leuven
Phone: +32 16 33 73 52
Fax: +32 16 33 73 40
Contract number: CT931691

Participants:
Anna KARLSSON
Biochemistry 1
Box 60400
SE 10401 Stockholm
Phone: +46 8 7286985
Fax: +46 8 305193

Carlo-Federico PERNO
Univ of Rome Tor Vergata
Dept. of Experimental
Medicine
Via Orazio Raimondo
IT 00173 Rome
Phone: +39 6 72592118
Fax: +39 6 7234793

Maria-José CAMARASA
Instituto de Quimica Médica
Calle Juan de la Cierva 3
ES 28006 Madrid
Phone: +34 1 4113155
Fax: +34 1 5644853

EUROPEAN NETWORK FOR THE TREATMENT OF AIDS

Key words
Clinical trials, HIV infection, opportunistic infections.

Brief description
The objective of the ENTA is to set up a coherent and independent network for clinical trials in Europe. This network will have as research priorities, clinical trials which are not funded by the industry such as:
- evaluation of drugs which are already licensed but whose indications are not well defined in the setting of HIV infection;
- prevention of opportunistic infections which are highly prevalent in Europe (i.e. toxoplasmosis, tuberculosis);
- prevention of infections which are frequently found in HIV patients and represent significant public health problems (i.e. pneumococcal infection).

These priorities have been defined in order to avoid duplication of trials already implemented in the United States or elsewhere in Europe and to cover areas which are not covered by national efforts or by the pharmaceutical industry.
In view of this specificity, EEC funding would be the only financial support and is requested for the coordination of the trials. This coordination will be generated by the following structures:
- a Coordinating and Data Centre, located in Brussels;
- National Coordinators, who constitute the Steering Committee of ENTA.
This Committee has already approved six protocols which are ready to start.

Project leader:
Professor N. CLUMECK
European Network for the Treatment of Aids
Coordinating and Data Centre
rue Haute 322
BE 1000 Bruxelles
Phone: +32 2 535 41 31
Fax: +32 2 539 36 14
Contract number: CT931222

Participants:
Prof. F. ANTUNES
Hospital de Santa Maria,
Serviçio de Doenças Infecciosas
Av. Egas Moniz
PT 1600 Lisbon
Phone: +351 1 797 62 42

Prof. M. DIETRICH
Bernhardt-Nocht-Institut für Tropenmedizin
Bernardt-Nocht-Strasse 74
DE 2000 Hamburg 36
Phone: +49 40 31 18 23 90
Fax: +49 40 31 18 23 94

Dr. J.M. GATELL
Hospital Clinic i Provincial de Barcelona,
Servicio Infecciones
Villarroel 170
ES 08036 Barcelona
Phone: +34 3 323 14 14
Fax: +34 3 451 44 38

Dr. R. HEMMER
Centre Hospitalier de Luxembourg,
Département des Maladies Infectieuses
Rue Barblé 4
LU 1210 Luxembourg
Phone: +352 44 11 30 91
Fax: +352 45 87 62

Dr. B. HIRSCHEL
Hôpital Cantonal Universitaire de Genève,
Division des Maladies Infectieuses
Rue Micheli-du-Crest 24
CH 1211 Geneva 4
Phone: +41 22 372 98 10
Fax: +41 22 372 98 20

Dr. C. KATLAMA
Hôpital de la Pitié-Salpêtrière,
Dépt. de Médecine Tropicale
Blvd. de l'Hôpital 83
FR 75651 Paris Cedex 13
Phone: +33 1 45 70 25 43
Fax: +33 1 44 24 04 50

Dr. J. KOSMIDIS
The General Hospital of Athens,
1st Dept. of Medicine
Messoghion Avenue 156
GR 11527 Athens
Phone: +30 1 777 66 88
Fax: +30 1 770 59 80

Dr. J.O. NIELSEN
Hvidovre Hospital,
University of Copenhagen,
Dept. of Infectious Diseases, 144
DK 2650 Hvidovre
Phone: +45 36 32 30 15
Fax: +45 31 47 49 79

Dr. S. VELLA
Istituto Superiore di Sanità,
Centro Operativo AIDS
viale Regina Elena 299
IT 00161 Rome
Phone: +39 6 445 27 61
Fax: +39 6 445 67 41

ONCOGENES, ANTISENSE OLIGODEOXYNUCLEOTIDES AND APOPTOSIS

Key words
Apoptosis, AIDS, oncogenes, anti-sense oligodeoxynucleotides.

Brief description
Apoptosis is a form of cell death in which the dying cell plays an active part in its own demise.

The process appears to be under genetic control and is quite distinct from necrosis.

Physiologically, apoptosis is the balancing mechanism by which multicellular organisms maintain relatively unwavering cell numbers following cell generation via mitosis.

Deregulation of the control mechanism of apoptosis appears to have a central role to play in the pathology of a number of human diseases of socioeconomic importance.

Two examples of this are the T cell deletion seen in AIDS patients and the development of a number of cancers, a specific example being follicular cell lymphomas.

An association between expression of a particular set of oncogenes including myc, bcl-2, P53 and deregulation of apoptosis has been demonstrated by a number of laboratories.

In this proposal we would like to clearly identify which oncogenes have a regulatory role to play in apoptotic cell death.

We would also like to determine whether we can manipulate oncogene expression in vitro with anti-sense oligodeoxynucleotides.

Such a manipulation may allow us to control whether a cell undergoes apoptosis or not.

Finally we would like to extend some of the more promising in vitro findings into in vivo models.

The main potential scientific benefits of this project are that we may be able to regulate expression of specific oncogenes involved in the control of apoptosis by the use of appropriate anti-sense oligodeoxynucleotides.

The proposal brings together most of the major European laboratories working in this field, in a concerted attempt to unravel some of the cell biology of this fundamental process.

Project leader:
Dr. Thomas G. COTTER
Dept of Biology, St. Patrick's College
IE Maynooth, Co.Kildare
Phone: +353 16 28 52 22
Fax: +353 16 28 94 32
Contract number: CT931530

Participants:

Prof. Chris HASLETT
Respiratory Medicine Unit, Dept. of Medicine
The Univ of Edinburgh Medical School
Teviot Place
UK Edinburgh EH8 9AG Scotland

Dr. Abelardo LOPEZ-RIVAS
Instituto Lopez Neyra de Parasitologia,
CSLIC
c/ Ventanilla 11
ES 18001 Granada

Dr. Mary COLLINS
The Insitute of Cancer Research
The Royal Marsden Hospital
Fulham Road
UK London

Dr. Michel LANOTTE
Insitut National de la Sante en de la Recherche
Medicale Unit 301 Inserm, Hospital Saint-Louis
1 av. Cl. Vellefaux
FR 75010 Paris

Dr. Peter KRAMMER
German Cancer Research Centre
Div. of Immunogenetics
Im Neuenheimer Feld 280
DE 6900 Heidelberg

Dr. Seamus MARTIN
Dept. of Immunology, Univ College &
Middlesex School of Medicine,
Arthur Stanley House
40-50 Tottenham St.
UK London W1P9PG

Dr. Wilfried BURSCH
Institut für Tumorbiologie-Krebsforschung
Universität Wien
Borschkegasse 8a
AT 1090 Vienna

Prof. Andrew WYLLIE
Dept. of Pathology,
Univ Medical School Edinburgh Univ
Teviot Place
UK Edinburgh EH8 9AG Scotland

Prof. J. DUMONT
Universite Libre de Bruxless
Campus Erasme, Bldg C
BE 1070 Brussels

Prof. S. DOSKELAND
Dept. of Cell Biology & Anatomy
Univ of Bergen
Arstadveien 19
NO Bergen

MONKEY MODELS FOR AIDS RESEARCH

Key words
AIDS research, experimental animals, SIV, HIV, pathogenicity, experimental therapy, vaccine development.

Brief description
Objectives: The programme will mobilize, coordinate, and focus resources available in ten individual European primate institutes equipped to house infected monkeys for AIDS research.

Coordination: The objectives will be achieved through improved communication, standardization of experimental procedures, and coordination of conce ted trials.

Results of common experiments as well as the know-how of the individual participants will freely be exchanged.

These joint experiments will optimize the resources for such type of work within Europe. The mobility of researchers is encouraged by the support of short-term visits to other participating laboratories.

Moreover, the intended pooling of valuable and limited resources will ensure its effective use, speed-up the development, increase the international competitiveness of European AIDS research, improve the well-fare of experimental animals, and reduce the overall number of monkeys required.

Areas of scientific cooperation: As in the past scientists from ten centres able to perform experiments with SIV- or HIV-infected macaques will cooperate in the three major areas of AIDS research:

i pathogenicity,
ii experimental therapy, and
iii vaccine development.

Experimental approach: In the first phase we will concentrate on vaccine development by initiating experiments to:
- identify the protecting immmunogen;
- develop sources for such immunogens (e.g. peptides, recombinant proteins, tissue culture grown virus);
- improve the antigen presentation (e.g. adjuvant selection, delivery systems, route of immunization);
- comparison of various challenge virus stocks (e.g. PBMC-grown virus);
- type of inoculation (e.g. mucosal versus intravenous application of challenge, cell-associated virus challenge);
- monitor the duration of protection in the different experiments;
- elucidate the nature of the protecting immune mechanism;
- examine the potentials of live recombinant vaccines and viral chimeras;
- search for and implement new experimental systems, in particular, the infection of pig-tailed macaques (Macaca nemestrina) with HIV-1 or rhesus and cynomolgus macaques with SIV recombinants carrying the HIV envelop.

First experimental protocol: Protection against PBMC-grown challenge virus with life recombinant SIV vaccines. Recently, a genetically attenuated SIV (SlVmac239 nef~)

was shown to replicate poorly in rhesus monkeys.

Animals infected with these recombinant SIV were, however, protected against high doses of a complete pathogenic SIVmac.

We will examine attenuated recombinant SIV immunogens deleted in their nef or vpr or rev genes or in several of these nonstructural genes.

The purpose is to find out whether protection against monkey PBMC-grown challenge viruses or challenge stocks derived ex vivo can be achieved.

Moreover, we want to elucidate the immune mechanisms by which infection with the challenge virus is abrogated.

Currently, we are concerned about the safety of potential recombinant life HIV-vaccines. The results of the planned experiment would help to define the protecting immune mechanisms which we then would try to induce with safer vaccines potentially applicable in humans.

In a first concerted experiment we will investigate the protective potential of an SIVmac239 nef~ recombinant against various titrated challenge viruses.

Project leader:
Professor Gerhard HUNSMANN
Deutsches Primatenzentrum GmbH
Kellnerweg 4
DE 37077 Göttingen
Phone: +49 551 385 11 55
Fax: +49 551 385 12 28
Contract number: CT931795

Participants:
Dr. Ab OSTERHEUS
National Inst. of Public
Health (RIVM)
A. van Leeuwenhoeklaan 9
NL 3720 Bilthoven
Phone: +31 30 742142
Fax: +31 30 742971

Dr. C. STAHL-HENNIG
Deutsches Primatenzentrum
GmbH Abteilung Virologie
und Immunologie
Kellnerweg 4
DE 3400 Göttingen
Phone: +49 551 3851 155
Fax: +49 551 3851 228

Dr. Jim STOTT
Blanche Lane, South Mimms,
Potters Bar
UK Hertfordshire EN6 3QG
Phone: +44 707 54753
Fax: +44 707 49865

Dr. Jonathan HEENY
Primate Center TNO
Lange Kleiweg 151
NL 2280 HV Rijswijk
Phone: +31 15 842842

Fax: +31 15 843998

Dr. Peter GREENAWAY
PHLS Centre for Applied
Microbiology and Research
Div. of Pathology
Porton Down, Salisbury
UK Wiltshire SP4 OJG
Phone: +44 980 610391
Fax: +44 980 611096

Dr.Dominique DORMONT
Centre de Recherches du
Service de Santé des Armées
Av de la Div. Leclerc 60-68
FR 92265
Fontenay-aux-Roses Cedex
Phone: +33 1 46548122
Fax: +33 1 46549180

Prof. Dr. Giovanni ROSSI
Istituto Superiore di Sanità
Roma Dipartamento di
Virologia
Viale Regina Elena 299
IT 00161 Rome
Phone: +39 6 445 71 61
Fax: +39 6 445 39 04

Prof. Dr. G. BIBERFELD
The National Bact.Laboratory
Lundagatan 2
SE 105 21 Stockholm
Phone: +46 8 735 10 00
Fax: +46 8 735 41 36

Prof. Dr. Kal KROHN
Univ of Tampere Dept. of
Pathology
P.O. Box 607
FI 33101 Finland
Phone: +358 31 156 666
Fax: +358 31 156 170

Prof. Dr. Reinhardt KURTH
Paul Ehrlich-Institut
Paul Ehrlilchstrasse 51-59
DE 6070 Langen
Phone: +49 6103 755 0
Fax: +49 6103 755123

Prof. Dr. V. ERFLE
Gesellschaft für Strahlen- und
Umweltforschung
Ingolstädter Landstrasse 1
DE 8042 Neuherberg
Phone: +49 89 31872416
Fax: +49 89 31873322

VAGINAL AND RECTAL IMMUNIZATION AGAINST AIDS IN NON-HUMAN AND HUMAN PRIMATES

Key words
Mucosal immunization, AIDS, SIV, HIV, primates.

Brief description
Mucosal immunization to prevent entry of the virus through the rectal mucosa in the homosexual and through the genital mucosa in the heterosexual subject is a rational and as yet untried approach in preventing AIDS. In view of the incidence of AIDS and the rate of spread of the epidemic, We propose to investigate the immunogenicity of SIV' and HIV antigens and the controlling T cell functions in primates. SIV envelope gpl2o and core P27 antigens Will be used, so as to elicit secretory Iga antibodies to both, and thereby prevent epithelial attachment by anti-9P120 siga, and intra-epithelial viral replication by anti-p27 siga.

The role oE immune complexes in enhancing mucosal immunogenicity will also be investigated. Macaques will be tested for protection against SIV infection by vaginal or rectal challenge with live SIV. The immunogenicity and safety of an HIV designer poly-peptide vaccine will first be tested in non-human primates and then in sero-negative and Sero-positive human subjects. The polypeptide consists of 4B cell neutralising epitopes and IT cell epitope. The efficacy of the polypeptide vaccine chemically linked to cholera toxin B subunit (CTB) will be compared With genetically Eused CTB. Quality control between the 4 laboratories will be an essential feature of this project.

The experimental basis of this proposal is to induce 3 immunological barriers to SIV/HIV in primates:

1 secretory Iga antibodies to HIV/SIV envelope and core antigens may prevent extracel-lular epithelial attachment of the virus and intracellular viral replication.

2 Failure of the epithelial siga barrier may result in the virus being carried to the region-al genital or rectal lymph nodes, where the second level of immunity Will be activat-ed, consisting of specific T and B cell functions.

3 A failure of both the mucosal and lymphoid barriers still leaves the circulating Igg and Iga antibodies and specifically sensitised T and B cells in preventing the viral infec-tion. The objective of effective mucosal immunization against Hiv can be achieved by concerted action of the 4 centers in England, France, Italy and Sweden with long-term expertise in mucosal immunity of primates.

Project leader:
Professor Thomas LEHNER
United Medical and Dental
School of Guy's and St.
Thomas' Hospital
Division of Immunology,
Guy's Tower (floor 28)
UK London SE1 9RT
Phone: +44 71 955 40 48
Fax: +44 71 407 66 93
Contract number: CT931210

Participants:
Dr. Fabrizio MANCA
Univ of Genoa, dept. Immu-
nology, San Martino Hospital
IT 16132 Genoa
Phone: +39 10 39 10354008
Fax: +39 10 39 10357582

Prof. Cecil CZERKINSKY
INSERM Unit 80, Hopital
Edouard Herriot, Pavillion P
FR Lyon
Phone: +33 78 53 8111/3821
Fax: +33 72 33 0044

Prof. Jan HOLMGREN
Medical Microbiology &
Immunology,
Univ of Goteborg
Guldhedsgatan 10A
SE 143 46 Goteborg
Phone: +46 10 46 31 604911
Fax: +46 10 46 31 820160

VERTICAL TRANSMISSION OF HIV INFECTION

Key words
Vertical transmission, paediatric HIV infection.

Brief description
The European Collaborative Study (ECS) on children born to HIV-infected women was set up in 1986, and to date more than 1300 mother-child pairs have been enrolled from paediatric and obstetric centres throughout Europe. The rate of vertical transmission has been estimated at 15%, and there is no significant difference over time or between centres. The natural history of early paediatric HIV infection has been described.

Some risk factors for vertical transmission (VT) have been identified and maternal clinical and immunological status, delivery before 34 weeks gestation and breastfeeding are associated with an increased risk of vertical transmission. More detailed pregnancy and delivery information is now being collected, and this and the linkage of maternal and infant samples (cell, plasma and serum) will enable further clarification of risk factors for VT.

Indirect evidence from the ECS and other sources now suggests that a substantial, but unquantified, proportion of VT occurs around the time of delivery. possibilities for intervention, such as the use of non-nucleoside reverse transcriptase inhibitors, passive and active immunisation and short-term use of AZT, are being explored. The evaluation of any such intervention will have to be carried out in the context of a vertical transmission study and this European network provides an ideal opportunity. It is essential that this unique paediatric cohort continues to be followed, to clarify the natural history at later ages and to monitor seroconversion. Additional mother/child pairs need to be enrolled to allow further risk factor analysis and the evaluation of intervention of VT.

Project leader:
Professor Catherine PECKHAM
Institute of Child Health, Department of Epidemiology
Guilford Street 30
UK London WC1N 1EH
Phone: +44 71 242 97 89
Fax: +44 71 18 31 04 88
Contract number: CT931553

Participants:
Dr. Antonio MUIR &
Hosni YASBECK
Deparamento de Pediatria Hospital del Mar
Passeig Maritim 25-29
ES 08003 Barcelona
Phone: +34 3 309 2208
Fax: +34 3 309 8936

Dr. Ann-Britt BOHLIN
Huddinge Hospital
S-141 86 Huddinge
SE 141 86 Huddinge
Phone: +46 8 746 1000
Fax: +46 8 774 1317

Dr. Antonio FERRAZIN &
dr. Andrea DE MARIA
Oespedale San Marino, I Clinica Malattie
Infettive Padiglione 9 Fondi
Viale Benedetto XV 10
IT 16132 Genova
Phone: +39 10 352 824
Fax: +39 10 353 7680

Dr. C. CANOSA
Dep of Medicine Pediatria, Instituto Nacional de la Salud Hospital de la Seguridad Social 'La Fe'
ES 46009 Valencia
Phone: +34 6 386 2791
Fax: +34 6 386 2791

Dr. C. GIAQUINTO
Universita Degli Studi di Padova
Instituto di Clinica Pediatrica
Via Giustiniani 3
IT 35100 PADOVA
Phone: +39 49 821 3585
Fax: +39 49 821 3510

Dr. F. Omenaca TERES
Servicio de Neonatologia Hospital 12 de Octubre
Carretera de Andalucia
ES Madrid 20041
Phone: +34 1 390 8272
Fax: +34 1 390 8272

Dr. H. SCHERPBIER
Academisch Ziekenhuis bij de Universiteit
van Amsterdam, Ac. Medisch Centrum
Meibergdreef 9
NL 1105 AZ Amsterdam Zuidoost
Phone: +31 20 566 9111
Fax: +31 20 566 4440

Dr. Ilse GROSCH-WÖRNER
Kinderklinik, Universitätsklinikum
Rudolf Virchow Standort Charlottenburg
Heubnerweg 6
DE 1000 Berlin 19
Phone: +49 30 3035 4631
Fax: +49 30 3035 4638

Dr. Jack LEVY
Hospital St Pierre Paediatric,
Infectious Diseases Unit
322 Reu Haute
BE 1000 Bruxelles
Phone: +32 2 538 0000
Fax: +32 2 535 4006

Dr. J.Y.Q. MOK
Infectious Diseases Unit
City Hospital
Greenbank Drive
UK Edinburgh EH10 5SB
Phone: +44 31 447 1001
Fax: +44 31 452 9720

Dr. GARCIA-RODRIQUEZ
Servicio de Immunologia Popital La Paz
Castellana 261
ES 28046 Madrid
Phone: +34 1 358 2600
Fax: +34 1 729 1179

Dr. Oriol COLL
Dept. of Obs/Gyn, Hospital Clinic
c/Villarroel 170
ES 08028 Barcelona
Phone: +34 3 454 6000
Fax: +34 3 454 6691

Prof. Giogio PARDI
Dept. Obs e Gin Ospedale San Paolo
vi di Rudini 8
IT 20142 Milano
Phone: +39 2 891 0746
Fax: +39 2 813 5662

APPLICATION OF A REPLICATION COMPETENT FOAMY VIRUS-BASED RETROVIRUS VECTOR TO STUDY THE PATHOGENECITY AND IMMUNOGENECITY OF RETROVIRAL PROTEINS

Key words
Animal model, human foamy virus (HFV), retro-viral vectors, oncogenes, lentivirus gene products.

Brief description
1 Establishment of a small laboratory animal model for human foamy virus (HFV) infection to analyse the requirements of accessory HFV Proteins for the efficient virus replication in vivo in order to elucidate the function of lentivirus gene products (NEF, VPR).

2 Use of recently constructed replication competent HFV -based retro- viral vectors to analyse the pathogenicity and immunogenicity of viral oncogenes (tax and others) and lentivirus gene products (NEF, VPR, TAT ENV etc) in rodents.

3 Use of these vectors to study the transforming potential of viral oncogenes in vitro.

4 Characterization of the HFV packaging sequence; knowledge of which is required for the establishment of an HFV packaging cell line to be used in experimental gene therapy.

Project leader:
Dr. Axel RETHWILM
Institute for Virology & Immunobiology,
University of Würzburg
Versbacher str. 7
DE 97078 Würzburg
Phone: +49 931 201 39 54
Fax: +49 931 201 39 34
Contract number: CT931142

Participants:
Dr. Adriano AGUZZI
Insitute of Neuropathology
Dept. of Pathology, Univ Hospital of Zürich
Sternwartstr. 2
CH 8005 Zürich

Dr. Myra McCLURE
Dept. of G.U. Medicine and
Communicable Diseases Jefferiss
Research Trust Wing
Pread Street
UK London W2 1NY

STRUCTURE, FUNCTION AND DYNAMICS
OF HIV-REGULATING PROTEINS

Key words
HIV.

Brief description
We propose the determination of the three-dimensional structure and the dynamics of three proteins that regulate the replication cycle of the human immunodeficiency virus (HIV), the causative agent of the human acquired immunodeficiency syndrome (AIDS), and their RNA complexes.

The three proteins concerned are transactivating protein (Tat), negative factor protein (Nef), and anti-repression transactivator protein (Rev).

These proteins are mandatory for HIV replication. Thus, the final goal of our proposal is the setting of a rational basis for the development of HIV-directed drugs.

For the structure determination procedure we will use the classical techniques, i.e. X-ray crystallography and nuclear magnetic resonance (NMR), which we will also use for the determination of the dynamics of the proteins and, in the case of Tat and Rev, their respective RNA complexes.

The size of the Tat and the Rev proteins of the HIV are well within the scope of current possibilities of NMR spectroscopy, whereas the HIV Nef protein with a molecular weight of 27 KD is currently beyond easy reach for NMR.

An additional problem is that for neither of these proteins an efficient expression system is available, so that we will have to resort to chemical protein synthesis to get the necessary quantities of material. Again, this will be feasible for the Tat and the Rev proteins of HIV, but not for the HIV Nef protein.

We thus propose to study the structure of the Nef protein of the feline immunodeficiency virus (San Diego isolate), a protein highly related to the HIV protein, but with a molecular weight of only 13 KD.

In addition to the structure and the dynamics of the free protein we suggest determination of the structure and the dynamics of the Tat and Rev recognition RNA complexes with the above methods.

To this end, we are planning to synthesize the RNA using the T7 polymerase system. This would also give us an opportunity to use 13C- and 15N-labeled RNA for high-resolution structure determination by multidimensional NMR.

Project leader:
Professor Dr. Paul ROESCH
Lehrstul für Struktur und
Chemie der Biopolymere
P.O. Box 101251
DE 95447 Bayreuth
Phone: +49 921 55 35 40
Fax: +49 921 55 35 44
Contract number: CT931175

Participants:
Dr. Rainer FRANK
Zentrum für Molekulare
Biologie, Univ. Heidelberg
Im Neuenheimer Feld 282
DE 69120 Heidelberg

Prof. Dr. Jens LED
The Protein-NMR
Research Group
Dept. of Chemistry,
Univ of Copenhagen
Universitetsparken 5
DK 2100 Copenhagen

Prof. Michael KOKKINIDIS
Inst. of Molecular Biology
and Biotechnology
Foundation for Research
and Technology
P.O. Box 1527
GR 71110 Heraklion, Crete

RATIONAL DESIGN OF ANTIVIRAL AGENTS INHIBITING THE FUSOGENIC ACTIVITY OF HIV

Key words
HIV, antiviral agents, HIV fusogenic activity.

Brief description
The first step in the retroviral HIV infection is a fusion between the retrovirus and the host cell. Inhibition of this process will block the entry of the virus into the cell and therefore the infectivity. Two processes have been shown to play a pivotal role in this fusion mechanism
- the insertion of the N-terminal domain of a viral envelope protein into the host cell lipid bilayer (1,2)
- the destabilization of the host cell membrane generating transient lipid species (inverted micelle structures) (4).

The objective of this proposal is to use these available molecular information about the fusion mechanism in order to design, on a rational basis, antiviral agents that block specifically the entry of HIV into the host cell.
Recently, we provided evidence that drugs inhibiting either the insertion of the N-terminal domain of HIV gp41 (3) or the inverted micelle formation (4) completely abolished the HIV fusogenic activity and consequently the viral infectivity. On the basis of this available experimental information new antiviral agents will be built, taking advantage of a conformational analysis procedure (5) especially tailored to calculate the structure of drugs in a lipid environment or the interaction between peptides. The selected drugs or peptides will be synthesized and tested for their in vivo or in vitro activity.

1 M. Horth, B. Lambrecht, M.C. Lay Khim, F. Bex, C. Thiriart, J.-M. Ruysschaert, A. Burny and R. Brasseur; EMBO Journal vol 10, 10, 2747- 2755 (1991).
2 V. Vonèche, D. Portetelle, R. Kettmann, L. Willems, E. Paoletti, J.M. Ruysschaert, A. Burny and R. Brasseur; proc. Natl. Acad. Sci. 89, 3810-3814 (1992).
3 I. Martin, M.C. Dubois, T. Saermark and J.M. Ruysschaert; Biochem. Biophys. Res. Commun. 186, 95-101 (1992).
4 I. Martin, F. Defrise-Quertain, E. Decroly, M. Vandenbranden, R. Brasseur and J.M. Ruysschaert; Biochim. Biophys. Acta 1145, 124-133 (1993).
5 R. Brasseur and J.-M. Ruysschaert; Biochem. Journal 238, 1-11 (1986).

Project leader:
Prof. J.M. RUYSSCHAERT
Laboratoire de Chimie Phy-
sique des Macromolécules
aux Interfaces
Bd du Triomphe CP 206/2
BE 1050 Brussels
Phone: +32 2 650 53 77
Fax: +32 2 650 51 13
Contract number: CT931429

Participants:
Dr. Torben SAERMARK
EEC Concerted Action HIV
Membrane Biology c/o
Neurosearch
Smedeland 26 B
DK 2600 Glostrup

Prof. Volker ERFLE
GSF-Forschungszentrum für
Umwelt und Gesundheit
GMBH Insititut für
Molekulare Virologie
Neuherberg, PO 11 29
DE 857558 Oberschleissheim

GENETIC MARKERS FOR THE EPIDEMIOLOGY
OF TUBERCULOSIS

Key words
Tuberculosis, epidemiology, DNA fingerprinting, AIDS, chemotherapy.

Objectives
1 The implementation of an international network for the epidemiology of tuberculosis, using standardised DNA fingerprinting of M. tuberculosis complex isolates.
2 The build up of a fingerprint data base, which is accessible for the scientific community.
3 The training and exchange of scientists in the field of tuberculosis.
4 The development of and distribution of of tools and reagents to set up the network.
5 The design of protocols for the investigation of risk factors for active transmission due to drug resistance and HIV infection and to particular settings such as hospitals, schools, shelters and prisons using DNA fingerprinting data in combination with epidiomiological data.
6 The formulation of new intervention strategies to limit the recent increase in tuberculosis observed in most European countries.

Brief description
Implementation of a network for the epidemiology of tuberculosis
A method will be implemented, which enables participants in the various countries to carry out DNA fingerprinting by a standardized method. This will be done by the training of scientists, the development of laboratory protocols, the production and the distribution of biologicals, the comparison of different methods of DNA typing of M. tuberculosis, the development of computerized methods to analyze and compare large numbers of DNA fingerprints and the development and distribution of software that enables participants to carry out epidemiological studies, which take advantage of finqerprint data.

Epidemiology of tuberculosis in the various countries
The new technique of strain differentiation of M. tuberculosis by DNA techniques will be applied by the various participants to:
1 Control the dissemination in hospitals, prisons, shelters and to facilitate actve case finding and active tracing of main sources of tuberculosis infection.
2 Evaluate the effect of druq resistance on the efficacy of treatment. DNA typinq allows to distinquish between relapse of a previous (non well treated) infection and reinfection with a newly aquired strain.
3 Determine wether dual infection with HIV and tuberculosis has an effect on the transmission of tuberculosis to the general population and on the development and dissemination of drug-resistant tuberculosis.
4 Formulate new intervention strategies to control tuberculosis more effectively and to halt the further and development and spread of drug resistant tuberculosis. The time schedule comprises 3 years of research.

Project leader:
Dr. J.D.A. VAN EMBDEN
National Institute of Public Health and Environmental Protection,
Unit of Molecular Microbiology
P.O. Box 1
NL 3720 BA BILTHOVEN
Phone: +31 30 742889
Fax: +31 30 292957
Contract number: CT931614

Participants:
Dr. Arthur P. AGUAS
Universidade do Porto,
Centro de Citologia
Experimental
R. Campo Alegre 823
PT 4100 Porto
Phone: +351 2 699154
Fax: +351 2 699157

Dr. Arend KOLK
Koninklijk Instituut
voor de Tropen
Wibautstraat 135
NL 1097 DN Amsterdam
Phone: +31 20 5665463
Fax: +31 20 6971841

Dr. Åse B. ANDERSEN
Statens Seruminstitut
Artillerivej 5
DK 2300 Copenhagen
Phone: +45 32 68 32 68
Fax: +45 32 68 38 68

Dr. Brigitte GICQUEL
Microbial Engineering Unit
Institut Pasteur
28, Rue du Dr. Roux
FR 75724 Paris, Cedex 15
Phone: +33 1 45688828
Fax: +33 1 45688843

Dr. David CATTY
Univ of Birmingham Dept. of
Immunology, Medical School
Vincent Drive
UK Birmingham B15 2TJ
Phone: +44 21 414 4065/7
Fax: +44 21 414 4036

Dr. G. KÄLLENIUS
The National Bacteriological
Laboratory
Lundgatan 2
SE 10521 Stockholm
Phone: +46 8 7351000
Fax: +46 8 7303248

Dr. Jeremy W. DALE
Univ of Surrey Dept. of
Microbiology
UK Guildford GU2 5 XH
Phone: +44 0483 300800

Dr. Jose Moniz PEREIRA
Universidade de Lisboa
Faculdade de Farmacie
PT 1699 Lisboa
Phone: +351 1 733064
Fax: +351 1 7934212

Dr. M. FAUVILLE
Institut Pasteur du Brabant
BE Bruxelles 1180
Phone: +32 2 3733208
Fax: +32 2 3733174

Dr. Neil G. STOKER
Dept. of Clinical Sciences,
London School of Hygiene
and Tropical Medicine
Keppel Street
UK London WC1E 7HT
Phone: +44 71 927 2425
Fax: +44 71 637 4314

Dr. Varerie SCHWOEBEL
Hospital National de
Saint Maurice
14 Rue de Val D'Osne
FR 944110 Saint Maurice
Phone: +33 1 43966545
Fax: +33 1 43965081

Prof. E. NUNZI
Università de Genova
Viale Benedetto XV, 7
IT 16132 Genova
Phone: +39 10 3538400
Fax: +39 10 3538427

Prof. Françoise PORTAELS
Inst. of Tropical Medicine
Prince Leopold Laboratory of
Microbiology
Nationale Straat 155
BE 2000 Antwerpen
Phone: +32 3 2476317
Fax: +32 3 2476333

Prof. Jacques H. GROSSET
Faculte de Medicine
Pitie-Salpetriere Bacteriologie
et Virologie
91, Boulevard de l'Hopital
FR 75634 Paris Cedex 13
Phone: +33 1 40779746
Fax: +33 1 40779596

Prof. Paul FINE
Univ of London, Dept. of
Epidemiology and Population
Sciences
Keppel Street
UK London WC1E 7HT
Phone: +44 71 636 8636
Fax: +44 71 436 5389

Prof. Peter F. SMITH
Univ of London, Dept. of
Epidemiology and Population
Sciences
Keppel Street
UK London WC1E 7HT
Phone: +44 71 636 8636
Fax: +44 71 436 5389

Prof. R. GOMEZ-LUS
Univ of Zaragoza, Faculty of
Medicine Area Microbiology
ES Zaragoza
Phone: +34 76 357916
Fax: +34 76 567015

ANALYSIS OF THE SIGNALLING PATHWAYS REGULATING HIV TRANSCRIPTION IN HUMAN T-LYMPHOCYTES AND MONOCYTES AS POTENTIAL TARGETS FOR ANTI-AIDS INTERVENTION

Key words

Anti-HIV therapies, cell systems, AIDS, HIV-1 proviruses, HIV genes or LTR luciferase expression vectors, cellular transduction pathways.

Brief description

We propose an integrated research approach on the molecular mechanisms linking cellular activation and reactivation of the integrated HIV provirus, with the aim of finding cellular targets for future anti-HIV therapies. New cell systems, as relevant as possible to the pathogenesis of AIDS, will be created for this investigation. They will include stable expression of HIV-1 proviruses, HIV genes or LTR luciferase expression vectors in human IL-2 dependent T cell clones and cultures of bone-marrow derived macrophages. Some specific questions will also be addressed in systems permitting micro injection, such as Fibroblasts and Xenopus oocytes.

We will analyse the cellular transduction pathways induced by antigen recognition and by lymphokines such as TNF and ILI. We will focus on a pathway that our preliminary results indicate as being common to these stimulations, and critical for activation of the HIV LTR. Using vectors able to induce or suppress the activity of single cellular genes, we will document the role or RAS/GAP, protein phosphatases, MAP kinases and phospholipases in NF-kB and HIV LTR activation. A unique PKC isotype (zeta PKC) is funnelling through these pathways. We will block the activity of this enzyme by transdominant negative vectors and pseudo-substrate peptides. We will analyse the patterns of phosphorylation induced by zeta pkc on the inhibitory proteins (IKB alpha and P105 precursor) normally retaining P50-P65 NF-kB complexes in the cytoplasm. Specific monoclonal antibodies raised to recombinant P50, P105, IKB alpha, P65 and BCL-3 will be used to analyse trafficking of these proteins and their interactions.

We will identify the HIV protein responsible for NF-kB activation and self-perpetuation of HIV genome transcription in monocytes, in order to find ways to block its postulated interaction with one cellular signalling protein along the transduction pathway described.

The long-term objective of this project is to design pharmacological agents which can interfere with the cellular transduction pathways) reactivating HIV in T lymphocytes and macrophages. The short-term objective is thus to identify the cellular proteins involved, the cascade of their functional interactions and the most efficient ways to block this pathway.

Project leader:
Dr. Jean-Louis VIRELIZIER
Unité d'Immunologie Virale,
Institut Pasteur
Rue du Dr. Roux 28
FR 75724 Paris
Phone: +33 1 45 68 82 63
Fax: +33 1 45 68 89 41
Contract number: CT931007

Participants:
Jorge MOSCAT
CSIC-UAM, Centro de Biologia Molecular
ES Madrid Canto Blanco 28049
Phone: +34 1 536 83 12
Fax: +34 1 586 83 12

José ALCAMI
Hospital 12 de Octubre,
Departamento de Microbiologia
ES Madrid 28041
Phone: +34 1 390 80 01
Fax: +34 1 390 80 89

Ronald T. HAY
Univ of St Andrews, Dept. of Biochemistry
and Microbiology
UK St Andrews fife KY 16 9 AL
Phone: +44 334 76161
Fax: +44 334 478721

ASSESSMENT OF AIDS/HIV GENERAL PREVENTION STRATEGIES IN EUROPE: PHASE II

Key words
AIDS prevention, preventive strategies.

Brief description
The project proposed here will build in and extend work completed in the EC Concerted Action 'Assessment of AIDS/HIV preventive Strategies' which has been concerned with documenting and comparing the experience of AIDS prevention mainly in Western Europe, and to extend it to Eastern European countries, in order to exploit to maximum advantage the materials collected and the insights gained. The CA has already been accepted for funding by the EC following its submission in January 1992. However, because of recent decisions taken relating to Switzerland's membership of the EC it is no longer possible to co-ordinate this CA from Lausanne as originally planned. Sanctions are therefore sought from the EC to co-ordinate it from London.

The aims of the general population group of the CA are to facilitate the selection and implementation of effective preventive strategies in Eastern European countries, to identify key programmatic factors which may lead to more successful implementation and sustainability, and to contribute to the stock of knowledge on evaluative techniques and procedures to disseminate examples of models of good practice. These will be achieved by means of the collection of country specific materials and consultation with those involved in their preparation and evaluation.

The main product will take the form of a Compendium of Case Studies of AIDS/HIV public Education Campaigns in Western Europe indicating their strengths and weaknesses and the specific relevance of their design features to the cultural contexts in which they occur.

Project leader:
Dr. Kaye WELLINGS
St Mary's Hospital Medical School,
Dept. of Public Health
Praed Street
UK London W2 1PG
Phone: +44 71 723 12 52
Fax: +44 71 724 73 49
Contract number: CT931665

Participants:
Mr. Kurt KRICKLER
Österreichisches AIDS-Informations und
Dokumentationszentrum (ÖAIDZ)
Blechturmgasse 7/9
AT 1050 Vienna

Dr. C.J.M. VAN EYK
National Committee on AIDS Control
Polderweg 92
NL 1093 KP Amsterdam

Dr. Elisabeth POTTS
Bundeszentrale für Gesundheitliche Aufklarung
Oostmerheimer Str 200
DE 5000 Köln 91

Dr. Froinçoise VARET
Agence Frençaise de Lutte Contre le Sida
2 Rue Auguste Comte
FR 92170 Vanves

Dr. James WALSH
Dept. of Health Hawkins House
IE Dublin 2

Dr. Kaye WELLINGS
London School of Hygiene and
Tropical Medicine Univ of London
Keppel Street
UK London WC1E 7HT

Dr. Manuela Santos PARDAL
General Dirictorate of Primary Health Care
Alameda D Afonso Henriques 45-3
PT 1056 Lisbon Codex

Dr. Odd Einar JOHANSEN
National Inst. of Public Health AIDS
Information and Awareness Centre
Geitmyrsveien 75
NO 0462 Oslo-4

Dr. Olli HAIKALA
Senior Medical Officer, National Agency
for Social Welfare and Health
FI Helsinki

Françiose DUBOIS-ARBER
Institut Universitaire de Medecine Sociale
et Preventive
Rue du Bugnon 17
CH 1005 Lausanne

Mr. Bjorn KNUDSEN
The National Board of Health AIDS Secretariat
P.O. Box 2020
DK 1012 Copenhagen K

Mr. D. HANSEN-KOENIG
Div. d'Epidemiologie Direction de la Sante
22 Rue Goethe
LU Luxembourg

Mr. Enrique Carcia HUETE
Spanish AIDS Foundation Complutense Univ
C/ Jose Ortega y Gasset 61
ES 28006 Madrid

Mr. Giovanni REZZA
Istituto Superiore di Sanita Centro operativo
Viale Regina Elena 299
IT 00161 Rome

Mr. G. PAPEVANGELOU
Greek Society for the Study and Control of
Papadiamantopoulou St 4
GR 115-28 Athens

Ms. Anne Lies Van MECHELEN
Interprovinciaal AIDS Coördinaat (IPAC)
(Inter-regional AIDS Coördination)
Nationalestraat 155
BE 2000 Antwerp 1

Ms. Bodil LANGBERG
AIDS Office Swedish National Board of Health
SE 10630 Stockholm

Ms. Doriana TORREIRO
Associazione Nazionale per la Lotte Contro
l'Via Barberini 3
IT 00187 Rome

Ms. Lilian KOLKER
Mass Media Campaigns AIDS/STDs
P.O. Box 9074
NL 3506 GB Utrecht

Ms. Lindsay NEIL
Health Education Officer Hamilton House
Mabdledon Place
UK London WC1H 9TX

Nikolai CHAIKA
Global Programme on AIDS WHO
Scherfigsvey 8
DK 2100 Copenhagen

PATHOGENESIS AND ALTERNATIVE THERAPY OF HIV/SIV ASSOCIATED LYMPHOMAS

Key words
AIDS, HIV, SIV, oncogenesis, Kaposi's sarcoma, malignant lymphoma.

Objectives
The proposed CA-program aims at improving research efforts by synergizing activities of several European laboratories and clinics with the following objectives:
1 To standardize procedures and methods as specimen collection, patient monitoring, pathological evaluation, laboratory assays.
2 To characterize HIV/SIV related malignant lymphomas ARL in man and monkey respectively, particularly with regard to a) the biology, immunology, EBV-association, retrovirology of human and monkey ARL, b) growth factors important for HIV/SIV induced persistent generalized B-cell hyperplasia and ARL development.
3 Development of alternative treatment protocols for ARL, particularly protocols based on immune intervention against cytokines/growth factors.
4 To characterize and compare AIDS-associated (AKS) and endemic (EKS) Kaposi's sarcoma, particularly with regard to a) characterization of angiogenic mechanisms/factors, b) various cell compartments during KS evolution and, c) to consider alterative treatment protocols, particularly targeting on the angiogenic factors.

Brief description
HIV-infected patients are at highly increased risk to develop AIDS related Kaposi's sarcoma (AKS) or malignant lymphoma (ARL) presumably due to increased expression of oncogenic factors and the effect(s) of immunodeficiency. Evidently, under the clinical conditions of AIDS these opportunistic tumours may have some oncogenic mechanism(s) in common.

Importance
The various research activities involved in this concerted action are expected to elucidate important biological and clinical aspects of oncogenesis in AIDS and possibly allow development of alternative of alternative treatment protocols for AIDS related lymphoma and Kaposi's sarcomas.

Project leader:
Dr. Peter BIBERFELD
Immunopathology Laboratory,
Karolinska Institute and Hospital
SE 17176 Stockholm
Phone: +46 8 729 4523/3595/4689
Fax: +46 8 34 58 20
Contract number: CT940947

Participants:

Prof. Hakan MELLSTEDT
Oncology Clinic, Karolinska Hospital
SE 17176 Stockholm
Phone: +46 8 729 4641
Fax: +46 8 31 15 85

Prof. Eric SANDSTROM
Dermatology Clinic, South Hospital
SE 11883 Stockholm
Phone: +46 8 616 2571
Fax: +46 8 616 2509

Dr. Dominique EMILIE
INSERM U131, Service de Pathologie
32 rue des Carnets
FR 92140 Clamart
Phone: +33 1 4632 1208/1213
Fax: +33 1 4632 7993

Dr. Hans FEICHTINGER
Institute of Pathology,
Leopold Franzens University of Innsbruck
Müllerstrasse 44
AT 6020 Innsbrock
Phone: +43 512 507 4236
Fax: +43 512 5820 8815

Dr. Carlo PARRAVICINI
Dept. of Pathology, Hospital L. Sacco
Via G.B. Grassi 74
IT 20157 Milano
Phone: +39 2 3579 9348
Fax: +39 2 3820 0385

Prof. Luigi CHIECO-BIANCHI
Institute of Oncology, Busonera Hospital
Via Gattamelata 64
IT 35128 Padova
Phone: +39 49 807 1859/1863
Fax: +39 49 807 2854

Dr. Adriana ALBINI
Laboratorio Cancerogenesi Chimica,
Istituto Nazionale per la Ricera sul Cancro
Viale Benedetto XV 10
IT 16132 Genova
Phone: +39 10 353 4212
Fax: +39 10 352 999

Prof. Helga RUBSAMEN-WAIGMANN
Georg-Speyer-Haus,
Chemotherapeutisches Forschungsinstitut
Paul-Erlich-Strasse 42-44
DE Frankfurt
Phone: +49 69 63 395 100
Fax: +49 69 63 395 297

Dr. Mikael STURZL & prof. HOFSCHNEIDER
Max-Planck-Institut für Biochemie,
Dept. of Virology
Am Klopferspiz 18a
DE 82152 Martinsried
Phone: +49 89 8578 2286
Fax: +49 89 8578 3777

Prof. Jean-Claude GLUCKMAN
Laboratoire de Biologie et Génétique des Déficits
Immunitaires, Bât. CERVI, Hôpital de la Pitié
83 Boulevard de l'Hôpital
FR 75651 Paris Cedex 13
Phone: +33 1 4217 7443
Fax: +33 1 4217 7441

Dr. Erwin TSCHACHLER
Dept. of Dermatology,
University of Vienna Medical School
Währinger Gürtel 18-20
AT 1090 Vienna
Phone: +43 1 408 1271
Fax: +43 1 403 4922

Dr. Alberto MANTOVANI
Istituto Mario Negri
Via Eritrea 62
IT 20157 Milano
Phone: +39 2 390 141
Fax: +39 2 354 6277

RISK FACTORS FOR AIDS ASSOCIATED KAPOSI'S SARCOMA: A EUROPEAN CASE-CONTROL STUDY

Key words
Risk factors, Kaposi's sarcoma (KS), HIV, AIDS.

Brief description
The general objective of this project is to identify possible genetic, biological, environmental or behavioral risk factors for the occurrence of Kaposi's sarcoma (KS) among HIV infected patients. This is an epidemiological project with a strong laboratory component. The study design is a case-control study, where cases are defined as any HIV infected patient presenting a KS diagnosed by clinical and - if possible - histological means.

Two different controls (Cl and C2) will be selected for each case. C1 controls are HIV infected patients without KS but with another AIDS indicative disease.

C2 controls are assimptomatic HIV infected patients.

Controls will be matched by sex, age, HIV transmission group and immunological status.

In both cases and controls demographic, sexual and drug use behavior, and clinical information will be collected by means of a standardized questionnaire implemented by interviewer; blood will be also drawn and tested for several viral serological markers; finally, HLA genotypes will be determined with DNA techniques.

If possible sarcoma tissue samples will be collected from cases. Data will be collected in an anonymous manner.

To achieve the necessary sample size and to gain in heterogeneity, this should be a multicenter/multinational project.

The analysis of the results will result in a better understanding of the ethiology of KS and therefore in cancer prevention.

Moreover, it will allow the creation of an European bank with the studied biological samples, for future analysis.

Project leader:
Dr. Jordi CASABONA
Dept. of Health,
Generalitat de Catalunya
Trav. de les Corts 131-159
ES 08028 Barcelona
Phone: +34 3 330 80 11
Fax: +34 3 411 11 14
Contract number: CT941385

Participants:
Dr. VALL & PODZAMCER
& dr. RUBIO
EMSKAS Group,
Dept. of Health,
Generalitat de Catalunya
Trav. de les Corts 131-159
ES 08028 Barcelona
Phone: +34 3 330 80 11
Fax: +34 3 411 11 14

Dr. HERMANS &
dr. CLUMECK
Saint-Pierre University
Hospital, Division of
Infectious Diseases
Rue Haute 322
BE 1000 Brussels
Phone: +32 2 538 91 91
Fax: +32 2 539 36 14

Dr. D.A. HAWKINS
Clinician HIV Services,
Dept. Genitourinary Medicine, John Hunter Clinic,
St. Stephen's Clinic
369 Fulham Road
UK London SW10 9TH
Phone: +44 81 846 61 58
Fax: +44 81 846 61 98

Dr. FRANCESHI &
dr. SERRAINO
Centro Regionale di
Riferimento Oncologico,
Servizio di Epidemiologia
Via Pedemontana Occ. 12
IT 33081 Aviano
Phone: +39 434 6591
Fax: +39 434 652 182

Dr. Brigitte CICQUEL
Unité de Génétique
Mycobactérienne
Rue du Dr. Roux 25
FR 75724 Paris Cedex

BETA-LACTAMASE AS A CARRIER FOR HIV AND SIV ENV MOTIFS. STUDY OF THEIR STRUCTURAL AND IMMUNOLOGICAL PROPERTIES

Key words
HIV, SIV, vaccines, hybrid proteins, vaccine vector, antigenic motifs, immunogenicity.

Brief description
A new, original approach is proposed for the preparation of anti HIV or SIV vaccines and for the determination of the three-dimensional structures of various potential antigenic motifs of the ENV protein. The method rests on the insertion of these motifs in a protein carrier, the beta-lactamase of Mycobacterium fortuitum. The hybrid proteins will be purified and their immunogenecity investigated.

A first hybrid protein has already been obtained. The V3 loop of the ENV protein of the HIV1 virus has been inserted between helices a2 and a3 of the beta-lactamase, a region pre-dicted to be on the surface of the protein. The fused gene has been transferred into the BCG where it was found to be expressed and the gene product was secreted in the culture medium. The chimeric protein retains a detectable beta-lactamase activity, which indicates that the structure of the enzyme has not been grossly modified. It will be crystallized and its structure determined by X-ray diffraction, a task which will be greatly facilitated by the fact that the structures of several homologous beta-lactamases are already known. Other hybrid proteins will be obtained and similarly studied. If the hybrid proteins are active, the structures of the antigenic loops will also be analysed by molecular modelling. Utilization of the BCG as a vaccine vector presents the advantage that it is a well-known, already widely utilized innocuous vaccinal strain. Hopefully, it will be possible to easily generalize the method for obtaining hybrid proteins containing various antigenic motifs to deter-mine the three-dimensional structure of the latters and to estimate their immunogenicity.

In the long term and besides the immediate benefits of the preparation of a potential original anti-HIV vaccine, the project will result in a better understanding of the correlations between the structure of antigenic motifs and their immunogenicity.

Project leader:
Dr. Brigitte CICQUEL
Unité de Génétique Mycobactérienne
Rue du Dr. Roux 25
FR 75724 Parix Cédex
Phone: +33 1 45 68 88 28
Fax: +33 1 45 68 88 43
Contract number: CT941171

Participant:
Dr. Jean-Marie FRERE
Laboratoire d'Enzumologie, Université de Liège,
Instituut de Chimie (B6) au Sart Tilman
BE 4000 Liège 1
Phone: +32 41 56 33 98
Fax: +32 41 56 33 64

PNEUMOCYSTIS AND PNEUMOCYSTOSIS. IMPACT OF THE BIO-DIVERSITY OF PNEUMOCYSTIS CARINII ON EPIDEMIOLOGY, PATHOLOGY, DIAGNOSIS, MONITORING AND PREVENTION OF PNEUMOCYSTOSIS. NEW THERAPEUTIC APPROACHES

Key words

Pneumocystic carinii, P. Carinii Pneumonia (PCP), PCP prevention, therapeutic strategies, pathogenicity markers.

Brief description

Since Pneumocystic carinii (which remains the most frequent parasitic agent in AIDS patients) stimulates CD4+ cells, it may increase HIV replication and contribute to AIDS pathogenesis. Thus, it appears essential to prevent P. Carinii Pneumonia (PCP) in HIV infected individuals.

Chimioprophylaxy is expensive, not fully successful and drugs often induce secondary effects.

New approaches for PCP prevention are therefore needed. The aim of the present Concerted Action is to regroup the complementary competences existing in 13 EC groups in order to generate new prevention approaches, based on the knowledge of the epidemiology of the disease and the definition of new therapeutic strategies.

The epidemiological studies will focus on determination of parasite reservoirs and pathogenicity studies of parasite isolates of different origins.

These objectives will be reached through the biotyping of P. Carinii isolates (using genomic, iso-enzymatic and antigenic markers), cross infection experiments and the identification of various pathogenicity markers (in vitro as well as in vivo).

The definition of new therapeutic strategies will be attempted on the basis of fundamental biochemical researches in order to define essential parasite target molecules.

Furthermore, a wider structural range of molecules will be in vitro and in vivo evaluated. Results could have consequences in terms of epidemiology, pathology, diagnosis, monitoring and prevention of pneumocystosis. In fact:

1 A better knowledge of the sources of human P. Carinii infection and how humans become infected could help the prevention of PCP.

2 The knowledge of the degree of pathogenicity of parasite strains should be useful for the monitoriny of the patients.

3 The parasite polymorphism should be considered for the development of specific probes for diagnosis.

4 New therapeutic concepts could be the bases of new prevention and treatment strategies.

Project leader:
Dr. Eduardo DEI CAS
Inserm (Unité 42),
Biologie et Biochimie Parasitaires et fongiques
Rue Jules Guesde 369
FR 59650 Villeneuve d'Ascq
Phone: +33 20 47 25 73
Fax: +33 20 05 91 72
Contract number: CT941118

Participants:
Dr. M. TIBAYRENC
Laboratoire de Génétique des parasites,
ORSTOM
BP 5045, Ave Agropolis 911
FR 34032 Montpellier Cedex
Phone: +33 67 617 497/572
Fax: +33 67 547 800

Dr. A.E. WAKEFIELD
Institute of Molecular Medicine, University
of Oxford, John Radcliffe Hospital
Headington
UK Oxford OX3 9DU
Phone: +44 865 222344/742555
Fax: +44 865 222626

Prof. A.F. PETAVY
Section Pharmacie, Dept. de Parasitologie
8 Avenue Rockefeller
FR 69373 Lyon Cedex 08
Phone: +33 78 77 70 58
Fax: +33 78 77 71 58

Prof. O.P. SETTNES
Institute of Medical Microbiology and
Immunology, University of Copenhagen
Blegdamsvej 3
DK 2200 Copenhagen N
Phone: +45 31 35 50 60
Fax: +45 31 37 66 22

Prof. Vivi BILLE-HANSEN
National Veterinary Laboratory
Bülowsvej 27
DK 1790 Copenhagen V
Phone: +45 31 35 45 44
Fax: +45 31 35 37 37

Prof. L. POLONELLI
Istituto di Microbiologia,
Via A. Gramsci 14
IT 43100 Parma
Phone: +39 521 99 2668/3620
Fax: +39 521 99 3620

Dr. P.M. GIRARD
INSERM U 13, Hôpital Claude Bernard
190 Boulevard Mac Donald
FR 75944 Paris
Phone: +33 1 1640 193030/353644
Fax: +33 1 1640 193040/361699

Dr. E. DELAPORTE
ORSTOM
BP 5045
FR 34032 Montpellier Cedex
Phone: +33 67 61 74 00
Fax: +33 67 54 78 00

Dr. H.C. JACKSON
GLAXO, Glaxo Group Research Limited
Greenford Road
UK Middlesex UB6 0HE
Phone: +44 81 422 3434/3126
Fax: +44 81 423 5579

Dr. M.C. PREVOST
INSERM U 326, Hôpital PURPAN
Place du Docteur Baylac
FR 31059 Toulouse Cedex
Phone: +33 61 491853/772441
Fax: +33 61 319752

Prof. J.W.M. VAN DER MEER
Dept. of Medicine, University Hospital
Nijmegen, St. Radboud
P.O. Box 9101
NL 6500 HB Nijmegen
Phone: +31 80 61 43 56
Fax: +31 80 54 02 16

Dr. B. POLACK
Ecole Nationale Vétérinaire d'Alfort
7 Avenue de Général De Gaulle
FR 97704 Maison-Alfort Cedex
Phone: +33 43 96 71 57
Fax: +33 43 96 71 25

Prof. P. COUDERT
Laboratoire de Pathologie du lapin, INRA
FR 37380 Nouzilly
Phone: +33 47 42 77 52
Fax: +33 47 42 77 74

Dr. Bettina LUNDGREN
Infectious Diseases Dept. 144,
University of Copenhagen, Hvidovre Hospital
DK 2650 Hvidovre
Phone: +45 36 32 24 29
Fax: +45 31 47 49 79 /36 32 33 57

Prof. Enrica TAMBURRINI
Dept. of Infectious Diseases, Catholic University
Largo A. Gemelli 8
IT 00168 Roma
Phone: +39 6 30 15 49 45
Fax: +39 6 30 51 343

Prof. Massimo SCAGLIA
Laboratory Clinical Parasitology,
University-IRCCS San Matteo
IT 27100 Pavia
+39 382 50 26 98
+39 382 42 33 20

TROPHOBLAST ALPHA, BETA AND GAMMA INTERFERON EFFECTS ON INFECTION BY DIFFERENT HIV ISOLATES FROM TROPHOBLASTS AND FETAL BLOOD

Key words

Transplacental transmission, HIV, 2'-5'oligoadenylate synthetase, protective effects, trophoblast, placental blood cells.

Brief description

Transplacental transmission of HIV comprises a major route for vertical infection. The lack of transmission from most infected mothers however points to strong local defence mechanisms which might be manipulated for preventive purposes. We here focus on the interferon (IFN)-related antiviral mechanisms.

Our aim is:

a to study the IFN and 2'-5'oligoadenylate synthetase of the trophoblasts;

b to define the in vitro protective effects of trophoblast IFNs against infection with relevant HIV variants.

To carry out this programme we will isolate and characterize trophoblasts and other placental cells, isolate and characterize trophoblast-produced IFNs and 2'- 5'. A synthetases, and isolate and characterize HIV from trophoblast and placental blood cells.

With this in place we will determine the effects of HIV on endogeneous tro-IFNs and finally quantificate the anti-HIV effects of exogenous tro-IFN with respect to the 2'-5'. A system and indirectly via modulation of local immune responses to HIV.

A growing collaborative network has been in effect for a few years. It now encompasses 8 groups.

We believe that the proposed work will lay a needed foundation for future clinical trials of tro-IFNs with the purpose of reducing vertical transmission of HIV.

Project leader:
Dr. P. EBBESEN
Danish Cancer Society,
Dept of Virus and Cancer
Gustav Wieds Vej, 10
DK 8000 Aarhus C
Phone: +45 86 12 73 66
Fax: +45 86 19 54 15
Contract number: CT941593

Participants:
Prof. J.C. CHERMANN
INSERM U 322,
Campus Universitaire de Muliny
BP 33
FR 13273 Marseille Cedex 9
Phone: +33 91 41 32 32
Fax: +33 91 41 92 50

Dr. Gottfried DOHR
Institut hur Histologie und Embryologie
der Universitat Graz
Harrachstrasse 21/6
AT 8010 Graz
Phone: +43 316 380 4230
Fax: +43 316 355 66

Prof. M.N. THANG
Institute National de la Sante
et de la Recherche Medical,
Unite 245, Centre INSERM
Hopital Saint Antoine
Rue du Faubourg 184
FR 75571 Paris Cedex
Phone: +33 1 43 34 42
Fax: +33 1 43 43 32 34

Prof. Andrease ZIEGLER
Institut fur Experimentelle Onkologie und
Transplantationsmedizin, Universitatsklinikum
Rudolf Virchow, Freie Universitat Berlin
Spandauer Damm 130
DE 1000 Berlin 19
Phone: +49 30 3035 2617
Fax: +49 30 3035 3778

Prof. Wolfgang ZSCHIESCHE
Max Delbruck Center of Molecular Medicine
Robert-Rissle-Strasse 10
DE 1115 Berlin
Phone: +49 30 9406 3366/3561
Fax: +49 30 9494 161

Prof. Ferenc TOTH
Institute of Microbiology,
University Medical School
HU 4012 Debrecen
Phone: +36 52 17 565
Fax: +36 52 17 565

Dr. Vladimir ZACHAR
Institute of Virology,
Dept. of Medical Virology
Dubravska Cesta 9
SK Bratislava
Phone: +42 7 374 468
Fax: +42 7 374 284

HIV VARIABILITY

Key words
HIV, antigenic variability, HIV expression.

Brief description
To study biologically important functional and antigenic changes of HIV, the underlying genetic and regulatory determinants and the molecular mechanisms responsible for variability.
The proposal consists of four main collaborative projects:
1 Phenotypic and genotypic analysis of HIV replicative capacity and cytopathogenicity (10 collaborating laboratories).

We propose to investigate how naturally occurring virus variation in HIV infected humans alters the properties of HIV and influences virus tropism for different cell types.
This will have implications for understanding disease progression and virus transmission.
2 Studies on antigenic variability of HIV as reflected by the neutralizing antibody response and inhibitory activity of CD8+ cells (8 collaborating laboratories).

We propose to map determinants responsible for virus neutralisation and to identify changes underlying resistance with the help of monoclonal antibodies and peptide reagents. These studies may shed light not only on the pathogenic process but may help to identify relevant immunogenic sites to be included in a candidate vaccine.
3 Molecular studies on the mechanism of HIV variation will be carried out in order to understand the molecular basis of HIV base misincorporation in general, and the details of G->A hypermutation, in particular (2 collaborating laboratories).

By studying enzyme cofactors, nucleoside analogues or simply some of the RT inhibitors and derivatives we hope to increase hypermutation to a point beyond which it is not possible to make a complete provirus.
4 Studies on the regulation of HIV expression as a possible determinant of HIV biologic variability will be carried out *in vitro* and *ex vivo* (3 collaborating laboratories).

Knowledge about the process of virus expression in infected cells/individuals may provide possibilities for therapeutic intervention.
The present proposal has been developed through scientific discussions during the yearly gatherings of the HIV variability group in the last five years.
These meetings have broadened our view and have increased our appreciation of the complexity of HIV variability.
The group now wishes to continue with a closer cooperation also on the experimental level.
The projects presented herein are all parts of nationally funded ongoing projects or continuation of projects developed in the collaborating key laboratories.
Building on this fundament we now wish to establish a European network of collaborations within the area of HIV variability.

Project leader:
Dr. Eva Maria FENYÖ
Karolinska Institute,
Department of Virology
c/o SBL
SE 105 21 Stockholm
Phone: +46 8 735 1204
Fax: +46 8 730 4407
Contract number: CT941395

Participants:
Dr. T. SCHULZ &
dr. R. WEISS
Chester Beatty Labs, Institute
of Cancer Research
UK London
Phone: +44 71 352 8133
Fax: +44 71 352 3299

Dr. Q. SATTENTAU
INSERM, Retrovirology and
Associated Diseases
FR Marseille
Phone: +33 91 26 94 94
Fax: +33 91 26 94 30

Dr. D. PIATIER-TONNEAU
& dr. C. AUFFRAY
CNRS, Molecular Genetics
and Biology of Development
FR Villejuif
Phone: +33 1 4958 1111
Fax: +33 1 4958 1122

Jane MCKEATING
University of Reading,
Dept. of Microbiology
UK Reading
Phone: +44 73 487 5123
Fax: +44 73 475 0140

Hagen VON BRIESEN
George-Speyer-Haus,
Chemotherapeutisches
Forschungsinstitut
DE Frankfurt
Phone: +49 69 633 95 100
Fax: +49 69 633 95 297

Dr. H. RUBSAMEN
WAIGMANN
Bayer AG, Inst. für Virologie
DE Wuppertal
Phone: +49 202 36 8413
Fax: +49 202 36 4162

Dr. P. VERANI
Instituto Superiore di Santitá,
Laboratorio di Virologia
IT Rome
Phone: +39 6 4457 888
Fax: +39 6 4453 369

Dr. A. JUNGBAUER
University of Agriculture,
Inst. of Applied Microbiology
AT Vienna
Phone: +43 222 3692 924402
Fax: +43 222 3692 924 400

Dr. B. WAHREN
Infections Disease Control,
Dept. of Virology
SE Stockholm
Phone: +46 8 735 1130
Fax: +46 8 272 231

Dr. P. BALFE
Middlesex School of
Medicine, Dept. of
Medical Microbiology
UK London
Phone: +44 71 380 9490
Fax: +44 71 580 5896

Dr. S. WAIN-HOBSON
Institute Pasteur, Laboratory
of Molecular Retrovirology
FR Paris
Phone: +33 1 4568 8821
Fax: +33 1 4568 8874

Dr. Brigitta ASJO
Bergen High Technology
Center, Virus and Immuno-
chemistry Laboratories
NO Bergen
Phone: +47 5 54 45 10
Fax: +47 5 54 45 12

Pauli LEINIKKI
National Public Health
Institute, Dept. of HIV
FI Helsinki
Phone: +358 0 4744403
Fax: +358 0 4744461

Dr. A. MEYERHANS
Inst. Medical Microbiology
and Hygene Dept of Virology
DE Freiburg
Phone: +49 761 203 2217
Fax: +49 761 203 2187

Dr. F. MIEDEMA &
dr. H. SCHUITEMAKER
Central Laboratory of the
Netherlands Red Cross Blood
Transfusion, Dept. of
Clinical Viro-Immunology
NL Amsterdam
Phone: +31 20 51 23 261
Fax: +31 20 51 23 310

Dr. J. GOUDSMIT &
dr. F. DE WOLF
University of Amsterdam,
Human Retrovirus Laboratory
NL Amsterdam
Phone: +31 20 566 4853
Fax: +31 20 691 6531

Jan ALBERT
Swedish Institute for
Infections Disease Control,
Dept. of Virology
SE Stockholm
Phone: +46 8 735 1064
Fax: +46 8 730 3248

Dr. F. AVILLEZ
Instituto Nacional Saude
PT Lisboa
Fax: +351 1 759 0441

Dr. L. CHIECO BIANCHI
Università degli studi
di Padova,
Instituto di Oncologia
IT Padova
Phone: +39 49 807 1850
Fax: +39 49 807 2854

Dr. A. LEIGH-BROWN
University of Edinburgh,
Division of Biological
Sciences
UK Edinburgh
Phone: +44 31 650 5523
Fax: +44 31 667 4507

Dr. Rob GRUTERS
CNRS Biomerieux
FR Lyon
Phone: +33 72 72 83 58
Fax: +33 72 72 85 33

PROTOCOL DEVELOPMENT FOR COMPARATIVE STUDIES ON SOCIAL AND CONTEXTUAL ASPECTS OF HETEROSEXUAL CONDUCT AND RISKS OF HIV INFECTION

Key words
HIV, risk related behaviours.

Brief description
There is a growing awareness of the limitations of survey based data concerning sexual behaviour, especially in their application to the design of culturally relevant and meaningful HIV preventive measures.

This proposal is aimed at coordinating comparative analyses of existing qualitative data from two countries on sexual activity of young adults, developing a protocol for comparative studies, and testing and refining this protocol by collecting data on the development of young adults' (16-30 yrs) sexual knowledge and interactional competencies in the context of the risk of HIV infection.

Individual interviews and focus group discussions will be used. Comparative analyses will permit the identification of dynamic factors in two countries (the Netherlands and the UK). Which differ considerably in terms of sexual 'openness' and other indices, including, for example, teenage pregnancy rates.

The comparative approach is essential if data and methods are to be produced which are culturally sensitive. It is intended that the resultant protocol can be used by research teams in other European countries and elsewhere in order to collect culturally specific data to complement their survey data. Amongst the issues to be explored are:

1 identification of understandings of risk related behaviours and the processes through which decisions are reached regarding the adoption of safer sexual techniques;

2 exploration of the personal and social contexts in which sexual activity amongst young adults takes place, and the ways in which such activities are explained and justified;

3 exploration of the sources and range of meanings of sexual activity and related issues amongst samples of young adults in particular contexts, and;

4 the development of culturally relevant explanatory models regarding sexual behaviour outcomes amongst young adults, and elaboration of the implications of these for the design of appropriate interventions.

Project leader:
Dr. Roger INGHAM
University of Southampton,
Department of Psychology
Highfield
UK Southampton SO9 5NH
Phone: +44 70 359 25 87
Fax: +44 70 359 39 39
Contract number: CT941338

Participant:
Drs. Gertjan VAN ZESSEN
NISSO
Postbus 5018
NL 3502 JA Utrecht
Phone: +31 30 94 62 46
Fax: +31 30 96 10 20

MULTINATIONAL SCENARIO ANALYSIS CONCERNING EPIDEMIOLOGICAL, SOCIAL AND ECONOMIC IMPACTS OF HIV/AIDS ON SOCIETY

Key words

Epidemiological, Social and Economic Impacts of HIV/AIDS, scenario analysis.

Brief description

The Concerted Action on Multinational Scenario Analysis concerning Epidemiological, Social and Economic Impacts of HIV/AIDS on Society aims at the development and application of a common frame for scenario analysis at a multinational level involving linkage of several research areas (epidemiology, public health, social sciences, health services research, economics) and quantitative methods (mathematical modelling). The main (interrelated) questions underlying the CA are:

- What future course of the epidemic can be expected in the EC in the short and medium term? What are the uncertainties and what implications does this have for the fight against AIDS?
- What has been the sociocultural and economic impact of the epidemic and what consequences for health care and preventive policies need to be anticipated in the future?

The objectives are:

- to stimulate the integration of relevant disciplines: epidemiology, social sciences, health services research and economics;
- to strengthen the link between data collection, mathematical modelling and impact assessment, and;
- to develop and to apply a common methodology for AIDS scenario analysis as an internationally useful frame for the assessment of present and future impacts.

The envisaged scenario analysis will use a well worked out methodology prepared by two EC activities, viz. the Concerted Action on Mathematical Modelling of HIV and the European Study on Economic Aspects of AIDS, the related co-operation with WHO and the Dutch AIDS Scenario Study initiated by WHO and coordinated by the Steering Committee on Future Health Scenarios.

An international study group started already with the development of methodologies to link routine AIDS surveillance data (collaboration with the European Centre for the Monitoring of AIDS), estimates about future AIDS-incidences, modelling of HIV-incidence behind these AIDS incidences and possible impacts by medical and preventive intervention. It also looked at possibilities for standardized multinational scenarios, beginning with three countries (France, the Netherlands, Germany). Recently it published preliminary scenarios on hospital care and costs for the whole of the EC.

Project leader:
Dr. Johannes C. JAGER
R.I.V.M., Rijksinstituut voor
Volksgezondheid en Milieuhygiene
P.O. Box 1
NL 3720 BA Bilthoven
Phone: +31 30 743074
Fax: +31 30 250740
Contract number: CT941723

Participants:
F.M.L.G. VAN DEN BOOM
National Committee on Chronically Ill People
NL Zoetermeer

M.J. POSTMA
Public Health Forecasting, R.I.V.M.
P.O. Box 1
NL 3720 BA Bilthoven

H. HOUWELING
Epidemiology, R.I.V.M.
P.O. Box 1
NL 3720 BA Bilthoven

S.H. HEISTERKAMP
Mathematical Methods, R.I.V.M.
P.O. Box 1
NL 3720 BA Bilthoven

R. LEIDL
Dept. of Health Economics,
University of Limburg
NL Maastricht

J. ROVIRA
SOIKOS
ES Barcelona

A.M. DOWNS
European Centre for the Epidemiological
Monitoring of AIDS/WHO,
Hôpital National de Saint-Maurice
FR Saint-Maurice

K. TOLLEY
Dept. of Economics,
University of Nottingham
UK Nottingham

J.D. GRIFFITHS & J.E. WILLIAMS
University of Wales,
School of Mathematics
UK Cardiff

B.C. DANGERFIELD & C.A. ROBERTS
University of Salford,
Centre for OR and Applied Statistics
UK Salford

K. DIETZ
Medical Biometry,
University of Tubingen
DE Tubingen

G. REZZA
AIDS National Italian Task Force,
Istituto Superiore di Sanita
IT Roma

N.T.J. BAILEY
Federal Office of Public Health Bern
CH Lauenen

J.A.M. VAN DRUTEN
Dept. of Medical Statistics,
University of Nijmegen
NL Nijmegen

M. LAGERGREN
Ministry of Health and Social Affairs,
Social Department
SE Stockholm

J. SANTOS LUCAS
Human and Social Sciences,
National School of Public Health
PT Lisboa

M. GYLDMARK
Dansk Sygehus Institut
DK Copenhagen

M.V. ZUNZENEGUI-PASTOR
Centro Universitario de Salud Publica
ES Madrid

D.P. REINKING
Netherlands Institute of Mental Health
NL Utrecht

E.J. RUITENBERG
Central Laboratory of the Netherlands Red
Cross, Blood Transfusion Service (CLB)
NL Amsterdam

R.A. COUTINHO
Dept. of Infectious Diseases,
Municipal Health Service
NL Amsterdam

J.C.C. BORLEFFS & M.G.W. DIJKGRAAF
Dept. of Internal Medicine,
Immunology and Infection,
University Hospital Utrecht (AZU)
NL Utrecht

PROSPECTIVE CLINICAL FOLLOW-UP OF HIV INFECTED PATIENTS IN EUROPE: PROAIDS 1994 - 1996 STUDY

Key words
Natural history of the HIV infection.

Brief description
The aim of PROAIDS is to prospectively collect demographic, clinical, therapeutic and laboratory data on some 4500 European HIV-infected individuals from 32 centres in 16 European countries.
PROAIDS will thus be able to describe the natural history of the HIV infection in Europe including the impact of therapeutic regimes on disease pattern and out-come. Proaids is the successor of the EC-sponsored concerted action *AIDS in Europe* - a multi-center study (official title: *Clinical manifestations and outcome of AIDS in Europe*), which retrospectively has collected similar data on some 6,600 European AIDS patients diagnosed between 1979 and 1989.
The AIDS in Europe study has recently been completed and the first report submitted for publication. Centres and the coordinating centre to be participating in proaids have all been participants of the AIDS in Europe study and thus the organization of the Proaids study is already established and the collaboration has proved to function excellently.

Project leader:
Dr. Jens D. LUNDGREN
Hvidovre Univ. Hospital,
Dept. Infectious Diseases 144
Kettegaard Alle 30
DK 2650 Hvidovre
Phone: +45 36 32 30 15
Fax: +45 47 49 79
Contract number: CT941637

Participants:
Prof. Nathan CLUMECK
Saint-Pierre Hospital, Division of Infectious Diseases
322 rue Haute
BE 1000 Brussels
Phone: +32 2 53 89 191
Fax: +32 2 53 93 614

Prof. Peter SKINHOJ
Epidemiafd., Rigshospitalet
Tagensvej 20
DK 2200 Kopenhagen N
Phone: +45 35 45 35 45
Fax: +45 35 45 66 48

Dr. Jan GERSTOFT
Medical Dept. B,
Frederiksberg Hospital
DK 2000 Frederiksberg C
Phone: +45 3834 7711
Fax: +45 3186 0556

Dr. Jens Ole NIELSEN
Dept. Infectious Diseases,
Hvidovre University Hospital
DK 2650 Hvidovre
Phone: +45 3632 2930
Fax: +45 3147 4979

Dr. S.E. BARTON
John Hunter Clinic,
St. Stephen's Clinic
369 Fullham Road
UK London SW10 9TH
Phone: +44 81 8466 184
Fax: +44 81 8466 198

Dr. Anne JOHNSON
Academic Dept. of Genito-Urinary Medicine, University
College, James Pringle House
UK London W1N 8AA
Phone: +44 71 3809 145
Fax: +44 71 3230 355

Dr. Anthony J. PINCHING
Dept. of Immunology,
Saint Bartholomew's Hospital
51-53 Bartholomew Close,
West Smithfield
UK London EC1A 7BE
Phone: +44 81 601 8428
Fax: +44 71 600 3839

Dr. Cristina KATLAMA
Dept. de Medicine Tropicale,
Hopital de la Pitie-Salpetiere
Boulevard de l'Hopital 83
FR 75013 Paris
Phone: +33 1 4570 2861
Fax: +33 1 4670 2045

Prof. M. DIETRICH
Bernard Nocht Institute
for Tropical Medicine
Bernard Nocht Strasse 74
DE 20359 Hamburg
Phone: +49 40 311 823 90
Fax: +49 40 311 823 94

Prof. F.D. GOEBEL
Medizinische Poliklinik der
Universität Munchen
Pettenkoferstrasse 8a
DE 80336 Munchen
Phone: +49 89 5160 3581
Fax: +49 80 5160 3581

Dr. J. KOSMIDIS
First Dept. of Medicine, The
General Hospital of Athens
Messogheion 156
GR 11527 Athens
Phone: +30 1 777 66 888
Fax: +30 1 883 07 47

Dr. George STERGIOU
1st IKA Hospital 'Penteli'
153 Third September Street
GR 11251 Athens
Phone: +30 1 804 2474
Fax: +30 1 804 1837

Dr. F. MULCAHY
St. James's Hospital, Dept.
of Genito-Urinary Medicine
P.O. Box 580
IE Dublin 8
Phone: +353 1 537 941
Fax: +353 1 544 494

Dr. Stefano VELLA
Centro Operativo AIDS,
Istituto Superiore di Sanita
Viale Regina Elena 299
IT 00161 Rome
Phone: +39 6 445 2761
Fax: +39 6 445 6741

Dr. Antonio CHIESI
Clinica e Terapia, Istituto
Superiore di Sanita
Viale Regina Elena 299
IT 00161 Rome
Phone: +39 6 445 6741
Fax: +39 6 445 6741

Prof. Adriano LAZZARIN
Ospedale San Raffaele, Dept.
of Infectious Diseases
Via Stamira d'Ancona 20
IT 20127 Milano
Phone: +39 2 26437 939
Fax: +39 2 26437 030

Dr. A. D'ARMINIO
MONFORTE
Clinica delle Malattie
Infettive, Ospedale L. Sacco
Via G.B. Grassi 74
IT 20157 Milano
Phone: +39 2 356 7031
Fax: +39 2 356 0805

Dr. R. HEMMER
Dept. des Maladies
Infectieuses, Centre
Hospitalier
Rue Barble 4
LU 1210 Luxembourg
Phone: +352 44 113 091
Fax: +352 44 458 762

Dr. Sven DANNER
Academisch Ziekenhuis
Universiteit van Amsterdam
Meibergdreef 9
NL 1105 AZ Amsterdam
Phone: +31 20 566 9111
Fax: +31 20 566 4440

Dr. F. ANTUNES
Dept. of Infectious Diseases,
Hospital Santa Maria
Av. Prof. Egas Moniz
PT 1600 Lisboa
Phone: +351 1 775 171
Fax: +351 1 797 6242

Dr. R. PROENCA
Hospital Curry Cabral,
Servicio de Doencas
Infecto-Contaglosas
Rua da Beneficiencia
PT 1000 Lisboa
Phone: +351 1 769 0886
Fax: +351 1 769 515

Dr. J.M. GATELL
Servicio Infecciones,
Hospital Clinic i Procincial
Villaroel 170
ES 08036 Barcelona
Phone: +34 3 323 1414/2181
Fax: +34 3 451 4438

Dr. B. CLOTET
AIDS Care Unit, Hospital
Universitari 'Germans
Trias i Pujol'
ES 08916 Barcelona
Phone: +34 3 465 1200
Fax: +34 3 395 4206

Dr. J. GONZALES-LAHOZ
Hospital del Rey, Institute
of Health Carlos III
c/ Sinesio Delgado 6
ES 28029 Madrid
Phone: +34 1 315 0040
Fax: +34 1 733 6614

Prof. Israel YUST
Dept. of Medicine A,
Ichilov Hospital
6 Weizman Street
IL 64239 Tel Aviv
Phone: +972 354 366 633
Fax: +972 354 695 80

Prof. Z. BENTWICH
R. Ben Ari Institute of
Clinical Immunology, Kaplan
Medical Center Jerusalem
IL 78100 Rehovot
Phone: +972 8441 211
Fax: +972 8410 461

Dr. Z. BEN-ISHAI
Rambam Medical Center
P.O. Box 9602
IL Haifa
Phone: +972 45 15688
Fax: +972 45 34887

Prof. T. SACKS
Dept. of Clinical Microbiol-
ogy and Infectious Diseases,
Hadassah Hospital
PO Box 12000
IL 91120 Jerusalem
Phone: +972 24 27 427
Fax: +927 24 34 434

Dr. B. LEDERGERBER
Schweizerische HIV-
Kohortenstudie,
Koordinationszentrum
Zurichbergstrasse 29
CH 8032 Zurich
Phone: +41 1 26 216 62
Fax: +41 1 26 216 74

Prof. R. LUTHY
Schweizerische HIV-
Kohortenstudie,
Koordinationszentrum
Zurichbergstrasse 29
CH 8032 Zurich
Phone: +41 1 255 1111
Fax: +41 1 255 3291

Dr. B. HIRSCHEL
Departement de Medecine,
Division des Maladies
Infectieuses, Hopital
Cantonal Universitaire
CH 1211 Geneve 14
Phone: +41 2 23 82 33 11
Fax: +41 2 23 72 98 20

Prof. M.P. GLAUSER
Medecine 2 - BH07, CHUV
CH 1011 Lausanne
Phone: +41 13 14 27 69
Fax: +41 13 14 45 60

DETERMINANTS OF DISEASE PROGRESSION IN HIV-1 INFECTED INFANTS

Key words
Vertical transmission of HIV-1, disease progression, virological and immunological determinants.

Brief description
Recent data have shown that vertical transmission of HIV-1 is occurring by transfer of a genotipically homogeneous virus population. In the infected infants, two distinct natural courses of the disease progression have been observed: the early presentation pattern with symptoms occurring within the first year of life and the late one with disease occurring with a median incubation period of 6.1 years. The virological and immunological determinants which are responsible for these distinct natural course of disease are still largely unknown.

The aims of the present proposal are the following:

- To characterise prospectively the genotypes of HIV-1 virus in children born to HIV-1 infected mothers in an attempt to correlate the rate of emergence of viral variants with biological properties and disease progression;
- To analyse the kinetics of infant antibody response to synthetic peptides representing gp 120 V3 sequences of autologous HIV-1 quasi species and to correlate it with neutralising activity to autologous and heterologous primary isolates in relation to disease progression;
- To analyse the kinetics of infant CTL response to autologous HIV-1 quasi species in correlation with disease progression;
- To measure constitutive and induced cytokine expression in lymphocytes from infants born to Hiv-1 infected mothers and correlated it with disease progression. About 200 HIV-1 infected infants are expected to be born to HIV-1 infected mothers in the 7 European Clinical centers involved as collaborative centers in this proposal. Each child will undergo to an early diagnosis of HIV-1 infection by shared diagnostic procedure which will include virus gene amplification by polymerase chain reaction, virus isolation, and detection of specific HIV-1 Iga. Blood sampling will be done at the following times: 1, 3, 6, 9, 12, 18 and 24 months of age. Clinical Centers will be responsible for diagnosis of infection, clinical and immunological follow up. Basic science groups will be responsible for molecular and biological characterisation of HIV-1 virus, detection and characterisation of neutralising antibodies, fine specificity and quantitation of cellular cytotoxicity to HIV-1 epitope as well as analysis of T cell v alfa, V beta chain usage.

Project leader:
Dr. Paolo ROSSI
Karolinska Institutet,
Department of Immunology
P.O. Box 60400
SE 10401 Stockholm
Phone: +46 8 32 88 78
Fax: +46 8 28 878
Contract number: CT941492

Participants:

Jan ALBERT
Dept. of Virology, Swedish Institute
for Infectious Disease Control
SE 10521 Stockholm
Phone: +46 8 735 1000
Fax: +46 8 272 231

Cipriano CANOSA
Dept. Pediatric Medicines,
La Fe Childrens Hospital
Avenida de Campanar 21
ES 46009 Valencia
Phone: +34 6 386 2791
Fax: +34 6 386 2791

Alfonso DELGADO RUBIO
Hospital Cicil de Basurto, Dept. of Pediatrics
Avda Montevideo 18
ES 48013 Bilbao
Phone: +34 4 441 9095
Fax: +34 4 442 5804

Andrea DE MARIA
Dept. of Infectious Diseases,
University of Genova, Ospedale San Martino
IT Genova
Phone: +39 10 3535 2366
Fax: +39 10 3537 680

Anita DE ROSSI
Institute of Oncology, University of Padova
Via Gattamelata 64
IT Padova
Phone: +39 49 807 1859
Fax: +39 49 807 2854

Marzia DUSE
Dept. of Pediatrics, University of Bresia
Via F.lli Ugoni 32/f
IT 25126 Brescia
Phone: +39 30 399 5716
Fax: +39 30 380 599

Elia LUIGI
Dept. of Pediatrics, Infectious Diseases,
Children's Hospital Bambino Gesu
IT Roma
Phone: +39 6 6859 2190
Fax: +39 6 6859 2498

Teresa ESPANOL
Immunology Unit
C.S. Valle Hebron
ES 08035 Barcelona
Phone: +34 3 4183 400
Fax: +34 3 4280 443

Frank MIEDEMA
Clinical Viro Immunology, Central Laboratory
of the Netherlands Red Cross Blood
Transfusion Service
PO Box 9190
NL 1006 AO Amsterdam
Phone: +31 20 512 3317/3110
Fax: +31 20 512 3310

Viviana MOSCHESE
Dept. of Pediatrics, St. Eugenio Hospital,
University II
Tor Vergata
IT Rome
Phone: +39 6 591 3603
Fax: +39 6 592 2077

Catherine PECKHAM
Institute of Child Health
30 Guilford Street
UK London WC1N
Phone: +44 71 829 8699
Fax: +44 81 831 0488

Nicola PRINCIPI
Dept. of Pediatrics, University of Milano
IT Milano
Phone: +39 2 3579 9269
Fax: +39 2 3567 346

Gabriella SCARLATTI
Laboratory of Immunobiology of AIDS, Dibit
Foundation, St. Raffaele Hospital
IT Milano
Phone: +39 2 2643 7986
Fax: +39 2 2643 7989

Pier Angelo TOVO
Dept. of Pediatrics, University of Torino
IT Torino
Phone: +39 11 6927 256
Fax: +39 11 6927 382

Hans WIGZELL
Micro & Tumorbiology Center, Karolinska
Institute
SE 17177 Stockholm
Phone: +46 8 735 1000
Fax: +46 8 730 3248

EUROPEAN NETWORKS FOR THE SURVEILLANCE OF HIV INFECTION IN SENTINEL POPULATIONS OF STD PATIENTS

Key words
HIV monitoring in STD patients, socio-cultural, behavioural factors.

Brief description
Whithin the framework of the programme medical and Health Research 1988-1991 of the EC (DGXII), a Concerted Action monitoring HIV seropositity in STD patients has been launched, with effective registration starting in June 1990.

Its main result has been to establish sentinel surveillance networks in 17 countries for HIV monitoring in STD patients, About 50,000 STD episodes have been registered during the two-year observation period using the surveillance networks set up during the previous CA, this proposal has the following objectives:

1 To be on the watch for significant changes in the HIV seroprevalence rate in each network, thanks to a long enough monitoring period.

2 To make reliable comparisons between the registered trends of the different networks.

3 To observe changes in the proportion and characteristics of HIV infected STD patients in the participating networks, including data about migration from outside and within the EC.

4 To provide on a regular basis some indicators of the effectiveness of prevention programmes, such as the percentage of known HIV seropositives among new STD cases.

5 To make a comparative analysis (between networks) of the socio-cultural and behavioural factors associated with HIV seropositivity. Monitoring will be performed on a continuous basis, or when impossible, during shorter periods at different moments of the year. In most networks, HIV testing is performed with informed consent in the English and Welsh, Scottish and French networks, unlinked anonymous testing is adopted. Blood specimens are tested for HIV-1 (HIV-2 remains optional) by an ELISA test and confirmed by western blot or immunofluorescence.

Each national coordinator has found the ressources needed for organizing and maintaining his network. Community support is required for:
- organization of workshops;
- meetings of the steering committee;
- exchange of staff;
- coordination.

Project leader:
Dr. André STROOBANT
Institute of Hygiene and Epidemiology
Rue J. Wytsman 14
BE 1050 Brussels
Phone: +32 2 642 50 29
Fax: +32 2 642 50 01
Contract number: CT941392

Participants:
Dr. M. CATCHPOLE
Communicable Diseases Surveillance Center
61 Colindale Avenue
UK London NW9 5EQ
Phone: +44 81 200 6868
Fax: +44 81 200 7868

Prof. H.J. VOGT
Dermatologische Klinik Technische Universität
Biedersteiner Strasse 29
DE 80802 Munchen
Phone: +49 89 38 49 32 34
Fax: +49 89 33 49 83

Dr. B. SULIGOI
Istituto Superiore di Sanita
Viale Regina Elena 299
IT 00161 Roma
Phone: +39 6 445 2761
Fax: +39 6 445 6741

Dr. J. CARDOSO
Centro de Saude da Lapa
Av 24 de Julho 120
PT 1300 Lisboa
Phone: +351 1 395 2115
Fax: +351 1 395 4957

Dr. R. DE ANDRES MEDINA
Centro Nacional de Biologia Celular
ES 28220 Majadahonda, Madrid
Phone: +34 1 63 40 648
Fax: +34 1 63 80 613

Dr. A.H. WORM
Bispebjerg Hospital,
Dept. of Dermato-Venereology
DK 2400 Copenhagen
Phone: +45 35 31 31 70
Fax: +45 35 31 39 50

Dr. L. MEYER
INSERM U292, Service d'Epidémiologie,
Hôpital de Bicêtre
78 rue du Général Leclerc
FR 94275 Le Kremlin Bicêtre
Phone: +33 1 4521 2334
Fax: +33 1 4521 2075

Dr. M. HADJIVASSILIOU-PAPPA
National University of Athens,
Dept. of Dermatology
Dragoumi Street 5
GR 16121 Athens
Phone: +30 1 72 43 579
Fax: +30 1 72 11 122

Dr. H. FENNEMA
Municipal Health Service,
Dept. of Public Health Service
P.O.Box 20244
NL 1000 Amsterdam
Phone: +31 20 5555 302
Fax: +31 20 5555 533

Dr. D. GOLDBERG
Communicable Diseases Unit, Ruchill Hospital
Bilsland Drive
UK Glasgow G20 9NB
Phone: +44 41 946 7120
Fax: +44 41 946 4359

Dr. I. DE LA MATA
Encomienda 10-1B
ES 28012 Madrid
Phone: +34 1 539 0147
Fax: +34 1 586 7723

Dr. B. KRIZ
National Institute of Public Health,
Centre of Epidemiology & Microbiology
Srobarova 48
CZ 10042 Praha 10
Phone: +42 2 6731 1874
Fax: +42 2 7469 47

Dr. A. HORVATH
State Institute for Dermato-Venereology
Maria Strasse 41
HU 1085 Budapest
Phone: +36 1 210 0314
Fax: +36 1 134 0566

Dr. C. ANAGRIUS
Falu Lasarett, Dept. of Dermatology
SE 79182 Falun
Phone: +46 23 820 00
Fax: +46 23 867 73

Dr. A. PONKA
Helsinki City Centre of the Environment
Helsinginkatu 24
FI 00530 Helsinki
Phone: +358 0 7099 2418
Fax: +358 0 7099 2401

Dr. A. GRANHOLT
Olafiaklinikken
Olafiagangen 7
NO 0188 Oslo
Phone: +47 2217 6100
Fax: +47 2217 1870

Dr. J. PAGET
Office Fédéral de la Santé Publique
Hess Strasse 27 E
CH 3097 Bern-Liebefeld
Phone: +41 31 970 8747
Fax: +41 31 970 8795

STUDIES ON THE 3D STRUCTURE, FUNCTION AND INHIBITION OF HIV-1 REVERSE TRANSCRIPTASE, AIMING AT RATIONAL DRUG DESIGN AGAINST HIV/AIDS

Key words
3-dimensional structure of HIV-1 Reverse Transcriptase (HIV-RT).

Brief description
The goal with this project is to determine the 3-dimensional structure of HIV-1 Reverse Transcriptase (HIV-RT) at highest possible resolution and to use this information as a base for rational drug design of specific inhibitors of the enzyme. Among the HIV-proteins RT is probably the most suitable target for design of specific inhibitors, the reasons being the vast accumulated knowledge of polymerases in general and the existence of such drugs as AZT with well established effects on AIDS through their inhibiting power of HIV-RT. However, long term use of AZT (and of other existing RT-inhibitors) is creating both side and resistance effects. Thus, there is a great need for design of more specific drugs - and in fact for design of several and quite different ones of these good drugs because of the very diffifult problem of resistance.

The proposing group has all necessary knowledge, experience and equipment as well as already obtained crucial achievements on HIV-1 RT for justification of a successful outcome of the research: Thus, (i) we have established well functioning procedures for large scale production and purification as well as for characterization and activity studies of the p66/p51 heterodimer molecule; (ii) we have produced good crystals of RT in complex with tRNA(Lys3), the natural primer of RT. These crystals diffract to at least 3.8-resolution using the synchrotron radiation at the EMBL out-station in Hamburg;

(iii) we have so far collected and processed 3-D data to 5.0-6.5-resolution from crystals of native RT and of three heavy atom derivatives; a 3-D structure has been calculated and interpreted to 6.5-resolution and will soon be extended to about 5.0-resolution;

(iv) we have recently done gene construction, expression, purification and the first crystallization experiment of the N-terminal half of the RT-molecule (two domains together), which ought to be non-flexible and thus has a possibility to lead to high quality crystals and diffraction. We are well aware of the research efforts done in this field by three other competent groups. However there are several good reasons for these parallel efforts:

a the present resolution is not allowing an interpretation of the protein side chains;

b different complexes are investigated, and;

c several and quite different good inhibitors are needed because of resistance problem.

Project leader:
Dr. Keith WILSON
European Molecular Biology
Laboratory,
Outstation Hamburg
Notkestrasse 85
DE 22607 Hamburg
Phone: +49 40 89 90 20
Fax: +49 40 89 90 21 49
Contract number: CT941224

Participants:
Prof. H. BUC
Unite de Physiochimie des
Macromolecules Biologiques
(URAI49 du CNRS),
Institut Pasteur
FR 75724 Paris Cedex 15

Prof. B. STRANDBERG
University of Uppsala, BMC
Box 590
SE 75124 Uppsala

PARTNER NOTIFICATION FOR HIV INFECTION IN EUROPE

Key words
Partner notification for HIV, data collection.

Brief description
Partner notification (formerly known as contact tracing) is vital in the control of sexually transmitted diseases (STD). Recent reports have shown that partner notification for HIV infection may be cost effective compared to screening programmes in diagnosing persons unaware of being HIV infected and that it may induce behaviour changes of the infected persons and thus break the chain of HIV transmission.

There is little information available about the cost effectiveness of existing programmes for partner notification in the different European countries and of which groups that would most benefit from counselling and support. The attitudes to, tradition for and policy of partner notification for HIV infection differ within the European countries. It is the aim of the study to evaluate the situation in each of the participating countries (Belgium, Denmark, England, Finland, Scotland, Sweden and Switzerland). Participating countries as well as other European countries may benefit from the results when implementing programmes of partner notification for HIV within the next years. A questionnaire will be developed by the coordinating center together with the Steering Committee. Each national coordinator will be responsible for the selection of data in their country and find their own ressources needed for organizing the data collection. The collected data will be coded and analyzed at the co-ordinating center, and the final report will be available for all HIV centers with partner notification programmes.

Community support is needed for:
- organization of workshops with invited experts;
- meetings of the Steering Committee;
- exchange of staff;
- coordination;
- computing;
- analyzing of data.

Project leader:
Dr. Anne-Marie WORM
Dept. of Dermato-Venereology,
Bispebjerg Hospital
Bispebjerg Bakke 23
DK 2400 Copenhagen NV
Phone: +45 35313170
Fax: +45 35313950
Contract number: CT941144

Participants:
Prof. N. CLUMECK
Saint-Pierre University Hospital,
Division of Infectious Diseases
322 Rue Haute
BE 1000 Brussels
Phone: +32 2 535 41 31
Fax: +32 2 539 36 14

Prof. W.M. ADLER
Academic Dept. of Genito-Urinary Medicine,
James Pringle House
73-75 Charlotte Street
UK London W1N 8AA
Phone: +44 71 380 9146/9145
Fax: +44 71 323 0355

Dr. David GOLDBERG
Communicable Diseases Unit,
Ruchill Hospital
UK Glasgow G20 9NB
Phone: +44 41 946 7120/1388
Fax: +44 41 946 4359

Dr. Sirkka-Liisa VALLE
Dept. of Dermatovenereology,
University Central Hospital
Meilahdentie 2
FI 00250 Helsinki
Fax: +358 0 752 4057

Dr. Harald MOI
Center for STD and HIV,
Ulleval University Clinic,
Olafiaklinikken
Olafiagangen 7
NO 0188 Oslo
Phone: +47 22 17 61 00
Fax: +47 22 17 18 70

Dr. Johan GIESECKE
Dept. of Infectious Diseases,
Huddinge University Hospital,
Karolinska Institute
SE 14186 Huddinge
Phone: +46 8 746 1000
Fax: +46 8 779 5173

Prof. A. EICHMANN
Städtische Poliklinik für Haut-
und Geslachtskrankheiten
Herman Greulich-Strasse 70
CH 8004 Zurich
Phone: +41 1 241 8832
Fax: +41 1 291 0522

II.2 CANCER RESEARCH

Introduction

During the past decade, the treatment of cancer has ceased to be separated into the interests of surgeons, chemotherapists and radiotherapists, and has become an integrated clinical discipline. Further improvement in cancer therapy requires integration of the fundamental and clinical approaches to research, with particular attention to building of necessary interactions between cellular, molecular and developmental genetics with oncology and epidemiology. This permits the development of new biological insights into the underlying causes of cancer and the ways in which they interact with normal cellular processes.

Clinical research aims at improving both diagnosis and treatment for cancers. In general, the earlier that cancers are diagnosed, the better the prognosis for treatment. There are still striking discrepancies for treatment outcomes in different regions or between countries, and while some of this may be due to fundamental biological or differences, much is due to unequal availability of best diagnosis or treatment; the aim should be to bring the same high standard of quality of care to all patients.

The specific areas addressed in the BIOMED 1 programme aim at research on preventing cancer by coordinating epidemiological research with a view to the identification of groups at risk, paying attention to environmental factors and the incidence of cancer with the aim of defining preventive approaches, and by evaluating the effectiveness of preventive approaches. They also aim at improving methods of earlier diagnosis by promoting fundamental cancer research, and by stimulating research aimed both at improving and extending anticancer screening and at identifying individuals with a genetic predisposition to cancer - including childhood cancers. The stimulation of research aimed at the improvement of therapy by promoting improvements of systemic treatments such as chemotherapy and immunotherapy through optimization of protocols, and by encouraging the improvement of local treatments through advances in conventional radiotherapy and through the exploration of newer radiotherapeutic modalities are addressed by the proceeding projects supported by the programme.

Dr. Bill Baig

ASSESSMENT OF THE IMPACT OF IMPROVED LOCAL CONTROL BY RADIOTHERAPY ON SURVIVAL IN CANCER PATIENTS

Key words
Primary tumour, tumour extension, tumour growth characteristics, irradiation, fractionation irradiation.

Brief description
The general objective of this project proposal is: to improve survival by a more effective treatment of the primary tumour, in head and neck and breast cancer.

This will be achieved by developing and consequently applying methods which allow adaptation, careful monitoring and intensification of the treatment regime according to the precise tumour extension and tumour growth characteristics of the individual patient.

This goal will be pursued by the execution of two clinical trials by the EORTC Radiotherapy Cooperative Group and the management and statistical analysis of the data obtained from these studies. The two trials aim at:

1 Increase of the irradiation dose to the primary tumour by delivery of a booster dose to patients who are treated for early breast cancer.

2 Individual adaptation of the fractionation irradiation scheme to the individually measured potential tumour doubling times of patients with head and neck cancer.

The final aim is to improve local control by 20-30%, thereby improving survival by 5-10% through tailored treatment regimes.

Project leader:
Dr. H. BARTELINK
Dept. of Radiotherapy, The
Netherlands Cancer Institute
Plesmanlaan 121
NL 1066 CX Amsterdam
Phone: +31 20 512 21 22
Fax: +31 20 669 11 01
Contract number: CT921615

Participants:
Dr. A. Biete SOLA
Hospital Clinic Y Provincial
ES 08036 Barcelona

Dr. A. RENAUD
C.H. de Tivoli
BE 7100 LA Louviere

Dr. B. JANCAR
Oncoloski Inst.
SI 61000 Ljubljana

Dr. C. LANDMANN
Kantonsspital Basel
CH 4000 Basel

Dr. D. v.d. WEIJNGAERT
Alg. Ziekenhuis Middelheim
BE 2020 Antwerp

Dr. D.A.L. MORGAN
General Hospital, Dept.
Radiotherapy & Oncology
UK Nottingham NG1 6HA

Dr. E. CALITCHI
C H U Henri Mondor
Ave. M. de Lattre de
FR 94000 Creteil

Dr. E. MONPETIT
Centre Saint Yves
FR 56000 Vannes

Dr. G.G. KHOURY
St Mary's Hospital
UK Portsmouth, PO3 6AD

Dr. H.P. HAMERS
Dr. B. Verbeeten Inst.
NL 5000 LA Tilburg

Dr. J. BERNIER
Ospedale San Giovanni,
Radioterapia Oncologica
CH 6500 Bellinzona

Dr. J. JASSEM
Med Academy of Gdansk,
Radiotherapy Clinic
PL 80-211 Gdansk

Dr. J.H. MEERWALDT
Dept. of Radiotherapy, Med
Spectrum Twente
NL 7513 ER Enschede

Dr. J.J. JAGERD
Radiotherapy Inst. Limburg
NL 6401 CX Heerlen

Dr. K.A. JOHANSSON
Dept. of Radiation Physics,
Sahlgren Hospital
SE 41 345 Goteborg

Dr. M.E. SYVESTRE
Hospital Santa Maria
PT 1699 Lisbon

Dr. P.C. LEVENDAG
Daniel den Hoed Kliniek
NL 3075 EA Rotterdam

Prof. A. HORWICH
Royal Marsden Hospital,
Dept. of Radiotherapy
UK Sutton Surrey SM2 5PT

Prof. D. GONZALEZ
Dept. of Radiotherapy, AMC
NL 1105 AZ Amsterdam

Prof. E. v. d. SCHUEREN
Dienst Gezwelziekten,
St Rafael's Kliniek
BE 3000 Leuven

Prof.· F. ESCHWEGE
Institut Gustav Roussy
FR 94805 Villejuif Cedex 05

Prof. G. STORME
Oncologisch Centrum, AZ,
BE 1090 Brussels

Prof. H. POURQUIER
Centre A C Montpellier,
Clin Val d'AUrelle
FR 34000 Montpellier

Prof. J. BATTERMAN
Radiotherapy Dept.,
A.Z. Utrecht
NL 3584 CX Utrecht

Prof. J.C. HORIOT
Unité de Radiothérapie,
Centre G F Leclerc
FR 21034 Dijon Cedex

Prof. J.M. COSSET
Inst. Curie
FR 75231 Paris Cedex 05

Prof. J.M. KURTZ
Dept. Radiation Oncology,
Univ Hosp
CH 1211 Geneva

Prof. J.P. GERARD
C H Lyon-Sud
Chemin du Grand Revoyat
FR 69310 Pierre Benite

Prof. J.W. LEER
Academisch Ziekenhuis, Afd
Klin Oncologie Geb 1 K1-P
NL 2300 RC Leiden

Prof. L. CIONINI
Radiological Inst.,
Radiotherapy Div.
IT 50134 Firenze

Prof. M. BOLLA
Serivce de Radiothérapie, C
H Regional et Universitaire
FR 38043 Grenoble Cedex 9

Prof. M. de VILHENA
Oncological Inst. F Gentil,
Dept. of Radiotherapy
PT 1093 Lisbon Codex

Prof. O. LEFLOCH
Hopital Bretonneau, Clin
D'Oncologie et Radiothérapie
FR 37044 Tours Cedex

Prof. P. BEY
Centre Alexis Vautrin
FR 54511 Vandoeuvre les
Nancy Cedex

Prof. P. van HOUTTE
Inst. Jules Bordet,
Dept. of Radiotherapy
BE 1000 Brussels

Prof. R. de FUR
Centre Henri Becquerel
FR 76038 Rouen Cedex

Prof. R.O. MIRIMANOFF
C H U Vaudois
CH 1011 Lausanne

Prof. R.P. MULLER
Stahlenklinik Univ Koln
DE 5000 Koln 41

Prof. S. ROTH
Universitäts Strahlenklinik
DE 4000 Dusseldorf

Prof. S. SCHRAUB
Hopital Jean Minjoz
FR 25030 Besancon

Prof. V. BUDACH
West German Tumour Inst.,
Abt Strahlentherapie,
Univ Klin Essen
DE 4300 Essen

Prof. W. van DAAL
Inst.ituut voor Radiotherapie,
Univ Hosp Nijmegen
NL 6500 HB Nijmegen

COLON CANCER PREVENTION: EVALUATION OF RESISTANT STARCH AND ASPIRIN IN CARRIERS OF FAMILIAL ADENOMATOUS POLYPOSIS

Key words

Bowel wall, mutation, apc gene, familial adenomatous polyposis, fatty acids, butyrate.

Brief description

Colon cancer is one of Europe's biggest killers. The difficulty in investigating preventive measures is the long time course of the disease. One of the early genetic faults in the bowel wall is mutation in the *apc* gene. Some people inherit a fault in this gene. They have the rare dominant disorder familial adenomatous polyposis. They usually develop colonic polyps in their teens and require removal of the colon to avoid early progression to cancer. They are keen to try preventive treatments but the rarity of such families means many centres must combine their resources.

Twenty-five genetic registries across Europe will form this Concerted Action, with Newcastle as a Resource Centre. Two treatments will be assessed; aspirin use has been associated with reduced colon cancer risk and the related drug Sulindac can make colonic polyps regress. Daily low dose aspirin will be compared to a placebo. Resistant starch is digested by bacteria in the bowel to fatty acids such as butyrate. In population studies, dietary resistant starch and colon cancer have an inverse relationship. Resistant versus digestible starch as food supplements will form the second study limb.

The CAPP Study will harmonise screening policies, disseminate genetic knowledge and demonstrate how European integration can enable families with a rare genetic disorder to assess cancer prevention for the whole population.

Project leader:
Professor J. BURN
Division of Human Genetics,
University of Newcastle-
Upon-Tyne
Claremont Place 19/20
UK Newcastle-Upon-Tyne
NE2 4AA
Phone: +44 91 222 73 86
Fax: +44 91 222 71 43
Contract number: CT921390

Participants:
Dr. A.C.M. ALMEIDA
Portugese Polyposis
Registry Groupria
PT 1200 Lisbon
Phone: +351 1793 46 18
Fax: +351 1355 74 20

Dr. Gabriella MOSLEIN
Heidelberg Polyposis Regis-
try, Chir Univ Klin
DE 6900 Heidelberg
Phone: +49 6221 566110
Fax: +49 6221 565504

Dr. A. ELLIS
Gastroenterology Unit,
Broadgreen Hospital
UK Liverpool L14 3LB
Phone: +44 51 228 4878
Fax: +44 51 254 2070

Dr. A. MULLER
Dept. Innere Medizin,
Gastroenterologie
CH 8091 Zurich
Phone: +41 1 255 2420
Fax: +41 1 255 4503

Dr. Carol McKEOWN
Clin Genetics Unit,
Birmingham Maternity Hosp
UK Birmingham B15 2TG
Phone: +44 21 6272632
Fax: +44 21 6272602

Dr. Christine
VERELLEN-DEMOULIN
Center of Human
Genetics, UCL
BE 5220 Tour Vesale bte
Phone: +32 2 7645221
Fax: +32 2 7645222

Dr. Ch. S. BARTSOCAS
First Dept. of Pediatrics,
P & A Kyriakou
Chrildren's Hospital
GR 115 27 Athens
Phone: +301 7709316
Fax: +301 7796461

Dr. David APPLETON
Div of Med Statistics,
Univ of Newcastle
UK Newcastle upon Tyne
NE1
Phone: +44 91 2226000
Fax: +44 91 2611182

Dr. Eamonn MAHER
Dept. of Clinical Genetics,
Addenbrook's Hospital
UK Cambridge CB2 2QQ
Phone: +44 223 216446
Fax: +44 223 217054

Dr. E. TIRET
Groupe D'Etude des
Polypose, Hopital
Saint-Antoine
FR 75012 Paris
Phone: +33 1 49282546
Fax: +33 1 49282548

Dr. Gareth EVANS
Medical Genetics, Whitworth
Park, St Mary's Hospital
UK Manchester
Phone: +44 61 2761234
Fax: +44 61 2743159

Dr. Gwen TURNER
Clinical Genetics,
Leeds General Infirmary
UK Leeds
Phone: +44 532 432799
Fax: +44 532 316336

Dr. Heikki JARVINEN
Second Dept. of Surgery,
Helsinki Univ Central
Hospital
FI 00290 Helsinki
Phone: +358 0 471 2320
Fax: +358 0 471 4675

Dr. H.F.A. VASEN
Foundation for the Detection
of Hereditary Tumours c/o
Univ Hosp Leiden
NL 2333 AA Leiden
Phone: +31 71 261955
Fax: +31 71 212137

Dr. John CUMMINGS
Dunn Nutrition Unit,
Univ of Cambridge
UK Cambridge
Phone: +44 223 312334
Fax: +44 223 460089

Dr. John MATHERS
Agricultural Biochemistry,
Univ of Newcastle
UK Newcaslte upon Tyne
NE1 7RU
Phone: +44 91 2226000

Dr. Juan HEBRERO
Hospital San Millan
ES 26004 Logrono
Phone: +34 941 246033
Fax: +34 941 259508

Dr. Julian SAMPSON
Inst. of Med Genetics,
Univ Hosp of Wales
Heath Park
UK Cardiff CF4 4YW
Phone: +44 222 744028
Fax: +44 222 747603

Dr. Lucio BERTARIO
c/o A I Stom, Associatione,
Italiana Stomizzati
IT 20133 Milano
Phone: +39 223 60274
+39 223 90508

Dr. Malcolm DUNLOP
MRC Human Genetics
Univ Registry, Western
General Hospital
UK Edinburg
Phone: +44 31 3322471
Fax: +44 31 3432620

Dr. NEVA HAITES
Medical Genetics,
Medical School
UK Fosterhill Aberdeen
Phone: +44 224 681818
Fax: +44 224 685157

Dr. Olav FAUSA
Dept. of Gastroenterology,
The National Hospital,
Rikshospitalet
NO 0027 Oslo
Phone: +47 2 867619
Fax: +47 2 201401

Dr. Rodney J. SCOTT
Humangenetik,
Dept. Forschung, Kantons-
spital Basel
CH 4051 Basel
Phone: +41 61 265 2362
Fax: +41 61 261 1500

Dr. Rolf HULTCRANTZ
Div of Gastroenterology,
Dept. of Med,
Karolinska Hosp
SE 104 01 Stockholm
Phone: +46 8 7292000

Dr. Steffen BULOW
Dept. of Surgical Gastroen-
terology, Hvidovre Hosp
DK 2650k Hvidovre
Phone: +45 31 471411
Fax: +45 31 473311

Dr. Susan HUSON
Clinical Genetics,
Churchill Hospital
UK Oxford
Phone: +44 865 226024

Dr. S. HODGSON
Paediatric Research Unit,
8th Floor Guys Tower
UK London SE1 9RT
Phone: +44 71 4077600

Dr. S. OLSCHWANG
Inst. Curie,
Lab Tumour Genetique
FR 75005 Paris
Phone: +33 1 40566806
Fax: +33 1 43268087

Dr. Tim BISHOP
ICRF Genetic Epidemiology
Lab, Univ of Leeds
UK Leeds
Phone: +44 532 423617
Fax: +44 532 340183

Mr. James THOMPSON
The Polyposis Registry,
St Mark's Hosp
UK London EC1V 2PS
Phone: +44 71 2531050
Fax: +44 71 2503741

Mr. J.M.A. NORTHOVER
The Polyposis Registry,
St Mark's Hospital
UK London EC1 2PS
Phone: +44 71 6082323
Fax: +44 71 2501478

Prof. Sir Walter BODMER
Imperial Cancer
Research Fund
UK London
Phone: +44 71 242 0200

Prof. T.G. PARKS
Queen's Univ,
Dept. of Surgery
UK Belfast BT9 7AB
Phone: +44 232 329241

MOLECULAR INTERACTIONS BETWEEN CANCER CELLS AND LAMININ: BASIS FOR THE DEVELOPMENT OF NEW DIAGNOSTIC AND PROGNOSTIC APPROACHES AND FOR NEW ANTI-NEOPLASTIC THERAPEUTIC STRATEGIES

Key words
Invasion, metastasis, basement menbranes, laminin, laminin receptors, 67LR, invasive phenotype, chemotherapeutic agents.

Brief description
Tumour invasion and metastasis are the main causes for morbidity and mortality in cancer patients. They resuLt from complex interactions between cancer cells and host tissues, particularly with basement membranes. Basement membranes are specialized extracelluar matrix that separate tissue compartments one from each other and represent real natural barriers that the cancer cells must cross several times during tumour invasion and metastases. Interactions between laminin, a main basement membrane glycoprotein, and malignant cells is crucial for successful penetration of the basement membrane. These interactions are mediated through a variety of cell surface proteins called laminin binding protein or laminin receptors among which the 67 kD laminin receptor (67LR) appears to play a major role and exhibit a high affinity to its ligand, laminin. Indeed, expression of the 67LR is significantly increased in a variety of cancer cells including, breast, colon, ovary and gastric carcinoma cells. Interestingly, the increased expression of 67LR is correlated with the metastatic aggressiveness of cancer cells. One of the goals of our concerned action is to determine the diagnostic and prognostic value of the detection of the 67LR in human cancer pathology, and particularly in breast, colon and ovary cancers. The 67LR being is one of the genes that participate to the acquisition of the invasive and metastatic phenotype of cancer cells. We also plan to study the molecular mechanisms that regulate its expression and determine its increased expression in metastatic cancer cells.

These studies could lead to the identification of new tools to repress the invasive phenotype. In addition, we plan to assess the potential therapeutic value of monoclonal antibodies directed against the 67LR to target cancer cells, in system in which these monoclonal antibodies are made cytotoxic or used with liposomes containing chemotherapeutic agents. The potential therapeutic value of synthetic peptides containing various functional domains of the 67LR will be also analyzed.

Project leader:
Dr. V. CASTRONOVO
Faculté de Médecine, Université de Liège
BAT B35 Tour de Pathologie
BE 4000 Liège
Phone: +32 41 66 88 23
Fax: +32 41 66 88 22
Contract number: CT920520

Participants:
Drs. Alfonso COMLOMBATTI,
Antonino CARBONE
Div di Oncologia Sperimentale 2,
Div di Anatomia Pathologica Centro
di Riferimento Oncologico
Via Pedemontana Occidentale 12
IT 33081 Aviano
Phone: +39 434 659 294
Fax: +39 434 659 370

Dr. Elias CAMPO
Lab of Anatomic Pathology,
Hosp Clin Provincial de Barcelona,
Univ of Barcelona
Calle Villarroel 170
ES 08036 Barcelona
Phone: +34 3 454 6818
Fax: +34 3 454 6691

Dr. Giulia TATABOLETTI
Laboratori Negro-Bergamo
Via Gavazzeni 11
IT 24100 Bergamo
Phone: +39 35 319 888
Fax: +39 35 319 331

Dr. G. BEVILACQUA
Inst. of Pathological Anatomy,
Univ of PISA
Via Roma 57
IT 56126 Pisa
Phone: +39 50 561 840
Fax: +39 50 592 706

Dr. Sylvie MENARD
Istituto Nazionale per lo Studio
e la Cura dei Tumori
Via Vebezian 1
IT 20 133 Milano
Phone: +39 2 239 0566
Fax: +39 2 236 2692

Dr. Vincent CASTRONOVO
Faculté of Medicine,
Univ of Liege, BAT B35
Tour de Pathologie
BE 4000 Sart Tilman
Phone: +32 41 66 88 22
Fax: +32 41 66 88 23

MOLECULAR TARGETING OF LEUKAEMIC DIFFERENTIATION THERAPY USING ACUTE PROMYELOCYTIC LEUKAEMIA AS MODEL

Key words
Promyelocytic leukaemia, oral therapy, retinoic acid, differentiation mechanism, t (15;17), translocation, PML/RAR fusion gene, hyperleucocytosis.

Brief description
Acute promyelocytic leukaemia has recently focused the attention of clinicians and researchers for two major discoveries:

1 Complete remission may be achieved in these patients through *oral therapy* with all-trans retinoic acid via a *novel differentiation mechanism.*
2 The t (15;17) translocation specific of this leukaemia alters the retinoic acid receptor in these cells and produces a *PML/RAR fusion gene.*

These clinical and fundamental findings open new possibilities of differentiation therapies in malignancies and in the understanding of the possible roles of PML or RAR genes in normal myeloid differentiation and of their alteration in the leukemogenetic steps leading to acute myeloid leukaemia. However in the relationship between the in-vitro and in-vivo efficacies of RA in these leukaemic cells has still to be clarified. Understanding the relationship will be of the utmost importance as it represents the first model in oncology of differentiation therapy and efficacy related to a specific molecular abnormality.

The aim of this Concerted Action in clinical and fundamental research of all-trans RA efficacy in acute promyelocytic leukaemia is:

a to achieve an understanding of a novel mechanism of cancer therapy via differentiation taking as model a leukaemia in which the action of the therapeutic agent is probably linked to the oncogenesis of the disease (mechanism of action of all-trans retinoic acid in APL cells, physiological role of RA in normal myeloid differentiation, dominant negative effect of PML/RARa on RA-induces granulocytic differentiation); and

b study the management of this novel method of therapy for maximal efficacy (dose, structure, schedule), little toxicity (hyperleucocytosis, secondary resistance), and minimal residual disease. Acute promyelocytic leukaemia is a rare disease (less than 10% of the Acute myeloid leukaemia) and the joint efforts of the participants of this Concerted Action is the guarantee of its success.

Project leader:
Dr. C. CHOMIENNE
Laboratoire de Biologie Cellulaire,
Institut d'Hématologie, Centre Hayen,
Hôpital Saint-Louis
av. Cl. Vellefaux 1
FR 75010 Paris
Phone: +33 1 42 40 97 45
Fax: +33 1 42 03 92 12
Contract number: CT921144

Participants:

Prof. CASTAIGNE
Hopital Saint-Louis
1 Avenue Claude Vellefaux
FR 75010 Paris
Fax: +33 1 42 00 01 60

Prof. FENAUX
Service Hémato,
Hopital Claude Huriez
Place de Verdun
FR 59037 Lille Cedex
Phone: +33 20 20 44 40 94

Prof. CHASTANG
Hopital Saint-Louis
1 Avenue Claude Vellefaux
FR 75010 Paris
Fax: +33 1 44 49 97 45

Dr. SCROBOHACI
Hopital Saint-Louis
1 Avenue Claude Vellefaux
FR 75010 Paris
Fax: +33 1 42 49 44 60

Prof. LEFEBRE
Hopital Saint-Louis
1 Avenue Claude Vellefaux
FR 75010 Paris

Dr. DANIEL
Hopital Saint-Louis
1 Avenue Claude Vellefaux
FR 75010 Paris
Fax: +33 1 42 49 44 60

Prof. MICHAUX
Clinique Universitaire,
Hopital Saint Luc
Avenue Hippocrate 10
BE 12000 Bruxelles
Fax: +32 27 64 3703

Prof. HOELZER
Abteilung Hématologie,
Klinikum der Goethe
Universitat
Teodor Stern Kai 7
DE Frankfurt
Fax: +49 69 63 017 326

Prof. SANZ
Servico di Hematologia,
Hopital La Fe
Avdar Campanar 21
ES 4600 Valencia
Fax: +34 6 340 8094

Dr. LO COCO
La Sapienza university
Via Benedeto 6
IT 00161 Roma
Fax: +39 39 230 1646

Dr. LARNY
Service d'Hématologie,
Hopital Pontchaillou
Rue Henri Louis Guilloux
FR 35033 Rennes Cedex
Fax: +33 99 28 41 61

Dr. BIONDI
University of Milan Sezionbe
di Hematologia 'HS' Gerardo
Via Donezetti 106
IT 20052 Monza
Fax: +39 39 230 1646

Dr. TILLY
Centre Henri Becquerel
FR 76038 Rouen Cedex

Dr. ARCHIMBAUD
Service d'Hématologie,
Hopital E. Herriot
Place d'Arsonval
FR 69437 Lyon Cedex
Fax: +33 72 34 46 25

Prof. BORDESSOULE
Service d'Hématologie,
Hopital Dupuytren
2 Avenue A. Carrell
FR 87042 Limoges Cedex
Fax: +33 55 06 66 45

Porf. COIFFIER
Service d'Hématologie,
Centre hospitalier
FR 69320 Lyon Sud

Prof. GUERCI
Service d'Hématologie,
Hopital de Brabois
Allée Morvan
FR 54511 Vandoeuvre Cedex
Fax: +33 83 15 35 58

Prof. REIFFERS
Service d'Hématologie,
Hopital de Haut Leveque
FR 33604 Pessac
Fax: +33 56 55 65 14

Prof. AUZANNEAU
Lab. d'Hématologie,
Hopital Val de Grace
68 bd, du Port Royal
FR 75005 Paris
Fax: +33 1 40 51 42 35

Prof. NAVARRO
Service d'Hématologie,
Hopital Lapeyronie
FR 34059 Montpellier
Fax: +33 67 33 89 63

Dr. MERLE BERAT
Hopital Pitié Pavillon
Laverant
47 bd. de l'Hôpital
FR 75651 Paris Cedex
Fax: +33 1 42 16 02 10

F. FARZANEH
Molecular Medcine Unit,
King's College
Denmark Hill
UK London SE 5 8RX
Fax: +44 71 733 3877

E. SALOMON
Imperial Cancer Res. Fund
Linclon's Inn Fields
P.O. Box 123,
UK London WC2A 3PX
Fax: +44 71 269 3469

Prof. PELICCI
Lab. Biol. Molecolare
Via Bunamonti
IT 06100 Perugia
Fax: +39 75 578 3444

Dr. Hughes DE THE
Inst. d'Hematologie, Hopital
St Louis, Univ Paris VII
1 Av. Claude Vellefaux
FR 75010 Paris
Phone: +33 1 42494949
Fax: +33 1 42039212

GENETICS IN EPIDEMIOLOGY OF HEREDITARY BREAST CANCER

Key words
BRCA1, breast-ovarian cancer families, p53 oncogene, Li-Fraumeni Syndrome, gene BRCA1, inherited predisposition.

Brief description
A family history of breast cancer is now a well established risk factor for the disease. It is conjectured that one or more predisposing genes confer a high risk of the disease and may account for approximately 5% of all breast cancer cases. Ovarian cancer is also known to have a familial component, and there is evidence that this is also at least partly the result of an autosomal dominant gene or genes with high penetrance. Moreover, the risk of breast cancer is increased in ovarian cancer relatives and vice-versa. This suggests the existence of a gene or genes predisposing to both breast cancer and ovarian cancer.

One such a gene, which has been labelled BRCA1, was recently localised to the chromosomal region 17q12-q21 by genetic linkage in several breast cancer as well as breast-ovarian cancer families. A collaborative group subsequently investigated the critical region in a total of 214 families, including 57 breast-ovarian families. The results were consistent with all breast-ovary families being linked. In contrast, there was significant evidence of genetic heterogeneity amongst the families without ovarian cancer, with an estimated 45% being linked. The cumulative risk associated with the 17q gene was estimated to 59% by age 50, and 82% by age 70.

Another gene known to confer high risk of cancer when mutated is the p53 oncogene, located on the short arm of chromosome 17. It then gives rise to the Li-Fraumeni Syndrome, a familial clustering of breast cancer, brain tumours, and soft tissue sarcomas.

The objectives of the Concerted Action are to investigate the implications of the carriership of the cancer predisposing gene BRCA1 in terms of cancer risk, and age of onset. Experience with carrier detection programmes and genetic counselling will be exchanged. Further, to identify factors (genetic or non-genetic - for example, use of the oral contraceptive pill) which may modify the genetic risk and which could be manipulated to minimise it, and to determine the contribution of inherited predisposition to total cancer incidence, not only high-risk families. Finally, a search for other predisposing genes will be initiated in those families that are not linked to BRCA1.

These studies will be supplemented by genetic characterizations of breast tumours, to advance our understanding of the relationship between inherited gene mutations and genetic changes that take place during tumour growth. This may provide hints for the localization of predisposing genes other than BRCA1, as well as more insight into the genetics of the tumorigenic process.

Project leader:
Dr. P. DEVILEE
Dept. of Human Genetics, Sylvius Laboratories
Wassenaarseweg 72
NL 2333 AL Leiden
Phone: +31 71 27 61 17
Fax: +31 71 27 60 75
Contract number: CT920890

Participants:

Dr. Adalgeir ARASON
Lab of Cell Biology,
Univ Hosp of Iceland
P.O. Box 1465
IS 121 Reykjavik
Phone: +354 1 601 906
Fax: +354 1 601 519

Dr. Ake BORG
Dep of Oncology, Univ Hosp
SE 221 85 Lund
Phone: +46 46 177 500
Fax: +46 46 147 327

Dr. Catherina LARSSON
Dept. of Clin Genetics,
Karolinska Hosp L6
SE 10401 Stockholm
Phone: +46 87 293 923
Fax: +46 83 27 734

Dr. Fatima GARTNER
Unidade Patologia Molec,
Fac de Med,
Hosp de S Joao
PT 4200 Porto
Phone: +351 2 490 591
Fax: +351 2 410 3940

Dr. Generoso
BEVILACQUA
Inst. di Anatomia Patologica,
Univ of Pisa
Via Rome 57
IT 56126 Pisa
Phone: +39 50 561 840
Fax: +39 50 592 706

Dr. Gilbert LENOIR
Inst. Agency Res Cancer
150 Cours Albert-Thomas
FR 69372 Lyon Cedex 08
Phone: +33 72 73 84 85
Fax: +33 72 73 85 75

Dr. Hagay SOBOL
Head Oncology-Genetic Unit,
Centre Léon Bérard
28 Rue Laennec
FR 69373 Lyon Cedex 08
Phone: +33 78 00 28 28
Fax: +33 78 74 46 15

Dr. Jean FEUNTEUN
Unité UA/1158 du CNRS,
ab d'Oncol Molec, Ins
Gustave Roussy
Rue Camille Desmoulins
FR 94805 Villejuif
Phone: +33 1 45 59 42 94
Fax: +33 1 45 59 64 39

Dr. Michael STEEL
MRC Human Genetics Unit,
Western General Hospital
Crewe Road
UK Edinburgh EH4 2XU
Phone: +44 31 332 2471
Fax: +44 31 343 2620

Dr. Niels HOLM
Dept. of Oncology, Odense
Univ Hosp
Sdr Boulevard 29
DK 5000 Odense
Phone: +45 66 113 333
Fax: +45 66 124 681

Dr. Niger SPURR
Imperial Cancer Research
Fund, Clare Hall
Laboratories
Blanche Lane, South Mimms
UK Herts EN6 3LD
Phone: +44 70 744 444
Fax: +44 70 749 527

Dr. Robert WINQVIST
Dept. of Med Genetics,
Oulu Univ Central Hosp
Kajaanintie 50
FI 90220 Oulu
Phone: +358 81 31 53 224
Fax: +358 81 31 54 499

Dr. S. VASSILAROS
Breast Clinic
4 Semitelou Street
GR 115 28 Athens
Phone: +30 1 77 88 698
Fax: +30 1 32 18 458

Dr. Tim BISHOP
ICRF Genetic Epidemiology
Laboratory,
3K Springfield House
Hyde Terrace
UK Leeds LS2 9LU
Phone: +44 53 242 3617
Fax: +44 53 234 0183

Dr. Yves-Jean BIGNON
Centre Jean Perrin,
Lab d'Oncologie Moleculaire
Place Henri Dunant,
P.O. Box 392
FR 63011 Clermont-Ferrand
Phone: +33 73 27 80 50
Fax: +33 73 26 34 51

A EUROPEAN CANCER CELL LINE RESOURCE

Key words
Cancer Resources Bank, characterisation methods, quality control, DNA Fingerprinting.

Brief description
This is a new Concerted Action to establish a European Cancer Resources Bank. It will involve the production of a Cancer Resources Catalogue which will detail the types and source of cell lines available through the participating organisations.

The project will aim to improve the information available on these cell lines by improving characterisation methods and providing extended bibliographies on each cell line. Also methods of quality control will be improved by the introduction of new technology such as DNA Fingerprinting.

As well as improving current resources the project aims to increase the range of specifically characterised material such as the rarer cancers and banks of familial cancer cell lines.

All material will be made available to scientists in the European Community for Research and should greatly enhance the resources available for research into cancer.

Project leader:
Dr. A. DOYLE
European Collection of
Animal Cell Cultures,
Division of Biologics, PHLS
Porton Down
UK Salisbury SP4 OJG
Phone: +44 980 61 03 91
Fax: +44 980 61 13 15
Contract number: CT920181

Participants:
Dr. B. BOLTON
Centre for Applied
Microbiology and
Research, ECACC
UK Salisbury SP4 OJG
Phone: +44 980 612512
Fax: +44 980 611315

Dr. B. PARODI
Instituto Nazionale
per la Ricera sul Cancro
Viale Benedetto XV, 10
IT 16132 Genova
Phone: +39 10 352823
Fax: +39 10 352888

Dr. D. DAIJA
Inst. of Organic Synthesis
21 Aizkraukles Street
LV 1006 Riga
Phone: +371 8828114
Fax: +371 2553493

Dr. K. WAYSS
Krebsforschungszentrum,
Tumourbank
Im Neuenheimer feld 280
DE 6900 Heidelberg
Phone: +49 6221 423205
Fax: +49 6221 401271

Dr. L. RECHAUSSAT
Centre Européen de Recherches et de Dévelopment en
Information et Communication Scientifiques
FR Sophia Antipolis
Phone: +33 92 942288
Fax: +33 92 942294

Dr. Barbara PARODI
Instituto Nazionale per las
Ricera sul Cancero (IST),
Banca Dati per La Ricerca
Biomedica
IT Genoa
Phone: +39 10 3534515
Fax: +39 10 355573

Dr. Bruce PONDER
Univ Cambridge,
CRC Human Cancer
Genetics Res Group
UK Cambridge
Phone: +44 223 333711
Fax: +44 223 333875

Dr. Klaus WAYSS
DKFZ, Abt Histodiagnostik
u Pathomorphologische
Dokumentation Tumourbank
Im Neuenheimer Feld 280
DE 6900 Heidelberg
Phone: +49 6221420

Dr. Louis RECHAUSSAT
Centre European de Recherches Documentaires sur les
Immunoclones (CERDIC)
FR Sophia-Antipolis
Phone: +33 92942288
Fax: +33 92942294

Prof. B. PONDER
CRC Human Cancer Genetics
Group, Univ of Cambridge
UK Cambridge
Phone: +44 223 333875
Fax: +44 223 333705

Prof. D. TODOROV
National Oncological Centre,
Medical Academy
BG 1156 Sofia
Phone: +359 2 720654

SEARCH FOR NEW PROTO-ONCOGENES AND ANTI-ONCOGENES OF DIFFERENTIATED EPITHELIAL CELLS: THE THYROCYTES

Key words
Proliferation, differentiation, thyroid cells, protooncogenes, antioncogenes, tumour markers, putative oncogenes, in situ hybridization, immunocytochemistry.

Brief description
Objectives:
1 To develop our knowledge of the control of proliferation and differentiation of thyroid cells, in order to identify new protooncogenes and antioncogenes which might constitute both tumour markers and pharmacological targets.
2 To develop new thyroid cell lines, especially human thyroid cell lines as a standardized tool to pursue research 1 and to identify putative oncogenes.
3 To compare these new cell lines (2) to available cell lines. To standardize their use in the various laboratories.
4 To create a collection of samples from human thyroid tumours to constitute:
- a bank of tumour DNAs.
- a bank of fixed tissues for use for in situ hybridization and in immunocytochemistry (development of new tumour markers).

Project leader:
Professor J.E. DUMONT
Institute of Interdisciplinary Research,
University of Brussels
Route de Lennik 808
BE 1070 Brussels
Phone: +32 2 555 41 33
Fax: +32 2 555 46 55
Contract number: CT920081

Participants:
Dr. G. BRABANT
Dept. of Clin Endocrinology,
Med Hoschule Hannover
Konstanty Gutschowstr. 8
DE 3000 Hannover 61
Phone: +49 511 5323899
Fax: +49 511 5323825

Dr. P.E. GORETZKI
Chirurgische klinik A,
Heinrich Heine Univ
Moorenstr. 5
DE 4000 Dusseldorf
Phone: +49 211 3117350
Fax: +49 211 342229

Prof. Aldo PINCHERA
Istituto di Endocriniologia,
Metodiologia Clin e Med,
Univ degli Studi di Pisa
Viale del Tirreno 64
IT 56018 Pisa
Phone: +39 50 32590
Fax: +39 50 33433

Prof. E.D. WILLIAMS
Dept. of Pathology,
Univ of Wales,
Coll of Med Health Park
UK Cardiff CF4 4XN
Phone: +44 222 747747
Fax: +44 222 371921

Prof. G. FAYET
Fac de Med,
Lab de Biochemie Med,
INSERM U38-CNRS
27 Boulevard Jean Moulin
FR 13365 Marseille Cedex 5
Phone: +33 91 834374
Fax: +33 91 797774

CLINICAL IMPLEMENTATION OF
NEUTRON CAPTURE THERAPY

Key words
Boron neutron capture therapy (BNCT), glioma, radiotherapy, High Flux Reactor.

Brief description
The Concerted Action *Clinical Implementation of Neutron Capture Therapy* has the objective to determine whether boron neutron capture therapy (BNCT) of glioma with BSH is a useful treatment alternative to conventional treatment. It will have to establish under which conditions BNCT can be administered safely, and it will then have to investigate whether BNCT or glioma is more effective for treatment of glioma than conventional treatment. The work is a combined Phase I/Phase II clinical study on patients with high-grade gliomas.

Gliomas are responsible for around 4% of all cancer deaths. The mean survival time after diagnosis is about eight months, and has not changed over the last forty years. Patients die not because of wide-spread disease, but because of local recurrence and intracranial metastases. The incidence of high-grade gliomas in adult patients peaks at around the age of 55-60.

BNCT is a radiotherapy modality where the selective accumulation of (non-toxic) compounds in tumours can be exploited to increase the radiation damage to tumour tissue over that of normal tissue. The compounds must contain boron, an element which can capture neutrons and undergo a nuclear reaction. It requires a neutron beam of suitable characteristics. Such a beam has been installed at the Joint Research Centre in Petten, The Netherlands, and is available for this treatment.

The High Flux Reactor in Petten is a European research centre, and therefore could (and should) develop into a European treatment facility. This is motivated by the complexity of the treatment, the costs associated with an advanced radiotherapy unit, and by the hope that this European centre could form a model for supranational medical therapy centres.

It is assumed that eventually approximately 1,000 to 2,000 new patients per year could be treated at one single treatment centre. This constitutes a substantial fraction (up to 20%) of all those patients in Europe whose medical situation would warrant a treatment with BNCT. Preconditions for successful therapy of glioma with BNCT are:
- the treatment must be associated with a minimal and acceptable risk to the patient;
- the treatment must have a reasonable change of being effective.

This requires knowledge in two areas:
a the tumour must accumulate enough boron, and the surrounding tissue must be sufficiently cleared from boron, when treatment is to start;
b it must be known whether the chosen neutron beam is able to deliver enough neutrons within a reasonable treatment time, with acceptable damage to healthy tissue due to contamination with fast neutrons and gamma rays. The risk assessed must include short and long-term damage to all tissues exposed.

In order to attain the objectives, the Concerted Action will derive from the data available from the Concerted Action *European Collaboration on Boron Neutron Capture Therapy* and from other sources, all parameters and networks necessary to implement treatment of high-grade glioma patients by the end of 1998. Fifteen countries of the EC and COST participate in the Concerted Action. Active collaboration with groups in other countries in Europe and elsewhere is pursued.

Project leader:
Professor D. GABEL
Dept. of Chemistry,
University of Bremen
P.O. Box 33 04 40
DE 28359 Bremen
Phone: +49 421 218 22 00
Fax: +49 421 218 28 71
Contract number: CT920859

Participants:
Dra. M.E. SILVESTRE
PT 1600 Lissabon

Dr. B. EAST
UK Glasgow G75 0QU

Dr. B.S. LARSSON
SE 751 24 Uppsala

Dr. C.B.T. ADAMS
UK Oxford OX2 6HE

Dr. D. CHIARAVIGLIO
IT 27100 Pavia

Dr. D. ORENSTEIN
FR 67098 Strasbourg

Dr. G. BRUCHELT
DE 7400 Tubingen

Dr. G. van den AARDWEG
NL 3075 EA Rotterdam

Dr. G.A.B. GIBSON
UK Oxfordshire OX11 ORA

Dr. H. BARTELINK
NL 1066 CX Amsterdam

Dr. H. FRANKHAUSER
CH 1011 Lausanne

Dr. H. RIEF
IT 21020 Ispra (VA)

Dr. John HOPEWELL
UK Oxford OX3 7LJ

Dr. J. CARLSSON
SE 751 21 Uppsala

Dr. J. MORRIS
UK Glasgow G1 1XL

Dr. J.H.C. VOORMOLEN
NL 2300 Leiden

Dr. LAWAZCECK
DE 1000 Berlin 65

Dr. L. HOLSTI
FI 00290 Helsinki

Dr. L.G. SALFORD
SE 221 85 Lund

Dr. R. HUISKAMP
NL 1755 ZG Petten

Dr. R. L. MOSS
NL 1755 ZG Petten

Dr. R. TAVONI
IT 40129 Bologna

Dr. Th. AUBERGER
DE 8000 Munchen 80

Dr. Th. LOUGHLIN
UK Southampton SO9 4XH

Dr. W. SAUERWEIN
DE 4300 Essen 1

Prof. ALCOBER
ES 46100 Burjassot Valencia

Prof. Dr. A. WAMBERSIE
BE Louvain

Prof. Dr. B. LARSSON
CH 8029 Zurich

Prof. Dr. E. DUHMKE
DE 3400 Gottingen

Prof. Dr. G. PENDL
AT 8036 Graz

Prof. Dr. J. KALEF-EZRA
GR 451 10 Ioannina

Prof. J.A.C. BROEKART
DE 4600 Dortmund 50

Prof. Dr. K. PISCOL
DE 2800 Bremen 33

Prof. Dr. T. SPALDING
IE Cork

Prof. J.C. ABBE
FR 67037 Strasbourg Cedex

Prof. M. THELLIER
FR 76134 Mont St Aignan

Prof. P. HIISMAKI
FI 02151 Espoo

DEVELOPMENT OF A DATABASE ON TRANSCRIBED SEQUENCES IN TUMOUR CELLS AND IDENTIFICATION OF CHANGES IN TRANSCRIPTION PATTERNS RELATED TO TRANSFORMATION AND OTHER TUMOUR CELL PROPERTIES FOR THE GLOBAL FINGERPRINTING ANALYSIS OF HUMAN PANCREATIC CARCINOMA cDNA LIBRARIES

Key words
Genome mapping, pancreatic cancer, pancreatic tissues, hybridisations, computerized image analysis.

Brief description
Our Concerted Action is based on the application of automated molecular techniques that proved successful for genome mapping purpose for the large scale analysis of transcribed sequences in pancreatic cancer. 20,000 clones of representative cDNA libraries from pancreatic cancer cell lines and human pancreatic tissues (cancer and control tissue) will be spotted as high density insitu library arrays on Nylon membranes using a robotic device. These CDNA library arrays will form part of a *European Pancreatic Cancer Reference Library System* (EPCRLS) and will be available to all European groups involved in pancreatic cancer research. Basic data to each CDNA library array will be generated in our own laboratories by a series of complex hybridisations (e.g. identification of highly abundant clones, oncogenes, housekeeping genes, repetitive sequence elements). Data obtained in our experiments and by groups making use of the EPCRLS will be analyzed with a computerized image analysis system and stored within different experimental approaches. Groups participating in the EPCRLS will be supplied with their clone of interest and any additional data available in the database to this particular clone (sequence, abundance, identity with already characterized clones). Newly generated information will form part of the database, and will be handled confidentially if required.
The basic idea of this approach is to co-ordinate and correlate the research work of European laboratories on the molecular biology of pancreatic cancer by generating representative cDNA library resources and by developing a central relational computer database for storage and analysis of data obtained by different experimental approaches.

Project leader:
Dr. T. GRESS
Medizinische Klinik I, University of Ulm
Robert Koch Strasse 8
DE 89081 Ulm
Phone: +49 731 502 43 11 or 34
Fax: +49 731 502 43 02
Contract number: CT920401

Participant:
Dr. Hans LEHRACH
Genome Analysis Laboratory,
Imperial Cancer Research Fund
44 Lincoln's Inn Fields
UK London WC2A 3PX
Phone: +44 71 269 3308
Fax: +44 71 405 4303

INHIBITION OF NUCLEAR ONCOGENES ACTIVITY BY STEROIDS AND VITAMIN HORMONE RECEPTORS

Key words

Transcription factors, micro-environment, dysregulation, AP-1 family, adenoviral onco-gene E1A, papilloma virus, cancerogenesis.

Brief description

Transcription factors in the nucleus determine which genes will be active and, consequently which properties the cell will possess. Most cells harbour large numbers of transcription factors in an inactive state, each one ready to address specific genes. The transcription factor family A-1, the major focus of this Concerted Action, comprises some 80 to 100 members, whose exact function and specifity are largely unknown. These transcription factors turn on gene cells are stimulated by their *micro-environment*. Various protein components transmit the stimulus from the plasma membrane to the nucleus in a process defined as signal transduction. Dysregulation at any one of these levels including aberrant levels and mutations of the transcription factors promotes cancerogenesis. Current objectives are to understand the complexity of the AP-1 family, their functions and interactions with other nuclear proteins. One important aspect concerns the crosstalk between transcription factors involved in proliferation and those regulating differentiation. Influencing such cross-talk towards differentiation will be attempted in order to 'normalize' cancer cells. Members of the AP-I family will be defined that the adenoviral oncogene E1A uses in order to transform, and those that participate in human papilloma virus expression, the yet only agent related to human cancerogenesis. Since various members of the Jun family can act both as transcriptional repressors and activators, it will be investigated whether specific Jun proteins exhibit tumour suppressing function by acting as a negative regulator during cell transformation.

Project leader:
Professor P. HERRLICH
Institut für Genetik und Toxikologie von Spalt-stoffen, Kernforschungszentrum Karlsruhe
P.O. Box 3640
DE 76149 Karlsruhe
Phone: +49 7247 82 32 92
Fax: +49 7247 82 33 54
Contract number: CT921037

Participants:
Dr. Alex van der EB
Dept. of Med Biochemistry,
Sylvius Laboratory, Univ of Leiden
Wassenaarseweg 72
NL 2333 AL Leiden
Phone: +31 71 276052
Fax: +31 71 142582

Dr. Moshe YANIV
Dept. of Biotechnology, Inst. Pasteur
25 Rue du Dr. Roux
FR 75724 Paris Cedex 15.F
Phone: +33 1 45688512
Fax: +33 1 45688790

Dr. Peter ANGEL
Kernforschungszentrum Karslruhe,
Inst. für Genetik und Toxicologie
P.O. Box 3640
DE 7500 Karlsruhe 1
Phone: +49 7247 823444
Fax: +49 7247 823354

EUROPEAN INTERGROUP COOPERATIVE EWING'S SARCOMA STUDY 1992 (EICESS 92)

Key words

Ewing's sarcoma, malignant bone tumour, childhood malignancies, chemotherapy, etoposide, vincristine, actinomycin D, ifosfamide, adriamycin.

Brief description

Ewing's sarcoma is the second commonest malignant bone tumour in children and adolescents and accounts for approximately 5% of all childhood malignancies. The annual incidence is estimated at 0.6 per million population. The natural course of the disease is rapid dissemination and death from metastases within one or two years from diagnosis. With the combination of local control with surgery and/or radiotherapy and aggressive systemic combination chemotherapy two out of three patients can now be cured of their disease.

Both a British and German working group on Ewing's sarcoma have previous experience in conducting co-operative trials for treatment of Ewing's sarcoma resulting in improved disease-free survival. The joint European project is aimed to tailor the intensity of systemic chemotherapy to the individual risk of relapse. For standard risk patients (tumour volume - 100 ml) it is to be determined whether the treatment related morbidity can be reduced without compromising survival by returning to a less intensive maintenance chemotherapy regimen following intensive induction chemotherapy. For high risk patients (tumour volume ≥ 100 ml) it is to be determined whether the addition of a fifth drug (etoposide) to the standard four-drug combination chemotherapy regimen (vincristine, actinomycin D, ifosfamide, adriamycin) can improve survival without unacceptable acute toxicity or late effects.

In addition, the impact of surgery and radiotherapy on local control, overall survival and morbidity is to be evaluated. Additional objectives include: to relate outcome of treatment to patient characteristics, histologic subtype at diagnosis and histologic response to treatment, and also to prospectively evaluate late effects such as chemotherapy-related organ toxicity.

Based on a large patient accrual from several European Countries, the statistical analysis will allow to define exact guidelines to develop future strategies for treatment of this rare disease for the benefit of the affected patients.

Project leader:
Professor H. JÜRGENS
Universitäts-Kinderklinik,
Abt. Hämatologie/Onkologie
Albert-Schweitzer-Strasse 33
DE 48149 Münster
Phone: +49 251 83 77 42
Fax: +49 251 83 78 28
Contract number: CT921341

Participants:
Dr. A. ROMANOWSKI (DE)

Dr. BUCSKY (DE)

Dr. Ch. NIEMEYER (DE)

Dr. Ch. TAUTZ (DE)

Dr. C. BAILEY (UK)

Dr. D.A. WALKER (UK)

Dr. D.J. KING (UK)

Dr. EWERBECK (DE)

Dr. E. SIGNER (CH)

Dr. E.N. THOMPSON (UK)

Dr. FAUSER (DE)

Dr. FRITZ (DE)

Dr. F. BREATNACH (IE)

Dr. F.J. GÖBEL (DE)

Dr. GEIB-KÖNIG (DE)

Dr. GNEKOW (DE)

Dr. GRÜNBERGER (AT)

Dr. G. MÜLLER (AT)

Dr. G. NESSLER (DE)

Dr. HELLER (DE)

Dr. H. BODENSTEIN (DE)

Dr. H. BREU (DE)

Dr. H. MESSNER (AT)

Dr. H.J. SPAAR (DE)

Dr. ISSELS (DE)

Dr. JOBKE (DE)

Dr. J. KÜHL (DE)

Dr. J. MARTIN (UK)

Dr. J. OTTE (DE)

Dr. J.A. KOHLER (UK)

Dr. J.R. MANN (UK)

Dr. KAESBERGER (DE)

Dr. KUSNIERZ-GLAZ (DE)

Dr. K. EBERHARDT (DE)

Dr. M. CORNBLEET (UK)

Dr. M. GERRARD (UK)

Dr. N. GRAF (DE)

Dr. O. SAUER (DE)

Dr. P.B. MORRIS JONES (UK)

Dr. REICHARDT (DE)

Dr. R. HAWLICEK (AT)

Dr. R. LUDWIG (DE)

Dr. R. MERTENS (DE)

Dr. R. PINKERTON (UK)

Dr. R. SHANNON (UK)

Dr. SCHMIDT (DE)

Dr. SCHRÖDER (DE)

Dr. S. MÜLLERWEIHRICH (DE)

Dr. S. DEMPSEY (UK)

Dr. Thomas ACHAMMER (AT)

Dr. Th. KLINGEBIELL (DE)

Dr. U. EXNER (CH)

Dr. U. HEISE (DE)

Dr. V.A. BROADBENT (UK)

Dr. W. STERN (DE)

Dr. ZINTL (DE)

Dr. Z. BARJAKTAREVIC (YU)

Prof. A. BARRETT (UK)

Prof. A.W. CRAFT (UK)

Prof. Dr. BECKER (DE)

Prof. BENDER-GÖTZE (DE)

Prof. B. KORNHUBER (DE)

Prof. Dr. Ch. URBAN (AT)

Prof. C. ESCHENBACH (DE)

Prof. Dr. DIEHL. (DE)

Prof. Dr. DRINGS (DE)

Prof. D.K. HOSSFELD (DE)

Prof. Dr. ENGELHARDT (DE)

Prof. F. BERTHOLD (DE)

Prof. Dr. GUTJAHR (DE)

Prof. Dr. G. HENZE (DE)

Prof. Dr. HAUSAMEN (DE)

Prof. Dr. HAUSWALDT (DE)

Prof. Dr. HAVERS (DE)

Prof. Dr. HEIDEMANN (DE)

Prof. Dr. HOTZ (DE)

Prof. Dr. H. GADNER (AT)

Prof. Dr. H. RIEHM (DE)

Prof. Dr. H. THEML (DE)

Prof. Dr. H. WEHINGER (DE)

Prof. Dr. H.J. SCHMOLL (DE)

Prof. Dr. J. BECK (DE)

Prof. Dr. J. TREUNER (DE)

Prof. Dr. J. Th. FISCHER (DE)

Prof. K. SCHUMACHER (DE)

Prof. Dr. K. WINKLER (DE)

Prof. Dr. LAKOMEK (DE)

Prof. Dr. LAMPERT (DE)

Prof. Dr. LÜDERS (DE)

Prof. Dr. M. BAMBERG (DE)

Prof. Dr. M. RISTER (DE)

Prof. Dr. M. SALZER (AT)

Pr. M. WESTERHAUSEN (DE)

Prof. Dr. NIETHAMMER (DE)

Prof. Dr. O.B. EDEN (UK)

Prof. Dr. P.A. VOUTE (NL)

Prof. Dr. R. KOTZ (AT)

Prof. Dr. R. SAUER (DE)

Prof. SCHULTE-WISSERMANN (DE)

Prof. Dr. SEEBER (DE)

Prof. Dr. U. BODE (DE)

Prof. Dr. U. GÖBEL (DE)

Prof. VOGT-MOYKOPF (DE)

Prof. Dr. W. ANDLER (DE)

Prof. Dr. W. RAUH (DE)

Prof. J.M. CHESSELLS (UK)

Prof. M.G. MOTT (UK)

Prof. R.L. SOUHAMI (UK)

PROTEIN PHOSPHATASES IN MALIGNANT TRANSFORMATION AND THE REGULATION OF THE CELL CYCLE: THEIR ROLE AS TUMOUR SUPPRESSORS

Key words

Protein phosphorylation, dephosphorylation, protein kinases, protein phosphatases, 2A (PP2A), Phosospho Tyrosyl Phosphatase Activator (PTPA), PP21, cell proliferation.

Brief description

Protein phosphorylation and dephosphorylation play a fundamental role in all aspects of cellular function, including cell division and differentiation. It is equally evident that inappropriate or defective operation of these regulatory events contributes to malignant cellular transformation. The control of cellular processes through phosphorylation is not a one-way process, but involves both protein kinases and protein phosphatases. In the dynamic aspect of protein desphosphorylation, the different forms of protein phosphatase 2A (PP2A) play an essential role. Over the past years, the major regulatory subunits as well as the Phosospho Tyrosyl Phosphatase Activator (PTPA) have purified and cloned. The holoenzyme of PP21 are assembled from at least eight different gene products. At this stage, the study of the type 2A phophatases as relevant in diagnosis, prognostic evaluation or therapeutic choice in the treatment of cancer requires:

- a clear understanding of their selective function(s) in cell proliferation and cell cycle control;
- a direct assessment of the expression of the type 2A phosphatase sub-units and regulators in transformed cells and neoplasms;
- the chromosomal localisation of the type 2A phosphatase subunits and regulatory subunits (including PTPA) in normal and in transformed cells.

Based on these findings, new criteria will be recommended and assessed for early diagnosis of cancer, high cancer-risk identification, predictive and evaluation tests for chemotherapy.

Project leader:
Professor W. MERLEVEDE
Afdeling Biochemie, Catholic
University of Leuven
Campus Gasthuisberg
BE 3000 Leuven
Phone: +32 16 34 57 00
Fax: +32 16 34 59 95
Contract number: CT921074

Participants:
Brian HEMMINGS
Friedrich Miescher Institut
P.O. Box 2543
CH 4002 Basel
Phone: +41 61 6974046
Fax: +41 61 6973976

E. VAN DER SCHUEREN
Centrum voor Gezwelziekten,
Univ. Ziekenhuis St Rafael
BE 3000 Leuven
Phone: +32 16 21 5705
Fax: +32 16 21 2228

Jozef GORIS
Afd. Biochemie,
Fac Geneeskunde
BE 3000 Leven
Phone: +32 16 21 5705
Fax: +32 16 21 5995

Kurt BALMER
Friedrich Miescher Institut
CH 4002 Basel
Phone: +41 61 6973596
Fax: +41 61 6973976

Peter PARKER
Imperial Cancer Research
Fund Laboratories
P.O. Box 123
UK London WC2A 3PX
Phone: +44 71 2693450
Fax: +44 71 4050190

René OZON
Laboratoire de Physiologie de
la Réproduction
Quai Saint-Bernard 9
FR 75005 Paris
Phone: +33 1 44273926
Fax: +33 1 44273472

COORDINATION OF A CENTRALIZED FACILITY FOR CLINICAL TRIALS IN ONCOLOGY

Key words

Therapeutic modalities, clinical trials, clinical research, infrastructure, co-ordination of cancer trials.

Objectives

The objectives of the European Organization for Research and Treatment of Cancer (EORTC) are to conduct, develop, co-ordinate and stimulate research in Europe on the treatment of cancer and related problems with the final goal being a reduction in the mortality rate.

Brief description

No research in molecular biology being done now will impact on the number of cancer deaths in the next 10 years. However, new strategies, new drugs and the development of more effective therapeutic modalities can have an immediate effect.

Progress in the treatment of cancer requires clinical trials. Convincing clinical trials require a large number of patients and an objective analysis. Therefore, clinical trials must be carried out on a very wide scale i.e. on a European level leading to results widely applicable. However, the design and preparation of such trials, the collection of patient data, the statistical analyses and the publication of results require a centralized facility composed of high qualified scientific personnel.

Clinical research is vital for offering highest standards of care of all Europe's cancer patients. Less than 10% of cancer patients go into clinical trials, yet those patients will have a better survival and quality of life than the 90% treated outside clinical research settings.

Existing knowledge and technology should be made available to cancer patients as widely and as quickly as possible. Effective clinical research in oncology should be supported by a central structure co-ordinating clinical trials, linking basic research to clinical practise.

The goal of the EORTC Data Centre is to provide an adequate infrastructure for the design, the analyze and the co-ordination of cancer clinical trials in Europe and to improve the quality of EORTC trials. Such centralized facility allows an increased collaboration between investigators and scientists and provides an optimal framework for the conduct of cancer clinical trials as well as for the dissemination of knowledge and expertise within the EEC. Such a goal requires full scientific and administrative support in order to harmonize and standardize techniques as well as patient care among physicians.

Project leader:
Professor F. MEUNIER
EORTC Central Office,
Data Center
Avenue Mounier 83
P.O. Box 11
BE 1200 Brussels
Phone: +32 2 774 16 30
Fax: +32 2 771 20 04
Contract number: CT921677

Participants:
Vicky MINAS
83 Av Mounier, Bte 11
BE 1200 Brussels
Phone: +32 2 774 16 41
Fax: +32 2 772 35 45

Vincent PIEDBOEUF
83 Av Mounier, Bte 11
BE 1200 Brussels
Phone: +32 2 774 16 19
Fax: +32 2 772 35 45

GENETIC STUDIES IN HERIDITARY NON-POLYPOSIS CANCER OF THE COLON (HNPCC) AND FAMILIAL ADENOMATOUS POLYPOSIS (FAP) FAMILIES FOR IDENTIFICATION AND CHARACTERIZATION OF THE HPNCC GENE(S) AND FOR FURTHER CHARTING OF THE SPECTRUM OF FAP-MUTANTS

Key words
Hereditary cancers, large intestine, Familial Adenomatous Polyposis, Colon, Hereditary Non-Polyposis Cancer, genetic analysis, genetic diagnostics, prophylactic examinations, colonoscopy.

Brief description
The targets of the concerted action EUROFAP2, grant PL92 1374, are two kinds of hereditary cancers which together make up 5-10% of all cancers of the large intestine. They are FAP, or Familial Adenomatous Polyposis of the Colon, and the several times more frequent HNPCC, or Hereditary Non-Polyposis Cancer of the Colon. For both these conditions the ultimate objective of the action is to reduce casualties from cancer-This objective is approached via genetic analysis and establishment of genetic diagnostics throughout the community, for the purpose of serving prevention and management. In quantitative terms: in the total Community population the yearly number of casualties from colorectal cancer (death occurs at an early age in these conditions if they are not properly managed) in FAP and HNPCC families may be essayed as 2,000-10,000. All new cases in these families with colorectal cancer are in principle preventable once the families have been identified and efficient methodology for genetic preclinical diagnosis developed. The importance of this approach is emphasized by the sharp contrast between a low cost of genetic diagnosis and a prohibitively high cost of currently recommended clinical measures of prophylactic examinations (including colonoscopy).

With these objectives, the concerted action comprises:
1 Genetic studies in families with cancer of the colon (FAP as well as HNPCC) with particular regard to charting the mutational spectrum of the FAP gene and recognition through linkage analysis of the HNPCC gene(s).
2 Studies concerning implementation of the genetic results towards improved management and prevention, to assay (- and thereby help implementing research results) the practical possibilities of reducing casualties from cancer of the colon- Participants are research groups from all countries in the Community as well as cost nations, a total of 27 groups.

Project leader:
Professor J. MOHR
Genome Group Panum,
Institute of Medical Genetics,
University of Copenhagen
Blegdamsvej 3b
DK 2200 Copenhagen
Phone: +45 31 35 79 00
Fax: +45 31 35 76 81
Contract number: CT921374

Participants:
Drs. L. VARESCO
Cristina Mareni,
Cattedra di Genetica Medica
Viale Benedetto XV 6
IT 16132 Genova
Phone: +39 10 35 32 264
Fax: +39 10 35 23 24

Dr.VERELLEN-
DUMOULIN
Ctr of Human Genetics UCL
Avenue Mounier 52
BE 1200 Brussels
Phone: +32 2 764 5220
Fax: +32 2 764 5322

Dr. Gillis THOMAS
Inst. Curie
FR 75 231 Paris
Phone: +33 1 43 29 12 42
Fax: +33 1 46 33 20 09

Dr. H.F.A. VASEN
Stichting Opsporing
Erfelijke Tumoren,
NL 233 AA Leiden
Phone: +31 71 261 955
Fax: +31 71 212137

Dr. H.J. MULLER
Lab of Human Genetics,
Dept. of the Res of the
Univ Clinics
CH 4031 Basel
Phone: +41 61 2652362
Fax: +41 61 261 15 00

Dr. Jean Jaques CASSIMAN
Center for Human Genetics
Campus Gasthuisberg O en n
BE 3000 Leuven
Phone: +32 16 215860
Fax: +32 16 215997

Dr. John BURN
Div of Human Genetics,
Univ of Newcastle upon Tyne
UK Newcastle upon Tyne
NE2 4AA
Phone: +44 91 232 5131
Fax: +44 91 261 1182

Dr. Joy D.A. DELHANTY
Galton Lab Univ Coll
UK London NW1 3HE
Phone: +44 71 380 7409
Fax: +44 71 387 3496

Dr. Jukka-Pekka MECKLIN
Central Hospital
FI 40620 Jyvaskyla
Phone: +358 41 691811
Fax: +358 41 691099

Dr. J.M.A. NORTHOVER
St Mark's Hospital
UK London ECIV 2PS
Phone: +44 71 2531050
Fax: +44 71 2501478

Dr. Lucio BERTARIO
Ist per lo Studio dei Tumori,
Milano Univ
IT 20133 Milano
Phone: +39 2 8392390
Fax: +39 2 8397058

Dr. Malcolm DUNLOP
MRC Human Genetics Unit,
Western General Hospital
UK Edinburgh EH4 3XU
Phone: +44 31 332 2471
Fax: +44 31 343 2620

Dr. M. PONZ DE LEON
Instituto Pathologica Medica,
Univ di Modena
IT Modena
Phone: +39 59 379 269
Fax: +39 59 379 124

Dr. Neva HAITES
Medical Genetics, Dept.
of Genetics & Microbiol,
Med School Univ Aberdeen
UK Aberdeen
Phone: +44 681 818
Fax: +44 224 685 157

Dr. Niall TIERNEY
Dept. of Health,
Hawkins House
IE Dublin 1
Phone: +353 1 714711
Fax: +353 1 711947

Dr. R. HULTCRANTZ
Medicinska Kliniken,
Karolinska Hospital
SE 10 401 Stockholm 60
Phone: +46 8 729 2000
Fax: +46 8 318 264

Dr. Steffen BÜLOW
Dept. Surgical Gastroenterol,
Hvidovre Hospital, Dept. 235
DK 2650 Hvidovre
Phone: +45 36 32 22 36
Fax: +45 31 47 33 11

Dr. Sverre HEIM
Univ Inst. of Genetic Pathol-
ogy, Odense Univ
DK 5000 Odense
Phone: +46 46 17 3369
Fax: +46 46 13 1061

Prof. C.S. BARTSOCAS,
A. KYRIAKOU
Dept. of Pediatrics,
Athen's Chidren's Hospital
GR 11527 Athens
Phone: +30 1 722 5828
Fax: +30 1 779 6461

Prof. Carlos SAN RAMON
Dept. of Med Genetics,
Hosp Ramon Y Cajal
ES 28034 Madrid
Phone: +34 1 72 90000
Fax: +34 1 33 69016

Prof. Erich GEBHART
Inst. fur Humangenetik &
Anthrop
DE 8520 Erlangen
Phone: +49 9131 85/23 19
Fax: +49 9131-20 92 97

Prof. Manfred SCHWAB
Deutsch Krebsforschungsctr.
DE 6900 Heidelberg 1
Phone: +49 6621 484 220
Fax: +49 6221 410097

Prof. P. MEERA KHAN
Human Genetics Inst.
NL 2300 RA Leiden
Phone: +31 71 27 6090
Fax: +31 71 27 6075

Prof. Tobias GEDDE-DAHL
Det Norske Radiumhospital,
Dept. Genet (Canc Res)
Radiumhospitalet
NO Norway
Phone: +47 83 42000
Fax: +47 83 56990

Prof. T.G. PARKS
Dept. of Surgery,
Belfast City Hosp
UK Belfast
Phone: +44 232 329 241
Fax: +44 232 326 614

Sir Walter BODMER
Imperial Canc Research,
Fund Laboratories
UK London WC2A 3PX
Phone: +44 71 242 0200
Fax: +44 71 269 3469

ACUTE PROMYELOCYTIC LEUKAEMIA: PATHOGENESIS AND MOLECULAR BASIS OF RETINOIC ACID DIFFERENTIATION TREATMENT

Key words

Acute promyelocytic leukaemia, malignant promyelocytes, retinoic acid (RA), chemotherapy, bone-marrow aplasia.

Brief description

Acute promyelocytic leukaemia (APL) accounts for 5-10% of all acute myeloid leukaemia (AML) cases. The malignant promyelocytes are highly sensitive to the differentiative action of retinoic acid (RA). In fact, oral administration of RA induces complete disease remission in almost all APL patients in first diagnosis. Unlike conventional chemotherapy, RA triggers differentiation and, consequently, does not cause bone-marrow aplasia. Unfortunately, remission is brief and relapse is RA-resistant.

APLs are also characterized by a reciprocal chromosome 15;17 translocation. The chromosome breakpoints lie within the PML gene on I5 and within the retinoic acid receptorα (RARα gene on 17. A chimeric gene, PML-RARα is formed as a result of the translocation. There is preliminary evidence that, paradoxically, the abnormal translocation product (the PML/RARα protein), may contribute both to the differentiation block of the leukaemic phenotype and to the unique sensitivity of APL blasts to the differentiating action of RA.

The general objectives of this Concerted Action are to determine:

1 the physiological role of PML,
2 the leukaemogenic potential of the PML/RARα protein,
3 the capacity of the PML/RARα a protein or normal RARα to mediate sensitivity of APLs to RA therapy,
4 the molecular mechanisms of promyelocytic-blast resistance to RA.

Project leader:
Professor P.G. PELICCI
Istituto Clinica Medica 1°
Policlinico Monteluce
IT 06100 Perugia
Phone: +39 75 578 36 88
Fax: +39 75 578 34 44
Contract number: CT920755

Participants:
Dr. Anne DEJEAN
Unité de Recombianaison et
Expression Genetique,
INSERM U 163
28 Rue du Docteur Roux
FR 75724 Paris Cedex 15
Phone: +33 1 45688824
Fax: +33 1 45688943

Dr. Clara NERVI
Ist di Istologia ed
Embriologia Generale,
Univ di Roma La Sapienza
Via Antonio Scarpa 14
IT Roma
Phone: +39 6 4462851
Fax: +39 6 4462854

Dr. Hughes DE THE
Inst. d'Hematologie, Hopital
St Louis, Univ Paris VII
1 Av. Claude Vellefaux
FR 75010 Paris
Phone: +33 1 42494949
Fax: +33 1 42039212

Dr. Solomon ELLEN
Comatic Cell Genetics
Laboratory,
Imperial Cancer Res Fund
P.O. Box 123
UK London WC2A 3PX
Phone: +44 71 2693426
Fax: +44 71 2693469

ONCOSUPPRESSION BY PARVOVIRUSES: ASSESSMENT OF ITS POTENTIAL USE FOR THE PREVENTION ˋAND/OR THERAPY OF HUMAN CANCER

Key words
Tumoral cells, parvoviral infection, oncosuppression, antineoplastic activity, heterologous cytotoxic factors.

Brief description
Some human tumoral cells may serve as targets for parvoviral attack since their growth in vitro (cultures) or in vivo (transplants in recipient animals) was inhibited by virus infection. Furthermore, epidemiological studies in humans have revealed a correlation between serological evidence of parvoviral infection and a lower incidence of certain cancers. Yet, the exploitation of parvoviruses to achieve a surveillance against cancer in humans remains to be validated.

The present project aims at meeting two of the prerequisites to the use of parvoviral as antitumour agents:

1 the elucidation of the mechanisms of parvoviral oncosuppression;
2 the assessment of possible side-effects and the optimalisation of the antineoplastic activity of parvoviruses in animal models transplanted with human tumour cells.

Parvoviral oncosuppression is likely to reflect, at least in part, the modulation of virus replication in relation to cell proliferation and differentiation. One can not expect such a modulation of parvovirus-host cell interaction to produce an universal all-or-nothing type of response. Nevertheless, the apparent harmlessness of certain paroviruses towards humans, combined with their oncotropism, seems to justify the hope of using these agents in conjunction with other treatments, to specifically express parvoviral or heterologous cytotoxic factors in human tumours.

Cell sensitization of parvoviral attack occurs early during stepwise oncogenesis and parallels changes in cellular proteins interacting with parvoviral DNA. Accordingly, a fundamental goal of this project consists of using parvoviral molecular probes to reveal early events of neoplasic transformation, in particular the (in)activation of cellular (anti)oncongenes.

Project leader:
Professor J. ROMMELAERE
Institut für Angewandte
Tumorvirologie,
Deutsches Krebsforschungs-
zentrum
Im Neuenheimer Feld 280
DE 69120 Heidelberg
Phone: +49 6221 42 49 60
Fax: +49 6221 47 03 33
Contract number: CT920629

Participants:
Dr. P. CAILLET-FOAQUET
Dept. de Biologie Moleculai-
re, Univ libre de Bruxelles
Rue des Chevaux 67
BE 1640 Rhode St Genèse
Phone: +32 2 6509733
Fax: +32 2 6509744

Prof. D. STEHELIN
Unite INSERM 186,
Oncologie Moleculaire,
Inst. Pasteur de Lille
FR 59019 Lille
Phone: +33 20 877729
Fax: +33 20 877908

Prof. J.M. ALMENDRAL
Univ Autonoma,
Fac de Ciencias
ES 28049 Madrid
Phone: +34 1 3974870
Fax: +34 1 3974870

INVESTIGATIONS ON THE EFFECTS OF RADIATION QUALITY AND LOCALIZATION OF RADIONUCLIDES ON TUMOUR GROWTH AS A PREREQUISITE FOR THE DEVELOPMENT OF NEW RADIO-PHARMACEUTICALS FOR CANCER THERAPY

Key words
Estrogen, somatostatin analogues, radionuclides, breast cancer, radioligands, receptor-rich tumour cells, alpha-, beta-, gamma-rays, radiopharmaceuticals.

Brief description
In recent years estrogen and somatostatin analogues have been tagged with radionuclides without affecting their high affinity and specificity for the receptors; the latter are expressed with varying frequency in tumours of various organs (i.e. breast cancer). Mediated by the binding of their specific receptors, there radioligands are efficiently associated at the cell surface (somatostatin) or incorporated into the cell nucleus (estrogen) of receptor-rich tumour cells. In addition metal complexes have been tagged with radionuclides and are accumulated with high affinity in the cytoplasm (lysosome fraction) of tumour cells.

The strategy of the proposed study is to use vehicles to target radionuclides with different qualities of radiation (alpha-, beta-, gamma-rays, Auger-and conversion electrons) to different compartments of cells (cell Surface, cytoplasm, cell nucleus). This will provide insight into:

1 the biological (especially tumoricidal) effects of different radiation qualities on tumour cells with respect to the subcellular localization of the radiation source, and
2 the potential of these radiopharmaceuticals for therapy.

To this end the radiopharmaceuticals are added to i) tumour cell cultures (in-vitro), and ii) injected into nude mice with xenografts of human tumours (in-vivo). The radiotoxicity in-vitro will be measured via the decrease of cell survival and the occurrence of structural DNA damage (chromosome breaks). The biological effects in-vivo on target and non-target cells will be assessed by chromosome analysis, light and electron microscopic examination and morphometry.

The significance of the proposed study is:

A to improve the understanding of mechanisms of action of open radionuclides in tumour therapy;
B to increase insight into the influence of chemical characteristics of the vehicles on their accumulation in tumours and the radiotoxic effects;
C to design new tumoricidal radiopharmaceuticals with higher specificity for tumour cells and therefore less side effects, and
D to prepare clinical studies utilizing new radiotherapeutic modalities against cancer.

Project leader:
Dr. K. SCHOMÄCKER
Nuclear Medicine Clinic and Policlinic,
Cologne University Clinics
Joseph-Stelzmann Strasse 9
DE 50937 Köln 41
Phone: +49 221 478 59 77
Fax: +49 221 478 43 95
Contract number: CT920402

Participants:

Dr. A. SCHARL
Frauenklinik der Universitatskliniken Koln
Joseph Stelzmann Strasse 9
DE 5000 Koln 41
Phone: +49 221 4784040
Fax: +49 221 4784929

Dr. G. LIMOURIS
Aretaieon Hospital,
Dept. of Nuclear Medicine
Vassilisis Sophias 76
GR 10676 Athens

Dr. J.C. SACCAVINI
CIS Biointernational
P.O. Box 32
FR 91192 Fif Sur Yvette Cedex
Phone: +33 1 69857216
Fax: +33 1 69857475

Dr. Klemens SCHEIDHAUER
Klinik und Poliklinik für Nuklearmedizin
der Universitätskliniken Koln
Joseph Stelzmann Strasse 9
DE 5000 Koln 41
Phone: +49 221 4786301
Fax: +49 221 4784395

Dr. M. BECKMANN
Zentrum fur Frauenheilkunde und Geburtshilfe
Johann Wolfgang Goethe Univ Frankfurt/Main
Theodor Stern Kai 7
DE 6000 Frankfurt/Main 70
Phone: +49 69 6301
Fax: +49 69 6301 6317

Dr. W. KONNE
Isotopendiagnostik CIS GmbH
Einsteinstrasse 9-11
DE 6072 Dreieich
Phone: +49 6103 34017
Fax: +49 6103 34874

Frau I. GROSSMANN
Isocommerz Handelsgesellschaft mbH,
Unternehmensbereich Isotopentechnik
P.O. Box 19
DE 8051 Dresden
Phone: +49 351 5910

Prof. Dr. J.F. CHATAL
Unité 211 INSERM,
entre René Gauducheau,
Univ Nantes, Fac de Med
FR Nantes

Prof. Dr. S.K. SHUKLA
Servizio di Medicina Nucleare,
Ospedale S Eugenio
Piazzale Umanesimo 10
IT 00165 Roma
Phone: +39 6 5904 2319
Fax: +39 6 5923 968

MOLECULAR CYTOGENETICS OF SOLID TUMOURS

Key words

Chromosome translocation, solid tumours, q13-q15, chromosome 12, myxoid liposarcoma, cytogenetic, neuroblastoma, paediatric tumour, postganglionic sympathetic neutrons, lung cancer, renal cell cancer, loci D3S2, THRB.

Brief description

The present state of knowledge about chromosome aberrations and cancer clearly emphasizes the important and direct contributions of molecular cytogenetics to the more detailed description and understanding of oncogenesis. Molecular cytogenetic studies of solid tumours reinforce the generally accepted assumption that cancers arise as a result of a progressive series of genetic events by which particular genes, oncogenes and tumour suppressor genes, are affected. Genetic alterations may be mediated by consistent chromosome aberrations, which can be detected by cytogenetic techniques and, subsequently, characterized at the molecular level. In this context, the research programme *Molecular Cytogenetics of Solid Tumours* consists of five projects, which focus on the following aspects:

1 *Molecular analysis of chromosome translocation in solid tumours involving region q13-q15 of chromosome 12*

Chromosome translocation involving segment q13-q15 of chromosome 12 are frequently observed in human myxoid liposarcomas and in cytogenetically abnormal lipomas, uterine leiomyoma and pleomorphic adenomas of the salivary gland. The chromosome breakpoint in myxoid liposarcoma has recently been characterized and the transcription factor encoding CHOP gene on chromosome 12 was found to be affected. The objective of this part of the programme is to identify and characterize the genes that are directly affected by the translocation and thus likely implicated in tumourigenesis.

2 *Cytogenetic and molecular biological analysis of tumour suppressor genes in neuroblastoma*

In neuroblastoma, a paediatric tumour of the postganglionic sympathetic neutrons, the most characteristic cytogenetic abnormality is deletion of genetic sequences of the short arm of chromosome 1. The size of the deletions may vary considerably. A commonly involved region was determined to be 1p34-pter. It is assumed that a tumour suppressor gene is located in this region and the objective of this part of the programme is to identify and characterize this cancer gene.

3 *Identification of tumour suppressor genes on the short arm of chromosome 3 involved in lung cancer and renal cell cancer*

There is a good evidence now that a series of genetic lesions are involved in the pathogenesis of human lung cancer and renal cell cancer. Cytogenetic and molecular studies revealed deletions of genetic sequences of the short arm of chromosome 3. Despite recent observations suggesting that three distinct regions on 3p are apparently frequently deleted in lung cancer, only limited data about the extent of the deletion in chromosome 3p are available, at present. As far as renal cell cancer is concerned, RFLP analysis of sporadic renal cell carcinoma has revealed that the region of common allelic losses is bordered by the loci D3S2 and THRB. In summary, results obtained so far indicate that when future work is focused on these particular regions of chromosome 3p, this may lead to the identification and isolation of tumour suppressor genes involved in the pathogenesis of lung cancer and renal cell cancer.

4 *Development of tumour-derived cell lines*

Crucial for the detailed molecular analysis of chromosome aberrations in solid tumours is the availability of cell lines from the tumours and of somatic cell hybrids retaining the derivative chromosomes; in most cases, such biological materials do not exist yet. A protocol has been developed according to which cell lines can be generated from primary solid tumours. It is the aim of the proposal outlined here to set up a European collaboration to obtain similar cell lines and hybrids for a variety of human solid tumours; in particular, paediatric tumours, breast cancer, soft tissue tumours, thyroid tumours, gastric tumours, seminomas, and pleomorphic adenomas of the salivary gland.

5 *Molecular diagnostics of solid tumours*

The purpose of this project is to develop new techniques for the analysis of complex karyotypes, such as are found in solid tumours, using a combination of flow sorting, PCR technology and non-radioactive *in situ* hybridization.

Project leader:
Prof. W.J.M. VAN DE VEN
Center for Human Genetics
Herestraat 49
BE 3000 Leuven
Phone: +32 16 34 59 87
Fax: +32 16 34 59 97
Contract number: CT920156

Participants:

H. Van den BERGHE (BE)	B.Dockhorn-Dworniczak (DE)	W. MOLENAAR (NL)
C. BUYS (NL)	J.P. DUMANSKI (SE)	O. MYKLEBOST (NO)
S. CASTEDO (PT)	A. EDWARDS (UK)	G. OPDENAKKER (BE)
P. DAL CIN (BE)	C.D.M. FLETCHER (UK)	J.W. OOSTERHUIS (NL)
G. DELLA PORTA (IT)	A. GEURTS-Van KESSEL (NL)	L. OSORIO ALMEIDA (PT)
B. DUTRILLAUX (FR)	S. GILGENKRANTZ (FR)	J.M. PARRINGTON (UK)
A. HAGEMEIJER (NL)	J. DE GREVE (BE)	G. PETERS (UK)
F. MITELMAN (SE)	B.A. GUSTERSON (UK)	A.K. RAAP (NL)
C. TURC-CAREL (FR)	S. HEIM (DK)	J.A. REY (ES)
B. YOUNG (UK)	A.H.N. HOPMAN (NL)	M. SCHWAB (DE)
K. ZANG (DE)	Th. HULSEBOS (NL)	S. SINGH (DE)
P. AMBROS (AT)	B. DE JONG (NL)	R. SLATER &
A. AURIAS (FR)	C. JUNIEN (FR)	R. VERSTEEG (NL)
A. BERNHEIM (FR)	S. KENNEDY (IE)	A.P. SOARES FERREIRA (PT)
S. BERTRAND (FR)	M. KIRSCH VOLDERS (BE)	D. SPANDIDOS (GR)
N. BLIN (DE)	A. DE KLEIN (NL)	F. SPELEMAN (BE)
M.G. BOAVIDA (PT)	P. LITTLE (UK)	G. STENMAN (SE)
J.M. BOYLE (UK)	C. LOPEZ-GINES (ES)	G. THOMAS (FR)
J. BULLERDIEK (DE)	R.A. LOTHE (NO)	E. VAMOS (BE)
R. CABALLIN (ES)	N. MANDAHL (SE)	R. VANNI (IT)
P. CABELLO-ALBENDEA (ES)	J. MARK (SE)	A. VERHEST &
B. CARRITT (UK)	P. MARYNEN (BE)	M. PETEIN (BE)
T. CREMER (DE)	D. MATTHOPOULOS (GR)	E. ZWARTHOF (NL)
H. VAN DEKKEN (NL)	E. MEESE (DE)	

EUROCARE-2: CANCER REGISTRIES BASED STUDY
ON SURVIVAL AND CARE OF CANCER

Key words
Cancer survival, communal data bank, lymphnodes, breast cancer, colorectal cancer.

Brief description
EUROCARE-2 is a collaborative project among European population based cancer registries (CRs). Its pricipal aims are:
- To monitor time trends of cancer survival in Europe.
- To explain the reasons for the observed cancer survival differences within Europe; in
  particular to help disentangle the effect of therapies from that of early diagnosis only,
  on cancer survival.
- To provide a description of patterns of care through the collection of some key indicators of diagnostic and therapeutic procedures.

The project will profit from the scientific, technical and secretarial organization of the
CRs network established by the previous project EUROCARE-1.

The present study is divided into two parts:
1 *Survival*. Monitoring of cancer survival will be achieved by updating the communal
  data bank of 31 CRs. Updating will be performed both by prolonging the period of
  follow-up of patients in order to study long-term survival, and enlarging the study
  period to study time-trends.
2 *Care*. Stage specific survival comparisons would be necessary for the interpretation of
  survival differences, but the definition of stage categories varies over time and countries, depending on the thoroughness of diagnostic investigation. It is proposed to
  carry out survival comparisons adjusting by a few determinants on staging (e.g. the
  number of lymphnodes examined for breast cancer, or the performance of a liver
  echography for colorectal cancer). This methodology was tested on clinical series of
  breast cancer at the Istituto Nazionale Tumori, Milan, where the number of examined
  lymph nodes during surgery increased with time. This apparent improvement in prognosis of patients diagnosed recently disappeared after adjusting for the number of
  lymphnodes examined.

Cases included in the study will be those diagnosed in 1990-1991, followed up for at
least 3 years. The registries will collect a little more information than usual on diagnostic and therapeutic procedures, for selected tumours, to be decided collectively. Data
will be sent to the coordinating centre, where checks and basic analyses will be performed.

Project leader:
Dr. Franco BERRINO
Div. Epidemiologia Istituto Nazionale Tumori
Via Venezian 1
IT 20133 Milano
Phone: +39 22 39 04 60
Fax: +39 22 236 26 92
Contract number: CT931616

Participants:

Alessandro BARCHIELLI
Via san Salvi 12
IT 50135 Firenze

Arduino VERDECCHIA
Viale Regina Elena 299
IT 00161 Roma

Carmen MARTINEZ
Apartado de Cordreos 2070
ES 18014 Granada

Charles JOSLIN
UK Leeds LF16 6QB

Corrado MAGNANI
Via Santena 7
IT 10126 Torino

Derek PHEBY
Whiteladies Road
UK BS8 2PR Bristol

Didier POTTIER
FR 14040 Caen

Franco BERRINO
Via Venezian 1
It 20133 Milano

Gillian LAWRENCE
UK B15 2TH Birmingham

Hartwig ZIEGLER
Hardenbergstr. 3
DE 66119 Saarbrucken

Jacques ESTEVE
Cours Albert Thomas 150
FR 69372 Lyon

Jan Willem COEBERGH
P.O. Box 231
NL 3000 DR Eindhoven

Janine BELL
15 Cotswold Road
UK Sutton Surrey SM2 5NL

Jean FAIVRE
Boulevard Jeanne D'Arc 7
FR 21033 Dijon

Jenifer SMITH
Romsy Road
UK Winchester SO22 5DH

Joachin TORHORST
Schonbeinstrasse 40
CH 4003 Basel

Jorg MICHAELIS
Langenbeckstrasse 1
FR 6500 Mainz

Judith YOUNGSON
P.O. Box 147
UK Liverpool L69 3BX

Lorenzo GAFA
Piazza Igea 2
IT 97100 Ragusa

Luc RAYM0ND
Bd. de la Cluse 55
CH 1205 Geneva

Mark McCARTHY
Hampstead Road
UK London NW1 2LJ

Michel HENRY-AMAR
Cente Regional F. Baclesse
Service de Recherche
Clinique
Route de Lion sur Mer
FR 14040 Caen

Nicole RAVERDY
Place Victor Pauchet CHU
Nord
FR 80054 Amiens

Pascale GROSCLAUDE
FR 81000 Albi

Pau VILADIU I QUEMADA
Caterina Pl. Hospital 5
IT 17001 Girona

Ronald DAMHUIS
P.O. Box 289
NL 3000 Dr. Rotterdam

Simon SCHRAUB
Centre Hospitalier Regional
Jean Minjoz Registre de
Tumeurs du Doubs
Boulevard Flemming
FR 25030 Besancon

Stefania RODELLA
Istituto Anatomia Patologica,
Universita di Verona
Via le Grazie 8
IT 37100 Verona

Sue WILSON
Centre for Cancer Epidemiol-
ogy Christie NHS Trust
Kinnaird Road
UK Manchester M20 9QL
Withington

Thomas DAVIES
Inst. of Public Health
Forvie Site -
Robinson Way
UK Cambridge CB2 2QQ

Timo HAKULINEN
Finnish Cancer Registry -
The Insitute for Statistical
and Epidemiolocal Cancer
Research
Liisankatu 21b
FI 00171 Helsinki

MARKERS OF DNA DAMAGE AND RISK OF SECOND MALIGNANCY FOLLOWING CHEMOTHERAPY

Key words
Hodgkin's disease, second malignancies, leukemia, non-Hodgkin's lymphoma, lung cancer, markers of DNA damage, mechlorathamine, p53, micronuclei, chromatid.

Brief description
A collaborative group of major hospitals treating Hodgkin's disease (HD) patients will be established, a central register will then be established of all patients diagnosed with HD at a participating hospital.

These patients will be prospectively followed up for response to therapy and occurrence of second malignancies, particularly leukemia, non-Hodgkin's lymphoma and lung cancer.

In parallel to the registration of index and second cancers, blood samples will be taken from each patient, immediately following diagnosis, during and subsequent to therapy.

The red and white blood cells will be separated and frozen. Two case-control investigations will then be carried out, on response to therapy and risk of second malignancy, respectively.

For patients who will not respond to therapy and for a sample of patients who will respond to therapy, as well as for patients who develop a second malignancy and for matched controls who remain free of a second malignancy, the samples will be analyzed for markers of DNA damage, and comparison made between cases and controls.

In the case that markers of DNA damage are linked to response to therapy or to risk of second malignancy, the frequency and the level of such markers will be increased among cases as compared to controls.

Markers of DNA damage that are currently available include DNA adducts of alkylating agents such as procarbazine, dacarbazine, and nitrogen mustards (mechlorathamine), mutation in ras oncogenes, activation of tumour suppressor genes such as p53. Unspecific markers of damage such as micronuclei and sister chromatid exchanges will be investigated in a subgroup of patients.

Project leader:
Dr. Paolo BOFFETTA
Unit of Analytical Epidemiology, International Agency for Research on Cancer
Cours Albert Thomas 150
FR 69372 Lyon Cédex 08
Phone: +33 72 73 84 85
Fax: +33 72 73 85 75
Contractnumber: CT931134

Participants:
Dr. A. SWERDLOW
Dept. of Epi. and Population
Sciences, London School of
Hygiene and Tropical
Medicine
Keppel Street
UK London WC1E 7HT

Dr. A.T. Van OOSTEROM
Univ Hospital
Wilrijkstraat 10
BE 2650 Edegem

Dr. B. KONOPASEK
Nemocnice 2
CZ 12808 Praha 2

Dr. D. SHUKER
MRC Toxicology Unit,
Hodgkin Building,
Univ of Leicester
Lancaster Road
UK LE1 9HN Leicester

Dr. D.G. ZARIDZE
Inst. of Carcinogenesis,
All-Union Cancer Research
Centre,
Academy of Medical Sciences
24 Kashirskoye Shaussee
USSR Moscow 115478

Dr. F. LEVI
Insitut Universitaire de
Médecine Sociale et
Préventive Registre Vaudois
des Tumeurs
Falaises 1
CH 1011 Lausanne

Dr. F. RILKE
Istituto Nazionale Tumori
Via Venezian 1
IT Milano

Dr. G. JULIUSSON
Karolinska Inst.,
Dept. of Medicine,
Huddinge Univ Hospital
SE 14186 Huddinge

Dr. J. WALEWSKI
Maria Sklodowska-Curie
Memorial Cancer Center and
Inst. of Oncology,
Marie-Sklodowska
Cancer Center
P.O. Box 47
PL 00973 Warsaw 22

Dr. J.J. LOPEZ
Head, Clinical Oncology
Service, Hospital San Pablo
M. Claret 167
ES 08025 Barcelona

Dr. K. HEMMINKI
Center for Nutrition and
Toxicology, Karolinska Inst.
Novum
SE 14152 Huddinge

Dr. K. KATSOUYANNI
Dept. of Hygiene and
Epidemiology, Univ of
Athens Medical School
Goudi
GR 11727 Athens

Dr. L. SIMONATO
Registro Tumori de Veneto,
c/o Direzione Sanitaria
Via Giustinian 2
IT 35100 Padova

Dr. L. VATTEN
Univ of Trondheim,
Dept. of Community Medi-
cine and General Practice
NO 7005 Trondheim

Dr. M. HENRY-AMAR
Centre François Baclesse
Route de Lion sur Mer
FR 14021 Caen Cedex

Dr. Paolo BOFFETTA
Unit of Analytical
Epidemiology,
International Agency for
Research on Cancer
Cours Albert Thomas 150
FR 69372 Lyon

Dr. P. BOYLE
Div of Epidemiology and
Biostatistics,
European Inst. of Oncology
Via Ripamonti 332/10
IT 20141

Dr. S. KARJALAINEN
Univ of Tampere,
Dept. of Public Health
P.O. Box 607
SE 33101 Tampere

Dr. S. MONFARDINI
Centro di Riferimento
Oncologico
Via Pedemontana Occidentale
IT 33081 Aviano

Dr. S.A. KYRTOPOULOS
National Hellenic Research
Foundation, Inst. of
Biological Research and
Biotechnology
48 Vassileos Constantinou
Avenue
GR 11635 Athens

Dr. S.A. PANGALIS
Hematology Unit, First Dept.
of Internal Medicine,
Laikon General Hosp
17 Aghiou Thoma, Goudi
GR 11527 Athens

Ms. F. Van LEEUWEN
The Netherlands Cancer
Inst., Antonie van
Leeuwenhoekhuis
Plesmanlaan 121
NL 1066 CX Amsterdam

Prof. I. PLESKO
Cancer Research Inst., Slo-
vak Academy of Sciences
Spitalska 21
SV 81232 Bratislava

Prof. MARTIN-MORENO
Dept. of Epidemiology,
Escuela Nacional de Sanidad,
Ministerio de Sanidad y
Consumo
Calle Sinesio Delgado 10
ES 28029 Madrid

Prof. M. DICATO
Département d'hémato-cancér
ologie, Centre Hospitalier
4 Rue Barble
LU 1210 Luxembourg

Prof. S. KVINNSLAND
The Radium Hospital
Montebello
NO 0310 Oslo

IDENTIFICATION OF NEW HUMAN TUMOR REJECTION ANTIGENS RECOGNIZED BY AUTOLOGOUS T-LYMPHOCYTES, AND PILOT THERAPEUTIC STUDIES WITH DEFINED ANTIGENS

Key words
Tumor immunology, antigens, autologous T lymphocytes, MAGE-1, immunotherapy, expression.

Brief description
Tumor immunology is coming to a decisive turning point because of the molecular identification of antigens that are recognized on human tumor cells by autologous T lymphocytes.

The coordinator center of this proposal contributed to this progress by cloning several genes coding for tumor rejection antigens on murine tumors and by cloning the first gene (named MAGE-1) responsible for the expression of such an antigen on human tumors.

The identification of tumor antigens allows to rationalize the various immunotherapy protocols that have been carried on, some of them with promising results, for the last years.

Namely it becomes possible to vaccinate cancer patients with defined antigens expressed on their tumors.

This proposal comprises two related parts, dealing each of them with a major problem to be solved before tumor immunotherapy with defined tumor rejection antigens can be put into clinical testing.

The first task is to identify other genes that code for antigens recognized on human tumors by autologous T lymphocytes. We feel that it is critical to carry on the effort to identify new tumor rejection antigens.

First because this will increase the number of patients who could benefit from anti-tumor therapeutic vaccines containing these antigens.

And second because vaccines containing several antigens will be necessary if tumor cell variants having lost the expression of a given antigen escape the immune response.

The second part of this proposal consists in trying to find the most effective ways to immunize cancer patients with known tumor rejection antigens, and to assess the efficacy of these immunizations by finding out whether immunized patients have an increased frequency of circulating T lymphocytes that specifically recognize their tumor cells.

Project leader:
Professor Thierry BOON
Ludwig Institute for Cancer Research
avenue Hippocrate 74, UCL 74.59
BE 1200 Brussels
Phone: +32 2 764 74 59
Fax: +32 2 762 94 05
Contract number: CT931193

Participants:

Dr. Alex KNUTH
Johann-Wolfgang-Goethe-
Universität Chefartz der
Oncologischen Klinik,
Krankenhaus Nord west
Steinbacher Hohl 2 - 26
DE 6000 Frankfurt/Main 90
Phone: +49 69 760 13 80
Fax: +49 69 769 99 32

Dr. Catia TRAVERSARI
H.S. Raffaele - Istituto di
Ricovero e Cura a
Dipartimento Ematologia
Sperimentale - DIBIT
Via Olgettina 60
IT 20132 Milano
Phone: +39 2 239 06 30
Fax: +39 2 236 26 92

Dr. Daniel OLIVE
Institut National de la Santé
et de la Recherche Médicale
INSERM Unité 119
Boulevard Lei Roure 27
FR 13009 Marseille
Phone: +33 91 758 415
Fax: +33 91 26 03 64

Dr. Elizabeth SIMPSON
Clinical Research Centre,
Transplantation Biology
Section
Watford Road
UK Harrow,
Middlesex HA1 3UJ
Phone: +44 81 869 33 78
Fax: +44 81 869 33 76

Dr. Thomas WÖLFEL
Innere Medizinische Klinik
und Poliklinik Johannes
Gutenberg Universität
Langenbeckstrasse 1
DE 6500 Mainz
Phone: +49 6131 17 33 82
Fax: +49 6131 17 33 64

Mme Rolande BOUCKAERT
International Inst. of Cellular
and Molecular Pathology
75 Avenue Hippocrate
BE 1200 Bruxelles
Phone: +32 2 764 75 50
Fax: +32 2 764 75 73

Prof. C. MELIEF
Dept. of Immunohaematology
and Blood Bank University
Hospital Bldg, E3-Q
P.O. Box 9600
NL 2300 RC Leiden
Phone: +31 71 26 38 00
Fax: +31 71 21 67 51

Prof. Federico GARRIDO
Hospital Virgen de las
Nieves,
Dept. of Analisis Clinicos e
Immunologia
Avda Fuerzas Armadas s/n
ES 18014 Granada
Phone: +34 58 28 31 47
Fax: +34 58 28 31 47

Prof. Ferdinand LEJEUNE
Centre Hospitalier
Univ. Vaudois,
Centre pluridisciplinaire
d'Oncologie
Rue du Bugnon 46
CH 1011 Lausanne
Phone: +41 21 314 39 58
Fax: +41 21 314 39 57

Prof. CEROTTINI
Ludwig Institute for
Cancer Research
Chemin des Boveresses 155
CH 1066 Epalinges
s/Lausanne
Phone: +41 21 316 59 90
Fax: +41 21 653 44 74

THE ROLE OF IL-2 RECEPTORS AS REGULATORS OF LYMPHOCYTE PROLIFERATION: SIGNAL TRANSDUCTION BY IL-2 AND IL-5 RECEPTORS AND REGULATION OF HIGH AFFINITY IL-2R EXPRESSION

Key words
Cytokines Interleukin 2, Interleukin 5, haematopoietic cells, IL-2R, IL-5R, growth regulation, T cell, pathways.

Brief description
The cytokines Interleukin 2 and Interleukin 5 are important growth factors for haematopoietic cells. The proposed experiments address issues relating to the mechanism used by these receptors to control gene expression and growth of haematopoietic cells.

The participants in this proposal are all working on different aspects of IL-2R and IL-5R structure and fuaction including studies on receptor structure and growth regulation (G.P); studies on the regulation and function of the transcriptional factors and genes that are targets for IL-2R and IL-5R (MN,Rc,JI) and investigations into the immediate biochemical-consequence's of IL-2R triggerin (Dc).

To coordinate the research of these different groups will concentrate this expertise and accelerate the evaluation of the signal transduction mechanisms used by the IL-2 and IL-5R to control T cell growth.

One major focus of the studies is to examine the signalling pathways that allow the IL-2 and ILI5 receptors to regulate the IL-2 a-gene. The role of IL-2R mutations in malignant transformation will also be analysed. The rationale for this focus on IL-2R a chain regulation is that it is clear that this gene is an important target of IL-2R signalling.

Project leader:
Dr. Doreen CANTRELL
Lymphocyte Activation Laboratory,
Imperial Cancer Research Fund
Lincolns Inn Fields 44
UK London WC2A 3PX
Phone: +44 71 269 33 07
Fax: +44 71 269 35 81
Contract number: CT931426

Participants:
Daniel OLIVE
Institut National de la Sante
et de la Recherche Medicale
Unite 119
27 Boulevard Lei Roure
FR Marseille 13009
Phone: +44 91 758415
Fax: +44 91 260364

Geert PLAETINCK
Roche Research Gent
22 Jozef Plateaustraat
BE 9000 Gent
Phone: +32 9 2257698

Jean IMBERT
27 Boulevard Lei Roure
FR Marseille 13009
Phone: +44 91 742547
Fax: +44 91 260364

Markus NABHOLZ
Institut Suisse de Recherches
Experimentales sur le Cancer
155 Chemin des Boveresses
CH Epalinges/Lausanne 1066
Phone: +44 21 653 3061
Fax: +44 21 652 6933

Rhodri CEREDIG
U184/INSERM-LGME/CNR
S/UPR A6520
11 Rue Humann
FR Strasbourg 67085
Phone: +33 88 371255
Fax: +33 44 370148

EUROPEAN FRANCONI ANEMIA RESEARCH (EUFAR): MOLECULAR AND CLINICAL SIGNIFICANCE OF THE FANCONI ANAEMIA GENE DEFECTS

Key words
Fanconi anaemia, chromosomal instability, cancer-proneness, antioncogenesis.

Brief description
The cellular defence capacity against genetic change is a major endogenous factor controlling oncogenesis. Fanconi anaemia (FA), a recessive disorder featuring chromosomal instability, hyper-sensitivity to cross-linking agents and cancer-proneness, is a model disease for unravelling the molecular basis of the FA pathway of antioncogenesis. FA is genetically heterogeneous, i.e. 4 complementation groups have recently been distinguished among 7 unrelated patients.

In view of the low prevalence of FA in the human population (1-5 per million) an internationally coordinated approach is required to trace all the genes involved and to elucidate their function.

Support from the European Community will allow the integration and coordination of the now rapidly emerging developments in Fanconi anemia research. Integration will be achieved by:
1 annual workshops;
2 exchange visits (mobility) for active scientists;
3 a EUFAR newsletter;
4 a centralized registry for European FA patients;
5 a centralized cell repository and fine diagnostics facility for all European FA families.

Project leader:
Professor Eliane GLUCKMAN
Unité de Greffe de Moelle, Hôpital Saint-Louis
Av. Claude Vellefaux 1
FR 75475 Paris Cedex 10
Phone: +33 1 42 49 96 44
Fax: +33 1 42 49 96 34
Contract number: CT931562

Participants:
Dr. Anna SAVOIA
Research Inst., I.R.C.C.S.,
Ospedale Casa Sollievo della
Sofferenza
IT 71013 San Giovanni
Rotondo
Phone: +39 882 410374
Fax: +39 882 411616

Dr. C. MATHEW
Pediatric Research Unit,
7th & 8th Floors,
Guy's Tower,
GUY'S HOSPITAL
UK London 8E1 9RT
Phone: +44 71 955 4653
Fax: +44 71 955 4644

Dr. F. ARWERT
Dept. Human Genetics,
Free Univ
Van der Boechorststraat 7
NL 1081 BT Amsterdam
Phone: +31 20 5482764
Fax: +31 20 5483329

Dr. H. JOENJE
Dept. Human Genetics,
Free Univ
Van der Boechorststraat 7
NL 1081 BT Amsterdam
Phone: +31 20 5482764
Fax: +31 20 5483329

Dr. M.DIGWEED
Freie Universität Berlin,
Institut für Humangenetik
Heubnerweg 6
DE 1000 Berlin 19
Phone: +49 30 30354377
Fax: +49 30 30354613

Dr. M.Z. ZDZIENICKA
MGC Dept. of Radiation
Genetics and Chemical
Mutagenesis RUL
Wassenaarseweg 72
NL 2333 AL Leiden
Phone: +31 71 276175
Fax: +31 71 221615

Prof. Dr. A. Westerveld
Dept. Human Genetics,
Academic Medical Centre
Meibergdreef 15
NL 1105 AZ Amsterdam
Phone: +31 20 5665166
Fax: +31 20 6918626

Prof. Dr. E. MOUSTACCHI
Institut Curie,
Sect. de Biologie
26 Rue d'Ulm
75231 Paris Cedex 05
Phone: +33 1 40516710
Fax: +33 1 46333016

Prof. Dr. H. HOEHN
Institut für Humangenetik,
Universität Würzburg,
Biozentrum Am Hubland
DE 8700 Würzburg
Phone: +49 931 888 40 70
Fax: +49 931 888 40 69

Prof. SCHROEDER-KURTH
Institut für Anthropologie u.
Humangenetik,
Universität Heidelberg
Im Neuenheimer Feld 328
DE 6900 Heidelberg
Phone: +49 6221 563877
Fax: +49 6221 563898

TRANSGENIC ANIMALS: A MODEL FOR STUDYING THE MOLECULAR BIOLOGY OF HEPATITIS B VIRUS (HBV) INDUCED PRIMARY HEPATOCELLULAR CARCINOMA

Key words
Hepatitus B virus (HBV), hepatocellular carcinoma.

Brief description
Cancer tops the list of diseases. Everyone has a friend or relative how has or died from cancer. The disease was given its name about 24 centuries ago by hippocrates but it is still unclear in most cases what its causes and what are the molecular biological mechanisms that convert a normal cell into a tumor cell. In this regard the hapatocellular carcinoma is an exception because there is a clear causal correlation between Hepatitis virus infection and tumor formation. Tumor epidemiology and in vitro experiments indicate that the cell transformation is a multi-step event involving various genetic and epigenetic alterations. In the case of the hepatocellular carcinoma the Hepatitis B virus (HBV) pX protein seems to be a necessary but not sufficient trigger of tumor formation.

There is experimental evidence that the PX protein is a transactivator that has the capability to increase the transcription rate of different Viral and cellular genes, but there is no proof that this function is involved in cell transformation. A unique opportunity for analysing the role of the PX protein in tumor formation is the generating of transgenic animals that express the pX gene in specific organs. Experiments so far have failed to establish transgenic animals as a model, because it has not been possible to obtain animals that express the transgene permanently in the liver cells. To overcome this problem of early switch-off of the transgene and foetal loss, transgenic animals Will be generated that selevtively express the pX gene in the mammary gland cells.

To achieve this goal the pX gene and truncated versions will be cloned under the transcriptional control of the Whey Acid protein (WAP) promoter and the hybrid-genes (WAP-HBV-X) Will be used to generate transgenic animals. The wap gene encodes for the major mouse milk protein. Expression of this gene is restricted to the mammary gland cells and it is not expressed during embryo genesis. These animals will serve as models for studying the molecular biology of the HBV-induced tumor formation in a joint venture between three laboratories from three EC contries. Understanding of the epidemiology and of the molecular biological mechanism responsible for cell transformation is a prerequisite for any specific.

Project leader:
Prof. A. GRAESSMANN
Institute of Molecular Biology
and Biochemistry,
Free University Berlin
Arnimallee 22
DE 14195 Berlin 33
Phone: +49 30 838 25 64
Fax: +49 30 838 37 02
Contract number: CT931515

Participants:
Prof. J. CELIS
Institute of Medical
Biochemistry,
Aarhus University
Ole Worms Allé 170
DK 8000 Aarhus
Phone: +45 86 12 93 99
Fax: +45 86 13 11 60

Dr. M. LEVRERO
Fondazione Andrea
Cesalpino,
I. Clinica Medica,
Universita La Sapienza
Viale del Policlinico 155
IT 00161 Rome
Phone: +39 6 446 33 01
Fax: +39 6 494 05 94

SYSTEMATIC OVERVIEWS OF RANDOMISED CONTROLLED TRIALS IN THE TREATMENT OF COLERECTAL CANCER, LEUKEMIA AND LYMPHOMA

Key words
Colorectal cancer, leukaemia, lymphoma, myeloma, immunotherapy.

Brief description
Over the next 5 years, 600,000 people in the European Community will die of colorectal cancer, leukaemia, lymphoma or myeloma. Because these cancers are so common, any widely practicable treatment that could be reliably demonstrated to reduce mortality by tens of thousands of lives; while a reliable demonstration of the inactivity of a particular therapy could avoid the unnecessary treatment of hundreds of thousands of patients. However, to detect moderate reductions in mortality several thousand patients need to be studied, and because most previous randomised trials have involved just hundreds of patients the true value of many widely practicable cancer treatments remains unclear. But the CTSU has developed the statistical techniques for combining individual patient data from many small trials and have shown the value of these systematic cancer and in vascular disease.

The CTSU has recently initiated collaborative overviews in colorectal cancer, Hodgkin's Disease, leukaemia and myelomatosis and international agreement to participate has been reached. This application seeks financial support for extra administrative stafe and to hold the meetings which are an essential component of such projects. This Concerted Action will bring together the results of clinical research on radiotherapy, systemic therapy and immunotherapy of both common (colorectal) and less common cancers (leukaemia, lymphoma and myelomatosis) and will then provide uniquely reliable data on the benefits - or lack of benefits - of these treatments that will allow them to be used more rationally. It will directly benefit the European Community by improving the treatment of cancer, stimulating further research, and developing a coordinated network for the collection of clinical trial data that will lead to earlier detection of future treatment advances and more rapid dissemination of information about these advances. Europe has led the world in clinical research methods, and almost all European countries collaborate in these overviews. Commercial funding is ruled out because it may lead to accusations of lack of objectivity. The most practical and appropriate source of non-commercial funding is therefore the BIOMED programme.

Projectleader:
Dr. R. GRAY
Clinical Trial Service Unit,
Oxford University,
Harkness Building,
Radcliffe Infirmary
UK Oxford OX2 6HE
Phone: +44 86 55 72 41
Fax: +44 86 55 88 17
Contract number: CT931247

Participants:
Dr. AL BENSON (US)
Dr. A. LAPLANCHE (FR)
Dr. Alberto RICCARDI (IT)

Dr. Aldo MONTUORO (IT)
Dr. Alfred REITER (DE)
Dr. Alice MANIATIS (GR)
Dr. PLANINC-PERAICA (HR)
Dr. A. ÖSTERBORG (SE)
Dr. Anders WAHLIN (SE)
Dr. Andrea PESSION (IT)
Dr. Anne BANCILLON (FR)
Dr. Anne LINDBLAD (US)
Dr. Ants VAAR (EE)
Dr. Arild HORN (NO)
Dr. A. GEZIN (IE)
Dr. A. VAN DER DOES-

VAN DEN BERG (NL)
Dr. ABRAHAMSEN (NO)
Dr. A.L.A. FIELDS (CA)
Dr. A.M. LIBERATI (IT)
Dr. Bengt GLIMELIUS (SE)
Dr. Beow Yong YEAP (US)
Dr. B. CHEVALLIER (FR)
Dr. B.J. CUMMINGS (CA)
Dr. Bjorn ANDERSEN (DK)
Dr. B. CEDERMARK (SE)
Dr. B. SPARSO (DK)
Dr. Branimir JAKSIC (HR)
Dr. B.D. CHESON (US)

Dr. Chris WILLIAMS (UK)
Dr. Christian GEISLER (DK)
Dr. Claudia CORRADO (AR)
Dr. Colin BEGG (US)
Dr. Csilla CSAKI (HU)
Dr. C. ERLICHMAN (CA)
Dr. C. FERME (FR)
Dr. C. FOCAN (BE)
Dr. C. MONTALBAN (ES)
Dr. C.J. VAN DE VELDE (NL)
Dr. Dan L. LONGO (US)
Dr. D. CUNNINGHAM (UK)
Dr. D. POPLACK (US)
Dr. David MACHN (UK)
Dr. D. HARRINGTON (US)
Dr. David RYDER (UK)
Dr. HASENCLEVER (DE)
Dr. D. PEEST (DE)
Dr. D.J. BRUINVELS (NL)
Dr. E. BUARQUE (BR)
Dr. Ehtesham A. ABDI (AU)
Dr. Elaine PAKURIS (US)
Dr. E. McFADDEN (US)
Dr. Emilio ARANDA (ES)
Dr. E. MONTSERRAT (ES)
Dr. Eric LEPANGE (FR)
Dr. Eric LEVY (FR)
Dr. Erik HIPPE (DK)
Dr. E. KJARSGAARD (DK)
Dr. E. ROSENBAUM (US)
Dr. Eva KIMBY (SE)
Dr. Francesco IZZO (IT)
Dr. F. MEUNIER (BE)
Dr. F. PANETTIERE (US)
Dr. F.S. MURIEL (AR)
Dr. F. HAGEMEISTER (US)
Dr. F. BONICHON (FR)
Dr. F. CAVALLI (CH)
Dr. F. MANDELL (IT)
Dr. F. ZOETMULDER (NL)
Dr. G. HIGGINS (US)
Dr. G. HUTCHISON & Dr.
G. VAUGHAN-HUDSON (UK)
Dr. G AVVISATI (IT)
Dr. G. ZELLER (DE)
Dr. G.A. PANGALIS (GR)
Dr. G. BAYSOGOLOV (RU)
Dr. H. MELLSTEDT (SE)
Dr. H.N. SATHER (US)
Dr. H. van TINTEREN (NL)
Dr. H. ISHIKAWA (JP)
Dr. H. ROCKETTE (US)
Dr. H. BLEIBERG (BE)

Dr. H. FUKUMORI (JP)
Dr. H. Sam WIEAND (US)
Dr. H.J. BRENNER (IL)
Dr. Ian M. HANN (UK)
Dr. I. GATTERER MENZ (AT)
Dr. I.B. BALSLEV (DK)
Dr. I.P. PALVA (FI)
Dr. J. WERELDSMA (NL)
Dr. Jacob J. LOKICH (US)
Dr. Jacques OTTEN (DE)
Dr. James C. COX (US)
Dr. James N. ATKINS (US)
Dr. Jan WESTIN (SE)
Dr. J. DUTCHER (US)
Dr. J.P. PIGNON (FR)
Dr. Jim CASSIDY (UK)
Dr. Ji-Yeul KIM (KP)
Dr. John LASZLO (US)
Dr. John SALZBERG (AU)
Dr. J.S. LILLEYMAN (UK)
Dr. John ZALCBERG (AU)
Dr. Jörg ISENBERG (DE)
Dr. Joseph D. BORSI (HU)
Dr. Joseph L. PATER (CA)
Dr. Juan J. ORTEGA (ES)
Dr. Jules HARRIS (US)
Dr. J. SAKAMOTO (JP)
Dr. BLADE PETHEMA (ES)
Dr. J. HERMANS (NL)
Dr. J. KLUGER (DE)
Dr. J. Milburn JESSUP (US)
Dr. J.A. Reis NETO (BR)
Dr. J.D. AHIGREN (US)
Dr. J.G.A. HOUBIERS (NL)
Dr. Kaneo KIKUCHI (JP)
Dr. Kanti R. RAL (US)
Dr. Karl LINK (DE)
Dr. Katsuki ITO (JP)
Dr. Keichi HOZYO (JP)
Dr. Keith D. WATERS (AU)
Dr. Kiyashi MIWA (JP)
Dr. Kozaburo KIMURA (JP)
Dr. K. SHIMIZU (JP)
Dr. L. HAFSTROM (SE)
Dr. Lena SPECHT (DK)
Dr. Leslie DALY (IE)
Dr. Lorraine M. LEVY (ZA)
Dr. Luis T. CAMPOS (US)
Dr. M. BJORKHOLM (SE)
Dr. Marc BUYSE (BE)
Dr. M. T. NOBILE (IT)
Dr. M.G. VALSECCHI (IT)
Dr. M. R. SERTOLI (IT)

Dr. Markus LÖFFLER (DE)
Dr. Martin HJORTH (SE)
Dr. M. YASUTOMI (JP)
Dr. M. BRUGIATELLI (IT)
Dr. M. WUNDERLICH (AU)
Dr. M.E.J. BEARD (NZ)
Dr. M.G. HANNA (US)
Dr. M.J. O'CONNELL (US)
Dr. Michael STEVENS (AU)
Dr. M. BACCARANI (IT)
Dr. Mike K. PALMER (UK)
Dr. M. FONTANILLAS (ES)
Dr. Motomichi TORISU (JP)
Dr. Murray BOLES (US)
Dr. F. DE RODRIGUEZ (DE)
Dr. M. HARDING (UK)
Dr. M. Mork HANSEN (DK)
Dr. Nancy E. KEMENY (US)
Dr. Nobuo ISHIDA (JP)
Dr. Norman ALLAN (UK)
Dr. N. WOLMARK (US)
Dr. N. HAIM (IE)
Dr. Kildahi-ANDERSON (NO)
Dr. O.P. HANSEN (DK)
Dr. Pascal PIEDBOIS (FR)
Dr. P.F. ENGSTROM (US)
Dr. Pedro C. LARA (ES)
Dr. P.A. CASSILETH (US)
Dr. Philippe TRAVADE (FR)
Dr. V. ASSENDELFT (NL)
Dr. P. MAZZA (IT)
Dr. P. REIZENSTEIN (SE)
Dr. P.W. DYKES (UK)
Dr. R.D. GELBER (US)
Dr. R. SYLVESTER (BE)
Dr. Robert MAYER (US)
Dr. Robert KYLE (US)
Dr. Robert MADER (AT)
Dr. Robert P. GALE (US)
Dr. Robert W. BEART US
Dr. R.W. MAKUCH US
Dr. R. CHLEBOWSKI (US)
Dr. R. HERRMANN (CH)
Dr. R. LABIANCA (IT)
Dr. S. BOULIS-WASSIF (UK)
Dr. S. PAMPALLONA (CH)
Dr. P. GATLA (AR)
Dr. Shan YI (CN)
Dr. Shao YONGFU (CN)
Dr. S. TAKASHIMA (JP)
Dr. Stefan SUCLU (BE)
Dr. S.E. SALLAN (US)
Dr. Susumu KODAIRA (JP)

Dr. Sydney SALMON (US)
Dr. S. MARSONI (IT)
Dr. S. TURA (IT)
Dr. Takashi HIRAI (JP)
Dr. Tarek SAHMOUD (BE)
Dr. Tetsuichiro MUTO (JP)
Dr. Tomoyuki KATO (JP)
Dr. Torbjörn HOLM (SE)
Dr. Torgil MÖLLER (SE)
Dr. Toshio MITOMI (JP)
Dr. Toshio SAWADA (JP)
Dr. T. WIGGERS (NL)
Dr. Uriel BOHN (ES)
Dr. U. LAFFER (CH)
Dr. Valter TORRI (IT)
Dr. Vita J. LAND (US)
Dr. V. PARISI (IT)
Dr. W. LAWRENCE (US)
Dr. William M. CRIST (US)
Dr. Wim van PUTTEN (NL)
Dr. Won CHOI (KR)
Dr. W. NIEBEL (DE)
Dr. Y. KOYAMA (JP)
Dr. Young-Jin KIM (KP)
Dr. Yu HONGTIAO (CN)
Dr. Zhen-Zhou SHEN (CN)
Dr. Z. MOLNAR (HU)
Dr.Dan KRISTENSEN (DK)
Fr. Franz-Martin FINK (AT)
Mrs Jean MOSSMAN (UK)
Mrs. Mary CROSS (UK)
Mr. H. JOHANSSON (SE)
Mr. John BANCEWICZ (UK)
Mr. J. NORTHOVER (UK)
Mr. M. HANCOCK (US)
Mr. Ric SWINDELL (UK)
Mr. Roger JAMES (UK)
Mr. R.G. SOUTER (UK)

Mr. Steve DAHLBERG (US)
Ms. Jill de ZWART (AU)
Ms. Joan Houghton (UK)
Ms. Phyllis GOODMAN (CA)
Prof. G.A. OMURA (US)
Prof. Alan BURNETT (UK)
Prof. Bruce N. GRAY (AU)
Prof. B. NORDLINGER (FR)
Prof. B.W. HANCOCK (UK)
Prof. C.A. COLTMAN (US)
Prof. Ching-Hon PUL (US)
Prof. C. CHASTANG (FR)
Prof. Cyril KARABUS (ZA)
Prof. DE-SEN WAN (CN)
Prof. D. CATOVSKY (UK)
Prof. D. BERGSAGEL (CA)
Prof. David KERR (UK)
Prof. D. CROWTHER (UK)
Prof. GRUENAGEL (DE)
Prof. Dr. H. RAINER (AT)
Prof. BOGUSLAWSKA-
JAWORSKA (PL)
Prof. Dr. HERMANEK (DE)
Prof. Dr. HEHLMANN (DE)
Prof. Dr. V. DIEHL (DE)
Prof. GORDON-SMITH (UK)
Prof. F. ZINTI (DE)
Prof. G. BONADONNA (IT)
Prof. G. MASERA (IT)
Prof. G. de PALO (IT)
Prof. G. BEN ARI (IL)
Prof. G. DIGHIERO (FR)
Prof. G. JANKA (DE)
Prof. G. SCHAISON (FR)
Prof. Von der MAASE (DK)
Prof. Heinz LUDWIG (AT)
Prof. H. PICHIMALER (DE)

Prof. Ian MacLENNAN (UK)
Prof. Irving TAYLOR (UK)
Prof. Jacques OTTEN (BE)
Prof. J.L. BINET (FR)
Prof. J.L. MISSET (FR)
Prof. J.M. ANDRIEU (FR)
Prof. J.M. CHESSELLS (UK)
Prof. Julian PETO (UK)
Prof. HARDCASTLE (UK)
Prof. L.E. RUTQVIST (SE)
Prof. Lars PAHLMAN (SE)
Prof. L.P. FLEIDING (US)
Prof. M.B. VIANA (BR)
Prof. HENRY-AMAR (FR)
Prof. Noel PHILIPPE (FR)
Prof. Olav DAHL (NO)
Prof. O. KRONBORG (DK)
Prof. O.B. EDEN (UK)
Prof. Paul GAYNON (US)
Prof. Peter JACOBS (ZA)
Prof. Peter Johan MOE (NO)
Prof. STRYCKMANS (BE)
Prof. P.L. FAGNIEZ (FR)
Prof. R.T. HOPPE (US)
Prof. S.V. KANAYEV (RU)
Prof. Takeo FUJIMOTO (JP)
Prof. Th.B. GRAGE (US)
Prof. T.J. HAMBLIN (UK)
Prof. Urs METZGER (CH)
Prof. Vaino RATSEP (EE)
Prof. W.R. BEZWODA (ZA)
Prof. W.A. KAMPS (NL)

ANTISENSE OLIGONUCLEOTIDES AS ANTICANCER AGENTS

Key words
Biological macromolecules, chemotherapy, oligonucleotides, nucleotide sequences, lipids, steroids, peptides.

Brief description
The programme approach treatment Normal drugs used to treat cancers are small molecules which interact with biological macromolecules i.e. proteins or nucleic acids.
They inhibit the function of these macromolecules. Most of these drugs, however, are very toxic.
A major breakthrough in cancer chemotherapy could come from new molecules which interact specifically with DNA or RNA sequences.
By blocking specific DNA sequences, we might be able to reverse the neoplastic transformation. This proposal is aimed at developing new constructs (oligonucleotides) which are directed to nucleotide sequences of oncogenes and which interfere selectively with the translation of the oncogene mRNA or the transcription of the DNA.
As natural oligonucleotides can not be used for this purpose, because of their instability, we will synthesize new constructs with a neutral backbone and with modified sugar moieties. This synthesis is based on molecular modelling predictions.
We will study their hybridisation capacity, their cellular uptake, their stability in vivo and their biological in vitro activity.
The second approach involves the conjugation of oligonucleotides with lipids, steroids, peptides and other reporter groups. These molecules will be incorporated in liposomes to improve their cellular uptake. Cell targeting and intracellular distribution of the conjugates will be studied.
The final goal is to synthesize enough material to be tested in vivo. Therefore a SCID mice model will be used.
This multidisciplinary work programme will be carried out by five laboratories located in four different European countries. These five laboratories have their own specific know-how and active collaboration is necessary to succeed in this program.

Project leader:
Professor P. HERDEWIJN
Laboratory of Medicinal
Chemistry, Rega Instituut
Minderbroederstraat 10
BE 3000 Leuven
Phone: +32 16 33 73 87
Fax: +32 16 33 73 40
Contract number: CT931669

Participants:
Ester TULA
SAISON-BEHMOARAS
Lab de Biophys, Muséum 43,
Rue Cuvier
FR 75231 Paris Cedex 05
Phone: +33 1 40 793686
Fax: +33 1 40 793705

Lee LESERMAN
Centre d'Immunologie
INSERM CNRS, de Marseille Luminy, Case 906
Parc Scientifique de Luminy
9067
FR 13288 Marseille 09
Phone: +33 91269400
Fax: +33 91269430

Ramon ERITJA
Dep Genetica Molec, Centro
de Investigacion y desarrollo
conseyo superior de
investigacions scientificas
Jordi Girona 18-26
ES 08034 Barcelona
Phone: +34 32040600
Fax: +34 32045904

Wolfgang PFLEIDERER
Fakult Chemie,
Universität Konstanz
Universitätsstrasse 10
DE 7750 Konstanz
Phone: +49 7531 882279
Fax: +49 7531 883138

DNA REPAIR AND CANCER

Key words
DNA repair.

Brief description
The DNA inside all cells is continually being exposed to a variety of damaging agents, either produced endogenously (e.g. active oxygen species) or exogenously (e.g. radiation, chemical carcinogens).

Organisms have evolved a complex and intricate series of interrelated repair pathways by which all types of DNA damage can be repaired or processed. A variety of highly cancer-prone human genetic disorders (e.g. xeroderma pigmentosum, ataxiatelangiectasia, Fanconi's anaemia and Bloom's Syndrome), the symptoms of which result from molecular defects in one or other of these DNA repair pathways, attest to the importance of DNA repair in cancer avoidance. Excellent progress has been made in the study of DNA repair in the last 3 years, especially in the cloning of human DNA repair genes, and much of it has been achieved in the laboratories of the participants of our previous Concerted Action. In the current proposal we aim to:

1 clone and characterize more human DNA repair genes, using a variety of approaches, and to analyze their protein products, in order to understand their function and role in DNA repair;
2 to develop transgenic mice deficient in different DNA repair genes, in order to study the role of DNA repair in the different steps of carcinogenesis, to provide animal models for cancer-prone disorders and to provide sensitive animal detectors of carcinogens;
3 to develop assays to detect a wide variety of DNA adducts in man using immunological and PCR-based procedures, in order to determine the nature of carcinogens to which populations are exposed, thereby assisting in cancer prevention;
4 to develop new procedures for measuring mutations in man or in experimental animals;
5 to develop and apply assays to measure repair at the level of individual genes, in order to study the intricate control mechanisms for repair processes. The insights gained into the early steps of carcinogenesis will lead to improvements in cancer prevention, therapy and diagnosis.

Project leader:
Dr. A.R. LEHMANN
MRC Cell Mutation Unit,
University of Sussex
Falmer
UK Brighton BN1 9RR
Phone: +44 273 67 81 23
Fax: +44 273 67 81 21
Contract number: CT931510

Participants:
Dr. A. ABBONDANDOLO
Istituto Nazionale per la
Ricerca sul Cancro
Viale Benedetto XV 10
IT 16132 Genova

Dr. A. SARASIN
Institut de Recherches
Scientifiques sur le Cancer
7 Rue Guy-Moquet
FR 94801 Villejuif Cedex

Dr. A. van der EB
Silvius Laboratory,
State Univ of Leiden
P.O. Box 9503
NL 2300 RA Leiden

Dr. A.R. COLLINS
The Rowett Research Inst.
Greenburn Road, Bucksburn
UK Aberdeen AB2 9SB

Dr. BIGNAMI
Istituto Superiore di Sanita
Viale Regina Elena 299
IT 00161 Roma

Dr. BOOTSMA
Dept. of Cell Biology and
Genetics, Erasmus Univ
P.O. Box 1738
NL 3000 Dr. Rotterdam

Dr. C. PUEYO
Dept.o de Genetica,
Facultad de Ciencias,
Universidad de Cordoba
Avd. de San Alberto Magno
ES 14071 Cordoba

Dr. E. MOUSTACCHI
Institut Curie - Biologie
26 Rue d'Ulm
FR 75231 Paris Cedex 5

Dr. E. SEEBERG
Div Environmental Toxicol,
Norwegian Defence Research
Establishment
P.O. Box 25
NO Kjeller

Dr. G. MARGISON
Paterson Inst. for '
Cancer Research
Wilmslow Road
UK Manchester M20 9BX

Dr. G. de MURCIA
Lab de Biochimie II,
IBMC du CNRS
15 Rue Rene Descartes
FR 67084 Strasbourg Cedex

Dr. G.P. van der SCHANS
P.O. Box 45
NL 2280 AA Rijswijk

Dr. I. HICKSON
ICRF Inst. of Molecular
Medicine,
John Radcliffe Hospital
UK Oxford OX3 9DU

Dr. J. ARRAND
UK Northwood, Middlesex

Dr. J. JIRICNY
Via Pontina KM 30.600
IT 00040 Pomezia, Rome

Dr. J. LAVAL
Rue Camille Desmoulins
FR 94805 Villejuif

Dr. J. RUEFF
R. de Junquerira 96
PT 1300 Lisbon

Dr. J. THACKER
Chilton Didcot
UK Oxon OX11 0RD

Dr. M. BLANCO
Amadeo de Saboya 4
ES 46010 Valencia

Dr. M. DEFAIS
205 Route de Narbonne
FR 31400 Toulouse

Dr. M. RAJEWSKY
Virchow-Strasse 173
DE 4300 Essen 1

Dr. M. STEFANINI
Via Abbiategrasso 207
IT 27100 Pavia

Dr. O. WESTERGAARD
C.F. Mollers Alle 130
DK 8000 Aarhus

Dr. P. van de PUTTE
Laboratory of Molecular
Genetics, Gorlaeus
Laboratoria
P.O. Box 9502
NL 2300 RA Leiden

Dr. P.A. HERRLICH
Institut für Genetik
und Toxikologie,
Kernforschungszentrum
Karlsruhe
P.O. Box 3640
DE 7500 Karlsruhe 1

Dr. P.H.M. LOHMAN
Dept. of Radiation Genetics
& Chemical Mutagenesis,
Sylvius Laboratories
Wassenaarseweg 72
NL 2333 AL Leiden

Dr. P.J. SMITH
MRC CORU, MRC Centre
Hills Road
UK Cambridge CB2 2QH

Dr. R. MONTESANO
International Agency for
Research on Cancer
150 Cours Albert Thomas
FR 69372 Lyon, Cedex 8

Dr. R. TYRRELL
Institut Suisse de Recherches
Experimentales sur le Cancer
Ch. des Boveresses
CH 1066 Epalinges,
Lausanne

Dr. R. WATERS
School of Biological
Sciences, Univ of Swansea
Singleton Park
UK Swansea SA2 8PP

Dr. R.P.P. FUCHS
IBMC du CNRS, GCMMS
15 Rue Rene Descartes
FR 67084 Strasbourg Cedex

Dr. R.T. JOHNSON
Dept. of Zoology,
Cambridge Univ
Downing Street
UK Cambridge CB2 3EJ

Dr. S.A. KYRTOPOULOS
Programme of Chemical
Carcinolgensis,
NHRF Inst. of Bio Research
48 Vassileos Constantinou
Avenue
GR Athens

Dr. T. LINDAHL
ICRF Clare Hall Laboratories
Blanche Lane
UK Hertfordshire EN6 3LD,
South Mimms

COST EVALUATION OF TREATMENT MODALITIES IN CANCER PATIENTS

Key words
Costs and benefits, multidimensional economic assessments.

Brief description
The proposal is to develop procedures and methodologies to enable the costs and benefits of cancer treatments for all common cancers to be evaluated and to apply them in large-scale clinical trials.

A Cost Evaluation Unit (comprising an Economist, a Computer Scientist and a Secretary) will be set up in the EORTC Data Center to prepare, as a first step, standard economic questionnaires and assessment methodologies for incorporation in the trials protocols of all large-scale clinical trials undertaken by - or in collaboration with EORTC.

Initially this will be done (in consultation with the relevant EORTC Clinical Cooperative Groups and with Member States' health services) for the most common cancers.

In a second stage the work will be extended to cover all cancers and multidimensional economic assessments will be routinely undertaken in all future largescale clinical trials.

In a final stage of the three-year project guidance on the economic assessments of cancer treatments - for use by clinicians but also governmental bodies, hospital administrations, etc. - will be developed and published.

Attempts will also be made to draw wider conclusions - of relevance in other health service area - on the assessment of costs and benefits in health care.

With health care costs soaring throughout the Community and with little in the way of economic assessment of different treatments so far undertaken, this project has high innovation potential, both in relation to cancer treatment and to health care more generally.

Project leader:
Professor Françoise MEUNIER
EORTC Data Center
Avenue Mounier 83, Bte 11
BE 1200 Bruxelles
Phone: +32 2 774 16 30
Fax: +32 2 771 20 04
Contract number: CT931671

Participants:
Dr. Jean-Louis LEFEBRE
Centre Oscar Lambret
Combemale 1
FR 59020 Lille
Phone: +33 20 29 59 59
Fax: +33 20 29 59 62

Dr. Nico Van ZANDWIJK
Netherlands Cancer Inst.
Plesmanlaan 121
NL 1066 CX Amsterdam
Phone: +31 20 512 91 11
Fax: +31 20 617 26 25

Dr. Sergio PECORELLI
Clinica Ostetrica e
Ginecologica,
Universita de Brescia
Piazzale Spedali Civili 17
IT 25124 Brescia
Phone: +39 30 399 54 93
Fax: +39 30 338 44 60

Dr. Silvio MONFARDINI
Centro de Riferimento
Oncologico
Via Pedemontana
Occidentale 12
IT 33081 Aviano
Phone: +39 434 65 92 82
Fax: +39 434 65 20 70

Dr. Umberto TIRELLI
Div. of Medical Oncology,
AIDS, Centro di Riferimento
Oncologico
Via Pedemontana
Occidentale 12
IT 33081 Aviano

Prof. Frans DEBRUYNE
Urological Oncological
Laboratory
Geert Grooteplein 16
NL 6500 HB Nijmegen
Phone: +31 80 61 37 35
Fax: +31 80 54 10 31

Prof. Harry BLEIBERG
Gastroenterology Dept.,
Institut Jules Bordet
Rue Heger Bordet 1
BE 1000 Bruxelles
Phone: +32 2 535 35 74
Fax: +32 2 538 08 58

Prof. H. BARTELINK
Radiotherapy Dept.,
Antoni van Leeuwenhoek
The Netherlands Cancer Inst.
Plesmanlaan 121
NL 1066 CX Amsterdam
Phone: +31 20 512 21 22
Fax: +31 20 669 11 01

Prof. J. HILDEBRAND
Head Dept. of Neurology,
Hôpital Erasme, Clinique de
l'Université Libre de
Bruxelles
808 Route de Lennik
BE 1070 Bruxelles
Phone: +32 2 555 33 46
Fax: +32 2 555 39 42

Prof. Robert RUBENS
Imp. Cancer Research Fund,
Clinical Oncology Unit,
Guy's Hospital
St. Thomas Street 7
UK London SE1 9RT
Phone: +44 71 955 45 41
Fax: +44 71 378 66 62

Prof. Robert ZITTOUN
Chairman Leukemia Coopera-
tive Group Hôtel Dieu
Place du Parvis
Notre Dame 1
FR 75181 Paris Cedex 04
Phone: +33 1 42 34 84 13
Fax: +33 1 42 34 84 06

Prof. Stein RAASA
Quality of Life Group,
Trondheim Univ Hospital,
Palliative Medicine Unit,
Dept. of Oncology
NO 7006 Trondheim
Phone: +47 7 99 80 00
Fax: +47 7 99 72 55

FUNCTIONAL ANALYSIS OF HUMAN PAIRED BOX GENES

Key words
Mammalian, homeobox (HOX), paired box (PAX), POU genes, congenital malformations, Pax3, splotch phenotype, Pax6, aniridia, PAX2, PAX8, Wilms' tumors,
transactivation, thyroid system, c-ret oncogene, renal gonadal malformations.

Brief description
A number of mammalian developmental control genes have recently been isolated and
characterized by reversed genetics. Most of these genes, such as homeobox (HOX),
paired box (PAX) and POU genes, encode transcription factors. Recent evidence indicates a crucial role for PAX genes in mouse and human embryogenesis. These findings
indicate that certain congenital malformations in mice and man are associated with PAX
mutations PAX3 mutations have been linked to the splotch phenotype in mice and with
Waardenburg syndrome in man. Muatations in PAX6 confer a semidominant mutant
small eye (sey) in mice and aniridia in humans. Thus at least in the case of PAX genes
mouse system seems to be very useful to model human disease. Two human genes of the
PAX gene family will be investigated in the present study - PAX2 and PAX8. These
genes are highly homologous and are expressed during kidney development. Both are
possibly involved in the genesis of a particular childhood cancer, so called Wilms'
tumors, that originate in the human embryonic kidney.
Furthermore PAX is expressed in the fetal and adult thyroid. Dedifferentiation of thyroid
cells upon transformation with an activated RAS oncogene correlates with suppression of
PAX expression. We have chosen several approaches to study the function of PAX *in
vivo* and its involvement in kidney and thyroid cancer. We will establish a bigenic
transgenic mouse system to overexpress PAX2 and PAX8 during kidney development
and investigate a possibility that such over expression is a direct cause of human Wilms'
tumors. Such system will be useful to study any deletirous human genes such as activated oncogenes.
We will investigate the human PAX8 promoter and its interactions with RAS and tumor
suppressor WTI gene products. We will investigate the transactivation abilities of PAX8
in thyroid system, its regulation by CAM P-dependent signal transduction and how these
signals are regulated by RAS In addition we will investigate a possible involvement of
PAX8 in development of certain thyroid carcinomas with activated c-ret oncogene we
will carry out a mutation anlysis of PAX2 and PAX8 as well as of the zink finger gene
WTI in Wilms' tumors and in individuals with renal gonadal malformations. In addition
we will investigate the possible developmental interactions between these genes which
may act in a developmental cascade.

Projectleader:
Dr. Dimitrij PLACHOV
Institut für Humangenetik
Vesaliusweg 12,
DE 48149 Münster
Phone: +49 251 83 54 14
Fax: +49 251 83 69 95
Contract number: CT931105

Participants:

Dr. Anna Maria MUSTI
CEOS del CNR
Via S. Pansini
IT Napoli

Dr. Enrico AVVEDIMENTO
Dipartimento de Biologia,
Il Facolta de Medicina
Via S. Pansini
IT Napoli

Dr. H. STORM
Danish Cancer Registry,
Inst. of Cancer Epidemiology
Rosenvaegngets Hovedvej 35
P.O. Box 839
DK 2100 Copenhagen

Dr. Nicholas HASTIE
MCR Human Genetics Unit
Crewe Road
UK Edinburgh

Dr. Van HEYNINGEN
MCR Human Genetics Unit
Crewe Road
UK Edinburgh
Phone: +32 2 762 94 05

CLINICAL RELEVANCE OF PROTEASES IN TUMOR INVASION AND METASTASIS

Key words
Metalloproteases, cathepsins, plasminogen activators, tumor invasion, metastasis, melanoma, leukemia, immunohisto-chemistry, histomorphological data, prognostic relevance, proteolytic factors.

Brief description
The overall objective of thls transnational proposal with the title at a basic and also at a clinical level with the soal to explore the potential role of proteases (metalloproteases, cathepsins and plasminogen activators), their receptors and inhibitors in tumor invasion and metastasis.

Major perspective of the proposed Concerted European Action, with respect to the role of proteases in tumor invasion and metastasis, is to coordinate the various European scientific and clinical activities and to promote rapid exchange of knowledge, technical expertise, reagents and personnel between 22 different teams from 11 European countries. The Concerted Action will therefore have a harmonizing character.

It is anticipated that coordinated European research on the basics and clinical relevance of proteases in tumors will lead to rapid increase in information about the biological and clinical significance of tumor-associated proteases, their receptors and inhibitors which could not be reached by individual activities alone.

Four major topics are addressed and will be explored together in this transnational Concerted European Action:

1 Increase of the knowledge of mechanisms by which proteases facilitate tumor invasion and metastasis in solid tumors, melanoma and leukemia (tumor/host cell interaction).

2 Standardization of reagents, antibodies, gene probes, kits and assay procedures to determine expression of proteolytic factors at the gene and protein level (quality assurance).

3 Quantitative assessment of proteases, their receptors and inhibitors in human tumor tissue specimens of various origin by ELISA, immunohistochemistry or molecular biological approaches and correlation of these findings with established clinical and histomorphological data.

4 Determination of the prognostic relevance of proteolytic factors for disease-free and overall survival by standardized statistical methods. Define impact on therapy decision.

5 Harmonization of European basic and clinic-oriented scientific activitie within the field of tumor/host cell interaction and proteolytic factors.

6 Promote rapid exchange of information, reagents, test kits, tumor material and personnel. Centralize data storage, handling and statistical analysis.

7 Organize accompanying measures such as seminars and workshops for all participants.

Projectleader:
Dr. Manfred SCHMITT
Frauenklinik der Technischen Universität München
Ismaningerstrasse 22
DE 81675 München
Phone: +49 89 41 40 24 49
Fax: +49 89 41 80 51 46
Contract number: CT931346

Participants:

Dr. Alain-Pascal SAPPINO
Hôpital Cantonal
Universitaire de Genève,
Départment de Médicine Div.
d'Onco-Hématologie 24,
Rue Micheli-du-Crest
CH 1211 Genève 4

Dr. Gillian MURPHY
Strangeways Research Labo-
ratory, Cell & Molecular
Biology Dept.Wort's Cause-
way
UK Cambridge CB1 4RN

Dr. Hein VERSPAGET
Univ Hospital Leiden, Dept.
of Gastroenterology and
Hepatolgy
P.O. Box 9600
NL 2300 RC Leiden

Dr. John FOEKES
Rotterdam Radi-Therapeutic
Inst., Dr. Daniel den Hoed
Cancer Center
P.O. Box 5201
NL 3008 AE Rotterdam

Dr. L. RONNOV-JESSEN
The Fibiger Inst. of the
Danish Cancer Society, Dept.
of Tumor Endocrinology
Ndr. Frihavnsgade 70
DK 2100 Copenhagen

Dr. M. Joe DUFFY
St Vincent's Hospital,
Nuclear Medicine Dept.
Elm Park
IE Dublin 4

Dr. Nils BRÜNNER
The Finsen Laboratory
49 Strandboulevarden
DK 2100 Copenhagen 0

Dr. Paul BASSET
Institut de Chemie
Biologique,
11 Rue Humann
FR 67085 Strasbourg Cedex

Dr. Pierre BURTIN
Assistance Publique,
Hôpitaux de Paris,
Hotel-Dieu de Paris,
Laboratoire Sainte-Marie
1, Place du Parvis
Notre Dame
FR 75181 Paris Cedex 04

PD Dr. M.D. KRAMER
Universität Heidelberg,
Institut für Immunologie
Im Neuenheimer Feld 305
DE 69120 Heidelberg

PD Dr. SCHWARZ-ALBIEZ
Deutsches Krebs-
forschungszentrum,
Institut für Immunologie
und Genetik
Im Neuenheimer Feld 280
DE 69120 Heidelberg

Prof. Dr. Antti VAHERI
Univ of Helsinki,
Dept. of Virology
Haartmaninkatu 3
FI 00290 Helsinki

Prof. Dr. Bernard SORDAT
Insitut Suisse de Recherches
Expérimentales sur le Cancer
(ISREC)
155, Ch. des Boveresses
CH 1066 Epalinges
S/Lausanne

Prof. Dr. Dirk RUITER
Academisch Ziekenhuis
Nijmegen, Pathologie
Geert Grooteplein 24
NL 6500 HB Nijmegen

Prof. Dr. D. STEHLIN
Centre National de la
Recherche Scientifique
URA 1160,
Inst. Pasteur de Lille Unité
d'Oncologie Moleculaire
1, Rue Calmette
FR 59019 Lille Cedex

Prof. Dr. Francesco BLASI
Università Degli Studi di
Milano, Dept. of Genetics
and Microbial Biology
Via Celoria 26
IT 20133 Milano

Prof. Dr. H. TSCHESCHE
Universität Bielefeld, Fakultät
für Chemie, Abt Biochemie I
P.O. Box 100131
DE 33501 Bielefeld

Prof. Dr. H. ROCHEFORT
Université de Montpellier 1,
INSERM Unité 148 Hormone
et Cancer Faculté
de Médicine
60 Rue de Navacelles
FR 34090 Montpellier

Prof. Dr. FOIDART
Université de Liège,
Lab of Biology,
Tower of Pathology (B23),
Sart Tilman
BE 4000 Liège

Prof. Dr. TRYGGVASON
Univ of Oulu,
Biocenter and Dept.
of Biochemistry,
Linnanmaa
FI 90570 Oulu

Prof. Dr. Theo BENRAAD
Academisch Ziekenhuis
Nijmegen,
Dept. of Experimental and
Chemical Endocrinology
P.O. Box 9101
NL 6500 HB Nijmegen

Prof. Dr. Vito TURK
Jozef-Stefan-Institut,
Dept. of Biochemistry
Jamovar 39
FI 611111 Ljubljana

A MULTICENTRIC CASE-CONTROL STUDY OF THE MAJOR RISK FACTORS FOR LUNG CANCER IN EUROPE WITH PARTICULAR EMPHASIS ON INTERCOUNTRY COMPARISON

Key words
Carcinogenic risk factors, diet constituents.

Brief description
Nine case-control studies on lung cancer are presently being conducted in eight European countries investigating carcinogenic risk factors from personal habits and outdoor, and indoor environment.

Potential protective action from diet constituents are also investigated.

The total number of cases included in the studies will exceed 5,000. It is proposed to constitute a common database after adequate processing and standardization of the information and to analyse the material collected using a collaborative approach.

Projectleader:
Dr. Lorenzo SIMONATO
European Lung Cancer Working Party,
Institut Jules Bordet
Rue Heger Bordet 1
BE 1000 Bruxelles
Phone: +32 2 539 04 96
Fax: +32 2 537 66 25
Contractnumber: CT931047

Participants:
D. TECULESCU
Inserm Unite 115,
Facultes de Medicin
FR Vandoevres-les-Nancy
Phone: +33 83 592595
Fax: +33 83 446112

Dr. Carlos A. GONZALES
Jordi Joan
ES 08301 Mataró
Phone: +34 3 7905513
Fax: +34 3 7906802

Dr. Franco MERLETTI
Via Santena 7
IT 10126 Torino
Phone: +39 11 678872
Fax: +39 11 6635267

Dr. Marianna PAESMANS
European Lung Cancer,
Working Party,
Institut Jules Bordet
Rue Héger Bordet 1
BE 1000 Bruxelles
Phone: +32 2 5355047
Fax: +32 2 5381811

Dr. Paola BOFFETTA
International Agency for
Research on Cancer
FR 69372 Lyon Cedex 08
Phone: +33 72 738485
Fax: +33 72 738575

Dr. Sarah DARBY
Imperial Cancer
Research Fund,
Cancer Epidemiology Unit,
The Radcliffe Infirmary
UK Oxford
Phone: +44 865 311933
Fax: +44 865 310545

Dr. Simone BENHAMOU
Institut Gustave Rousy
FR 94805 Villejuif
Phone: +33 1 45594909
Fax: +33 1 46787430

Prof. Cristian VUTUC
Alser Str. 21/12
AT 1080 Wien
Phone: +43 1 427694 334
Fax: +43 324 1 438790

Prof. Göran PERSHAGEN
Dept. of Epidemiology
P.O. Box 60206
SE 104 01 Stockholm
Phone: +46 87287460
Fax: +46 8313961

Prof. Karl-Heinz JOECKEL
Bremen Inst. for Prevention,
Research & Socila Medicine
Grunenstr. 120
DE 2800 Bremen 1
Phone: +49 4215959651
Fax: +49 4215959668

A COMPREHENSIVE STUDY ON THE BIOLOGY OF MULTIPLE MYELOMA AND ITS CLINICAL APPLICATIONS IN PROGNOSIS AND THERAPY

Key words

Multiple Myeloma, B cell lineage, neoplastic bone marrow, monoclonal immunoglobulin, osteolytic lesions, monoclonal gammopathy, lymphokines, IL-6.

Brief description

Project Multiple Myeloma (MM) is a malignancy of the B cell lineage, in which a clone of neoplastic bone marrow (BM) plasma cells secretes a monoclonal immunoglobulin (IG) and produces factors which induce osteolytic lesions.

A benign counterpart, monoclonal gammopathy of undetermined significance (MGUS), results from the stable expansion of a plasma cell clone, which is not associated with bone destruction or significant proliferation among the plasma cells.

Although the predominant cell type in MM is the bone marrow Plasma cell, some of the genetic changes leading to the neoplastic transformation may take place at earlier stages of B cell differentiation.

The precursors of marrow plasma cells which are potential targets for these genetic changes are the memory cell during activation in the germinal centre or the pre B cell.

Regulation of MM qrowth may relate to input from precursors of the neoplastic plasma cells and/or functional interactions between these plasma cells and the bone marrow environment.

Various lymphokines, particularly IL-6, are involved in this growth control and their action may be supported by adhesion mechanisms.

The clinical evolution of the disease seems to be associated with an increase in genetic alterations and might also be aggravated by impaired immunosurveillance.

Each from a different angle, several European groups (Nantes, Brussels, Birmingham, Hannover, Torino, Utrecht) have been studying the pathogenesis of MM and MGUS, They are internationally competitive and offer together a unique multidisciplinary collaboration which ranges from basic research towards clinical applied sciences.

They dispose of a large amount of myeloma cell lines, several animal models and an impressive bank of frozen serum and cell samples from well documented patients with myeloma.

Project leader:
Professor Benjamin VAN CAMP
Academic Hospital V.U.B. Hematology
Laarbeeklaan 101
BE 1090 Brussels
Phone: +32 2 477 62 11
Fax: +32 2 477 67 27
Contract number: CT931407

Participants:

B. KLEIN
Laboratory for
Immunological and
Oncological Hematology
Quai Moncousu 9
FR 44035 Nantes

D. PEEST
Abteilung Immunologie und
Transfusionsmedizin,
Zentrum Innere Medizin
und Dermatology
Konstanty-Gutschow-Str. 8
DE 3000 Hannover

E. BAST
Dept. of Immunology,
Univ Hospital Utrecht
NL 3508 GA Utrecht

F.K. STEVENSON
Lymphome Research Unit,
Southampton General
Hospital,
Tenovous Laboratory
UK Southampton S09 4XY

H. MELLSTEDT
Dept. of Oncology,
Karolinska Hospital
P.O. Box 6050
SE 104 01 Stockholm

I. MAC LENNAN
Dept. of Immunology,
Univ of Birmingham
UK Birmingham B15 2TT

J. BLADE
Hospital Clinic I Provincial
de Barcelona
Villarroel 170
ES 08036 Barcelona

J. ECONOMIDOU
Evangelismos Hospital,
Dept.of Immunology-
Histocompatibility
45, Ipsilontou Str
GR 10676 Athens

M. BOCCADORO
Laboratorio Div. e di
Ematologia dell'Universita di
Torino Ospedale Molinette
Via Genova 3
IT 10126 Torino

P. SONNEVELD
Dept. of Hematology,
Room L407,
Univ Hospital Rotterdam
Dr. Molewaterplein 40
NL 3015 GD Rotterdam

EUROPEAN RANDOMISED TRIAL OF
OVARIAN CANCER SCREENING

Key words
Sreening, ovarian cancer, transvaginal ultrasound examination, colour Doppler ultrasound.

Brief description
The study is a randomised controlled trial of screening for ovarian cancer in women aged 55-64 years taking place in eight European centres in Denmark, Norway, Sweden and the UK.

Because a randomised trial based on ovarian cancer mortality is a long term commitment (taking about 10 years), it is an advantage to obtain evidence sooner than this that could indicate whether screening might be so ineffective that the trial should be stopped. An appropriate way of achieving this is to conduct a pilot trial lasting 4 years in which surrogate outcome measures of screening eeeicacy were used.

The European multicentre trial of ovarian cancer screening is such a trial which could later be expanded to a full mortality study if it were justified. The study design is the same as the full mortality study that would be needed to investigate the central question but is scheduled to last 4 years instead of 10, and uses surrogate measures of screening outcome. These are:

a stage distribution of ovarian cancer;

b prevalence and incidence of ovarian cancer;

c interval cancers and;

d screening uptake.

The design incorporates an examination of the effect of screening interval, and includes two study groups with screening intervals of 1.5 years and 3 years as well as a control group who are not screened. 80,000 women are required over 4 years; 20,000 to be randomised each year.

The screening method under investigation is transvaginal ultrasound examination, followed by colour Doppler ultrasound as a secondary screening test if ultrasound is positive.

Project leader:
Professor N.J. WALD
Dept. of Environmental and Preventive Medicine,
Wolfson Institute
St Bartholomew's Hospital Med. College
Charterhouse Square
UK London EC1M 6BQ
Phone: +44 71 982 62 69
Fax: +44 71 982 62 70
Contract number: CT931741

Participants:

Dr. Ann TABOR
Dept. of Obstetrics and Gynaecology,
Rigshospitalet
Blegdansvej 9
DK 2100 Copenhagen
Phone: +45 35 453 545
Fax: +45 35 454 285

Dr. Bruno CACCIATORE
1st Dept. of Obstetrics
and Gynecology,
Helsinki Univ Hospital
Haartmaninkatu 2
FI 00290 Helsinki
Phone: +358 0479102

Dr. Ian SCOTT
Consultant in Obstetrics & Gynaecology,
Derbyshire City Hospital
Uttoxeter Road
UK Derby DE3 3NE
Phone: +44 332 401 31
Fax: +44 332 290559

Dr. Sturla EIK-NES
National Center for Fatal Medicine,
Dept. of Gynaecology and Obstetrics,
Trondheim Univ Hospital
NO 7006 Trondheim
Phone: +47 7998307
Fax: +47 7997696

Prof. Stuart CAMPBELL
King's College Hospital, Dept. of
Obstetrics & Gynaecology, 9th Floor,
New Ward Block
Denmark Hill, Camberwell
UK London SE5 9RS
Phone: +44 71 326 3020
Fax: +44 71 737 4609

TUMOUR CELL HETEROGENEITY AND ITS IMPLICATION FOR THERAPEUTIC MODALITIES STUDIES IN HUMAN TUMOUR CELLS GROWN IN MULTICELLULAR SPHEROID CULTURE

Key words
Disseminated metastatic cells, monoclonal antibodies, fragments, antigens, ligand conjugates, avascular micrometastases, phenotypic, neuroblastoma, 13II-mIBG, EGF receptor.

Brief description
The treatment of disseminated metastatic cells is the biggest challenge in cancer research for the next decades.

The approaches to therapy will be many but the common denominator will be that some kind of tumour cell-seeking principle will be tried. Examples of cell-seeking substances are monoclonal antibodies or fragments of monoclonal antibodies for tumour cells with well characterized antigens. Ligand conjugates might be applied when receptor amplification is a characteristic feature of the tumour cells and it might in some cases, be possible to use low molecular weight agents such as catecholamine precursor analogues like 13II-mIBG for targeting of neuroblastomas. Tumour cells grown in multicellular spheroids seem to be the ideal model to study heterogeneity-related questions.

Spheroids simulate in vitro the formation of avascular micrometastases and display their typical variations in phenotypic appearances. The four groups combined in this concerted action like to approach the problem of tumour cell heterogencity and cell seeking with the aid of multicellular spheroids from different directions.

The group from Norway is specialized in tumour cell invasion and is able to visualize this process by transfecting tumour cells by a receptor gene lac-z fascilitating the identification of tumour cells in normal tissue. The group from England is experienced in targeting neuroblastoma cells with 13II-mIBG and to remodel mathematically the heterogeneity of 13II-mIBG uptake caused by variations in local environmental factors. The group from Germany has developed microelectrodes and photometric devices to monitor differences in the microenvironment of spheroids and to construct different metabolic situations by specifically changing enzyme activities.

The group from Sweden studied EGF receptor - as well as E4 antigen-expression and used this to guide tumour-seeking substances to the corresponding tumour cell.

Using the expertise of the different laboratories it should be possible to work out optimized therapy schemes for different tumour cell lines by mapping the degree of tumour cell heterogeneity in multicellular spheroids regarding their invasion capacity, receptor and antigen expression as well as metabolism.

Modelling mathematically the results will be useful to predict clinical efficacy of different tumour therapy modalities.

Project leader:
Professor Dr. H. ACKER
Max Planck Institut für
Systemphysiologie
Rheinlanddamm 201
DE 44139 Dortmund 1
Phone: +49 231 120 65 30
Fax: +49 231 120 64 64
Contract number: CT941068

Participants:
Dr. T. WHELDON
UK Glasgow G61 1BD
Phone: +44 41 3304126
Fax: +44 41 3304127

Prof. Dr. J. CARISSON
SE 75121 Uppsala
Phone: +46 18 183841
Fax: +46 18 183833

Prof. Dr. R. BERKVIG
Anatomisk Institut
Arstadveien
NO 5009 Bergen
Phone: +47 55 206349
Fax: +47 55 206360

CLUSTERING OF CHILDHOOD LEUKAEMIA IN EUROPE

Key words
Childhood Leukaemias.

Brief description
To determine whether *Childhood Leukaemias* show a general tendency to Cluster within small areas, and, if so, to note where, which ages and which diagnostic groups. The answers will be derived using community wide research and expertise and therefore valid throughout the EC. This (the primary) objective will be achieved by applying a uniform protocol and conducting centralised statistical analyses of data from at least 12 member and COST states.

Estimates of the background frequency of childhood leukaemia clusters will be used to formulate improved *Guidelines for public health specialists* who are required to advise on many reported clusters - a time consuming and often inconclusive task.

SUBSIDIARY ANALYSES will aim to test and refine current competing hypotheses for the cause of childhood leukaemia and the explanation of clusters. These are:

i one or more common infectious agents: unusual timing of exposure and/or viral dose occupational;

ii environmental exposure or paternal pre-conception exposure to low levels of ionising radiation and other leukaemogens.

The diverse skills of the participants will be used in the specification of detailed proto-cols, the collection of data of uniform quality, and, particularly, forming a *Consensus Interpretation* of the results. The conclusions will be widely disseminated in peer review journals, EC reports and workshops. Recommendations for further research are expected.

Extensive travel between centres and to meetings and workshops will ensure maximum contribution from all participants.

Project leader:
Dr. F.E. ALEXANDER
Leukaemia Research Centre for Clinical Epidemiology,
Royal South Hants Hospital
Graham Road
UK Southampton SO9 4PE
Phone: +44 703 825 836
Fax: +44 703 825 836
Contract number: CT941785

Participants:
Dr. A. VAN DER DOES-VAN DEN BERG
DCLSG, Julian Children's Hospital
Postbus 60604
NL 2506 LP Den Haag
Phone: +31 70 365 7930
Fax: +31 70 361 7427

Dr. E. PETRIDOU
Dept. of Hygiene and Epidemiology,
Univ of Athens
GR 11527 Athens
Phone: +30 1 77 71 165
Fax: +30 1 77 04 225

Dr. F. LEVI
Institut Universitaires de Medicine CHUV
Falaises
CH 1011 Lausanne
Phone: +41 21 314 39 08
Fax: +41 21 323 03 03

Dr. H. STORM
Div. for Cancer Epidemiology,
Danish Cancer Society
Strandboulevarden 49, P.O. Box 839
DK 2100 Kobenhaven
Phone: +45 35 26 88 66
Fax: +45 35 26 00 90

Dr. H.O. ADAMI
Cancer Epidemiology Unit,
Univ Hospital
SE 75185 Uppsala
Phone: +46 18 665 045
Fax: +46 18 503 431

Dr. L. TEPPO
Finnish Cancer Registry
Liisandatu 21B
FI 00170 Helsinki
Phone: +358 0 135 331
Fax: +358 0 135 5378

Dr. L. VATTEN
Inst. of Community Medicine,
Univ Medical Centre
NO 7005 Trondheim
Phone: +47 73 59 87 87
Fax: +47 73 59 87 89

Dr. P. BOYLE
Div. of Epidemiologu & Biostatistics
Via Ripamonti 332/10
IT 20141 Milan
Phone: +39 2 574 08795
Fax: +39 2 574 08883

Dr. C.S. MUIR
Cancer Registration
23 Hill Street
UK Edinburgh EH 3JP
Phone: +44 31 225 1333
Fax: +44 31 225 9395

Dr. G. DRAPER
Dept. of Paediatrics,
Univ of Oxford
57 Woodstock Road
UK Oxford OX2 6HH
Phone: +44 865 310030
Fax: +44 865 514254

Dr. R. PERIS-BONET
Registro Nacional de Tumores Infantiles
Avandia Blasco Ibanez 17
ES 46010 Valencia
Phone: +34 6 369 2466
Fax: +34 6 361 3975

Prof. B. TERRACINI
Dept. of Biological Sciences &
Human Oncology, Univ of Turin
IT Turin
Phone: +39 11 678 872
Fax: +39 11 663 5267

Prof. J. MICHAELIS
Institut fur Med. Statistik und Dokumentation
Langenbeckstrasse 1, Postfach 3960
DE 55101 Mainz
Phone: +49 6131 17 73 69
Fax: +49 6131 17 29 68

Prof. P.M. CARLI
Laboratoire D'Hematolgie, Hopital Du Bocage
2 Bd Marechal-de-Lattre-de Tassigny
FR 21035 Dyon
Phone: +33 8065 8123
Fax: +33 8039 3421

PARACRINE GROWTH STIMULATION IN ORGAN METASTASIS: THE ROLE OF HEPATOCYTE GROWTH/SCATTER FACTOR AND MET ONCOGENE

Key words

Paracrine growth stimulation, Hepatocyte Growth Factor/Scatter Factor (HGF/SF), metastasis, angiogenetic factor, teratocarcinoma, M5076 reticulum, sarcoma.

Brief description

One of the limiting steps in the Organ colonization pattern of malignanant cells is their ability to grow efficiently in the target organ. In this respect, the production cf autocrine growth factors, or the ability to respond to paracrine growth stimulation, can strongly contribute to the successful establishment of a metastatic colony.

Hepatocyte Growth Factor/Scatter Factor (HGF/SF) is indeed a pleiotropic factor which might be helpful in tumor and metastasis formation: it is a growth and angiogenetic factor, it can stimulate motility and UPA production. The hypothesis that we want to test is the following. Since HGF/SF has been implicated in the regenerative growth response (mainly in liver and kidney) it is possible that the presence of tumor cells in the liver produce a local damage and thus induce the expression of regeneretive growth factors such as the HGF/SF. If tumor cells can respond to these factors (if they have a functional receptor), they will gain a growth advantage which c2n favour metastatic colonization in an organ specific manner.

We intend to investigate this possibility by using syngeneic murine model systems in which liver-specific cell lines have been identified (namely the B16 melanoma the F9 teratocarcinoma, the M5076 reticulum cell sarcoma and the Lewis Lung carcinoma).The first step will be the study of the expression (both in vitro and in vivo) of the c-met cncogene (receptor for the HGF/SF), and the factor itself, by these cell lines, and test their susceptibility to the factor's effects.

In parallel, we will determine the inducibility of the HGF/SF by the presence of tumor cells in the liver (in vivo), or in aco-culture system in vitro with tumor cells and liver cells. We will also artificially induce liver damage and regeneration (in order to induce the expression of the regenerating factors, including the HGF/SF) to see to what extent the production of regenerating factors can influence bodies and thereby see to what extent we can prevent metastatic growth in target.

Project leader:
Professor Walter BIRCHMEIER
Max-Delbrück-Center for Molecular Medicine,
MDC Berlin-Buch
Robert-Rössle-Strasse 10
DE 01115 Berlin-Buch
Phone: +49 30 940 60
Fax: +49 30 949 41 61
Contract number: CT941651

Participants:
M.M. BURGER
The Friedrich Miescher Inst.
P.O.Box 2543
CH 4002 Basel
Phone: +41 61 69 722 01
Fax: +41 61 650 91 05

P.M. COMOGLIO
Dipartimento Di Scienza Biomediche
e Oncologia Umana Sezione
di Istologia e Embriologia
C.so Massimo D'Azeglio 52
IT 10126 Torino
Phone: +39 11 652 77 39
Fax: +39 11 650 91 05

ANALYSIS OF THE IMPACT OF INFECTION BY HEPATITIS B AND C VIRUSES ON PRIMARY LIVER CANCER IN EUROPE AND OF THE MOLECULAR MECHANISMS OF THE LIVER CARCINOGENESIS

Key words
HBV and HCV related carcinogenesis, polynerase chain reaction.

Brief description
The aim of the proposal is to investigate, on a significant number of patients from both South and North Europe, the association between hepatitis B and C viral chronic infections and primary liver cancer. In addition, the proposal will allow to collect serum and liver samples in good conditions to investigate the molecular mechanisms of the HBV and HCV related carcinogenesis.

It is important to realise that, despite a number of studies on these issues, several questions still remain unanswered or debated. The development of new technical approaches, such as the polynerase chain reaction, together with a concerted action from six representative centres in South and North Europe will allow to address the following issues:
- The prevalence of HBV and HCV serological markers in patients with primary liver cancer (alcoholics or not).
- The prevalence of HBV DNA and HCV RNA genomes persistence in serum and tissues in seropositive and negative individuals.
- The mechanisms of liver carcinogenesis and the importance of viral genetic variations.

These issues would provide for the first time a comprehensive view of the extent of viral factors in liver cancer in Europe and thus would have major implications for prevention.

Project leader:
Prof. Christian BRÉCHOT
INSERM Unité 370
Rue de Vaugirard 156
FR 75730 Paris Cédex 15
Phone: +33 1 40 65 99 12
Fax: +33 1 40 61 55 81
Contract number: CT941789

Participants:
Dr. R. WILLIAMS
King's College School of
Medicine and Dentistiry,
Inst. of Liver Studies
Bessemer Road 7
UK London SE5 9PJ
Phone: +44 71 13263254
Fax: +44 71 13263167

Dr B. MOUREN
INSERM U. 370
Rue de Vaugirard 156
FR 75730 Paris
Phone: +33 1 40 65 99 12
Fax: +33 1 40 61 55 81

Dr. F. SOLEY
Fundacio Clinic per
a la Recerca Biom
Villaroel
ES Barcelona
Phone: +34 3 4516286
Fax: +34 3 4515272

Prof J. RODES
Hospital Clinic i Provincial,
Liver Unit
Villaroel 170
ES 08036 Barcelona
Phone: +34 3 4546000
Fax: +34 3 4515272

Prof. M. COLOMBO
Università di Milano;
Istituto di Medicina Interna
Via Pace 9
IT 20122 Milano
Phone: +39 2 55035431
Fax: +39 2 55181725

Prof. N. NAOMOV
King's College School of
Medicine and Dentistry,
Inst. of Liver Studies
Bessemer Road 7
UK London SE5 9PJ
Phone: +44 71 13263254
Fax: +44 71 13263167

Prof. P. MANTEGAZZA
Università degli Studi
di Milano
Via Festa del Perdono 7
IT 20122 Milano
+39 2 58303824

DESCRIPTIVE AND MOLECULAR EPIDEMIOLOGY
OF NON-HODGKIN'S LYMPHOMA IN EUROPE

Key words
Non-Hodgkin's Lymphoma, NHL, diagnostic protocol, molecular epidemiology.

Brief description
Currently there are roughly 26,000 new cases of non-Hodgkin's Lymphoma occurring annually in community countries. It is known that non-Hodgkin's Lymphoma (NHL) is increasing in incidence in several European countries. In a decade NHL could be in the top 5 commonest cancers. This phenomenon cannot be properly investigated, however, without specific concerted European action to harmonise procedures for:
a collecting good quality data on NHL over a span of years in defined geographical areas;
b agreeing a common diagnostic protocol for light microscopy;
c using new methods to investigate the molecular epidemiology of the disease. This action will enable specific questions to be answered and lead to future analytic studies.

These questions include:
a are the NHL rates increasing in all participant countries?
b are the rates of increase the same?
c which type of NHL is increasing?
d what is the influence of HIV infection?
e can the increase be accounted for by pesticide use in different countries?

The aims and objectives therefore of this proposal cover several aspects of the work programne of Biomed I, but are particularly pertinent to the cancer research tasks in epidemiology on 'less common cancers' and 'exploiting geographical differences in cancer incidence'.

Project leader:
Dr. Ray A. CARTWRIGHT
Leukaemia Research Fund Centre
for Clinical Epidemiology,
University of Leeds
Springfield Mount 17
UK Leeds L3 9NG
Phone: +44 532 333 909
Fax: +44 532 42 60 65
Contract number: CT941769

Participants:
Dr. J.W. COEBERGH
Comprehensive Cancer
Centre (South)
P.O. Box 231
NL 5600 AE Eindhoven
Phone: +31 40 455775

Dr. L. TEPPO
Finnish Cancer Registry
Liisankatu 21B
FI 00170 Helsinki
Phone: +358 0 135331
Fax: +358 0 1355378

Dr. RAZENBERG
Medical Director
Schipholweg 5, P.O. Box 231
NL 2316 XB Eindhoven

Prof. P.M. CARLI
Laboratoire d'Hematologie
Hopital du Bocage ,
2 Bd. Morechal de Lattre
de Tassigny
FR 21034 Dijon
Phone: +33 80293314
Fax: +33 80293660

Dr. A. NAUKKARINEN
Dept. of Clinical Pathology
Kuopio Univ Hospital
P.O. box 1777
FI 70211 Kuopio
Phone: +358 71 173477

Dr. A.S. JACK
Algernon Firth Building
Leeds Genral Infirmary
Great George Street
UK Leeds LS1 3EX
Phone: +44 0532 333534
Fax: +44 0532 347662

Dr. E. PUKKALA
Finnish Cancer Registry,
Inst. for Statiscal and
Epidemiological Cancer
Research
Liisankatu 21 B
FI 00170 Helsinki
Phone: +358 0 135331
Fax: +358 0 1355378

Dr. F. d'AMORE
Danish Cancer Registry Inst.
of Cancer Epidemiology
Strandboulevarden 49
DK 2100 Kobenhavn
Phone: +45 35268866
Fax: +45 35260090

Dr. G. MORGAN HMDS
Algernon Firth Building
Leeds General Infirmary
UK Leeds LS1 3EX
Phone: +44 0532 333974
Fax: +44 0532 347662

Dr. H.J. KRUYFF
Comprehensive Cancer
Centres - West and South
Schipholweg 5, P.O. Box 231
NL 2316 XB Eindhoven
Phone: +31 40 259759
Fax: +31 40 259759

Dr. J.H. OLSEN
Danish Cancer Registry Inst.
of Cancer Epidemiology
Stransboulevarden 49
DK 2100 Kobenhavn
Phone: +45 35 26 88 66
Fax: +45 35 26 00 90

Dr. J. PUITTINEN
Dept. of Pathology
Savonlinna Central Hospital
FI 57120 Savonlinna
Phone: +358 57 5811
Fax: +358 57 51476

Dr. J.W. COEBERGH
Comprehensive Cancer
Centre (West)
Schipholweg 5A
NL 2316 ZD Leiden
Phone: +31 71 55775
Fax: +31 71 259700

Dr. K. SYRJANEN
Dept. of Clinical Pathology
Kuopio Univ Hospital
FI Kuopio
Phone: +358 71 173477

Dr. L. DARDONANI
Registro Tumori Ragusa
Centro Tumori 9
Piazza Igea 2
IT Ragusa

Dr. M. VORNANEN
Dept. of Clinical Pathology
Kuopio Univ Central Hospital
P.O. Box 6
FI 70211 Kuopio

Dr. P. VINEIS
Dept. of Biomedical Sciences
and Human Oncology,
Univ of Turin
Via Santena 7
IT 10126 Turin
Phone: +39 11 638484
Fax: +39 11 635267

Dr. R.J.Q. McNALLY
Leukaemia Research
Fund Centre
17 Springfield Mount
UK Leeds, West Yorkshire
LS2 9NG
Phone: +44 0532 333909
Fax: +44 0532 426065

Dr. S. RODELLA
Istituto Anatomia Patologica
Policlinico Borgo Roma
IT 37134 Verona
Phone: +39 45 8098137
Fax: +39 45 8098136

Dr. S.S. BAIG
Medical Research
Commission of the
European Communities
Rue de la Loi 200
BE 1049 Brussel
Phone: +32 2 2963437
Fax: +32 2 2955365

NEPHROBLASTOMA CLINICAL TRIAL AND STUDY: SIOP 93-01

Key words
Wilms' tumour, histological morphology, toxicity, Sequelae, nephroblastoma.

Brief description
The main objective of the SIOP Wilms' tumour study is to collect detailed information on unselected patients, recruited from many centres. In this way it is possible to obtain knowledge of the characteristics of the total population of Wilms' tumour to be treated in the co-operative Siop centres. The information includes initial extension of the disease, surgical procedures, gross and histological morphology, treatments, clinical outcome and late consequences of therapy.

A second objective is to refine methods of treatment. This in order to reduce the costs of recovery in terms of toxicity and late Sequelae, expenditures, aefective and social costs i.e. to prevent relapses and subsequent treatments. Also to adapt therapy to the risk, to find new drugs or new modalities of administration: less toxic, more active or of shorter duration.

Furthermore to test treatment hypothesis according to prognostic factors by multicehtric randomized prospective clinical trials When the accrual of the patients allows for it.

SIOP 93-01 is based on the previous Siop studies and on the results of the NWTS protocols.

Project leader:
Dr. Jan DE KRAKER
SIOP Nephroblastoma Trial
and Study Office,
Soc. Intern. d'Oncologie
Pediatrique
Meibergdreef 9
NL 1105 AZ Amsterdam
Phone: +31 20 566 56 97
Fax: +31 20 691 22 31
Contract number: CT941144

Participants:
Prof. P.J. MOE
Barneklinikken
Regionsykehuset 1
NO 7006 Trondheim
Phone: +47 73 998 000
Fax: +47 73 997 322

Dr. J. SANCHEZ
Clinica Vall d'Hebron
Paseo Vall d'Hebron s/n
ES 08035 Barcelona
Phone: +34 3 427 20 00
Fax: +34 3 428 21 71

Dr. NAVAJAS
Seccion de Oncologia,
Hospital de Cruces
Plaza de Cruces
(Cruces-Baracaldo)
ES Bilbao
Phone: +34 4 485 00 86
Fax: +34 4 499 29 45

Dr. P. GARCIA-MIGUEL
Servico de Oncologia
Pediatrica, Hospital La Paz
Paseo de Castellana 261
ES 28046 Madrid
Phone: +34 1 358 26 00
Fax: +34 1 358 25 45

Dr. N. SCHOUTEN
Dept. of Pediatrics,
Academisch Ziekenhuis der
Vrije Universiteit
Postbus 7057
NL 1007 MB Amsterdam
Phone: +31 20 548 22 87
Fax: +31 20 548 22 89

Dr. J.P.M. BÖKKERINK
Kinderoncologisch Centrum,
Sint Radboud Ziekenhuis
Postbus 9101
NL 6500 HB Nijmegen
Phone: +31 80 616 928
Fax: +31 80 540 576

Dr. PEREIRA
Claraziekenhuis
Olympiaweg 350
NL 3078 HT Rotterdam
Phone: +31 10 432 01 00
Fax: +31 10 432 88 09

Dr. MADSEN
Dept. of Pediatrics,
University Hospital,
Haukeland Sykehus
NO 5021 Bergen
Phone: +47 55 975 200
Fax: +47 55 975 147

Dr. T.STOKLAND
Barneavdelingen,
Regionsykehuset i Tromso
NO 9012 Tromso
Phone: +47 77 626 000
Fax: +47 77 626 369

Dr. O. LEJARS
Service Hématologie,
Hôpital Clocheville
49 Boulevard Béranger
FR 37044 Tours
Phone: +33 47 47 47 51
Fax: +33 47 47 37 03

Dr. M.F. TOURNADE
Service de Pédiatrie,
Institut Gustave-Roussy
39 rue Camille Desmoulins
FR 94805 Villejuif
Phone: +33 1 45 59 41 80
Fax: +33 1 45 59 64 51

Dr. W. STERNSCHULTE
Kinderkrankenhaus
Amsterdamer Strasse 59
DE 5000 Köln
Phone: +49 221 7774 1
Fax: +49 221 7774 240

Dr. N. GRAF
Universitätsklinik für
Kinder- und Jugendmedizin
DE 6650 Homburg/Saar
Phone: +49 6841 16 40 20

Prof. A. DONFRANCESCO
Servizio Oncologia Pediatrica
Piazza S. Onofrio 4
IT 00165 Roma
Phone: +39 6 68 59 22 42
Fax: +39 6 68 77 693

Prof. M. CARLI
Centro Leucemie Infantili,
20 Clinica Pediatrica
Via Giustiniani 3
IT 35128 Padova
Phone: +39 49 821 35 79

Dr. F. MECHINAUD
Unité Oncologie Pédiatrique,
CHR de Nantes
FR 44035 Nantes
Phone: +33 40 08 36 10
Fax: +33 40 08 36 08

Dr. A. THYSS
Service d'Hématologie-
Oncologie,
Centre Antoine-Lacassagne
36 Voie Romaine
FR 06054 Nice
Phone: +33 93 81 71 33
Fax: +33 93 53 09 01

Dr. ZUCKER
Service de Pédiatrie
Oncologique, Institut Curie
26 rue d'Ulm
FR 75231 Paris
Phone: +33 1 44 32 45 63
Fax: +33 1 44 32 40 05

Dr. G. LEVERGER
Service de Pédiatrie,
Hôpital Trousseau
26 Av. A. Netter
FR 75012 Paris
Phone: +33 1 44 73 60 62
Fax: +33 1 44 73 65 73

Dr. P. LUTZ
Hospices Civils de
Strasbourg, Pédiatrie 4,
Inst. de Puériculture
Boite Postale 426
FR 67091 Strasbourg
Phone: +33 88 16 10 10

Dr. H. RUBIE
Unité d'Hémato-Oncologie,
CHU Purpan
Avenue de Grande Bretagne
FR 31059 Toulouse
Phone: +33 61 77 20 96
Fax: +33 61 77 77 06

Dr. PLANTAZ
Clinique Médicale,
CHR de Grenoble
BP 217 X
FR 38043 Grenoble
Phone: +33 76 76 55 37

Dr. M.C. DEMAILLE
Centre Oscar Lambret
B.P. 307
FR 59020 Lille
Phone: +33 20 29 59 20
Fax: +33 20 29 59 62

Dr. B. NELKEN
Service de Pédiatrie,
Hôpital Huriez
FR 59037 Lille
Phone: +33 20 44 42 24

Prof. L. DE LUMLEY
Service de Pédiatrie I,
CHU Dupuytren
2 Av. Alexis Carrel
FR 87042 Limoges
Phone: +33 55 05 68 01

M. BRUNAT-MENTIGNY
Service de Pédiatrie,
Centre Léon Bérard
28 rue Laënnec
FR 69373 Lyon
Phone: +33 78 78 26 42
Fax: +33 78 78 27 15

Dr. J.C. GENTET
Service d'Oncologie
Pédiatrique, Hôpital
d'Enfants de la Timone
Boulevard Jean-Moulin
FR 13385 Marseille
Phone: +33 91 38 68 21
Fax: +33 91 38 76 92

Dr. B. PAUTARD
Immunohématologie et
Oncologie Pédiatrie I
Place Victor Pauchet
FR 80000 Amiens
Phone: +33 22 66 80 00

Dr. X. RIALLAND
Service de Pédiatrie A,
CHU Angers
FR 49000 Angers
Phone: +33 41 35 38 63
Fax: +33 41 35 52 91

Dr. E. PLOUVIER
Service de Pédiatrie,
CHU de Besançon
FR 25030 Besançon
Phone: +33 81 66 81 38
Fax: +33 81 66 97 41

Dr. V. PEREL
Service de Pédiatrie,
Hôpital des Engants,
CHU de Bordeaux
168 Cours de l'Argonne
FR 33077 Bordeaux
Phone: +33 56 79 59 62

Dr. BERTHOUC
Service d'Hématologie-
Oncologie, CHU Morvan
FR 29200 Brest
Phone: +33 98 22 33 33

Dr. P. BOUTARD
Service Pédiatrie B,
CHU de Caen
Avenue Georges Clemenceau
FR 14033 Caen
Phone: +33 31 06 44 88

SEARCH FOR GENETIC ALTERATIONS IN RELATION TO THE STEPS OF HUMAN COLORECTAL CARCINOGENESIS

Key words
Genetic alterations, colorectal tumours, precancerous lesions, cytogenetics, karyotypes, c-DNA expression library, immunohistochemistry.

Brief description
Several genetic alterations have been described in colorectal tumours. Despite these significant findings, some of the key events in the process of malignant transformation of the colorectal tissue remain to be defined, since cancer lesions with none of the known genetic alterations have been described and some precancerous lesions may show several of these genetic alterations.

The early stages of colorectal carcinogenesis will be studied by a different approach compared to those that have been followed until now. Based on the identification by cytogenetics of colorectal cancers with normal karyotypes, we plan to construct a c-DNA expression library from those tumours which can be assumed to present the minimal number of genetic alterations. Several of these cancers have already been established as nude mice xenografts and the absence of the known genetic alterations has been verified in some of them. From the absence of deletion it can be hypothesised that there is no recessive loss of function, but potentially the strong expression of a dominant gene, either normal or mutated. The library will be used for differential hybridisation relative to normal mucosa, in order to detect highly expressed genes, specifically in cancers. The screening can then be refined by studying also the differential expression in precancerous adenomatous tissue for a better characterisation of the events involved in the transformation from non invasive to invasive lesions.

Finally, we plan to map the genes by in situ hybridisation on chromosomes and produce monoclonal antibodies to synthetic peptides which will help in the study of tissue expression by immunohistochemistry.

Project leader:
Dr. Bernard DUTRILLAUX
Institut Curie, Section de Biologie
CNRS, URA 620
rue d'Ulm 26
FR 75321 Paris Cédex 05
Phone: +33 1 40 51 66 71
Fax: +33 1 40 51 66 74
Contract number: CT941619

Participants:
Dr. D. SPANDIDOS
Inst. of Biological Research and Biotechnology
National Hellenic Research Foundation
48 Vas. Constantinou Avenue
GR 11635 Athens
Phone: +30 30 1 7241505
Fax: +30 30 1 7241505

Dr. D. LANE
Cancer Research Campaign Laboratories,
Dept. of Biochemistry and Anatomy and
Physiology-Medical Sciences Inst.
The Univ of Dundee
UK Dundee DD1 4HN
Phone: +44 382 231 81 ext 4921
Fax: +44 382 241 17

ANTICANCER DRUG ACTION ON TOPOISOMERASE II: ROLE OF THE TERNARY DNA COMPLEX IN ` DRUG SENSITIVITY AND RESISTANCE

Key words
Antitumour agents, cytotoxic effects, topoisomeraseassociated DNA, anthracyclines, etoposide, teniposide, mitoxantrone, amsacrine, solid tumours, leukaemias, DNA-topo II-drug.

Brief description
Many clinically important antitumour agents are thought to exert their cytotoxic effects by promoting topoisomeraseassociated DNA breakage. The nuclear enzyme topoisomerase II is of particular interest being the target of anthracyclines, etoposide, teniposide, mitoxantrone and amsacrine, agents widely used in the treatment of both solid tumours and leukaemias.

Topo II acts by a double strand DNA break mechanism and we have recently shown is expressed in human cells as two genetically distinct isoforms, a and B.

Anticancer topo II-targetting drugs are known to induce DNA breakage by forming a ternary DNA-topo II-drug complex.

However, the molecular basis of DNA breakage by the ternary complex, the role of a and B isoforms and the subsequent events leading to tumour cell death are poorly understood.

This proposal tackles these areas with the aim of defining the nature of the topo II-drug-DNA complex formed *in vivo* and *in vitro* by known antitumour drugs and by new experimental agents.

This knowledge will be of seminal importance in the rational design of more selective and more potent agents, and in the circumvention of acquired cellular resistance to topo II-inhibitors.

We plan to utilize recombinant human topo IIa and B proteins that we have recently successfully overexpressed in active form.

These proteins together with bacterial topo II (DNA gyrase) provide the basis for detailed studies of the role of drug-sequence specificity in topo Il associated DNA breakage.

Work will focus both on clinically established agents such as etoposide, teniposide, doxorubicin and amsacrine and on quinolone and flavonoid inhibitors.

Methods will be established to examine the mechanism of topo II inhibitors such as ICRF 193 that do not promote topo II-dependent DNA breakage. Drosophila and yeast model systems will be used to examine drug interactions in vivo particularly whether B can function as an intracellular target.

Human topo II proteins bearing candidate resistance mutations will be expressed in yeast to establish their phenotypic effects on yeast growth in the presence of drugs.

The mutant topo II proteins will be purified to allow studies of ternary complexes involving resistant topo II.

Completion of the work will significantly advance understanding of sensitivity and resistance to topo II-directed drugs.

The proposal brings together a consortium of three European groups with diverse and complementary experience that can rival work in the United States in this key therapeutic area.

This will provide a strategic base for joint projects with European companies with intcrests in developing antitumour agents.

Project leader:
Dr. Larry Mark FISHER
St. Georges Hospital Medical School,
Cellular and Molecular Sciences
Cranmer Terrace
UK London SW17 ORE
Phone: +44 81 672 99 44
Fax: +44 81 784 70 92
Contract number: CT941318

Participants:
Dr. C.A. AUSTIN
Dept. of Biochemistry and Genetics,
The Medical School of the University
UK Newcastle upon Tyne NE2 4HH
Phone: +44 91 222 8864
Fax: +44 91 222 7424

Dr. G. CAPRANICO
Div. of Experimental Oncology,
Istituto Nazionale per lo Studio
e la Cura dei Tumori
Via G. Venezian 1
IT 20133 Milano
Phone: +39 2 2390203
Fax: +39 2 2362692

THE USE OF SINGLE CHAIN-FV RECOMBINANT ANTIBODIES CONJUGATED WITH RADIOACTIVE TRACERS AND PHOTOSENSITIZERS IN RADIOIMMUNOIMAGING AND SELECTIVE IMMUNO-PHOTODYNAMIC THERAPY OF INTRAOCULAR TUMOURS: APPLICATIONS TO OCULAR MELANOMA AND RETINOBLASTOMA

Key words
Radioactive tracers, uveal melanoma, retinoblastoma, laser photocoagulation, ocular melanoma, antimelanoma, antiretinoblastoma single chain Fv, radioimmunoimaging.

Brief description
Monoclonal antibodies tagged with radioactive tracers and drugs have been widely used, in the past, for diagnostic and therapeutic purposes against cancer, with a variable but still unsatisfactory success rate. The recombinant DNA technology has recently made available new promising antibodies or antibody fragment molecules, such as single chain-Fv, that show a number of advantages when compared to the old monoclonal antibodies. Furthermore, single chain-Fv antibodies can be easily tagged with different molecules such as radiolabeled tracers and photosensitisers. This aspect is particularly appealing if we consider some of the most important intraocular tumors, such as uveal melanoma and retinoblastoma, together with the currently available therapeutic modalites. The theoretical framework behind the present proposal is represented by the possibility of using the advantages of the currently available antibody production technologies in order to get new, powerful carriers that, by exploiting the antibody specificity for selected tumor antigens, can deliver different molecules directly into the tumor site for both diagnostic and therapeutic purposes.

Furthermore, since Laser photocoagulation is one of the currently used therapeutic procedures for both ocular melanoma and retinoblastoma, the conjugation of specific antimelanoma and/or antiretinoblastoma single chain Fv antibodies, with photosensitisers, could theoretically open new appealing prospectives in the conservative treatment of both tumors by allowing an extremely selective intervention with laser activation of the photosensitisers brought into the tumor site by the specific single chain Fv antibody.

The main aim of the present project is, therefore, to exploit the new antibody production technology in order to:

a improve the current radioimmunoimaging techniques for the detection and monitoring of intraocular melanoma;

b improve the therapeutic approaches against the two most common tumors of the eye (melanoma and retinoblastoma) in terms of preservation of visual function, reduction of complications, implementation of safe and less invasive anticancer therapies, increasing of the quality of life.

Because of its innovative potential, the objective in section (b) will be considered high-priority.

Project leader:
Professor Renato FREZZOTTI
Institute of Ophthalmological
and Neurosurgical Sciences,
Nuovo Policlinico "Le Scotte"
Viale Bracci
IT 53100 Siena
Phone: +39 577 284 183
Fax: +39 577 289 331
Contract number: CT941266

Participants:
E. BALESTRAZZI
Eye Clinic Univ of L'Aquila
San Salvatore Hospital Viale Nizza
IT 67100 L'Aquila
Phone: +39 862 778427
Fax: +39 862 433333

G. WINTER
Cambridge Centre for Protein Engineering,
Medical Research Council Centre
Hills Road
UK Cambridge CB2 2QH
Phone: +44 223 402110
Fax: +44 223 402140

M. NARDI
Inst. of Ophthalmology
Via Roma 65
IT 56100 Pisa
Phone: +39 50 553431
Fax: +39 50 592018

P.NERI
Dept. of Molecular Biology
Nuovo Policlinico Le Scotte, Viale Bracci
IT 53100 Siena
Phone: +39 577 41121
Fax: +39 577 263302

S. LIARIKOS
Eye Dept. St. Savvas Hospital,
Greek Anticancer Inst.
Alexandras Ave. 171
GR Athens
Phone: +30 1 6430811
Fax: +30 1 6420146

OPTIMIZATION OF PROCEDURES FOR TREATMENT OF HAEMATOLOGIC MALIGNANCIES BY BONE MARROW TRANSPLANTATION FROM VOLUNTEER DONORS

Key words
Bone marrow transplantation (BMT).

Brief description
Bone marrow transplantation (BMT) has proved to be the most promising method for treatment of patients with malignant and premalignant haematologic disorders. More than 50 percent of patients with otherwise lethal haematological malignancies, are alive and well free of disease 10 years after BMT. In 1990, 2000 allogenic bone marrow transplants using matched sibling donors were performed in Europe. Since about 65 percent of patients with an indication for BMT lack sibling donors, several thousand searches have been made in order to find matched unrelated volunteers. Despite an impressive search activity only 180 unrelated-donor BMTs were performed in Europe in 1990 and 220 in 1991. This contrasts with the potential of many thousands, at least as many as are now receiving sibling-donor BMT, if an unrelated volunteer donor had been available through a more effective search process. The Project Managing Group of the Concerted Action programme "Treatment of Haematological Malignancies by BMT from Volunteer Donors" has addressed several of the problems involved and has recently provided means to speed up donor searches and co-ordinate donor pools. New methods for rapid HLA matching have been developed. However, there are still numerous problems to be solved in order to maximize the number of patients that can receive an allogenic bone marrow graft from an unrelated donor. The following problems have been identified:

1 Problems concerning donor pools:
- The chance of finding a donor depends on the frequency and distribution of recipient phenotypes within the donor pool. As an example, minorities do not benefit from a large pool of donors if they are not represented in the pool.
- The total number of volunteer donors available in Europe is insufficient to meet demand.
- Of the techniques in routine use serology lacks precision on class splits identified biochemically, and class II-alleles identified DNA methods.
- The access to donor pools varies. There are different ethical, legal and financial requirements.

2 Problems with coordination of search and lack of search prognosis index
- Currently, a search starts with access to a national donor registry. An international search cannot easily be initiated by simultaneously contacting all existing registries.
- There is no common language in all donor registries, neither has documentation been standardised.
- There is no standardisation for criteria for initiating or terminating searches. Searches for rare HLA phenotypes are time-consuming for registry staff, slowing down other searches that may be successful.
- A search prognosis index which could predict a successful search for individual patients has not been established.
- The lack of total computerised coordination slows down the process, which in turn increases the risk for patients to succumb before a donor is identified.

3 Problems in clinical evaluation
- It is uncertain who are ideal candidates for unrelated BMT. Therefore, unsuccessful transplants use up too much time of the resources for the transplant teams.
- Clear guidelines have yet to be established for disease type, stage and subtype.
- A number of BMT treatment protocols are available and it remains to be established which are best for unrelated donor BMT. The optimal conditioning regimens and optimal approaches to GVHD prevention still need to be defined.
- The influence and precision of matching for class I, II and III HLA antigens are poorly defined. It is necessary to obtain information on suitability of different matching techniques with emphasis on speed and on the influence of level of HLA matching on BMT survival, engraftment, GVHD and relapse.
- Socio-economic factors for and consequences of BMT are not sufficiently known.

Project leader:
Professor Gösta GAHRTON
Karolinska Institutet,
Huddinge University Hospital
SE 14186 Huddinge
Phone: +46 8 746 10 00
Fax: +46 8 774 87 25
Contract number: CT940300

Participants:
Prof. John GOLDMAN
Haematology Department,
Royal Postgraduate
Medical School
Ducane Road
UK London W12 0H2
Phone: +44 81 740 3238
Fax: +44 81 740 9679

Prof. W. HINTERBERGER
Interconvention Kongress-
organisationsge. m.b.H.
Am Hubertusdamm 6
AT 1223 Wien
Phone: +43 222 23 69 640
Fax: +43 222 23 69 648

Prof. Norbert-Claude GORIN
Hématologie, Unité de Auto-
greffes de Moelle, Centre
Hospitalier Saint-Antoine
184 Rue du Faubourg Saint-
Antoine
FR 75571 Paris Cedex 12
Phone: +33 1 434 433 33
Fax: +33 1 434 455 01

Prof. Alain FISCHER
Dépt. de Pédiatrie, Hôpital
Necker Enfants Malades
FR 75015 Paris
Phone: +33 1 4273 8302
Fax: +33 1 4273 2896

Dr. Andrea BACIGALUPO
Dept. of Hematology,
Ospedale San Martino
IT 16132 Genova
Phone: +39 10 3535 2148
Fax: +39 10 355583

Prof. A. H. GOLDSTONE
Dept. of Haematology,
University College Hospital
Gower Street
UK London WC1E 6AU
Phone: +44 71 387 6424
Fax: +44 71 380 9911

Dr. Fulvio PORTA
Dept. of Pediatrics,
University of Brescia
c/o Spedali Civili
IT 25123 Brescia
Phone: +39 30 399 5712
Fax: +39 30 303 658

Prof. A. E. GLUCKMAN
Hopitaux de Paris, Hopital
Saint-Louis, Centre Hayem
2 Place du Doc. A. Fournier
FR 75010 Paris
Phone: +33 1 42499644
Fax: +33 1 42492699

Dr. Colette RAFFOUX
Association Greffe de Moelle
France Transplant, Siège
Social, Hopital Saint-Louis
2 Place du Doc. A. Fournier
FR 75475 Paris Cedex 10
Phone: +33 1 4249 4070
Fax: +33 1 4803 0202

Prof. Ben BRADLEY
UKTS
Southmead
UK Bristol BS10 5ND
Phone: +44 272 50 77 77
Fax: +44 272 50 89 78

Dr. Jill M. HOWS
Immuno-Haematology,
Blood Transfusion,
Hammersmith Hospital
Du Cane Road
UK London W12 0NN
Phone: +44 81 743 2030
Fax: +44 81 740 3169

Prof. Jon J. VAN ROOD
Dept. of Immunohaematology
and Bloodbank, Academisch
Ziekenhuis Leiden
Postbus 9600
NL 2300 RC Leiden
Phone: +31 71 26 3802/9111
Fax: +31 71 21 6751

Dr. Louis ERRAZQUIN
Hospital Universitas
V. Macaraena
Avenida Dr. Edriani
ES 410071 Sevilla
Phone: +34 54 378 400
Fax: +34 54 377 573

Prof. Alois GRATWHOHL
Dept. Innere Medizin,
Abteilung Haematologie,
Kantonspital Basel
Petergraben 47
CH 4031 Basel
Phone: +41 61 265 2525
Fax: +41 61 265 4450

DEVELOPMENT OF MOLECULAR CYTOGENETIC DIAGNOSTICS FOR HEMATOLOGICAL MALIGNANCIES WITH IMPLICATIONS FOR THERAPY

Key words
Molecular cytogenetic diagnostics, hematological malignancies, chromosomal aberrations, t(11q23), t/inv(16), PCR/FISH.

Brief description
The main objective of the present CA is to develop molecular cytogenetic diagnostics in hematological malignancies, and as a consequence improve patient therapy.

The emphasis is on the characterization of specific molecular genetic rearrangements caused by chromosomal aberrations and their detection using highly sensitive techniques, such as PCR, PFGE, Southern blot, or interphase cytogenetics (FISH) with cosmids or YAC probes which lay in the vicinity of the breakpoints.

Three interacting and complementary approaches will be followed:

1 Creation or exploitation of infrastructural facilities: firstly, making molecular clones of various sizes available for research and routine diagnosis, and secondly, developing a data base of the many tumor cell banks of the participating laboratories, in order to provide research scientists with samples of rare chromosomal abnormalities.

2 Fundamental molecular investigations focussed on specific chromosomal aberrations, in particular t(11q23), t/inv(16), and various other chromosomal deletions or translocations. The analysis of rare recurrent translocations and other aspects of leukemogenesis such as genomic risk factors, the role of imprinting, etc., can only be addressed in multinational studies with a large intake of well characterized patient material.

3 Screening of cohorts of patients with molecular techniques (PCR/FISH) in conjunction with cytogenetics and evaluation of diagnostic efficiency based on large international treatment trials.

The 11 participants to the CA are from prominent cytogenetics laboratories, involved in karyotyping of hematological malignancies and major referral centers for national programs.

They carry on research into molecular rearrangements of genes in a number of tumor specific chromosome aberrations, their role in leukemogenesis as well as the development of alternative diagnostic tools and their clinical application.

The expected results are a major improvement of genetic diagnosis, new insight in leukemogenesis and in the role of new oncogenes, new data on risk factors, and improvement of the EC tumor cell bank resources.

Project leader:
Dr. A. HAGEMEIJER
Institute of Genetics, Medical Faculty,
Erasmus Universiteit Rotterdam
Dr. Molewaterplein 50
NL 3015 GE Rotterdam
Phone: +31 10 408 71 96
Fax: +31 10 436 02 25
Contract number: CT941703

Participants:

Dr. A. BIONDI
Clinica Pediatrica Universitá di Milano,
Hospital St. Gerardo
106 Via Donizetti
IT 20052 Monza
Phone: +39 39 363 3525
Fax: +39 39 230 1646

Dr. F. BIRG & Dr. M. LAFAGE
Unité 119 INSERM,
Institut Paoli-Calmette
27 Bd. Leï Roure
FR 13009 Marseille
Phone: +33 91 758 419
Fax: +33 91 260 364

Dr. G. ALIMENA
Univ of Roma La Sapienza, Dept. of
Human Biopathology, Section Hematology
Via Benvenuto 6
IT 00161 Roma
Phone: +39 6 44 230 920
Fax: +39 6 44 241 948

Dr. H. LEHRACH
Imperial Cancer Research Fund (ICRF),
Laboratory of Genome Analysis
44 Lincoln's Inn Fields, P.O. Box 123
UK London WC2A 3PX
Phone: +44 71 269 3308
Fax: +44 71 269 3068

Dr. M.H. BREUNING
State Univ Leiden, Dept. of
Human Genetics, Sylvius Laboratory
Wassenaarseweg 72
NL 2333 AL Leiden
Phone: +31 71 276 048
Fax: +31 71 276 075

Dr. O. HAAS
Children's Cancer Research Inst. (CCRI),
St. Anna Children's Hospital
Kinderspital Gasse 6
AT 1090 Vienna
Phone: +43 1 404 70 406
Fax: +43 1 408 72 30

Dr. R. BERGER
Unité 301 INSERM, Institut
de Génétique Moléculaire
27 Rue Juliette Dodu
FR 75010 Paris
Phone: +33 1 4249 9266
Fax: +33 1 4206 9531

Prof. B.D. YOUNG
Imperial Cancer Research Fund (ICRF),
Dept. of Medical Oncology
45 Little Britain
UK London EC1A 7BE
Phone: +44 71 600 8814
Fax: +44 71 796 3979

Prof. Dr. C FONATSCH
Medical Univ of Lübeck,
Inst. of Human Genetics Section,
Tumor Cytogenetics
Ratzeburger Allee 160
DE 23538 Lübeck
Phone: +49 451 500 2629
Fax: +49 451 500 2995

Prof. F. PASQUALI
Univ of Pavia, Dept. of
Human Pathology and Genetics
14 Via Forlanini
IT Pavia
Phone: +39 382 507 519
Fax: +39 382 525 030

EUROPEAN FIBREOPTIC SIGMOIDOSCOPIC TRIAL: IMPROVING THE SENSITIVITY OF SCREENING FOR COLORECTAL CANCER

Key words

Faecal occult blood, sigmoidoscopy, colorectal cancer.

Brief description

The European Multi-centre randomised control trial for faecal occult blood testing alone compared with faecal occult blood testing and flexible sigmoidoscopy was commenced in 1992. In each participating Centre persons aged 50-74 living in the local community and eligible for colorectal cancer screening have been identified.

Permission of the local Ethical Committees have been obtain and the subjects randomised into two groups:

Group 1 will be offered flexible sigmoidoscopy and a faecal occult blood test.

Group 2 will be offered a faecal occult blood test alone. In the Group offered flexible sigmoidoscopy, the measurement of interest is the proportion of neoplasia detected in people where faecal occult blood tests have been negative, so enabling the sensitivity of faecal occult blood test relative to sigmoidoscopy to be estimated and thereby show the additional yield obtained by adding sigmoidoscopy to the existing screening procedure. If the yield of neoplasia in the flexible sigmoidoscopy group is sufficiently great to suggest mortality advantage the design of the study is such that it could be expanded into a randomised trial to measure the size of such a gain. This trial has been supported by the European Community. It is essential, if it is to be successful, that the participants meet on a regular basis and this Application is for funding to enable six monthly meetings of the participants to take place.

Project leader:
Professor J.D. HARDCASTLE
Dept. of Surgery,
University of Nottingham,
Queen's Medical Centre
UK Nottingham NG7 2UH
Phone: +44 602 709245
Fax: +44 602 709428
Contract number: CT941502

Participants:

Mr. J.R. REYNOLDS
Consultant Surgeon
Derbyshire Royal Infirmary
London Road
UK Derby DE1 2QY
Phone: +44 0332 347141

Mr. K. VELLACOTT
Consultant Surgeon Royal
Gwent Hospital
Cardiff Road - Newport
UK Gwent NP9 2UB
Phone: +44 0633 252244

Mr. V. MOSHAKIS
Consultant Surgeon George
Eliot Hospital
College Street
UK Nuneaton CV10 7DJ
Phone: +44 0203 351351

Prof. J. CHAMBERLAIN
CSEU, Inst. of Cancer
Research, D Block
15 Cotswold Road, Belmont
UK Sutton, Surrey SM2 5NG
Phone: +44 081 643 8901
Fax: +44 081 770 7876

Prof. O. KRONBORG
Dept. of Surgical
Gastroenterology,
Odense Univ Hospital
DK 5000 Odense C
Phone: +45 6611 3333
Fax: +45 6613 2854

Prof. S. BESBEAS
Hellenic Cancer Society
18-20A, Tsoha Street
GR Athens 115 21
Phone: +30 1 689 7478
Fax: +30 1 642 1022

THE RAT AS A MODEL ORGANISM IN
HUMAN BIOMEDICAL RESEARCH

Key words
Polymorphic genetic markers, rat physical map, rat linkage map, rat chromosome 5, FISH, PFGE.

Brief description
The proposal is focused on further development of the rat as an experimental model organism for human polygenic diseases, such as hypertension, diabetes, obesity, mental disorders and cancer. Recent advances have already shown that the rat has great potential as a model organism, but full exploitation of the system is hampered by the lack of a well-developed integrated gene map and the limited availability of informative polymorphic genetic markers. However, now there is remedies for both of these drawbacks, and considerable progress has already been made.

The proposed research includes the development of both the rat physical map and the rat linkage map, as well as the amalgamation of the two. We will attempt to sublocalize anchor marker to each chromosome. These anchor loci will be selected in such a way to provide the best possible foundation for comparative mapping, ie the comparison of rat genome structure with other species such as mouse and man. Available data on comparative mapping indicate that there is a high degree of conservation of genome structure among mammals. This is important when studying model systems, because comparative mapping is the key to ascertaining that the genes studied in the model system, really correspond to specific genes in humans.

Within the present project We also want to apply the rat model system to some specific scientific questions involving the rat tumor suppressor gene Sail. Using deletion mapping this suppressor gene has been sublocalized to a specific region of rat chromosome 5. We want to use FISH and PFGE analysis, as well as insertion mutagenesis to try to finely map the region around the Sail gene, in order to ultimately isolate and characterize it. Comparative mapping studies clearly suggest that this important tumor suppressor gene has homologs both in the mouse and in man.

We have collaborations with numerous groups in Europe and elsewhere, who are using the rat as a valuable tool in human biomedical research. The usefulness of this tool would greatly increase oE the proposed research is carried out.

Project leader:
Professor Göran LEVAN
Department of Genetics,
University of Gothenburg
Guldhedsgatan 23
SE 413 90 Gothenburg
Phone: +46 31 773 32 90
Fax: +46 31 82 62 86
Contract number: CT941742

Participants:
Prof. Claude SZPIRER
Dept. of molecular biologie,
Université Libre de Bruxelles
67 Rue des Chevaux
BE 1640 Rhode-St-Genese
Phone: +32 2 650 9623
Fax: +32 2 650 9625

Prof. Hans J. HEDRICH
Institut für Versuchstier-
kunde und Zentrales Tier-
laboratorium, Medizinische
Hochschule Hannover
DE 30623 Hannover
Phone: +49 511 532 6567
Fax: +49 511 532 3710

FUNCTION OF TUMOUR GENES IN DROSOPHILA AND XIPHO-PHORUS AND THEIR HOMOLOGUES IN MAMMALIAN CANCER

Key words
Drosophila, xiphophorus, genes controlling cell proliferation, melanoma, Tu, autosomal locus Differentiation, tumour Suppressor gene, membrane receptor tyrosine kinase, EGF-receptor.

Brief description
The proposed Concerted Action takes aim to develop a network of researchers studying cancer genetics in animal model systems such as the fruitfly Drosophila and the fish xiphophorus so that the knowledge gained from the analysis of the cancer qenes-isolated in these organisms can be used for unraveling the mechanisms leading to human oncogenesis. Neoplams are not limited to humans but occur throughout the animal kingdom, from the most primitive metazoa to invertebrates and vertebrates. In higher vertebrates, cancer can arise in any organ of the body, whereas further down the phylogenic scale neoplasia seems to affect far fewer tissues. Some of these organisms, such as the fruitfly Drosophiila and the fish Xiphophorus, are very suitable for genetic analysis-and for-studying genes controlling cell proliferation and differentiation. Because of their relatively short life span and ease of rearing in laboratory these animals have proven to be useful for studying genetic mechanisms of neoplasia.

Genetic and molecular studies of Drosophila have shown that tumorigenesis may arise from inactivation of sin genes. Currently 40 genes causing tissue overgrowth are known in Drosophila and recent saturation mutagenesis of the 2nd chromosome-of drosophila performed by the applying investigators have led to the identification-of 17 new tumour genes. These genes are presently under genetic, biological and molecular studies among the cooperating research groups. Melanomas of genetic origin develop in interspecies hybrids of the fish Xiphophorus. The melanoma appears when a sex-linked chromosomal gene (Tu) is present among the progeny animals lacking an autosomal locus Differentiation, which acts as a tumour Suppressor gene. A sequence encoding a membrane receptor tyrosine kinase, similar to the EGF-receptor, has been shown to correspond to the Tu gene.

The long-term purpose of the present co-operation is to use the cloned Drosophila sequences for isolating evolutionary conserved sequences in the xiphophorus and human genomes With the perspective that the homologous Sequences may play equally important role in the etiology of human diseases, such as cancer. In addition, the study in xiphophorus of genes related to tumour suppressor genes of Drosophila may-help to understand the function of these genes during vertebrate-development and their

Project leader:
Professor Bernard MECHLER
Dept. of Developmental Genetics,
Deutsches Krebsforschungszentrum
Im Neuenheimer Feld 280
DE 69120 Heidelberg
Phone: +49 622 1424502
Fax: +49 622 1474623
Contract number: CT941572

Participants:

Dr. A. GARCIA-BELLIDO
Centro de Biologia Molecular,
Universidad Autonoma Facultad de Ciencias
Canto Blanco
ES 28049 Madrid
Phone: +34 1 397 41 29
Fax: +34 1 397 87 32

Dr. I. KISS
Dept. of Genetics, Biological Research Center,
Hungarian Academy of Sciences
Temesvari krt. 62, P.O. Box 521
HU Szeged 6701
Phone: +36 62 43 22 32
Fax: +36 62 43 35 03

Dr. I. RASKA
Academy of Sciences of Czech Republic,
Inst. of Experimental Medicine
Albertov 4
CZ 128 000 Praha 2
Phone: +422 29 45 90
Fax: +422 29 45 90

Dr.C. BRACK
Biozentrum der Universität Basel
Klingelbergstrasse 70
CH 4056 Basel
Phone: +41 37 22 96 22
Fax: +41 61 267 20 78

Monsieur le Docteur R. OLLO
Institut Pasteur
24 rue du Docteur Roux
FR 75724 Paris Cedex 15
Phone: +33 1 45 68 85 19
Fax: +33 1 45 68 85 21

Prof. Dr. J.B. MONJO
Departemento de Genétics, Facultad de Biologia,
Universidad de Barcelona
Av. Diagonal 645
ES 08071 Barcelona
Phone: +34 402 14 98
Fax: +34 411 09 69

Prof. Dr. M. SCHARTL
Theodor-Boveri-Institut für Biowissenschaften,
Biozentrum, Universität Würzburg,
Physiologische Chemie I
Am Hubland
DE 97074 Würzburg
Phone: +49 931 888 41 57
Fax: +49 931 888 41 50

Prof. D.M. GLOVER
CRF Laboratories, Dept. of Biochemistry
Medical Sciences Inst.
UK Dundee DD1 4HN
Phone: +44 382 30 77 93
Fax: +44 382 34 42 13

EVOLUTION OF THE STOMACH WITH CHRONIC GASTRITIS WITH A PARTICULAR EMPHASIS ON DISEASE MARKERS FOR PEPTIC ULCER AND PREMALIGNANT CONDITIONS

Key words

Helicobacter pylori, chronic gastritis, peptic ulcer, atrophic gastritis, gastric cancer, paucisymptomatic, immune response, pathogenic characteristics, cytotoxins, adhesins.

Brief description

Recent literature described the causal association between a newly discovered bacterium, helicobacter pylori, and chronic gastritis. Chronic gastritis is a life-long process which can:

1 evolve towards peptic ulcer disease, atrophic gastritis - a precursor of gastric cancer - or;

2 stay asymptomatic or paucisymptomatic. H. Pylori is a condition necessary but not sufficient for the evolution toward the disease previously mentioned.

The objective of this project is to study the natural history of the stomach with chronic gastritis and, in particular to identify markers of an evolution toward peptic ulcer or atrophic gastritis. The factors explored will be environmental (H. Pylori infection, smoking, diet, etc.), host dependent (immune response in igg, iga, igm, and response to different anti-gens, antral metaplasia in the duodenum, change in gastric physiology) or dependent on the pathogenic characteristics of H. Pylori strains (cytotoxins, adhesins, etc.).

The method will consist of a 3 year cohort study with a nested case-control study. Inclusion will concern successive out-patients (30-60 y) consulting for non ulcer dyspepsia. At inclusion they will have a panel of tests on biopsy specimens, blood samples, and a breath test and a questionnaire will be filled out. There will be a yearly follow-up. The expected number of patients to be included is 2,700 (100/centre) during a 6 month period in order to analyze the results of 2,000, with an expected number of peptic ulcer of 75 to 100 and 150 to 200 cases of atrophic gastritis. Twenty-seven centres distributed in 15 countries will include patients in order to have an adequate representation of europe (1 centre per 15 million inhabitants of less for smaller countries). Several tests will be performed in centralized facilities also in different countries : detection of cytotoxins (Italy), adhesins (Sweden), gastrin hormones (Germany), H. Pylori serology (France) and breath test (UK). A panel of histo-pathologists will review the slides when necessary.

The coordination will be handled from bordeaux. A steering committee will be formed with some of the participants. The data will be analyzed as soon as they arrive in order to provide updated summaries.

Peptic ulcer and gastric cancer are still frequent diseases in Europe. The possibility of eradicating H. Pylori with antimicrobial agents does exist and would lead to a dramatic decrease in the morbidity and mortality due to these diseases. however, it is not conceivable to treat everyone suffering from chronic gastritis and, therefore, it is important to determine the subpopulation which could benefit from such a treatment because of additional factors present. It is, a unique situation where an intervention would be possible only by changing the guidelines currently used by physicians regarding the dyspeptic patient. This would be an important achievement in relation to the health of the european population and an important social and economic benefit taking into account the loss of work, cost of treatment (antiulcer agents are among the most sold drugs in the world) and hospitalisations. Because of the large number of patients needed, such a study cannot be performed under another form than a multicentre study.

Project leader:
Professor F. MEGRAUD
INSERM U330, Université
de Bordeaux 2
146 rue Léo Saignat
FR 33076 Bordeaux
Phone: +33 567 959 10
Fax: +33 567 959 87
Contract number: CT941569

Participants:
Dr. A.B. PRICE
Dept. of Pathology, North-
wick Park Hospital and CRC
UK Middlesex HA1 3UJ

Dr. A.F. MENTIS
Bacteriology Dept.,
Hellenic Inst. Pasteur
GR 115 21 Athens

Dr. A.M. HIRSCHL
Abt. f. Klinische Mikrobiolo-
gie des Hygiene Inst. AKH
AT 1090 Wien

Dr. B.J. RATHBONE
Gastroenterology Leicester
UK Leicester LE1 5WW

Dr. E.A.J. RAUWS
Dept. of Gastroenterology
Academic Medical Center
NL 1105 AZ Amsterdam

Dr. G. BÖRSCH
Dept. of Internal Medicine
Elisabeth Hospital
DE 4300 Essen

Dr. J. Claude DEBONGNIE
Dept de Gastroentérologie,
BE St. Pierre d'Ottignies

Dr. L. ANDERSEN
Dept. of Clinical Microbio-
logy, Statens Serum Inst.
DK 2300 Copenhagen S

Dr. N. FIGURA
Instituto di Patologia Speciale
IT 53100 Siena

Dr. P. MICHETTI
Div. of Gastroenterology
CH 1011 Lausanne

Dr. P. SIPPONEN
Dept. of Pathology,
Jorvi Hospital
FI 02740 Espoo

Dr. R.I. RUSSEL
Gastroenterology Unit,
UK Glasgow G31 2ER

Dr. H. LAMOULIATTE
Service des Maladies de
l'Appareil Digestif,
Hôpital Saint André
FR 33075 Bordeaux

Dr. K. TAMASSY
Semmelweis Medical Univ
HU 1125 Budapest

Prof. H. BOSSECKERT
Clinic of Internal Medicine
DE 6902 Jena

Prof. A. BLASI
Instituto di Medicina,
Interna Ospedale Garibaldi
IT 95123 Catania

Prof. BRETAGNE
Service de Gastroentérologie
Hôpital Ponchaillou
FR 35000 Rennes

Prof. B. FIXA
2nd Dept. of Internal
Medicine, Charles Univ
CZ Hradec Kralove

Prof. C. O'MORAIN
Consultant Clinic,
Charlemont Mall
IE Dublin 2

Prof. G. GASBARRINI
Instituto de Clinica Medica
Universita Catolica
IT 0032 Roma

Prof. H.I. MAAROOS
Dept. of Internal Medicine
EE 2400 Tartu

Prof. I. A. MIRAVE
Hospital Virgen de Azanzaru
ES San Sebastian

Prof. J. D. de KORWIN
Service de Médecine D,
Hôpital de Brabois
FR 54511 Vandoeuvre Cédex

Prof. J. GUERRE
Service d'Hépato-Gasto-
Entérologie, CHU Cochin
FR 75674 Paris Cedes 14

Prof. J. MONES
Hospital Santa Creu i
Sant Pau Autonomous Univ
ES 08025 Barcelona

J.M. PAJARES GARCIA
Gastroenterologia Hospital
de la Princesa
ES 28006 Madrid

Prof. KNAPIK
Dept. and Clinic of
Gastroenterology Medical
Univ of Wroclaw
PL 50-326 Wroclaw

Prof. M.G. QUINA
Hospital de Pulido Valente
PT 1799 Lisboa

Prof. P. MALFERTHEINER
Universitätsklinik Bonn
DE 5300 Bonn 1

Prof. R. NACCARATO
Divisone di Gastroenterologia
Cattedra Malattie Apparato
IT 35128 Padova

Prof. T. WADSTRÖM
Dept. of Med. Microbiology
Univ of Lund
SE 22 362 Lund

STUDY FOR THE EVALUATION OF NEUROBLASTOMA SCREENING IN EUROPE (SENSE)

Key words
Neuroblastoma, epidemiological evaluation, infant screening.

Brief description
This proposal is concerned with an application for funds for the coordination and development of a European study to evaluate the effectiveness of screening infants for neuroblastoma, the most common solid tumour of childhood.

Whole population screening for neuroblastoma was introduced in Japan in 1985. following favourable pilot studies in Kyoto and Sapporo cities. Unfortunately, however. because of the lack of an appropriate epidemiological evaluation of the infant screening the question as to whether neuroblastoma screening has saved lives in Japan remains unanswered.

An evaluative study is currently under way in Quebec, Canada, in which children are being screened at both 3 weeks and 6 months of age. The results of this study will be available in 1996, though it is now widely considered that screening children at over the age of 1 year will have a greater impact on mortality, and it is with the evaluation of this later screening that the current proposal is principally concerned. All the European screening groups involved have extensive experience of screening for neuroblastoma within their own regions. However, the implementation of an International controlled trial of neuroblastoma screening requires considerable planning and development. Since evaluation is only possible with a very large screened population (approx. 1000,000 babies) a European collaborative trial is clearly essential. The group has been meeting twice a year for the past 2 years and aims to begin the screening phase of the project in 1994.

Project leader:
Dr. Louise PARKER
Univ. of Newcastle-upon-
Tyne, Children's Cancer Unit
(Child Health),
The Medical School
Framlington Place
UK Newcastle-upon-Tyne
NE2 4HH
Phone: +44 91 222 69 58
Fax: +44 91 222 62 22
Contract number: CT941398

Participants:
Dr. A. JENKNER
Div.e di Oncologia Pediatrica
and Laboratorio di Analisi
e Microbiologia
Ospedale Pediatrico Bambino
Gesü
IT Rome

Dr. F.H. SCHILLING
Pilot Center Olg-Hospital,
Pediatric Center
Bismarckstr 8
DE 7000 Stuttgart

Dr. R. ERTTMAN
Dept. Pediatric Hematology
and Oncology,
Univ Children's Hospital
Martinstrasse 52
DE 2000 Hamburg 20

Dr. R. KERBI
Graz Laboratory,
Dept. of Pediatrics
Univ of Graz
AT Graz

Prof. F. BERTHOLD
Children's Hospital
of Cologne
DE Koln

Prof. S.O. LIE
Bameklinikken
Rikshopitalet
NO Oslo

Prof. T. PHILIP
Association pour le Depistage
du Neuroblastome Service
de Biologie du CHS
95 Boulvard Pinel
FR 69677 Broncedex

CHROMOSOMAL ABNORMALITIES AND ALTERED EXPRESSION OF HOMEOBOX CONTAINING GENES IN HUMAN CANCERS: ARE THESE PATTERNS COORDINATED?

Key words
Epigenetic alterations, oncogenes, tumour suppressor genes, chromosome aberrations, HOX (homebox) genes, cytogenetics, lung cancers, colorectal cancers, melanomas, gliomas, karyotype, IICB, neoplastic, cytogenetic, S-phase fraction.

Brief description
Genomic changes are the most common feature of cancer cells. Epigenetic alterations may also contribute to change the expression of genes. In several cases, the role of oncogenes, and/or tumour suppressor genes can be demonstrated.

However, in the majority of tumours, there is no specific genetic change, but complexe patterns of alterations, making it difficult to assign them a precise role in the tumourigenesis.

The aim of this project is to improve our understanding of two types of alterations observed in human tumours:

1 chromosome aberrations, and;

2 changes in the expression of the HOX (homeobox) genes, a network of developmentally regulated genes.

Both events can independently be linked to the stage of tumour progression (localized or metastasized).

Our two laboratories arrived independently at the same interpretations, using different approaches (HOX genes, Naples, cytogenetics, Paris): cancers evolve according to determined patterns which involve non random genetic events.

Given the organization of the HOX gene family in restricted regions of 4 chromosomes (7, 17, 12, 2) often affected by alterations, we intend to study, in 4 human tumours (small cell lung cancers, colorectal cancers, melanomas, gliomas) the relationships between chromosomal rearrangements and the changes of HOX gene expression, as a function of their chromosomal location and to determine whether HOX gene methylation is involved in these events.

The tumours will be collected at Institut Curie, established in short-term cultures for karyotype, amplified by grafting into nude mice, for RNA and DNA extractions.

First analyses of the expression of a panel of 38 HOXgenes (IICB, Naples) from normal tissues and their neoplastic counterparts indicate that overall patterns of HOX gene expressions could be characteristic for each tissue, more HOX gene expression may lead to identify specific pattern(s) of alterations in tumours.

Chromosome alterations correlate with the stage of tumour progression, demonstrating in some tumours a close relationship between cytogenetic evolution, increase of S-phase fraction and histological data (Institut Curie, Paris).

Chromosome alterations do not occur at random, accumulate during tumour progression following a limited number of paths which may delineate tumour subsets, with different prognoses.

The exact meaning of these chromosome changes remains to be deciphered. The HOX genes have the particularity to form multiple gene clusters, with a fairly well organized cascade of expression.

A chromosome loss or gain could lead to extinction or increase of transcription units. Therefore, it is particularly interesting to look for a possible coordinated modification of chromosome numbers and HOX gene expression. The C5 methylation of the cytosine plays an important role in the regulation of the expression of several genes by modulating the DNA/regulatory protein interactions or through its function in the changes of chromatin structure (demethylated/open/active or methylated/closed/inactive). Using the same tumours, used for karyotype and the study of HOX gene expression, we intend to determine whether the concerted activation/inactivation of the HOX genes is related to DNA methylation.

Project leader:
Dr. Marie-France POUPON
Laboratoire de Structure et Mutagenèse
Chromosomiques, URA 620 CNRS,
Institut Curie, Section de Biologie
16, rue d'Ulm
FR 75231 Paris Cédex 05
Phone: +33 1 40 51 66 67
Fax: +33 1 40 51 66 74
Contract number: CT941595

Participants:
Dr. Bernard MALFOY
Structure et Mutagenès Chromosomiques,
Institut Curie, Pavillon Trouillet R
16, rue d'Ulm
FR 75231 Paris Cédex 05
Phone: +33 1 40 51 66 72
Fax: +33 1 40 51 66 74

Dr. Clemente CILLO
Istituto Internazionale di
Genetic e Biofisica
Via G. Marconi 10
IT Napoli
Phone: +39 81 725 72 63
Fax: +39 81 593 61 23

DECISION-MAKING IN A CELL: PROLIFERATION DIFFERENTIATION, APOPTOSIS?

Key words

Intracellular infrastructure, signal-transduction, proliferation, differentiation, quiescence, apoptosis, Nerve growth factor (NGF), pheochromocytoma cell, PC 12, fibroblasts, Epidermal growth factor (EGF), neurodegenerative diseases.

Brief description

Cells respond to selected external stimuli in a manner that is dependent upon the status of the intracellular infrastructure necessary for signal-transduction.

This, in turn, is a function of the cell type and its totipotency. Exposure to external stimuli obliges the cell to take decisions concerning its fate i.e. resulting in proliferation, differentiation, quiescence or apoptosis.

Perturbation of any of these processes will have very grave consequences on the organism as a whole.

This proposal addresses certain aspects of the decision-making processes of the cell, using model systems for neuronal development and apoptosis. The project is designed to identify components of the Nerve growth factor (NGF) signal-transduction pathways specific for the differentiation, neuronal survival and proliferative responses, using the pheochromocytoma cell line PC12 as principal model.

Fibroblasts transfected with expression vectors for key proteins (NGF receptors, c-myc, bc12, mutants and combinations thereof) will also be used for comparison of their roles in a non-neuronal system. The effects of selected

(IGF1) and Epidermal growth factor (EGF) are to be studied in the light of their potential roles as modulators of apoptosis.

This is approached by the observation and subsequent manipulation of selected pathways of signal transduction during the cell cycle and identification of genes and regulatory factors implicated in the differentiation and survial programs.

Industrial interest for this project is probable, in the area of anti-cancer related agents but also in the area of neurodegenerative diseases.

This is expected from the potential identification of a link between cell cycle regulatory proteins and the action of a neurotrophic factor for the triggering of differentiation and the maintenance of the neuronal state. Indeed, due to the novelty of the ideas to be tested in this program, the results of these studies should offer fertile ground for development of novel pharmacologically-active agents. We expect these studies to open the way for a more precise understanding of how decisions are made within a cell and how they relate to the cell cycle at various stages of its life: proliferation, differentiation, and maintenance of the differentiated state in a neuronal model.

The three groups involved are located in Great Britain, Spain, and France.

Each group in this project is relatively small (less than six people). All are managed by experienced researchers, early in their carreer. No single group is in a position to undertake all of the experiments described herein.

To be able to freely interact, exchanging tools, know-how, culture as if the three labs were one, will indeed offer the synergism necessary to implement and achieve this program.

Project leader:
Dr. Brian RUDKIN
Laboratoire de Biologie Moléculaire & Cellulaire,
CNRS/ENS UMR49, Cell Cycle & Differentiation Group
Allée d'Italie 46
FR 69364 Lyon Cedex 07
Phone: +33 72 72 81 96
Fax: +33 72 72 80 80
Contract number: CT941471

Participants:
D.M. ZANCA
Instituto de Microbiologia Bioquimica,
C.S.I.C. Universidad de Salamanca,
Edificio Interdepartamental
Campus Miquel de Unamuno
ES 37007 Salamanca
Phone: +34 23 12 16 44
Fax: +34 23 26 79 70

G. EVAN
Imperial Cancer Research Fund Laboratories
44 Lincoln's Inn Fields
UK London WC2A 3PX
Phone: +44 71 269 30 27 (28 Lab)
Fax: +44 71 269 35 81

INVESTIGATION OF MINIMAL DISEASE (MRD) IN ACUTE NON-LYMPHOCYTIC LEUKAEMIA (ANLL): INTERNATIONAL STANDARDIZATION AND CLINICAL EVALUATION

Key words

Acute non-lymphocytic leukemia (ANLL), cytomorphological techniques-minimal residual disease (MRD), immunological marker analysis, immunophenotypes, leukemic cells, polymerase chain reaction (PCR), leukemia-specific nucleotide, t(15;17), t(9;22), t(6;9).

Brief description

Despite the high rate of morphological complete remissions achieved in acute non-lymphocytic leukemia (ANLL), most of these patients relapse due to the persistance of low numbers leukemic cells (<1-5%) which are undetectabe by conventional cytomorphological techniques-minimal residual disease (MRD). Whereas major progress has been obtained in MRD detection in acute lymphoblastic leukemia patients, at present sensitive techniques for MRD detection in ANLL have not been well established. The final goal of this project is the development of internationally standarized techniques for detection of MRD in ANLL patients and evaluation of their clinical impact on treatment and management of these patients.

Two different types of techniques will be used:

a Immunological marker analysis, which is based on detection of uncommon or aberrant immunophenotypes of the leukemic cells by double and triple antigen combinations at flow cytometry. According to the immunophenotypic and scatter characteristics of blast cells at diagnosis a phenotype/scatter pattern will be established for each patient to be used during follow-up;

b Polymerase chain reaction (PCR) analysis of leukemia-specific nucleotide (DNA and RNA) sequences i.e. junctional regions of rearranged immunoglobulin (Ig) and T-cell receptor (TCR) genes as well as fusion regions of chromosome aberrations such as t(15;17), t(9;22); t(6;9).

The study is planned to last three years and each centre will include at least 25 ANLL patients in the study. The major innovations and achievements wich are expected to be reached by this Concerted Action are:

1 Adaptation of basic scientific technology for clinical applications.

2 Exchange and international standarization of techniques for MRD detection in ANLL patients.

3 Application of identical sets of antibodies gene probes, and oligonucleotide primers in all participating centers.

4 Elucidation of the reported interlaboratory discrepancies in aberrant antigen expression and crosslineage Ig/TcR gene rearrangements in ANLL.

5 Clinical evaluation of the MRD techniques for monitoring the effectiveness of ANLL treatment. The close colaboration with regular exchange of experience and techniques together with centralized production.

Project leader:
Professor Dr. J.F. SAN MIGUEL
Departamento de Hematología,
Hospital Clínico Universitario
Paseo de San Vicente 58-182
ES 37007 Salamanca
Phone: +34 23 29 13 84
Fax: +34 23 26 47 43
Contract number: CT941675

Participants:
Prof. Dr. A. PARREIRA
Departamento Hematología
Instituto Portugués de Oncología
PT Lisboa
Phone: +351 1 726 78 50
Fax: +351 1 726 15 29

Prof. Dr. B. WORMANN
Zentrum der Inneren Medizin,
Univ of Göttingen
Robert Kochstrasse 40
DE 3400 GÖTTINGEN
Phone: +49 551 39 63 25
Fax: +49 551 39 29 14

Prof. Dr. C.R. BARTRAM
Dept. of Pediatrics II, Section of
Mócular Biology Universitatsklinik ULM
DE 7900 Ulm
Phone: +49 731 15 01 68
Fax: +49 731 15 01 75

Prof. Dr. G. JANOSSY
Dept. of Immunilogy,
Royal Free Hospital
UK London
Phone: +44 71 794 0500
Fax: +44 71 431 08 79

Prof. Dr. J.J.M. VAN DONGEN
Dept. of Immunology,
Erasmus University
P.O. Box 1738
NL 3000 Dr. Roterdam
Phone: +31 10 408 80 94
Fax: +31 10 436 76 01

MOLECULAR ANALYSIS OF GENOMIC ALTERATIONS IN TUMOURS FROM MAMMARY CARCINOMA FAMILIES: A WHOLE-GENOME SCREEN USING SIMPLE SEQUENCE POLYMORPHISMS ON MICRODISSECTED ARCHIVAL MATERIAL

Key words

Breast cancer, susceptibility genes, screening, prevention, treatment, genome screen, genomic alterations, microdissected histological specimens, cell bank, heterozygosity, LOH, polymorphic markers, tumourigenesis, epidemiology.

Brief description

Breast cancer, currently the most common cancer among women in European industrialized countries, has a strong genetic component. The identification of susceptibility genes has therefore great relevance for screening, prevention and treatment of this disease of great socio-economic impact.

A whole genome screen for genomic alterations in microdissected histological specimens obtained from the tumour carriers of thirty breast cancer families is proposed. The program comprises:

- Building a comprehensive collection of archival material from tumour carriers matched to an already established cell bank.
- Screening pathologically defined microdissected regions of archival material and for loss of heterozygosity (LOH) using approximately 150 highly polymorphic markers selected for strategic coverage of the whole human genome. This novel methodologic approach will increase accuracy and specificity in the diagnosis of genomic alterations and highlight chromosomal regions potentially involved in tumourigenesis in individual families.
- Checking each region of loss for genetic linkage with the markers showing allelic imbalance in all members of the index family. Such an individualised linkage approach is aimed at identifying genomic regions relevant for susceptibility which previously may have been missed on the basis of pooled data from different families.

The project will generate a unique data set integrating somatogenetic, linkage, and clinical information and will be entered into the European Breast Cancer Consortium database, currently focused on chromosome 17 linkage and epidemiology. The comprehensive approach proposed herein will therefore complement and extend the scope of an existing European collaboration towards understanding the genetic complexity of mammary cancer.

Project leader:
Dr. Siegfried SCHERNECK
Tumourgenetik, Max-Delbrück-Centrum
für Molekulare Medizin
Robert-Rössle-Strasse 10
DE 13125 Berlin
Phone: +4930 940 62 226
Fax: +49 30 940 63 842
Contract number: CT941423

Participants:
Dr. Kenneth B. REID
Univ of Oxford
UK Oxford

Dr. K. KÖLBE
Freie Universität Berlin
DE Berlin

METABOLIC POLYMORPHISM OF DRUG METABOLISING ENZYMES AS MARKERS OF SUSCEPTIBILITY IN CANCER AND NEUROLOGICAL DISORDERS

Key words
Genetic polymorphisms, drug metabolising enzymes, neurological diseases, Parkinson's disease, cytochrome P450s (CYPA1, CYP2E1 and CYP2D6) glutathione S-transferase (GSTM1), N-acetyl transferase (NAT), carcinogenicity, toxins, mutagens, lung, stomach, colon, bladder, prostate, oesophagus, leukaemia, lymphomas, myelomas, Motor Neurone disease.

Brief description
The aim of this project is to establish whether genetic polymorphisms in drug metabolising enzymes are associated with susceptibility to cancer and neurological diseases for example Parkinson's disease.

Should this prove to be the case it will allow for the identification of individuals at risk and, based on the known substrate specificity's of the enzymes to be studied, should provide important clues about the environmental agents involved in the disease process.

The enzymes to be studied are three members of the cytochrome P450s (CYPA1, CYP2E1 and CYP2D6), the glutathione S-transferase (GSTM1) and N-acetyl transferase (NAT) where there is evidence of genetic polymorphism in man.

All of these enzymes have been shown to play a central role in the metabolism and carcinogenicity of important chemicals, toxins and mutagens. To eliminate problems associated with drug phenotyping we will use genotyping assays for mutations in the genes coding for these enzymes. A number of assays have been developed using polymerase chain reaction amplification to identify the disabling mutations in the CYPA1, CYP2D6, GSTM1 and NAT genes.

We aim to develop further assays for the other genes.

These assays will be used to genotype individuals from control populations in the region of each participant and compare the observed allele frequencies with those seen in groups of individuals with various diseases. The disease groups to be studied will be; cancers of the lung, stomach, colon, bladder, prostate, oesophagus, leukaemia, lymphomas and myelomas and neurological disorders including Parkinson's, Alzheimer's and Motor Neurone disease.

Each participant will be involved in the collection of blood samples from these groups of individuals and will carry out the genotyping in their own laboratories.

The development of new genotyping assays and data analysis will be conducted by selected participants who already have considerable experience in these areas.

In addition to the study of disease susceptibility, this collaboration should yield other important information on the population distribution of these polymorphisms in different regions of the European Community that will allow us to evaluate whether the genetic tests, we have developed and will be developing further, are able to identify individuals at risk of drug side-effects.

Project leader:
Dr. N.K. SPURR
Imperial Cancer Research Fund,
Clare Hall Laboratories,
Human Genetic Resources
Blanche Lane
UK South Mimms Herts EN6 3LD
Phone: +44 71 269 38 46
Fax: +44 71 269 38 02
Contract number: CT941608

Participants:
Dr. M. LANG & Dr. H. BARTSCH
International Agency for Research on Cancer
150 Cours Albert-Thomas
FR 69372 Lyon Cedex 8
Phone: +33 727 38485
Fax: +33 727 38575

Dr. A. HAUGEN
Dept. Of Toxicology, National Inst.
of Occupational Health
P.O. Box 8149
NO 0033 Oslo
Phone: +47 22 466850
Fax: +47 22 609032

Prof. A. RANE
Depart. of Clinical Pharmacology,
Akademiska Hospital
SE 75185 Uppsala
Phone: +46 18 664261
Fax: +46 18 519237

Prof. C.R WOLF
Biomedical Research Centre,
Ninewells Hospital
UK Dundee DD1 9SY
Phone: +44 382 632621
Fax: +44 382 69993

Prof. H. AUTRUP
Steno Inst., Univ of Aarhus
Ole Worms Alle
DK 8000 Aarhus
Phone: +45 894 22943
Fax: +45 894 22970

PRECLINICAL EVALUATION OF TWO TUMOUR ASSOCIATED ANTIGENS AS POTENTIAL IMMUNOGENS FOR THE IMMUNOTHERAPY OF BREAST AND OVARIAN CANCER

Key words
Tumour associated antigens, breast, ovarian cancer, p53, polymorphic epithelial mucin (PEM), glycosylated, MUCI gene, humoral response, cytotoxic T cells, proliferative, cytolytic response.

Brief description
The project involves preclinical studies designed to investigate immune responses to two tumour associated antigens with a view to introducing novel therapies in breast and ovarian cancer patients and possibly developing preventative treatments. The antigens to be focussed on are p53 and a polymorphic epithelial mucin (PEM), the glycosylated product of the MUCI gene. The p53 antigen is mutated and overexpressed in a high proportion of breast and ovarian cancer patients (of the order of 50%) while PEM is overexpressed, and aberrantly glycosylated in more than 90% of these patients. Evidence for a humoral response to these antigens in breast cancer patients is already available. In addition cytotoxic T cells reactive with PEM expressing cells have been isolated from these patients. The proliferative and cytolytic response to immunogens based on the two antigens will be examined using:
a lymphocytes taken from patients or normal individuals, and;
b rodent model systems.

This will involve working with peptides as well as cells expressing the antigens. A detailed analysis of the specificity of the antibodies found in some breast and ovarian cancer patients will also be performed. Additionally, the problem of antigen presentation will be addressed since cancers which express the antigens have clearly not mobilised an immune response which results in tumour rejection. In this context, molecules involved in co-stimulation, which are absent from tumour cells, and certain cytokines will be expressed in cells used for antigen presentation and the effect on immune responses examined in human lymphocytes. In the rodent models, the effect on rejection of tumours expressing the antigen can also be examined. These experiments analyzing the response to different forms of the anti-gens, presented in vapious ways, should help in deciding on the mode of antigen delivery which we hope will subsequently be used in the clinic.

Project leader:
Dr. Joyce TAYLOR-PAPADIMITRIOU
Epithelial Cell Biology Laboratory,
Imperial Cancer Research Fund
Lincoln's Inn Fields 44
UK London WC2A 3PX
Phone: +44 71 269 33 62
Fax: +44 71 269 30 94
Contract number: CT941462

Participants:

Dr. C. HANSKI
Universitatsklinikum Steglitz,
Medizinische Klinik Und Poliklinik
Hindenburgdamm 30
DE D12200 Berlin

Dr. F.X. REAL
Institut Municipal d'Investigacio Medica,
Dept. d'Immunologia
Passeig Maritim 25-29
ES 08003 Barcelona

Dr. J. HILGERS
Academisch Ziekenhuis,
Vrije Universiteit
De Boelelaan 1117
NL 1081 HV Amsterdam

Dr. J.M. MELIEF
Dept. of Immunohaematology and Blood Bank,
AZL, Bldg.1, E3-Q
Postbus 9600
NL 2300 RC Leiden

Dr. M. NUTI
Dipartimento di Medicina Spoerimentale, Policli-
nico Umberti I, Universita Degli Studi Di Roma,
La Sapienza
Viale Regina Elena
IT 00161 Roma

Sir W. BODMER
Imperial Cancer Research Fund
44 Lincoln's Inn Fields
UK London WC2A 3PX

HTLV EUROPEAN RESEARCH NETWORK (HERN)

Key words
Human T-cell Leukaemia viruses (HTLV-I, HTLV-II), oncogenic retrovirus, HAM, tropical spastic paraparesis (TSP).

Brief description
This multi-disciplinary concerted action proposes to coordinate and extend research into the Human T-cell Leukaemia viruses types I and II (HTLV-I, HTLV-II) in the EC.
HTLV-I is an infectious human oncogenic retrovirus, aetiologically associated with Adult T-cell leukaemia/lymphoma (ATLL) and with diverse non-malignant sequelae including a demyelinating disease known as HTLV-associatedmyelopathy (HAM), or tropical spastic paraparesis (TSP). The full clinical Spectrum and public health significance of these viruses are unknown. HTLV-I/IIare transmitted both vertically and horizontally, the latter by sexual intercourse, whole blood transfusion and useof contaminated equipment for IV drug use.
HTLV-I is endemic in West/Central Africa, the Caribbean, parts of North and South America, and in Japan and Melanesia; HTLV-I exists in the EC in migrants from these endemic areas, and is transmitted within the EC both vertically and horizontally. It is likely that HTLV-I/II viruses are widely disseminated throughout the EC, but no concerted information is available, and information from blood donor screening is limited.

The specific objectives of HERN are firstly to standardise the diagnosis of HTLV-I/II infection by serology and by DNA PCR amplification, to allow uniform epidemiological information to be collected in the EC, and to begin formal sero-surveillance projects.
Secondly, to establish clinical definitions of ATLL for surveillance purposes, to create national registries of ATLL cases, and to prospectively study the clinical implications of HTLV infection.
Thirdly, to characterise the molecular epidemiology of HTLV-I/II in the EC, and to establish a repository of cells and DNA from cases and carriers. Fourthly, to coordinate research into the phenotypic and genotypic characteristics of HTLV-transformed and malignant cells, and fifthly to coordinate European research into the immunological control of HTLV infection. The epidemiological goals will involve new collaborative European research, while the cellular and molecular goals will involve the coordination and exchange of reagents between existing research groups.

Project leader:
Professor Jonathan WEBER
Department of Medicine,
Communicable Diseases Unit,
St. Mary's Hospital
Medical School
Praed Street, Paddington
UK London W2 1NY
Phone: +44 71 725 1539
Fax: +44 71 725 6645
Contract number: CT941116

Participants:
Dr. A. BARACCO
Epiunit, HIV Center IRCCS,
San Raffaele
Via Stamira d'Ancona 20
UT 20127 Milano
Phone: +39 2 264 37993
Fax: +39 2 264 37989

Dr. A. MOONE
Communicable Disease
Surveillance Centre
61 Colindale Avenue
UK London NW9 5EQ
Phone: +44 81 200 6868
Fax: +44 81 200 7868

Dr. A.M.L. LEVER
Dept. of Medicine, Univ of
Cambridge, Clinical School
Addenbrooke's Hospital
Hills Road
UK Cambridge CB2 200
Phone: +44 223 336747
Fax: +44 223 336846

Dr. B. GUILLEMAIN
Inserm 328,
Fondation Bergonie
229 cours de l'Argonne
FR 33076 Bourdeaux Cedex
Phone: +33 56 91 16 61
Fax: +33 56 91 18 35

Dr. Ch.R.M. BANGHAM
Molecular Immunology
Group, Inst. of
Molecular Medicine,
John Radcliffe Hospital
Headington
UK Oxford OX3 9 DU
Phone: +44 865 222336
Fax: +44 865 222502

Dr. J.G. HUISMAN
Central Laboratory of the
Netherlands Red Cross Blood
Transfusion Service
Plesmanlaan 125
NL 1066 AD Amsterdam

Dr. O.E. VARNIER
Laboratory of Virology AIDS
Center San Luigi,
Hospital San Raffaelo
Via Stamira d'Ancona 20
IT 20127 Milano
Phone: +39 2 264 37985
Fax: +39 2 264 37985

Dr. Ph.P. MORTIMER &
Ms J.H.C. TOSSWILL
Central Public Health
Laboratory,
Virus Reference Laboratory
61 Colindale Avenue
UK London NW9 5HT
Phone: +44 81 200 4400
Fax: +44 81 200 7874

Dr. P. EBBESEN
The Danish Cancer Society
Dept. of Virus and Cancer
Gustav Wiede Vej 10
DK 8000 Aarhus C
Phone: +45 86 127366
Fax: +45 86 195415

Dr. P. GOUBAU
Rega Instituut Katholieke
Universiteit Leuven
Minderbroedersstraat 10
BE 3000 Leuven
Phone: +32 16 33 21 60
Fax: +32 16 33 21 31

Dr. S. OZDEN &
Prof. M. BRAHIC
Unite des Virus Lents,
Institut Pasteur
28 rue du Dr. Roux
FR 75724 Paris Cedex 15
Phone: +33 1 45 68 87 70
Fax: +33 1 45 68 88 85

Dr. V. SORIANO
Instituto de Salud Carlos III,
Centre Nacional de
Investigation, Clinica
Y Medicina Preventive
Sinesio Delgado 10-12
ES 28029 Madrid

Dra F. AVILLEZ
National Inst. of Health
AIDS Reference Laboratory
Av. Padre Cruz
PT 1699 Lisboa
Phone: +351 1 758 1729
Fax: +351 1 758 1729

Dr. Marie-Ch. DOKHELAR
Laboratoire d'Immuno-
Biologie Cellulaire,
Institut Gustave Roussy
39 rue Camille Desmoulins
FR 94805 Villlejuif Cedex
Phone: +33 1 45 59 48 71
Fax: +33 1 45 59 64 94

Prof. A.G. DALGLEISH
Div. of Oncology,
St. George's Hospital
Medical School
Cranmer Terrace
UK London SW17 ORE
Phone: +44 81 672 9944
Fax: +44 81 784 7092

Prof. D. CATOVSKY &
Dr. E. MATUTES
Academic Dept. of
Haematology, The Royal
Marsden Hospital
Fulham Road
UK London SW3 6JJ
Phone: +44 81 352 8171

Prof. G. de THE
Institut Pasteur
28 rue du Dr. Roux
FR 75728 Paris Cedex 15
Phone: +33 1 45 68 89 30
Fax: +33 1 45 68 89 31

Prof. K. von den HELM
Max von Pettenkofer Institut
Ludwig-Maximilians Univ.
Pettenkoferstrasse 9a
DE 8000 München 2
Phone: +49 89 51 60 5200
Fax: +49 89 5 38 0584

Prof. L. CHIECO-BIANCHI
Director Inst. of Oncology
Via Gattamelata 64
IT 35128 Padova
Phone: +39 49 807 1859
Fax: +39 49 807 2854

Prof. R. WEISS &
Dr. T. SCHULZ
Chester Beatty Laboratories
The Inst. of Cancer Research
Fulham Road
UK London SW3 6JB

Prof. U. BERTAZZONI
Inst. of Genetics,
Biochemistry and Evolution
Via Abbiategrasso 207
IT 27100 Pavia
Phone: +39 382 527967/8
Fax: +39 382 422286

Prof. V. LISO
Cattedra di Ematologia
Universita Degli Studi
Piazza G. Cesare 11
IT 70124 Bari
Phone: +39 80 536 9973
Fax: +39 80 228 978

ORGANIZATION OF PRECLINICAL AND CLINICAL RESEARCH ON ANTICANCER THERAPY WITH BIOLOGICAL RESPONSE MODIFIERS (BRMs)

Key words
Biological response modifiers'(BRMs).

Brief description
The chance of influencing malignant growth by biological therapy with 'biological response modifiers'(BRMs) is presently revolutionizing cancer therapy. However, BRMs are a completely new approach for oncologists and force us to adapt our research procedures originally tailored to cytotoxic agents. The limited availability of reliable predictive in vitro or animal models for BRMs on the one had and the ethical need for promising candidates to proceed rapidly to the clinic on the other implies that:
1 Preclinical testing of BRMs needs to be well organized and must be relevant for possible future clinical application.
2 As the final therapeutic potential of a BRM and its network interactions within the integral human body can only be assessed following careful studies in man, the effectiveness of clinical trials must be improved by closely relating them to research programmes utilising material from BRM-treated patients (= "ex vivo" research).

Therefore, close cooperation and regular exchange of knowledge among preclinical and clinical researcher is essential. Rapid progress is not feasible on a purely national basis, as experts in preclinical BRM research and clinicians experienced in the coordination of clinical trials with BRMs are spread throughout Europe. Therefore, the Task Force Biologicals (chairman: H. Zwierzina) has been created by the European Organization for Research and Treatment of Cancer (EORTC).
The structure of the EORTC has proven to be an excellent basis for preclinical and clinical investigation of anticancer therapy. A broad spectrum of expertise in test systems for in vitro, in vivo and "ex vivo" investigation of biological anticancer agents is available through the participants of this BIOMED 1 application. Participating researchers are able to specifically address scientific problems in cooperation with the members of their groups on the one hand, or are experienced in coordinating early clinical trials with biological agents on the other. Thus, the EORTC is principally prepared to face the new situation caused by the challenges of biological therapy. Financial support, however, is an essential requirement to organize the facilities of preclinical and clinical research available but spread throughout Europe. Non-critical application of the usually very expensive BRMs carries the risk of a cost explosion of our health care system. Well designed and well-organized clinical trials in combination with "ex vivo" research are ethically inevitable and will reduce costs by preventing non-critical application. In conclusion, this grant application aims to: (i) improve treatment of cancer; (ii) strengthen the European position in BRM research; (iii) consider the ethical need for "ex vivo" research; and (iv) reduce costs or our health care systems.

Project leader:
Dr. Heinz ZWIERZINA
Universitätsklinik für Innere Medizin
Anichstrasse 35
AT 6020 Innsbruck
Phone: +43 512 504 32 55
Fax: +43 512 504 33 40
Contract number: CT941587

Participants:
Dr. F. CALIGARIS-CAPPIO
Universita di Torino,
Dipartimento die Scienze Biomediche
Via Genova 3
IT 10126 Torino

Prof. T. CONNORS
Institute of Cancer Research,
Royal Cancer & Royal Marseden Hospital
15 Cotswold Road, Sutton
UK Surrey SM2 5NG

Dr. M.D'INCALCI
Instituto Mario Negri
Via Eritrea
IT 20157 Milano

Dr. J. DOUBLE
Clinical Oncology Unit,
University of Bradford
UK Bradford BD7 1DP

Dr. R. LEAKE
University of Glasgow,
Dept. of Biochemistry
UK Glasgow G12 8QQ

Dr. H. HENDRIKS
EORTC New Drug Development Office,
Acedemisch Ziekenhuis
De Boelelaan 1117
NL 1081 HV Amsterdam

Dr. H. NEWELL
Cancer Research Unit,
University of Newcastle Medical School
Framlington Place
UK Newcastle upon Tyne NE2 4HH

Prof. R. WILLEMZE
Acedemisch Ziekenhuis Leiden
Postbus 9600
NL 2300 Leiden

Prof. W. WILMANNS
Medizinische Universitaetsklinik III,
Klinikum Grosshadern
Marchioninistrasse 15
DE 81377 Munich

II.3 RESEARCH ON CARDIOVASCULAR DISEASES

Introduction

In the last decades, major achievements in the field of cardiovascular diseases have been obtained. Among the reasons for such an improvement are a better understanding of the physiopathological mechanisms leading to cardiovascular diseases, a better knowledge of risk factors and the establishment of broader prevention programmes in most countries, and the development of diagnostic methods and treatment modalities for these diseases. Nevertheless, cardiovascular disease is a leading cause of disability, morbidity and early mortality in the European countries.

The European Union, conscious of the social needs and sensitive to the suggestions of scientist, physicians and industrialists has been involved since 1990 in cardiovascular research through different activities, among them within the BIOMED 1 Programme.

This part of the BIOMED 1 Programme had as ultimate goal to contribute to the understanding of the pathogenic mechanisms leading to cardiovascular disease development and to translate these findings into prevention and treatment. In this context, the following objectives were addressed; to promote the basic understanding of the pathogenic mechanisms leading to cardiovascular diseases development, to provide support for the development of clinical research and to promote research on new methods for diagnosis and therapy and to contribute to the knowledge on disease control and prevention.

Transnational collaboration, multidisciplinarity and complementarity represent relevant issues which must be addressed in order to improve the knowledge on cardiovascular diseases. They also constitute the main strenghts of the project supported in this area.

A few examples can be mentioned as the creation of an European registry on past and current randomised trials on three key categories of cardiovascular disease treatment and prevention, which will contribute to the harmonisation of therapies across Europe. Clinical trials have made a major contribution to improving the treatment and prevention of cardiovascular diseases. This is an area where the EU can still give an important contribution.

Also, succesful action was started in the creation of an European network for transgenic animals development, a fairly extensive technique and where few teams have mastered this technique yet. Establishment of such a network led to the production of the first monogenetic model of hypertension.

At present there are 1383 research groups participating in 40 concerted actions as part of the BIOMED 1 Programme. Furthermore, a large number of these networks extend beyond the frontiers of the European Union. COST (Cooperation in the field of scientific and technical research) countries -Austria, Finland, Iceland, Norway, Sweden and Switzerland and Turkey- are actively participating in many of the ongoing projects.

Maria Vidal, MD

VASCULAR NITRIC OXIDE SYNTHESIS: PHYSIOLOGICAL AND PATHOPHYSIOLOGICAL IMPLICATIONS

Key words

Nitric oxide, nitric oxide synthase, endothelium, vascular smooth muscle, mesangial cells, circulatory shock, arteriosclerosis, ADP-ribosylation, bacterial lipopolysaccharide.

Objectives

The joint project aims to co-ordinate and facilitate investigations into the basic mechanisms of vascular and renal nitric oxide (NO) biosynthesis by combining a variety of different methods and approaches from fields as diverse as cellular physiology, biochemistry, cardiovascular pharmacology and molecular biology. Particular emphasis will be given to studies on the physiologically important shear stress-induced release of NO by cultured and native endothelial cells, intact vascular preparations and isolated organs from different species as well as in experimental animals. Another important objective of the group is to investigate the development of cardiovascular complications associated with arteriosclerosis, hypercholesterolemia, hypertension and sepsis. Experimental studies will be designed to evaluate potential changes in endothelial cell, smooth muscle cell, mesangial cell and macrophage NO synthase expression in these clinical conditions. A further objective is to investigate actions of NO not mediated by stimulation of soluble guanylyl cyclase in the target cell, i.e. the NO-mediated activation of ADP-ribosyltransferases and the possible role of this process in modulating NO biosynthesis in endothelial, smooth muscle or mesangial cells. Any leads for drug development arising from these studies will be tested further in animal models to provide a basis for a better understanding, treatment and/or prevention of cardiovascular diseases associated with an impaired or exacerbated synthesis/release of NO in the vascular system.

Brief description

The demonstration in 1957 of the formation of a potent vasodilatory autacoid, subsequently identified as NO, by vascular endothelial cells has opened up a new area of biological research. The vascular endothelium continuously produces NO in the absence of any external stimulus, and this so-called basal release represents a significant proportion of the total NO releasing capacity of native endothelial cells. The synthesis of NO can however be enhanced by receptor-dependent stimuli as well as by mechanical and chemical stimuli, such as shear stress or low arterial pO_2. Indeed the shear stress exerted on the endothelium by the circulating blood is the major stimulus for the sustained production of NO *in vivo*, and represents a highly effective and sensitive system for the local control of vascular resistance. The endothelium therefore plays a pivotal role in the maintenance of an adequate blood flow by continuously adjusting the fine balance between vasoconstriction and vasodilation. The collaborative project will pay particular attention to the effect of shear stress on the expression and activation of the endothelial NO synthase.

Recent evidence has linked disturbances in the regulation of NO production within the vascular tree with the cardiovascular complications associated with atherosclerosis, diabetes, hypertension and sepsis. A common feature in the onset and/or development of these diseases seems to be a failing or an exacerbated synthesis of NO within the vascular tree. These pathological changes occur not only in endothelial cells, but also in smooth muscle cells and leukocytes in which the induction of an NO producing pathway is initiated following exposure to bacterial lipopolysaccharide and/or various cytokines. The Concerted Action aims to gain insight into mechanisms involved in the regulation of vascular NO formation, thereby providing a basis for the development of more effective therapeutic agents for the treatment and/or prevention of these cardiovascular complications. The joint research will focus mainly on the changes in the expression or activity of the various NO synthase isoforms in endothelial cells, smooth muscle cells and macrophages in experimental models of atherosclerosis, hypertension or endotoxaemia *in vivo*, *ex vivo* and *in vitro*. Additional projects will investigate the role of NO in the renal circulation, especially in glomerulonephritis, and address actions of NO not mediated by stimulation of soluble guanylyl cyclase in the target cell.

Project leader:
Professor R. BUSSE
Klinikum der Johan Wolfgang Goethe Universität,
Zentrum der Physiologie
Theodor Stem kai 7
DE 60590 Frankfurt am Main
Phone: +49 69 6301 6049
Fax: +49 69 6301 7668
Contract number: CT921893

Participants:
Dr. Berhard BRUNE
Lehrstuhl für Biologische Chemie,
Universität Konstanz
Universitätsstrasse 10
DE 78464 Konstanz
Phone: +49 7531 88 2286
Fax: +49 7531 88 2966

Prof. Jim PARRATT
Dept. of Physiology and Pharmacology,
University of Strathclyde
204 George Street
UK Glasgow G1 1XW
Phone: +44 41 552 4400/2858
Fax: +44 41 552 2562

Prof. Jean-Claude STOCLET
Laboratoire de Pharmacology Cellulaire
et Moléculaire,
URA CNRS 600, Faculté de Pharmacie
74 route du Rhin, B.P. 24
FR 67401 Illkirch
Phone: +33 88 67 69 33
Fax: +33 88 66 46 33

Prof. Josef PFEILSCHIFTER
Dept. Pharmakologie,
Biozentrum der Universität Basel
Klingelbergstrasse 70
CH 4056 Basel
Phone: +41 61 267 2223
Fax: +41 61 267 2208

Dr. Christoph THIEMERMANN
The William Harvey Research Institute,
St. Bartholomew's Hospital Medical College
Charterhouse Square
UK London EC1M 6BQ
Phone: +44 71 982 6119
Fax: +44 71 251 1685

PREVENTION FROM THROMBOSIS BY UROKINASE ENHANCEMENT (ECAPTURE)

Key words
Preventive medicine, prophylactics, thrombosis, fibrinolysis, urokinase, plasminogen activator, single-chain urokinase-type plasminogen activator (scu-PA).

Objectives
The objectives of the project are:
1 to assess the efficacy of enhancement of the blood scu-PA level in preventing the vessel wall from thrombosis (the efficacy of the preventive measure).
2 to identify the functional sites and cell types involved in the regulation of the blood scu-PA level (the potential drug targets).
3 to trace leads for compounds that are potentially effective in enhancing the blood scu-PA level (leads for new prophylactics).

Brief description
In most westernized societies cardiovascular diseases are the leading cause of death over the age of 45 and a quarter of all these deaths in males occur before the age of 65. Therefore it is all-important to arrive at a universal form of prophylaxis that would accomplish a general delay of the fatal, occluding thrombosis. The *European Concerted Action on Prevention from Thrombosis by Urokinase Enhancement* (ECAPTURE) aims at prophylaxis by reinforcing the natural defence mechanism against thrombosis, the vascular fibrinolysis, specifically by chronic pharmacological enhancement of the endogenous level of single-chain urokinase-type plasminogen activator (scu-PA) in the blood. This is a novel approach of prevention from thrombosis.
The objectives of the project are:
1 to assess the efficacy of the preventive measure.
2 to identify the potential drug targets.
3 to trace leads for new prophylactics.

The efficacy of enhancement of the blood scu-PA level will be assessed *in vitro* (static and perfusion systems), and *in vivo* by: (i) artificially enhancing the blood scu-PA level (infusion) and monitoring the delay of onset of thrombosis upon provocation (experimental animals, prospective randomized clinical trials in patients who are temporarily at high risk for thrombosis), by (ii) constructing transgenic mice expressing a non-activatable scu-PA mutant and monitoring the tendency to thrombosis, and by (iii) analysing whether patients at risk for thrombosis with a relatively high blood scu-PA level have a coronary event less frequently (prospective epidemiological investigations).
The functional sites and cell types involved in the regulation of the blood scu-PA level will be identified, respectively, by measuring the scu-PA concentration gradients in the circulation over the various organs and vascular beds (blood sampling during catheterization), and by analysis of scu-PA and scu-PA receptors in tissue biopsies taken from the functional sites intraoperatively.
Leads for potentially-effective compounds will be obtained from any significant correlations between the blood scu-PA level of patients at risk for thrombosis and their various drug use on admission (cross-sectional investigations), and from experiments with the cell types significant to the regulation, in culture.

Project leader:
Dr. G. DOOIJEWAARD
Gaubios Laboratory
IVVO-TNO,
Dept. of Fibrinolysis
and Proteolysis
P.O. Box 430
NL 2300 AK Leiden
Phone: +31 71 18 14 99
Fax: +31 71 18 19 04
Contract number: CT920392

Participants:
Dr. E. ANGLES-CANO
INSERM U. 143, Institut de
Pathologie Cellulaire,
FR 94275 Bicêtre cedex

Dr V. VAN HINSBERGH
Dept. of Lipids and
Endothelium, Gaubius
Laboratory IVVO-TNO
NL 2300 AK Leiden

Dr. W.A. GUNZLER
Dept. of Biotech. Control,
Grünenthal GmbH
DE 5100 Aachen-Eilendorf

Dr. P.J. GAFFNEY
Division of Haematology,
National Institute for
Biological Standards and
Control
Blanche Lane South Mimms
Potters Bar
UK Hertfordshire EN6 3QG

Dr. M. SPANNAGL
Medizinische Klinik,
Ludwig-Maximillians-Univ.,
Klinikum Innenstadt
DE 8000 Munich 2

Prof. B.R. BINDER
Lab. clin. Exp. Physiology,
University of Vienna
AT 1090 Vienna

Prof. T. MANDALAKI &
dr. C. MARKAKIS
Second Regional Blood
Transfusion Centre,
University Hospital LAIKON
GR 11527 Goudi-Athens

Prof. M. SAMANA
Laboratoire Central d'Héma-
tologie, Hôpital-Dieu
FR 75181 Paris-Cedex 04

Dr. J. JESPERSEN
Section for Thrombois
Research, Ribe County
Hospital, South Jutland
University Centre
DK 6700 Esbjerg

Porf. A. MASERI &
dr. F. ANDREOTTI
Istituto di Cardiologia,
Universita Cattolica
del Sacro Cuore
IT 00168 Roma

Dr. J. PHILIPPE
Coagulation Laboratory,
University Hospital Gent
BE 9000 Gent

Prof. L.A.H. MONNENS
Dept. of Nephrology,
Univ. of Nijmegen,
Sint Radboud Hospital
NL 6500 Nijmegen

Dr. E. ROCHA &
dr. J.A. PARAMO
Servicio de Hematologia,
Clinica Universitaria,
Universidad de Navarra
ES 31080 Pamplona

Porf. B. Risberg
Dept. of Surgery,
Lund University,
Malmö General Hospital
SE 21401 Malmö

Dr. H. RIESS &
dr. G. HIMMELREICH
Dept. of Internal Medicine,
Univ. Hosp. Rudolf Virchow
DE 1000 Berlin 19

Dr. J.J. MICHIELS &
dr. M. KAPPERS-KLUNNE
Dept. of Hematology,
University Hospital
NL 3015 GD Rotterdam

Prof. D. KEBER
University Clinical Centre,
Trnovo Hospital of
Internal Medicine
SL 61000 Ljubljana

Dr. F.H.M. DERKX
Dept. of Internal Medicine I,
University Hospital
NL 3015 GD Rotterdam

Dr. M.B. DONATI &
dr. L. IACOVIELLO
Istituto di Ricerche
Farmacologische, Mario
Negri Sud, Laboratory of
Thrombosis Pharmacology
IT 66030 Santa Maria Imbaro

Dr. V. ELLIS &
dr. M. PLOUG
The Finsen Laboratory,
University Hospital
DK 2100 Copenhagen

Dr. D. DEPREZ
Dept. of Cardiology
and Angiology,
University Hospital
BE 9000 Gent

Dr. L. MOENS &
dr. R. VAN HOLDER
Dept. of Internal Medicine,
University Hospital Gent
BE 9000 Gent

Prof. G.D.O. LOWE
Dept. of Medicine,
Royal Infirmary
UK Glasgow G31 2ER

Prof. H.C. KWAAN
Hematology/Oncology sect.,
Veterans Adm.
Lakeside Hospital,
US Chicago IL 60611

Dr. Z. ARNEZ
Dept. of Plastic Surgery and
Burns, Univ. Clinical Centre
SL 61000 Ljubljana

PREVENTION OF MYOCARDIAL REPERFUSION DAMAGE BY PHARMACOLOGIC CONTROL OF CONTRACTILITY

Key words
Myocardial infarction, ischemic heart disease, reperfusion, infarct size, contractility, isolated myocytes, hypercontracture, cell-to-cell interaction, cardioprotection, osmotic swelling.

Objectives
The aim of the proposed project is to develop a new therapeutic approach to limit myocardial reperfusion injury. This is based on the understanding that reperfusion causes an important mechanical overload to the sarcolemma of ischemic myocytes and that this stress, secondary to hypercontraction and cell-to-cell mechanical interaction may cause the death of viable myocytes. Ways will be investigated which allow to inhibit the development of hypercontracture by a direct interference with its myofibrillar mechanism. The potential beneficial effects of drugs able to desensitize troponin C to Ca2+ or to inhibit cross-bridge formation will be investigated. The effects of these drugs on intracellular Ca2+ handling, cellular metabolism will be characterized and their cardiac side effects analyzed.

Brief description
The aim of the proposed project is to develop a new therapeutic approach to limit reperfusion injury. This approach would be based on the hypothesis that reperfusion causes an important mechanical overload to the sarcolemma of ischemic myocytes and that this stress, secondary to hypercontraction, cell swelling and cell-to-cell mechanical interaction may cause the death of viable myocytes. The role of and the interactions between these mechanisms will be investigated by modifying the initial reperfusate in different models of transient hypoxia and ischemia, mainly by adding substances able to selectively and reversibly inhibit myocardial contractility and by modifying the osmotic and oncotic pressures of the reperfusion fluids.

In the proposed project, therefore, ways are investigated which allow to inhibit the development of hypercontracture by a direct interference with its myofibrillar mechanism. The potential beneficial effects of drugs able to desensitize troponin C to Ca2+ or to inhibit cross-bridge formation will be investigated.

The methods will include the isolated myocyte, the isolated perfused heart and the in situ coronary occlusion with selective perfusion of the area at risk. In these models, different end points will be used. Cardiomyocytes from myocardium of adult rats are isolated and studied in 24-h short, term culture, in which preparations of 100% intact cells can be obtained. In the isolated cell model, cell morphology (phase contrast microscopy, electron microscopy), energy metabolism (CrP, ATP, cytosolic phosphorylation potential), and cytosolic cation homeostasis (using fluorescent indicators for Ca2+, Na+, pH) can be investigated strictly in parallel. The isolated working heart model will be used to optimize the effects of contractile blockade after global ischemia and to optimize the beneficial effects of this therapeutic approach on cardiac preservation. The interaction between contractile inhibition, osmotic and oncotic pressure, pH and Ca2+ concentration will be analyzed and cardiac side effects assessed in the in situ pig heart model. In addition to ECG and hemodynamics, regional wall function and electrophysiology, instantaneous and regional blood flow, platelet function and hemostasis will be monitored in this model, and infarct size, histology and ultrastructure will be used as main end points.

The project will be subdivided in three consecutive phases. During the first phase, characterization of contractile blocking agents will be carried out, and the effects of regional and global contractile blockade will be analyzed. During the second phase, the effects of transient contractile inhibition during reperfusion following acute coronary occlusion or global ischemia will be assessed. The third phase will be devoted to optimization of contractile inhibition therapy and analysis of interactions with other approaches to limit reperfusion injury and infarct size.

It is expected that the global approach used in this study (from the molecular level to the *in vivo studies in large animals*), with standardized methods and coordinated designs, will allow a much more rapid and efficient development of new treatments for reperfusion/reoxygenation injury in different clinical situations. These situations could include myocardial infarction, cardiac surgery or heart transplantation. These developments could ultimately result in the economical exploitation of the results. The potential clinical relevance of the results of the proposed investigation is underscored by the fact that they may open new ways for causal therapy of ischemic-reperfused myocardium acting specifically at the time of reperfusion. For this important clinical problem so far specific therapeutic approaches are lacking.

Project leader:
Dr. D. GARCIA-DORADO
Servicio de Cardiología,
Hospital General Vall d'Hebron
Vall d'Hebron 119-129
ES 08035 Barcelona
Phone: +34 3 428 04 96
Fax: +34 3 428 04 95
Contract number: CT921501

Participants:
Prof. H.M. PIPER
Physiologisches Institut,
Klinicum der Justus-Liebig-Universität
Aulweg 129
DE 35392 Giessen
Phone: +49 641 702 4551
Fax: +49 641 702 4575

Dr. Valdis MIKAZHAN
Dept. of Pharmacology,
Latvian Institute of Cardiology
Pilsonou str. 13
LV 1002 Riga
Phone: +0132276445
Fax: +0193348210

APPLICATION OF IN-VIVO GENE TRANSFER TO CARDIOVASCULAR RESEARCH (TRANSGENEUR)

Key words
Molecular genetics, gene transfer, hypertension, cardiovascular disease.

Objectives
1 The isolation, breeding and dissemination of new genetic models of hypertension using gene constructs supplied by participants in the concerted action.
2 Training scientists and technicians from the participating institutes in technical aspects involved in the projects, including cryopreservation techniques.
3 Organisation of a yearly scientific meeting to which all the participants are invited to attend and present data.
4 The development of cryopreservation techniques to facilitate the storage and shipment of strains to participating institutes.

Brief description
Cardiovascular morbidity and mortality accounts for about 50% of deaths in industrialised countries and is one of our primary health care concerns. Primary hypertension is multigenic in origin and is affected by environmental factors such as lifestyle and diet. In order to further our understanding of the genetic basis of this disease, new informative models are required.

The concerted action *Transgeneur* has been active for three years and comprises of a dual centre facility (Edinburgh and Berlin) for in-vivo gene transfer, with participating researchers able both to visit the centres for collaborative work and to be directly supplied with experimental materials and reagents. The participants provide an integrated range of expertise ranging from gene cloning methodology to complex physiological and pharmacological analyses.

Project leader:
Dr. J.J. MULLINS
AFRC Centre for Genome Research,
University of Edinburgh,
King's Buildings
West Mains Road
UK Edinburgh EH9 3JQ
Phone: +44 31 650 58 46
Fax: +44 31 667 01 64
Contract number: CT921436

Participants:
Dr. Niels KORSGAARD
Dept. of Pharmacology,
University of Aarhus
DK Aarhus
Phone: +45 86 19 56 87
Fax: +45 86 19 12 77

Dr. Michael MULVANY
Dept. of Pharmacology,
University of Arhuus
DK Aarhus
Phone: +45 86 19 56 87
Fax: +45 86 19 12 77

Dr. Nilesh SAMANI
School of Medicine,
Clinical Science Building,
University of Leicester,
Leicester Royal Infirmary
PO Box 65
UK Leicester
Phone: +44 0533 523 182
Fax: +44 0533 523 107

Dr. Pierre CORVOL
INSERM, U36,
Collège de France
3 rue d'Ulm
FR 75005 Paris
Phone: +33 1 44 27 16 70
Fax: +33 1 44 27 16 91

Dr. Florent SOUBRIER
INSERM U36,
Collège de France
3 rue d'Ulm
FR 75005 Paris
Phone: +33 1 44 27 16 70
Fax: +33 1 44 27 16 91

Prof. Jean SASSARD
Dept. Pharmacologie et
Physiologie Clinique ,
8 Avenue Rockefeller
FR 69008 Lyon
Phone: +33 78 77 70 00
Fax: +33 78 00 97 07

Dr. Madeleine VINCENT
Laboratoire de Physiologie,
Faculté de Medecine Lyon
Grange-Blanche,
Université Claude Berbard
(Lyon I)
8 Avenue Rockefeller
FR 69373 Lyon Cedex 08
Phone: +33 78 77 70 78
Fax: +33 78 77 71 58

Dr. Rainer RETTIG
Pharmakologische Institut
der Universität
Im Neuenheimer Feld 366
DE 6900 Heidelberg
Phone: +49 6221 563 856
Fax: +49 6221 563 901

Dr. Jürgen FINGERLE
Pharma Division,
Preclinical Research,
F. Hoffmann-la Roche Ltd.,
Dept. PRPV
CH 4002 Basel
Phone: +41 688 8013
Fax: +41 688 4943

Dr. Eric CLAUSER
INSERM U36, Laboratoire
de Médecine Expérimentale,
College de France
3 rue d'Ulm
FR 75005 Paris
Phone: +33 1 44 27 16 75
Fax: +33 1 44 27 16 91

Dr. Kjell FUXE
Dept. of Histology and
Neurobiology,
Karolinska Institute
Box 60 400
SE 104 01 Stockholm
Phone: +46 728 6400
Fax: +46 33 79 41

Prof. H.A.J. STRUIJKER
BOUDIER
Dept. of Pharmacology,
University of Limburg
PO Box 616
NL 6200 MD Maastricht
Phone: +31 43 882 222
Fax: +31 43 470 613

Dr. Alfred HAHN
ZLF Kantonsspital Basel
Hebelstrasse 20
CH 4031 Basel
Phone: +41 265 2358/2525
Fax: +41 261 1500

Dr. C. SANCHEZ-FERRER
Dept. de Farmacologia
y Terapeuttica,
Facultad de Medicina
Autonoma de Madrid
c/ Arzobispo Morcillo 4
ES 28029 Madrid
Phone: +34 1 3975 470
Fax: +34 1 3150 075

Dr. Kenneth GROSS
Dept. of Molecular and
Cellular Biology,
Roswell Park Cancer Institute
Elm and Charlton Streets
US Buffalo New York 14263
Phone: +716 845 5859
Fax: +716 845 8169

Prof. E. HACKENTHAL
Dept. pf Pharmacology,
University of Heidelberg
Im Neuenheimer Feld 366
DE 6900 Heidelberg
Phone: +49 6221 56 39 19
Fax: +49 6221 56 39 44

Dr. Giuseppe BIANCHI
Dipartimento di Scienze e
Technologie Biomediche,
Ospedale San Raffaele,
Università di Milano
Via Olgettina 60
IT 20132 Milano
Phone: +39 2 3350 0371
Fax: +39 2 3350 0408

Dr. Sebastian BACHMANN
Institut für Anatomie
und Zellbiologie I
Im Neuenheimer Feld 307
DE 6900 Heidelberg
Phone: +49 6221 56 3986
Fax: +49 6221 56 4951

Dr. Kazuo MURAKAMI
Institute of Applied
Biochemistry,
University of Tsukuba
JP Tsukuba City 305
Phone: +298 53 4628
Fax: +298 53 4605

Dr. John MULLINS
AFRC Centre for Genome
Research,
University of Edinburgh
King's Buildings
West Mains Rd.
UK Edinburgh
Phone: +44 31 650 5890
Fax: +44 31 667 0164

Dr. Giuseppe MANCIA
Università Degli Studi
di Milano,
Cattedra de Medicina Inter.II,
Osp. San Gerardo Dei Tintori
Via Donizetti 106
IT 20052 Monza
Phone: +39 3633 357
Fax: +39 2545 7666

Dr. Martin PAUL
Dept. Pharmacology
Im Neuenheimer Feld 366
DE 6900 Heidelberg
Phone: +49 6221 563905
Fax: +49 6221 562944

Dr. Detlev GANTEN
Centrum für Molekulare
Medezin, Berlin-Buch
Robert-Rössle Strasse 10
DE 13122 Berlin
Phone: +49 30 9406 3278
Fax: +49 30 9406 2681

APPLICATION OF NOVEL IN VITRO TECHNOLOGY TO HUMAN RESISTANCE ARTERY DISEASE

Key words
Arteriole, biology, cell physiology, cell receptors, coronary circulation, glaucoma hyperlipidaemia, hypertension, myography, peripheral resistance, pre-eclampsia, therapeutics, two dimensional gel electrophoresis, vascular resistance.

Objectives
The following sub-projects are being performed:
1 The role of genetic factors, mitogens and physical forces as determinants of resistance artery abnormalities in hypertension.
2 Changes in resistance arteries in pregnancy-induced hypertension.
3 Changes in resistance arteries in secondary hypertension.
4 Effects of antihypertensive therapy on resistance arteries in patients with essential hypertension.
5 Endothelial dysfunction in resistance arteries from young subjects with familial hyperlipidaemia.
6 Association of low-pressure glaucoma with hyper-activity of the resistance vasculature.
7 The effects of atherosclerosis, cardiac myopathy, Eisenmenger's syndrome on coronary resistance arteries.

Brief description
The main aim of this Concerted Action is to exploit a novel, European developed technique for determing the characteristics of human resistance arteries. The resistance arteries (pre-capillary vessels with diameters less than about 300 μm) are the blood vessels which are primarily responsible for the distribution of the blood from the heart. By controlling the diameter of the resistance arteries, the vascular control system can ensure that each capillary receives blood at the optimal pressure and the optimal amount. Furthermore, the total hydrodynamic resistance presented by the resistance arteries is a major determinant of systemic blood pressure. Disturbances of the resistance arteries can thus have profound effects on the body, both locally (e.g. ischaemia) and generally (e.g. hypertension). The ensuing diseases are major health risks in Europe, and represent a major drain on European health resources.
The technique is based on a so-called *microvessel myograph* and is used in conjunction with new molecular biology and genetic techniques. This allows the investigation of the role of human resistance arteries in a range of diseases, and to develop rational methods of treatment. The necessity for Concerted Action is that the patient base in any one laboratory is too small to obtain sufficient material, and the aims can only be achieved by co-ordination of effort between a number of laboratories. The project is based around a collaboration between 11 laboratories in 6 countries, who are grouped together as a European Working Party on Resistance Artery Disease (EURAD). In addition, six other European laboratories, which also use the microvessel myograph technique, or who have relevant specialized techniques, are associated with EURAD.
The microvessel myograph technology for examination of human resistance arteries is based on the in vitro investigation of small arteries taken from small biopsies. The technique allows measurement of vascular function and structure under closely defined conditions of extension.

Other techniques which are used include: microbiochemical measurements, genetic analysis, growth factors and organ culture, histomorphometric techniques, measurement of cytoplasmic calcium and pH, measurement of membrane potential.

Project leader:
Dr. M.J. MULVANY
Department of Pharmacology,
Aarhus University
University Park 240
DK 8000 Aarhus
Phone: +45 89 42 17 26
Fax: +45 86 12 88 04
Contract number: CT920777

Participants:
Dr. A. HOSTE
Dept. of Physiology,
Univ of Antwerp
BE 2020 Antwerp

Dr. C. AALKJAER
Dept. of Pharmacology,
Aarhus Univ
DK 8000 Aarhus C

Dr. D. PRUNEAU
Dept. Cardiovascular,
Laboratoire Founier
Fr 21121 Daix
Phone: +33 8044 7500

Dr. E. KEVELAITIS
Dept. of Physiology and
Pathophysiology,
Medical Academy
3000 Kaunas

Dr. H. THURSTON
Dept. of Medicine, Leicester
Univ, Clinical Sciences
UK Leicester LE2 7LX

Dr. J.G.R. DEMEY
Dept. of Pharmacology,
Faculties II.4.,
Univ of Limburg
NL 6200 MD Maastricht

Dr. J.R. DOCHERTY
Dept. of Clinical Pharma-
cology, Royal College of
Surgeons in Ireland
St. Stephens Green
IE Dublin 2

Dr. L. POSTON
Dept. of Physiology,
St. Thomas' Hospital
UK London SE1 7EH 2247

Dr. M. PFAFFENDORF
Dept. Pharmacotherapy,
AMC
NL 1105 AZ Amsterdam

Dr. N. SAMANI
Dept. of Medicine,
Clinical Sciences Building
UK Leicester LE2 7LX

Dr. N.C.B. NYBORG
Dept. of Pharmacology,
Aarhus Univ
DK 8000 Aarhus C

Dr. S.M. THOM &
Prof. P.S. SEVER
Clinical Pharmacology,
St. Mary's Hospital
Medical School
Uk London W2 1NY

Dr. U. SIMONSEN
Departamento de Fisiologia,
Facultad de Veterinaria
Universidad Complutense
ES 28040 Madrid

Ms. V. DAHL NIELSEN
Dept. of Pharmacology,
Aarhus Univ
DK 8000 Aarhus C

Prof. A.M. HEAGERTY
Univ Hospital of
South Manchester
UK Manchester M20 8LR

Prof. Dr. D.L. BRUTSAERT
Dept. of Physiology,
Univ of Antwerp
BE 2020 Antwerp

Prof. Dr. W. ZIDEK
Westfälische Wilhelms-Univ.
DE 4400 Münster

Prof. D. GANTEN
Centrum für Molekulare
Medizin
DE O-1115 Berlin-Buch

Prof. D.D. BRANISTEANU
Dept. of Physiology, Univ
of Medicine and Pharmacy
RO 6600 Iasi

Prof. E. AGABITI ROSEI
Università degli Studi di
Brescia, Scienze Mediche
IT 25100 Brescia

Prof. J.C. McGRATH
Autonomic Physiology Unit,
Inst. of Physiology
UK Glasgow G12 8QQ

Prof. M. YACOUB &
Dr. A. CHESTER
Thoracic and Cardiac
Surgical Unit,
Harefield Hospital
UK Harefield UB9 6JH

Prof. P.A. Van ZWIETEN
Dept. Pharmacotherapy,
AMC
NL 1105 AZ Amsterdam

Prof. R.J. GRYGLEWSKI
Dept. of Pharmacology,
Jagiellonian Medical
Research Center
PL 31531 Cracow

Prof. T. LÜSCHER
Div. of Cardiology,
Univ Hospital
CH-3010 Bern

MECHANISMS UNDERLYING CORONARY ARTERIAL THROMBOSIS AND ON THE MEANS FOR DISPERSION AND INHIBITION OF SUCH THROMBI

Key words
Thrombosis, anticoagulation, coronary artery disease.

Objectives
Cardiovascular disease is the major cause of death and morbidity in Europeans of working age. Our first priority is an attempt to establish the role of thrombosis as the common denominator for risk factors in coronary artery disease. Concurrently, the efficacy of antithrombotic prophylactic and therapeutic measures in the control of coronary artery disease will be explored.

Brief description
Activation of blood coagulation is a central event in the development of arterial occlusive disease. That thrombosis is involved in the late states of coronary artery disease (CAD) is now accepted and increasing attention is being paid to therapeutic intervention with antigoagulant and fibrinolytic drugs to prevent/reduce coagulation activation. The inadequacies of present approaches are now emerging, but it remains a goal to identify patients at risk of developing thrombosis early in the pathogenesis of the disease, and to find effective anti-thrombotic prevention and treatment. Thus effective antithrombotic prevention is predicted to lead to prevention of the development of coronary artery disease in susceptible persons. The four centres involved will provide interdependent research and data relevant to the single problem. Blood sample exchange, data exchange, interpretation and publication will be made jointly. All blood samples whether from human subjects or experimental preparations will be analysed for various markers of thrombosis, namely platelet factors, endothelin and activation fargments of coagulation. All coronary angiograms will be quantified by the same digital analytical system. The response of the variables measured in each centre will then be studied with various interventions such as serotonin antagonism, thromboxane receptor antagonism, or inhibition of cyclo-oxygenase and thrombin.

Project leader:
Professor M. NOBLE
Academic Unit of Cardiovascular Medicine,
Charing Cross and Westminster
Medical School
369 Fulham Road
UK London SW10 9NH
Phone: +44 81 746 85 53
Fax: +44 81 746 81 82
Contract number: CT920055

Participants:

Prof. D.A. LANE
Dept. of Haematology,
Charing Cross & Westminster Medical School
Fulham Palace Road
UK London W6 8RF
Phone: +44 81 846 7127
Fax: +44 81 846 7111

Prof. H. POULEUR
Cardiology Division,
St. Luc University Hospital
Av. Hippocrate 55/5560
BE 1200 Brussels
Phone: +32 2 764 5560
Fax: +32 2 764 5569

Dr. C. HANETEUR
Cardiology Division,
St. Luc University Hospital
Av. Hippocrate 10
BE 1200 Brussels
Phone: +32 2 764 2881
Fax: +32 2 764 2811

Prof. P. SERRUYS
The Catheterization Laboratory,
Thoraxcenter
P.O. Box 1738
NL 3000 DR Rotterdam
Phone: +31 10 408 8046/8047
Fax: +31 10 436 5192

Dr. K. MEETER
Thoraxcenter
P.O. Box 1738
NL 3000 DR Rotterdam
Phone: +31 10 463 3907
Fax: +31 10 436 2995

Prof. G. FITZGERALD
Dept. of Medicine, Mater Hospital
IE Dublin
Phone: +353 1 307 419
Fax: +353 1 307 704

Dr. I.M. GRAHAM
The Charlemont Clinic,
Charlemont Mall
IE Dublin 2
Phone: +353 1 536 555
Fax: +353 1 781 392

THE IMPORTANCE AND INTERACTION OF GENETIC AND ENVIRONMENTAL FACTORS IN THE PATHOGENESIS OF ATHEROSCLEROSIS (EARS II)

Key words
Atherosclerosis, insulin, glucose, triglyceride, genetics, males, obesity, lifestyle, environment, nutrition.

Objectives
The objectives of the study are:
1 Within populations, to test the hypothesis that insulin resistance is a risk factor for coronary heart disease (CHD), common to different populations in Europe, and which differentiates the male offspring of men with proven premature CHD from age and gender-matched controls randomly selected from the same population.
2 To test the hypothesis that the degree to which insulin resistance manifests itself varies between different populations throughout Europe.
3 To test the hypothesis that the variability to which insulin resistance is manifested is due to environmental factors, lifestyle, nutrition and physical exercise, thus reflecting genetic and environmental interaction.

Brief description
The EARS Group are cardiologists, epidemiologists, clinical and basic scientists with an interest in atherosclerosis. The group was formed to study the interaction of genetic and environmental factors in the pathogenesis of atherosclerosis. The EARS I study looked at the male and female offspring of men with a history of proven myocardial infarction before the age of 55 years and compared them with age and gender-matched controls recruited from the same student populations throughout Europe. In an attempt to standardise on the social background of the different populations groups it was decided to confine the study to university students.

Among the major findings of the EARS I study were that the male, but not the female, offspring of men with premature coronary heart disease differed from age and gender-matched controls in that they were not as tall, had increased body mass indices, increased waist/hip ratio and fasting plasma triglyceride. Their fasting plasma glucose also tended to be higher though this failed to reach statistical significance. It was of interest that the fasting plasma triglyceride was more powerful than cholesterol in discriminating cases from controls, though plasma apoB was the most powerful factor in discriminating cases from controls. These features were consistent across the 14 population groups studied. While significant regional differences existed with regard to lifestyle and diet, within the different regions of Europe the diet and lifestyle of cases was no different from that of their age and gender-matched controls.

These findings suggest that insulin resistance would appear to be a major genetic factor in Europeans with a predisposition to coronary heart disease. The EARS II study was set up to investigate this hypothesis further. The EARS II study will only recruit males. The male cases and their gender-matched controls will be studied with regard to their, and their families, medical history, lifestyle, dietary habits and clinical physical examination according to the protocols drawn up for the EARS I study. In addition, their insulin sensitivity will be assessed by a standardised fat and carbohydrate load with subsequent triglyceride, lipase, glucose and insulin measurements, and a glucose tolerance test with glucose and insulin measurements.

Plasma and DNA will also be collected for other biomarkers and genetic markers associated with the development of coronary heart disease.

The recruitment and subject assessment phase of this study began in October 1993 and will be completed April 1994. It is anticipated that approximately 800 subjects will be assessed from 13 university student populations covering all regions within Europe. The laboratory analyses for the entire study will be done in centralised specialist laboratories so that valid comparisons can be made between the different regions within Europe for all parameters. It is anticipated that the results of the study will be available in 1995/1996.

Project leader:
Dr. D. O'REILLY
European Atherosclerosis
Research Study Group
(EARS),
Institute of Biochemistry
Royal Infirmary
UK Glasgow G4 0SF
Phone: +44 41 304 46 31
Fax: +44 41 553 17 03
Contract number: CT920206

Participants:
Dr. B. MARTIN
Inst. of Social and Preventive
Medicine, Univ of Zurich
CH 8006 Zurich

Dr. D. STANSBIE
Dept. of Chemical Pathology,
Bristol Royal Infirmary
UK Bristol BS2 8HW

Dr. F. CAMBIEN &
Dr. L. TIRET
INSERM SC7
FR 75005 Paris

Dr. Hans-Jurgen MENZEL
Inst. for Med. Biology and
Genetics, Univ of Innsbruck
AT 6020 Innsbruck

Dr. L. HAVEKES
IVVO-TNO Gabius
Laboratory
NL 2300 AK Leiden

Dr. L. TIRET
INSERM U.258
FR 75674 Paris Cedex 14

Dr. M. ROSSENEU
Dept. of Clin. Biochemistry,
Algemeen Ziekenhuis St. Jan
BE 8000 Brugge

Dr. M. SAAVA
Dept. of Nutrition
and Metabolism
EE Tallinn 0001

Dr. P. TALMUD &
Prof. S. HUMPHRIES
Dept. of Medicine,
The Rayne Inst.
Uk London WC1 6JJ

Dr. S. VISVIKIS
Centre de Medecine
Preventive
FR Vandoeuvre-les-Nancy

Dr. U. BEISIEGEL
Medizinische Klinik,
Universitatskrankenhaus
DE 2000 Hamburg 20

Prof. A. EVANS &
Dr. F. KEE
Dept. of Epidemiology and
Public Health,
The Queen's Univ of Belfast
IE Belfast BT12 6BJ

Prof. A. KESANIEMI
Dept. of Internal Medicine,
Univ of Oulu
SF 90200 Oulu

Prof. C. EHNHOLM
National Public Health Inst.
SF 00300 Helsinki

Prof. E. FARINARO
Inst. of Internal Medicine
and Metabolic Disease,
IT 80121 Naples

Prof. G. DE BACKER
Dept. of Hygiene and Social
Medicine, Univ Hospital
BE 9000 Ghent

Prof. G. TSITOURIS
Dept. Medicine/Cardiology
Evangelismos Hospitals
GR Athens 10676

Prof. J. Charles FRUCHART
Service de Recherche sur les
Lipoproteines et l'athero-
sclerose, Inst. Pasteur
FR 590119 Lille Cedex

Prof. J. SHEPHERD
Inst. of Biochemistry,
Royal Infirmary
UK Glasgow G4 0SF

Prof. L. MASANA &
Dr. P. TURNER
Unitat Recerca Lipids,
Facultat Medicina Reus,
Universitat Barcelona
ES 43201 Reus

Prof. M.J. HALPERN
Inst. o Superior de
Ciencias da Saude
PT 2825 Monte de Caparica

Prof. O. FAERGEMAN
Dept. of Medicine and
Cardiology A, Univ Hospital
Tage Hansens Gade 2
DK 8000 Aarhus C

EUROPEAN INITIATIVE FOR IDENTIFYING GENETIC LOCI RESPONSIBLE FOR SPONTANEOUS HYPERTENSION (THE EURHYPGEN PROGRAM)

Key words
Hypertension, genetics, cardiovascular diseases, molecular biology.

Objectives
1 To identify the major genes responsible for genetic hypertension in rat models of human hypertension.
2 To understand the mechanisms by which these genes influence blood pressure.
3 To apply the data towards understanding the genetic basis of human hypertension.

Brief description
Primary hypertension (prevalence = 20%) is the main known risk factor for stroke, and significantly influences the risk of ischaemic heart disease, heart failure and peripheral vascular disease. Thus it is a major health problem with significant economic and social impact. Family studies have demonstrated that hypertension is a multifactorial trait with a strong genetic component. Defining the elements of this genetic component is the primary goal of this Concerted Action. The identification of the major genetic determinants of hypertension would: (a) enable preventive and therapeutic manoeuvres to be directed at high risk individuals; (b) define heterogeneous groups of patients with high blood pressure so that more specific forms of treatment could be matched to each group; (c) enable us to dissect the pathophysiological processes responsible for high blood pressure, and thereby develop more effective forms of management (both pharmacological and non-pharmacological).

The plan of investigation which brings together the major European group studying experimental hypertension rests on two foundations:
1 The availability of inbred strains of genetically hypertensive rats which serve as models of human essential hypertension.
2 The ability to systematically analyze the rat genome to localise genes involved in blood pressure regulation and hypertension as a result of advances made in the development and mapping of genetic markers by laboratories participating in the Concerted Action.

The main task of the Concerted Action will be to develop markers to cover the rat genome and to determine precise chromosomal localisations of major genes of blood pressure regulation in five of the principal models of experimental hypertension:
(1) the spontaneously hypertensive rat (SHR); (2) the stroke-prone spontaneously hypertensive rat (SHRSP); (3) the Lyon hypertensive rat (LH); (4) the Milan hypertensive rat (MHS); (5) the hereditary hypertriglyceredemic hypertensive rat (HTG).
The later will be done by looking for co-segregation of genetic markers with blood pressure. For each of the strains, crosses have been established with normotensive control strains in order to produce F2 generation, or backcross animals suitable for genetic studies in different centres associated with the network. Once genetic linkage has been established, knowledge of the chromosome localisation of a gene involved in blood pressure regulation will be applied in several areas: (1) construction of crosses for high resolution linkage mapping of genes involved in hypertension; (2) development of con-

genic lines to analyze the effect of a locus at the cellular, tissue, organ and whole body levels; (3) positional cloning of the genes utilising tools such yeast artificial chromosomes; (4) studies of the homologous regions as candidate chromosomes regions in human hypertension.

Project leader:
Dr. N.J. SAMANI
Dept. of Medicine,
Clinical Sciences Building,
Leicester Royal Infirmary
P.O. Box 65
UK Leicester LE2 7LX
Phone: +44 533 52 31 89
Fax: +44 533 52 32 73
Contract number: CT920869

Participants:
Prof. J.D. SWALES, Dr. D. LODWICK
Dept. of Medicine, Clinical Sciences Building.
Leicester Royal Infirmary,
University of Leicester
P.O. Box 65
UK Leicester LE2 7LX
Phone: +44 533 523 189
Fax: +44 533 523 273

Dr. M. VINCENT, Prof. J. SASSARD
URA CNRS 606, Dept. de Physiologie et
Pharamacologie Clinique
8 avenue Rockefeller
FR 69373 Lyon Cedex 08
Phone: +33 78 77 70 78
Fax: +33 78 77 71 58

Dr. M. LATHROP
Centre d'Etude de Polymorphisme Humain
27 rue Juliette Dodu
FR 75010 Paris
Phone: +33 1 42 49 98 71
Fax: +33 1 40 18 01 55

Dr. B. CORMAN
Service de Biologie Cellulaire,
Centre d'Etudes Nucleaires de Saclay
FR 91191 Gif-sur-Yvette Cedex
Phone: +33 1 69 08 63 99
Fax: +33 1 69 08 80 46

Prof. BIANCHI
Dipartimento di Scienze e
Technologie Biomediche,
Universita di Milano,
Ospedale San Raffaele
Via Olgettina 60
IT 20132 Milano
Phone: +39 2 33 50 03 70
Fax: +39 2 33 50 04 08

Dr. A.F. DOMINICZAK, Prof. J. REID
Dept. of Medicine & Therapeutics,
Gardiner Institute, Western Infirmary
UK Glasgow G11 6NT
Phone: +44 41 211 2000
Fax: +44 41 339 2800

Dr. Iwar KLIMES
Institute of Experimental Endocinology Vlasrska,
Slovak Academy of Sciences
SK Bratislava
Phone: +427 372 687
Fax: +427 374 247

Dr. J. KUNES, Dr. J. ZICHA
Institute of Physioligy,
Czech Academy of Sciences
Videnska 1083
CZ 142 20 Prague 4
Phone: +42 2 472 1151
Fax: +42 2 471 9517

CELLULAR REMODELLING ASSOCIATED WITH CARDIAC GROWTH, HYPERTROPHY AND FAILURE

Key words
Myocardium, smooth muscle cell, hypertrophy, phenotype, molecular biology, cell biology, transcription factors, growth factors, catecholamines.

Objectives
Definition of the molecular and cellular mechanisms involved in the development of cardiac hypertrophy and failure. This research will provide a deeper understanding of the process of hypertrophy and failure and will allow the development of new approaches to therapy and prevention of human cardiac diseases.

Brief description
The program which is mainly devoted to the experimental animal models includes both *in vivo* and *in vitro* experiments. The main outlines are to define:

1 *the triggers responsible for changes in cardiac gene expression.* The role of catecholamines during *in vivo* ischemic disease has been studied but their specific role in the development of the myocyte remodelling process as well as during the phase of chronic adaptation have to be elucidated. Combining *in vivo* and *in vitro* models the effects of ß- and α-adrenergic stimulation on gene expression and the physiological properties of cardiac myocytes will be analyzed. The increase in catecholamine levels may act directly on the myocyte or induce a cascade of events resulting in local synthesis of growth factors such as TGF ß or FGFs. The expression, the subcellular distribution of these growth factors as well as the binding to their respective receptors will be studied in the mammalian heart during ontogenic development, in hemodynamically overload and in ischemic situations. An *in vitro* study of the effects of growth factors on cardiac gene expression in adult myocytes maintained in culture will be performed.

2 *factors specifically involved in regulating the transcription of cardiac genes.* In contrast to skeletal muscle, the factors responsible for cardiac myocyte differentiation and the expression of cardiac genes are yet unknown. In an attempt to address this issue the isolation of potential transcription factors through molecular cloning will be undertaken.

3 *the role of heat shock proteins (HSP) in the adaptation of the heart to new hemodynamic conditions.* Failing hearts show a pronounced sensitivity to both ischemic and reperfusion damage as compared to non-hypertrophied heart. HSPs have been shown to be rapidly expressed after imposition of an hemodynamic overload or ischemia. Preconditioning of normal heart (synthesis of HSPS prior to a 2nd aggression) was demonstrated to have a remarkably positive effect on the degree of the post-ischemic functional recovery.

Thus the proposal is: 1) to investigate whether preconditioning of the hypertrophied heart can improve the post ischemic outcome of the hypertrophied and/or failing heart; 2) to determine how HSPs interfere with protein folding, transport and binding.

4 *specific changes in the cardiac phenotype.* The expression of fetal isoforms either the product of a gene family or the result of alternative splicing of the primary transcript from a single gene, has been described for many of the main contractile proteins which are expressed by myocytes, and for glycoproteins of the extracelluar matrix synthetised by smooth and non muscle cells. Important gaps exist concerning the

expression of the regulatory proteins (troponin complex) during both the early stage of adaptation of the heart to an increased hemodynamic load and the phase of cardiac failure. In addition there is little information about the differention state of coronary smooth muscle cells when they are submitted to a severe arterial hypertension. One aim of this concerted action is to extend the analysis of the striated myocyte phenotype to the study of the putative changes in smooth muscle cell phenotype.

Project leader:
Dr. J.L. SAMUEL
INSERM, Unité 127,
Hôpital Lariboisière
41, Boulevard de la Chapelle
FR 75010 Paris
Phone: +33 1 49 95 84 80
Fax: +33 1 48 74 23 15
Contract number: CT921171

Participants:
Dr. Saverio SARTORE
Dept. of Biomedical Sciences,
University of Padova
Via Trieste 75
IT 35121 Padova
Phone: +39 49 828 6516
Fax: +39 49 828 6576

Dr. Stefano SCHIAFFINO
Unit for Muscle Biology and
Physiopathology,
University of Padova
Via Trieste 75
IT 35121 Padova
Phone: +39 49 828 6538
Fax: +39 49 828 6576

Dr. Luc SNOECKX
Dept. of Physiology,
University of Limburg,
North lob level 3
University Teitssingel 50, area 29
NL 6229 ER Maastricht
Phone: +31 43 881 203
Fax: +31 43 671 028

Dr. Heinz-Gerd ZIMMER
Physiologgisches Institut
Universität München
Pettenkofferatstesse 12
DE C8000 München 12
Phone: +49 88 58 88
Fax: +49 89 59 96 378

Dr. Peter CUMMINS
Dept. of Physiology,
British Herat Foundation Molecular
Cardiology Research Group,
Birmingham School of Medicine
Edgbaston
UK Birmingham B15 sTT
Phone: +44 21 414 6896
Fax: +44 21 414 6924

Dr. CHARLEMAGNE
Unite 127 INSERM, Unit on the
Metabolism of Heart and Vessels,
Hopital Lariboisière
41 Bld de la Chapelle
FR 75010 Paris
Phone: +33 1 42 85 80 65
Fax: +33 1 49 95 84 80

Dr. SCHWARTZ
Unit 153, Pavillon Rambuteau,
Hopital Pitié Salétrière
41 Bd de l'Hopital
FR 75013 Paris
Phone: +33 1 4217 6802
Fax: +33 1 4217 6811

Dr. BOHELER
Molecular Biology Group,
National Heart Institute
Dovehouse Street
UK London SW 36LY
Phone: +44 71 3528121 ext3031
Fax: +44 71 3763442

THE INTERNATIONAL STROKE TRIAL

Key words
Cerebrovascular disorders, random allocation, aspirin, heparin, cerebral infarction, cerebral haemorrhage.

Objectives
To determine, in patients with acute ischaemic stroke, whether early antithrombotic treatment with aspirin and/or heparin, started as soon as possible (and no later than 48 hours after onset) and continued for two weeks is safe and effective.

Brief description
The International Stroke Trial will evaluate the safety and efficacy of antithrombotic therapy in patients with acute ischaemic stroke by means of a randomised controlled trial. The trial will enrol 20,000 patients from over 600 hospitals in 43 countries worldwide. Fourteen EC/COST countries are participating. The treatment policies to be compared are: 'give aspirin immediately' and 'avoid aspirin for the first two weeks'; 'give subcutaneous heparin 12,500 units subcutaneously twice daily for two weeks'. A 3 x 2 factorial design will allow each policy to be tested separately and in combination.

The study will have sufficient statistical power to provide reliable evidence on the effects of treatment on a number of outcomes, the most important of which are: death within 2 weeks, the proportion of patients dead or dependent at six months and fatal or disabling cerebral bleeding. The accumulating data will be reviewed in confidence by an independent data monitoring committee.

Project leader:
Dr. P.A.G. SANDERCOCK
Department of Clinical
Neurosciences,
Western General Hospital,
University of Edinburgh
Crewe Road
UK Edinburgh EH4 2XU
Phone: +44 31 3436639
Fax: +44 31 3325150
Contract number: CT921723

Participants:
Royal Perth Hospital (AU)
Queen Elizabeth Hospital,
Adelaine
Ballarat Base Hospital
Flinders Medical Centre,
Bedford Park
Princess Alexandra Hospital,
Brisbane
St Vincent's Hospital,
Darlinghurst
General Repatriation Hosp.,
Daw Park
Austin Hospital, Heidelberg
University of Tasmania Clinical
School, Hobart

Wimmera Base Hospital,
Horsham
Royal Melbourne Hospital
Westmead Hospital
Krankenhausen Amstetten (AT)
Krankenhaus der Stadt Baden
Landeskrankenhaus Bregenz
LKH-Oberwart
Landeskrankenhaus Gmunden
University of Graz
University Hospital, Innsbruck
General Hospital of Linz
Krankenhaus d. Barmh Bruder,
Linz
KH D. Elisabethinen, Linz
Landesnervenkl. Gugging
Krankenhaus Schwarzach
IKH Steyr
Hanusch Krankenhaus, Vienna
LKH Villach
Neurologisches Krankenhaus
der Stadt Wien-Rosenhugel
Krankenhaus Floridsdorf
University of Vienna
Fensblafeuf Hospital (BE)
University Hospital Gasthuisberg
Clinique St. Joseph, Mons
Mont-Godinne Hospital, Yvoir
Victoria General Hospital (CA)

Hospital del Salvador,
Santiago de Chile (CL)
University Hospital,
Hradec Kralove (CZ)
City Hospital, Ostrava
Nemocnice Pardubice
University Hospital, Plzen
FN Motole, Praha
General Hospital. Prostejov
Orlicka Nemocnice,
Rychnov nad Kneznou
The Outpatients Clinic,
Rychnov nad Kneznou
Hviodovre Hospital (DK)
St Columcille's Hospital,
Dublin (IE)
Regional General Hospital,
Limerick
Royal Victoria Hospital,
Belfast (IE)
The Ulster Hospital, Belfast
Whitla Medical Building, Belfast
Royal Infirmary of Edinburgh
Erne Hospital, Co. Fermanagh
Central Hosp., Jyvaskyla (FI)
Kymenlaakson Kaskussairaala,
Kotka
Satakunnan Keskussairaala, Pori
CHU de Grenoble (FR)

Univ. of Athens School
of Medicine (GR)
Aigion General Hospital
3rd Hospital I.S.S. of Athens
Dept of Internal Medicine,
Heraklion
Trikala General Hospital
Kwong Wah Hospital,
Hong Kong (HK)
The Prince of Wales Hospital,
Hong Kong
University of Debrecen Medical
School (HU)
B.A.Z. County Hospital,
Miskolc
Carmel Hospital, Haifa (IS)
Wolfson Hospital, Holon
Meir Hospital, Kfar-Saba
Ichilov Hospital, Tel Aviv
Ospedale Torrette, Ancona (IT)
Ospedale Geriatrico U. Sestilli,
Ancona
Ospedale di Arezzo
Ospedale di Ascoli Piceno
Ospedale di Assisi
Policlinico di Bari
Ospedale Civile Bassano
del Grappa
Ospedale Civile di Belluno
Ospedali Riuniti, Bergamo
Ospedale S. Orsola Malpighi.,
Bologna
Ospedale di Borgo San Lorenzo
Piallale Spedali I, Brescia
Ospedale Civile P. Cosma,
Camposampiero
Ospedale Ramazzini, Carpi
Ospedale di Cascia
Ospedale di Cento
Ospedale Bufalini, Cesena
Ospedale Civile, Ancona
Ospedale Valduce, Como
Ospedale di Cortona
Ospedale S.M. Annunziata,
Bagno a Ripoli
Ospedale S. Giuseppe, Empoli
Ospedale San Giovanni Battista,
Foligno
Via dell'Ospedale, Foligno
Ospedale Pierantoni, Forli
Universita di Genova
Ospedale di Imola
Stabilimento Ospedaliero
di Latisana
Ospedale di Lavagna
Ospedale SM Collemaggio,
L'Aquila
Ospedale San Martino, Mede
Policlinico Universitario,
Contesse Messina
Ospedale Civile di Mestre
Ospedale Niguarda Ca Grande,
Milano

Ospedale S. Raffaele, Milano
Ospedale Civile, Modena
Ospedale Santa Croce,
Mancalieri
Ospedale Monsedice
Ospedale S. Francesco, Nuoro
Presidio Ospedal P.L. Annibaldi,
Offida
Ospedale Civile di Orvieto
Ospedale di Orzinuovi
Ospedale di San Benvenuto
e Rocco, Osimo
Universita di Padova
Ospedale Maggiore, Parma
Fondazione C. Mondino, Pavia
Ospedale Policlinico, Perugia
Ospedale Silvestrini, Perugia
Ospedale Civile Piacenza
Ospedale di Pistoia
Ospedale San Carlo, Potenza
Ospedale Riuniti Neurologia,
Salerno
Ospedale di Sarnico
Ospedale di Sassari
Osp Civile S. Matteo degli
Infermi, Spoleto
Ospedale Civile S. Maria, Terni
Ospedale Civile di Todi
Ospedale S. Salvatore, Tolentino
Piazza Ospedale 1, Trieste
Ospedale di San Benedetto
del Tronto
Ospedale San Bortolo, Vicenza
Policlinico San Marco, Zingonia
Medisch Centrum Alkmaar (NL)
AMC, Amsterdam
St. Ziekenhuis Lievensberg,
Bergen op Zoom
St. Deventer Ziekenhuizen
Merwedeziekenhuis Dordrecht
Ziekenhuis Gelderse Vallei, Ede
Diaconessenhuis Eindhoven
Medisch Centrum Twente,
Enschede
Oosterschelde Ziekenhuis, Goes
Diaconessenhuis, Leiden
Ac. Ziekenhuis Maastricht
Ziekenhuis Canisius Wilhelmina,
Nijmegen
Sint Franciscus Gasthuis,
Rotterdam
Ac. Ziekenhuis Rotterdam
Ikazia Ziekenhuis, Rotterdam
Academisch Ziekenhuis Utrecht
Holyziekenhuis, Vlaardingen
Auckland Hospital (NZ)
Nelson Hospital
Tauranga Hospital
Wellington Hospital
Sentralsjukehuset I More Og
Romsdal, Alesund (NO)
Berum Sykehus
Haukeland Hospital, Bergen

Nordland Sentralsykehus, Bodo
Central Hospital Forde
Gjovik fylkessykhus
Hamar Sykehus
Harstad Sykehus
Fylkessykeuset I Haugesund
Ringerike sykehus, Honefoss
Vest-Agder Sentralsykehus,
Kristiansand
Fylkessjukehuset i Kristiansund
Lillehammer fylkessykehus
Fylkessjukehuset I Molde
Sentralsykehuset I Akershus,
Nordbyhagen
Notodden Sykehus
Aker University Hospital, Oslo
Diakonhjemmets Sykehus, Oslo
Lovisenberg Diakonale sykehus,
Oslo
Ulleval Hospital, Oslo
Ostfold Sentralsykehus,
Sarpsborg
Telemark Sentralsykehus, Skien
Vestfold Sentralsykehus,
Tonsberg
Regionsykehuset I Tromsö
Specjalistyczny Szpital ZOZ,
Gdansk (PO)
Klinika Neurologiczna AM,
Katowice
Institute of Psychiatry and
Neurology, Warsaw
Klinika Neurologiczna AM,
Zabrze
Centro Hospitalar de
Coimbra (PT)
Hospital Egas Moniz, Lisboa
Hospital de Sao Jose, Lisboa
Hospital Santa Maria, Lisboa
Hospital Militar Principal,
Lisboa
Hospital de St Antonio, Porto
F.D. Roosevelt Hospital,
Banska Bystrica (CZ)
Comeniu University, Bratislava
(SK)
Spolsan Bolnisnica Celje (CZ)
Medical Centre Ljubljana (SI)
Teaching Hospital Maribor (SI)
Groote Schuur Hospital,
Capetown (ZA)
St. Aiden's Hospital, Durban
Addington Hospital, Durban
St Augustine's Hospital, Durban
Entabeni Hospital, Durban
Port Shepstone Hospital
Hospital San Juan de Dios,
Barcelona (ES)
Hospital Mutua de Terrassa,
Barcelona
Hospital de Valle Hebron,
Barcelona
Hospital Clinico, Barcelona

Consorcio Sanitario de Mataro,
Barcelona
Hospital San Pau, Barcelona
Hospital del Mar, Barcelona
Hospital de Bellvitge, Barcelona
Hospital General de Cataluna,
Barcelona
Hospital General Yague, Burgos
Hospital Fernando Zamacola,
Cadiz
Hospital Josep Truet, Girona
Hospital Provincial, Girona
Hospital General de Huelva
Clinica Puerta de Hierro,
Madrid
Hospital 12 de Octubre, Madrid
Hospital Severo Ochoa, Leganes
Hospital Clinico San Carlos,
Madrid
Hospital La Paz, Madrid
Hospital General Gregorio
Maranon, Madrid
Hospital de Getafe, Madrid
Hospital Clinico Universitario,
Malaga
Hospital Son Dureta,
Palma de Mallorca
Hospital Central Asturias
Clinica Universitaria de
Navarra, Pamplona
Hospital Virgen Aranzazu,
San Sebastian
Hospital Marques de Valdecilla,
Santander
Hospital Virgen del Rocio,
Sevilla
Hospital Universitario Valme,
Sevilla
Hospital de Tarragona
Juan XXIII
Hospital General, Valencia
Hospital De Cruces, Vizcaya
Hospital Clinico Universitario,
Zaragoza
Medicinkliniken Alingsas
Lasarett (SE)
Med. Klin Avesta Las
Medicinkliniken Bollnas Sjukhus
Neurologiska Kliniken
Lasarettet, Boras
Enkoping Hospital
Medicinkliniken Lanssjukhuset,
Halmstad
Sjukhuset Med Kliniken,
Harnosand
Medicinkliniken Harnosands
Sjukhus
Med. Klin. Hassleholm Sjukhus
Karolinska Institut, Huddinge
Hudiksvalls Hospital
Kiruna Hospital
Lasaretter Med. Kliniken,
Koping

Hospital of Koping
Medicinkliniken
Centralsjukhuset, Kristiansand
Medicinkliniken Sjukehuset,
Kristinehamn
Med Klin. Kungalns Sjukhus
Med Kliniken Lindesberg
Med Kliniken Ljungby
University Hospital, Lund
Malmo General Hospital
Med Kliniken Motala
Nacka Sjukhus
Med. Kliniken, Norrtalje
Nykoping Hospital
Med. Kliniken Ornskoldsvik
Medicinska Kliniken
Oskarshamns Sjukhus
Med kliniken, Pitea
Med kliniken, Sandviken
Soder Hospital, Stockholm
Karolinska Sjukhuset, Stockholm
Sundsvalls Sjukhus
Med. Klin. Sjukhuset, Torsby
Neurologiska Kliniken, Uppsala
Varnamo Hospital
Neurologische Klinik,
Aarau (CH)
Kantonsspital Basel
Ospedale San Giovanni,
Bellinzona
Bezirksspital Belp
Lindenhofspital, Bern
Inselspital, Bern
Regionalspital Biel
Spital Brig
Kreisspital Bulach
Regionalspital Burgdorf
Kantonsspital Chur
Kantonsspital Frauenfeld
Bezirksspital Frutigen
Spital Grenchen
Kantonales Spital Heiden
Regionalspital Interlaken
Regionalsspital Langenthal
Kantonsspital Liestal
Ospedale Regionale la Carita,
Locarno
Kantonssptial Luzern
Kreisspital Mannedorf
Ospedale Beata Vergine
Mendrisio
Kantonsspital Munsterlingen
Kantonsspital Olten
Burgerspital Solothurn
Kantonsspital St Gallen
Burgerspital St. Gallen
Bezirksspital Sumiswald
Regionalspital Thun
Kantonales Spital Uznach
Regionalspital Sta Maria, Visp
Spital Wadenswil
Med. Klinik, Winterthur
Universitatsspital Zurich

Stadtspital Triemli, Zurich
Istanbul Medical Faculty (TR)
Marmara University Hospital,
Istanbul
Bakirkoy Ruh Ve Sinir
Hastaliklari, Istanbul
Royal Infirmary of Edinburgh
(UK)
Woodend Hospital,
Aberdeen
Aberdeen Royal Infirmary
William Harvey Hospital,
Willesborough Ashford
Ashford Hospital
Stoke Mandeville Hospital,
Aylesbury
Waveney/Braid Valley Hospital,
Ballymena
North Devon District Hospital
Clatterbridge Hospital,
Bebington
Selly Oak Hospital, Birmingham
General Hospital, Birmingham
Queen Elizabeth Hospital,
Birmingham
General Hospital Bishop
Auckland, Co.Durham
Queen's Park Hospital,
Blackburn
Bolton General Hospital
Bronllys Hospital, Powys Wales
Royal Sussex County Hospital,
Brighton
Frenchay Hospital, Bristol
Burnley General Hospital
Cardiff Royal Infirmary
Cumberland Infirmary, Cumbria
Countess of Chester Hospital
Chester Royal Infirmary
Castle Hill Hospital, Cottingham
Dewsbury & District Hospital,
Dewsbury
Dorset County Hospital,
Dorchester
Buckland Hospital, Dover
District General Hospital,
Dumbarton
Dumfries and Galloway Royal
Infirmary
Royal Infirmary of Edinburgh
Royal Devon & Exeter Hospital
Falkirk and Royal Infirmary
Western Infirmary, Glasgow
Princess Alexandra Hospital,
Harlow
Hartlepool & Easington Health
Care Unit
Hereford General Hospital,
Hereford
Hertford County Hospital
Queen Elizabeth II Hospital,
Hertford

Raigmore Hospital NHS Trust,
Inverness
The Ipswich Hospital
St James's University Hospital,
Leeds
Leicester Royal Infirmary
Leicester General Hospital
The Glenfield Hospital, Leicester
Leigh Infirmary,
Leigh Lancashire
Royal Liverpool Hospital
Fazakerley Hospital, Liverpool
St John's Hospital, Livingston
West Lothian
Greenwich District Hospital,
London
St George's Hospital Medical
School, London
King's College Hospital, London
The Dulwich Hospital, London
Guy's Hospital, London
Whittington Hospital, London
St Andrew's Hospital, London
Whipps Cross Hospital, London
Lewisham Hospital, London
Lurgan Hospital,
Lurgen Co Armagh
Luton & Dunstable Hospital
Macclesfield District Gen.
Hospital
Trafford General Hospital,
Manchester
Newark General Hospital
Hawtonville Hospital,
Newark Notts

Newcastle General Hospital
The Royal Victoria Infirmary,
Newcastle upon Tyne
School of Clinical Medical
Science, Newcastle upon Tyne
Freeman Hospital,
Newcastle upon Tyne
City Hospital, Nottingham
Ormskirk District General
Hospital
Radcliffe Infirmary, Oxford
Poole Hospital NHS Trust,
Dorset
Whiston Hospital,
Prescot Merseyside
Rush Green Hospital,
Romford Essex
Hope Hospital, Salford
Scarborough General Hospital,
North Yorkshire
Northern General Hospital,
Sheffield
Royal Hallamshire Hospital,
Sheffield
Royal Shrewsbury Hospital
South Tyneside District Hospital,
Tyne and Wear
H.M. Stanley Hospital, Clywd
Stirling Royal Infirmary
North Tees General Hospital,
Cleveland
Wordsley Hospital Stourbridge
Corbett Hospital, Amblecote
Sunderland General Hospital

Musgrove Park Hospital,
Taunton
Trinity Hospital, Taunton
Royal Cornwall Hospital, Truro
Pinderfields General Hospital,
Wakefield
South Warwickshire Hospital
Weston General Hospital,
Weston-Super-Mare Avon
Bassetlaw District Hospital,
Notts
Northwestern Memorial
Hospital, Chicago (US)
Southwestern Med Centre,
Dallas, Texas
Long Island Jewish Medical
Center, New York
Neurological Institute,
New York
Rochester General Hospital,
Rochester
Strong Memorial Hospital,
Rochester NY
Bowman Gray School of
Medicine, Winston Salem

UNEXPLAINED CARDIAC ARREST
REGISTRY OF EUROPE (U-CARE)

Key words
Sudden cardiac death, arrhytmias, idiopathic ventricular fibrillation.

Brief description
The primary objective of U-CARE is to collect cases of idiopathic ventricular fibrillation
and to follow for at least 10 years the enrolled patients with yearly check-up visits to
acquire information on:
1 recurrence of malignant arrhythmias or cardiac arrest,
2 development of a previously non obvious organic cardiac disease,
3 differences in outcome among patients treated with different drugs or devices.
U-CARE is a Registry. Therefore, at variance with clinical studies, there are no protocols to be followed and physicians are free to decide if any treatment is required and, in
the positive case, which medication or device is the most apporopriate in their judgment.
Criteria have been selected to define Idiopathic Ventricular Fibrillation (IVF).
Idiopathic Ventricular Fibrillation is defined as an episode of out-of-Hospital cardiac
arrest requiring defibrillation or CPR, (defined in accordance to the guidelines set by the
Task Force of the European Resuscitation Council, the American Heart Association, the
Heart and Stroke Foundation of Canada and the Australian Resuscitation Council, and
published on the British Heart Journal, 1991, 67:325-333) occurring in an indivicual in
whom no underlying cardiac disease which could be responsible for the cardiac arrest
can be detected.
The following examinations are mandatory in order to support the absence of underlying
cardiac disease: normal cardiac physical exam, normal ECG, normal echocardiogram, no
ventricular tachycardia at Holter monitoring or exercise stress test, normal exercise
stress test, no evidence of cardiac ischemia during a stresss test or during ST segment
analysis at Holter monitoring, no preexcitation as assessed by invasive EPS, normal
coronary arteries as assessed by angiography, normal ventricular wall motion and size of
both ventricles as assessed by ultrasound and angiography, no signs of right ventricular
dysplasia, no history of cardiac surgery. The following examinations are not mandatory
for enrollment, but are encouraged: myocardial biopsy, signal averaged ECG, heart rate
variability and baroreflex sensitivity assessment, inducibility of ventricular arrhythmias
at EPS.
The following data have been considered important for the evaluation of patients; there-
fore, they have to be reported and will be collected on standardized forms:
Patient characteristics:
- Sex, age, previous drug treatment, previous medical history, family history or cardiac
  disease;
- Circumstances of cardiac arrest;
- Resuscitation details;
- Conditions after resuscitation;
- Results of all clinical exams;
- Pharmacologic therapy;
- Implantation of defibrillator.
In order to follow the patients' natural history, each individual will be followed with a
yearly follow-up.

Project Leader:
Professor P.J. SCHWARTZ
Centro di Fisiologia Clinica e Ipertensione,
Clinica Medica Generale e Terapia Medica,
Università di Milano
Via F. Sforza, 35
IT 20122 Milan
Phone: +39 2 5513360
Fax: +39 2 5457666
Contract number: CT920132

Participants:
Dr. M. BORGGREFE
Med. Klinik und Poliklinik, Innere Medizin C
Westfalische WilhelmsUniversität Münster
Albert Schweitzer Strasse 33
DE 48129 Münster
Phone: +49 251 86 88 21
Fax: +49 251 821 45

Prof. A.J. CAMM
St. George's Hospital
Medical School, Dept. of Cardiological Sciences
Cranmer Terrace
UK London SW17 0RE
Phone: +44 81 672 99 44
Fax: +44 81 767 71 41

Dr. R.N.W. HAUER
University Hospital of Utrecht,
Heart Lung Institute
Heidelberglaan 100
P.O. Box 85500
NL 3508 GA Utrecht
Phone: +31 30 50 61 84
Fax: +31 30 54 21 55

Dr. H. KLEIN
Med. Akademie, Haus 3/5
Abt. Kardiologie
Leipziger Strasse 44
DE 39120 Magdeburg
Phone: +49 391 67 32 03
Fax: +49 391 67 32 02

Dr. K.H. KUCK
Universitätsspital Eppendorf
Kardiologische Abt.
2 Med. Klinik
Martinistrasse 52
DE 2000 Hamburg 20
Phone: +49 40 471 729 71
Fax: +49 40 471 741 25

Dr. P. TOUBOUL
Hôpital Cardiovasculaire et Pneumologique
Louis Pradel
B.P. Lyon Montchat
FR 69394 Lyon Cedex 03
Phone: +33 7 854 24 17
Fax: +33 7 235 73 41

Dr. H.J.J. WELLENS
Academisch Ziekenhuis Maastricht,
Dept. of Cardiology, Rijksuniversiteit Limburg
Postbus 5800
NL 6202 AZ Maastricht
Phone: +31 43 875 093
Fax: +31 43 875 104

CELL-CELL, CELL-MATRIX INTERACTIONS IN ATHEROSCLEROTIC PLAQUE AND SMOOTH MUSCLE DIFFERENTIATION

Key words
Smooth muscle cells, endothelial cells, integrins, matrix.

Objectives
The long-term goal of this project is to understand the mechanisms by which smooth muscle cells undergo a conversion that allows them to migrate from the medial layer and form intimal thickening (atheroma), and to determine the role of endothelial cells and cells of immune system in modulation of smooth muscle cell function during atheroma formation. The functions and regulation of expression of integrins ($\alpha1\beta1$, $\alpha4\beta1$), VCAM-I, the cytoskeletal protein, vinculin, and extracelluar matrix components (fibronectin, laminin, collagens) and its role in the smooth muscle cells and endothelial cells of normal vessel, and during development and atherogenesis will be studied. Another important point which will be investigated is the mechanism controlling the differentiation of smooth muscle cells.

Brief description
The aim of the project is to understand the mechanisms by which smooth muscle cells (SMC) migrate from the medial layer and form intimal thickening (atheroma), and to determine the role of endothelial cells (EC) and cells of immune system (IC) in modulation of SMC function during atheroma formation. The functions and regulation of expression of integrins ($\alpha1\beta1$, $\alpha4\beta1$), VCAM-I, the cytoskeletal protein, vinculin, and extracelluar matrix components (fibronectin, laminin, collagens) and their role in the SMC, EC and IC of normal vessel, during development and atherogenesis will be studied.

Another important point which will be investigated is the mechanism controlling the differentiation of SMC. The tasks of each participants are the following: regulation of integrin expression and function in EC (G. Tarone); analysis of the role of the cytoskeletal protein vinculin in adherens-type junctions: disruption of the mouse vinculin gene by homologous recombination in ES cells (D.R. Critchley); smooth muscle development (J.P. Thiery and V.E. Koteliansky), role of matrix components and their receptors on function of leucocyte in atherosclerotic lesions (A. Garcia-Pardo). The tasks of each participant are closely interdependent: antibodies to different integrins and cDNA probes for al integrin will be provided by G. Tarone to all participants. cDNA probes for fibronectin variants will be provided by J.P. Thiery; antibody and cDNA probes for vinculin will be provided by D. Crithley and V. Koteliansky; analysis of cell motility for all participants will be performed in Paris, micro-injection technique from laboratory in Paris also will be available for all participants; the disruption gene technology by homologous recombination developed in D. Critchley laboratory will be available for G.Tarone laboratory for knockout of integrin genes; developmental biology systems will be concentrated in Paris and available for all participants; antibodies and CDNA probes to active sites of IIICS region of fibronectin will be provided by A.Garcia-Pardo. The points at which major achievements should be reached are the following:
1 the role and regulation of $\alpha1\beta1$ integrin expression in EC and SMC will be established;

2 the promoters of α1 subunit of integrin and vinculin will be identified and characterized;

3 the spectrum of fibronectin isoforms synthesized by resting and activated EC will be analyzed;

4 the spectrum of laminin variants synthesised by SMC during development and atherogenesis will be established;

5 the mechanisms of α4β1 integrin, VCAM and fibronectin interrelations during interaction of leucocytes with activated EC will be determined;

6 the regulation of α4β1 integrin expression and function by cytokines and growth factors will be studied;

7 the structure of human and mouse vinculin genes will be established;

8 the role of different integrins and extracelluar matrix components on differentiation and motility of SMC will be analyzed;

9 the precursors of vascular SMC will be identified. Each laboratory has a unique research experience: the laboratory in Paris is very experienced in embryology in general and in SMC development and differentiation in particular; the laboratory in Torino has a strong background in integrin function and EC biology. The laboratory in Madrid has a long standing experience in leucocyte integrin biology, and the laboratory in Leicester has extensive experience in the molecular biology of major contractile proteins involved in cell-matrix interactions. The possibility to coordinate and support the scientific activities of these laboratories on the research projects described above represents an unique opportunity to develop an integrated approach to investigate the molecular mechanisms of atheroma formation and role of adhesion molecules in pathogenesis of vascular diseases. An outstanding aspect of the submitted projects is, in fact, that the three major cell types of atherosclerotic plaque, leucocytes, EC and SMC will be studied in coordinate manner by laboratories with high scientific potential.

Project leader:
Dr. J.P. THIERY
Dept. of Biology, CNRS and
Ecole Normale Supérieure 1337
46, rue d'Ulm
FR 75230 Paris Cédex 05
Phone: +33 1 43 26 88 77
Fax: +33 1 43 26 90 26
Contract number: CT920376

Participants:
Dr. A. GARCIA-PARDO
Centro de Investigaciones
Biologicas
Velazques 144
ES 28006 Madrid
Phone: +34 1 564 4562

Dr. Guido TARONE
Dept. of Genetics,
University of Torino
Via Santena 5 bis
IT 10126 Torino
Phone: +39 11 696 3106
Fax: +39 11 663 4788

Dr. David CRITCHLEY
Dept. of Biochemistry,
University of Leicester
University Road,
Adrian Building
UK Leicester LE1 7RH
Phone: +44 533 523 477
Fax: +44 533 523 369

Dr. Victor KOTELIANSKI
Laboratoire de Physiopathology de Dévelopement. CNRS-
Ecole Normale Supérieure
46 rue d'Ulm
FR 75230 Paris Cedex 05
Phone: +33 1 44 32 39 19
Fax: +33 1 43 26 90 26

THE USE OF EFFECTIVE SECONDARY PREVENTIVE TREATMENTS AFTER MYOCARDIAL INFARCTION: A MULTINATIONAL STUDY

Key words
Myocardial infarction, drug utilisation, data collection, adrenergic beta receptor blockaders, aspirin, thrombolytic therapy, smoking cessation.

Objectives
1 To obtain accurate representative and comparable data on the pattern of use of proven secondary preventive treatments after acute myocardial infarction in the participating countries;
2 To identify and measure differences in practice in the context of the shared clinical trials evidence upon which practice is based;
3 To identify possible reasons for international divergences in practice, in order to propose measures which would encourage the best possible application of current knowledge to reduce secondary mortality and morbidity after acute myocardial infarction.

Brief description
This Concerted Action examines the extent to which measures which have been proved to reduce mortality and risk of re-infarction are being applied in the routine care of patients with acute myocardial infarction (AMI).
The measures of interest are:
1 Thrombolytic treatment as early as possible in the acute phase;
2 Aspirin in the acute phase;
3 Aspirin for long term prophylaxis;
4 A beta-blocker for long term prophylaxis;
5 Cessation of smoking.

Data are being gathered in representative regions throughout Europe so that the effects of national differences in patterns of health care on the adoption of effective methods of secondary prevention can be examined.
The proportion of patients with AMI currently receiving the benefit of these measures is being estimated in the participating centres. A sampling frame of representative hospitals has been defined in a suitable region of each country. From this is being drawn an unbiased sample of patients admitted with AMI within a defined time window. Data on clinical characteristics and secondary prevention given are being gathered both for the acute episode and at 4-6 months after AMI. Analysis of the international data will be carried out at Leicester University, UK.
Sample sizes have been calculated to give standard errors of the order of 2-3% for the estimates of rates of secondary prevention. The total study recruitment will be approximately 3,000 subjects.
Secondary sources of information will also be used where available. The final analysis will provide a broad-based picture of current European practice. Divergence between countries and from optimum standards derived from available knowledge (recent large scale clinical trials) will be measured and, wherever possible, reasons identified.

Project leader:
Dr. K.L. WOODS
Department of Medicine & Therapeutics,
Clinical Sciences Building, University of Leicester
Leicester Royal Infirmary
UK Leicester LE2 7LX
Phone: +44 533 523125
Fax: +44 533 523108
Contract number: CT921819

Participants:

Prof. Franz DIENSTL
Cardiology, Univ Klinik
für Innere Medzin
Anichstrasse 35
AT 6020 Innsbruck
Phone: +43 512 577 663
Fax: +43 512 579 720

Dr. Alain LEIZOROVICZ
Unite de Pharmacologie
Clinique
162 Avenue Lacessagne
FR 69424 Lyon Cedex 3
Phone: +33 72 11 52 56
Fax: +33 78 53 10 30

Dr. Declan O'CAALGHAN
Beaumont Hospital
P.O. Box 1297,
Beaumont Road
IE Dublin 9
Phone: +353 1 37 7755
Fax: +353 1 37 6740

Dr. R. SEABRA-GOMES
Instituto Do Corsaacao
Av. Prof. Reynaldo Dos
Santos 27 Carnaxide
PT 2795 Linda-A-Velha
Phone: +351 1 418 8030
Fax: +351 1 418 6291

Porf. Felix GUTZWILLER
Institute of Social &
Preventive Medicine,
University of Zurich
Sumatrastrasse
CH 8006 Zurich
Phone: +41 92 252 927
Fax: +41 92 252 003

Prof. D. VASILIAUSKAS
Laboratory for Cardio-
vascular Rehabilitation
3007 Sukileliu 17
Kaunas Lithuania
Phone: +370 7 734 586
Fax: +370 7 732 286

Dr. Risto KALA
Maria Hospital
FI 00180 Helsinki
Phone: +358 0 609 9222
Fax: +358 0 694 0624

Prof. Nick KARATZAS
Maria Hospital
D Soutsou 9
GR 11521 Athens
Phone: +30 1 646 4184
Fax: +30 1 646 4678

Dr. Asmund REIKVAM
Research Forum (FUS),
Ulleval University Hospital
Midtblokka Kirkevn 166
NO 0407 Oslosinki
Phone: +47 22 11 81 94
Fax: +47 22 11 84 79

Dr. Lars WILHELMSEN
Dept. of Medicine,
Ostra Hospital
SE 41685 Goteborg
Phone: +46 31 374 081
Fax: +46 31 259 254

THE EUROPEAN STROKE DATABASE PROJECT

Key words
Stroke, cerebrovascular disorders, classification, case mix, comorbidity, prognosis, process assessment, outcome assessment, clinical trials, health services research.

Objectives
1 To create a common clinical language for epidemiological studies and clinical trials in stroke and to publish a *European Manual of stroke Assessments*.
2 To collect baseline information needed for planning future trials of service organisation, medical treatment and rehabilitation, and to identify clinical issues to be addressed in such trial.

Brief description
Progress in clinical stroke research has been hampered by a lack of standardisation in clinical terminology, classification, assessments and outcome measures. Stroke registers have been set up in many countries but basic information has been recorded in different ways, often using incompatible computer systems so that it is impossible to make meaningful comparisons between centres or countries, or to combine the data from different studies.

The Concerted Action aims to remedy this situation over the next 3 years in the following ways:
a by standardising clinical assessments and simple measurement scales (for neurological impairment, disability, handicap etc.) and testing them for validity and inter-rater reliability;
b by agreeing on a standard, simple clinical classification of stroke (to be validated by clinico-radiological comparisons);
c by standardising methods of functional, cognitive, perceptual and emotional assessment of stroke patients and simple measures of rehabilitation input;
d by developing better methods of predicting the outcome of stroke which can be used to stratify patients in future trials.
The above information will be incorporated into a European Stroke Database, using standardised computer software. The proposal will co-ordinate and build on work already begun in several European countries, setting up a programme of collaborative clinical research, and will provide all the information needed to plan the large-scale international controlled clinical trials which will be essential for improving the treatment and prevention of stroke.

Project leader:
Dr. David H. BARER
Dept. of Clinical Geriatric Medicine,
Newcastle General Hospital
westgate Road
UK Newcastle upon Tyne NE4 6BE
Phone: +44 91 27 38 81 ext. 22 410
Fax: +44 91 272 26 89
Contract number: CT931439

Participants:

Dr. Armandio VEIGA (PT)

Dr. A. Ch. SANCHEZ (ES)

Dr. A. FORSTER (UK)

Dr. A. INDEKEU (BE)

Dr. A. MAIN (UK)

Dr. A. MAMOLI (IT)

Dr. A. MARTIN (UK)

Dr. Bo NORRVING (SE)

Dr. B. SADZOT (BE)

Dr. Castro LOPES (PT)

Dr. Cecily PARTRIDGE (UK)

Dr. Charles WOLFE (UK)

Dr. Christos PASCHALIS

Dr. David BLACK (UK)

Dr. Derick WADE (UK)

Dr. D. INZITARI (IT)

Dr. D. MacMAHON (UK)

Dr. D. SASTRY (UK)

Dr. E. BOTTACCHI (IT)

Dr. Feliciana CORTESE (IT)

Dr. F. Chiodo GRANDI (IT)

Dr. F. PEZZELLA (IT)

Dr. F. RUBIO (ES)

Dr. G. BOYSEN (DK)

Dr. G. VENABLES (UK)

Dr. Henrique BARROS (PT)

Dr. James BARRETT (UK)

J.F. FERREIRA PALMEIRO &
Dr. G. GONCALVES (PT)

Dr. Jose A. EGIDO (ES)

Dr. José M. FERRO (PT)

Dr J. BOGOUSSLAVSKY (CH)

Dr. J. YOUNG (UK)

Dr. J.J. MURPHY (UK)

Dr. J.J.M. Driesen (NL)

Dr. J.M. BAMFORD (UK)

Dr. J.M. CANDIDO (PT)

Dr. Kjell ASPLUND (SE)

Dr. L.M. LAINEZ (ES)

Dr. Med. C.R. HORNIG (DE)

Dr. Miquel LEAO (PT)

Dr. M. DENNIS (UK)

Dr. M. GIROUD (FR)

Dr. M. GUIDOTTI (IT)

Dr. Nadina LINCOLN (UK)

Dr. Nuno Sousa FONTES (PT)

Dr. Paul E. BRIET (NL)

Dr. Pedro Gil GREGORIO (ES)

Dr. P.J. STEPHEN (UK)

Dr. Rosario MARTIN (ES)

Dr. R. LODWICK (UK)

Dr. S. HAMILTON (UK)

Dr. V. LARRUE (FR)

Ms. Victorine WOOD (UK)

Prof. A. CAROLEI (IT)

Prof. B. MIHOUT (FR)

Prof. Cesare FIESCHI (IT)

Prof. Dr. G. FRANCK (BE)

Prof. Dr. Jose CASTILLO (ES)

Prof. U.A. BESINGER (DE)

Prof. D.L. McLELLAN (UK)

Prof. G. MULLEY (UK)

Prof. H. CARTON (BE)

Prof. ORGOGOZO (FR)

Prof. Jean-Yves GOAS (FR)

Prof. J.M. CALHEIROS (PT)

Prof. J. van GIJN (NL)

Prof. J.R. CASADO (ES)

Prof. L. Provinciali (IT)

Prof. CHAIMBERLAIN (UK)

Prof. M.J.G. HARRISON (UK)

Prof. O.F.W. JAMES (UK)

Prof. P. KOUDSTAAL (NL)

Prof. LANGTON HEWER (UK)

Prof. R.C. TALLIS (UK)

Prof. Shah EBRAHIM (UK)

Prof. Willy DE WEERDT (BE)

CHARACTERIZATION OF THE MOLECULAR EVENTS RESPON
SIBLE FOR CELLULAR UPTAKE OF LIPOPROTEINS

Key words
Lipoproteins, receptors, LDL-receptor, apoprotein B, apoprotein E, fatty acids, endocytosis, lipases, hepatocytes, arteriosclerosis.

Objectives
The overall objective of this proposal is to allow five of the most prominent research laboratories to reach a consensus regarding the molecular mechanism responsible for the removal of lipoproteins. Towards this goal, four specific aims have been selected:
1 To determine the relative contribution of the 3 new candidate lipoproteins receptors, the LDL-receptor related protein (LRP), the lipolysis stimulated receptor (LSR) and the remnant receptor (RR) to the clearance of chylomicron remnants.
2 To define the respective contributions of the 4 receptors (LDL-R, LRP, LSR and RR) to the removal of VLDL, IDL, LDL and chylomicron remnants.
3 To characterize mechanisms that coordinate the action of these 4 receptors.
4 To define the influence of mutation of the LDL-R gene on the variation in the penetrance of type II hyperlipidemia.

Brief description
Regulation of the catabolism of lipoproteins has proven to play a key role in determining their plasma concentration and hence their potential atherogenicity. In human subjects, the hepatocyte is responsible for most of lipoprotein clearance. The LDL-Receptor plays an important role in this removal process; however, the extent of its contribution remains highly disputed. The overall goal of this proposal is to shed new light on the molecular mechanisms that are responsible for cellular uptake of apoB containing lipoproteins.
Our primary objectives are:
1 to biochemically characterize the 4 receptors - LDL-Receptor (LDL-R), LDL-Receptor Related protein (LRP), Remnant Receptor (RR) and Lipolysis Stimulated Receptor (LSR) - that are likely to take part in the removal of lipoproteins subfractions in both normal and hyperlipidemic human subjects.
The specific aim of this proposal is to create a structure that will allow European laboratories with established leadership in this area of research:
1 to benefit from the specific expertise achieved by each member of this group;
2 to rapidly and efficiently exchange specific information and;
3 to share with each other:
a the biochemical probes prepared during characterisation of the three new candidate receptors (e.g. monoclonal and polyclonal antibodies, DNA and/or protein sequences, bacterial vectors, purified native or chemically modified lipoprotein subfractions as well as cell lines from subjects with genetic defects of candidate receptors);
b the specialized instruments needed to complete these studies (e.g. BIAcore and microsequencer). We are confident that coordinating the efforts of the five most prominent European teams focusing their attention towards this area of research will considerably enhance our chances of tackling this issue and favor the development of a consensus on this highly controversial topic.

Project leader:
Professor Bernard BIHAIN
Laboratoire de Biochimie des Sciences
Pharmaceutiques et Biologiques,
Université de Rennes I
av Professor Léon Bernard 2
FR 35043 Rennes
Phone: +33 99 33 69 40
Fax: +33 99 33 68 88
Contract number: CT931088

Participants:
Dr. James SHEPHERD
Dept. of Pathological Biochemistry,
Royal Infirmary
UK Glasgow G4 0SF
Phone: +44 41 552 3335
Fax: +44 41 553 1703

Dr. Peter R. TURNER
Facultat de Medicina,
Universitat Rovira I Virgili
C/Sant Llorenç 21
ES 43201 Reus
Phone: +34 77 31 89 22
Fax: +34 77 31 91 47

Dr. Theo C. van BERKEL
Sylvius Laboratories
P.O. Box 9503
NL 2300 RA Leiden
Phone: +31 71 276216
Fax: +31 71 276292

Dr. W.J. SCHNEIDER
Dept. of Molecular Genetics,
Univ and Biocenter Vienna
Dr. Bohr-Gasse 9/2
AT 1030 Wien
Phone: +43 1 79515 2113
Fax: +43 1 79515 2013

SYSTEMATIC OVERVIEWS ('META-ANALYSES') OF RANDOMISED CONTROLLED TRIALS IN THE TREATMENT AND PREVENTION OF VASCULAR DISEASES

Key words
Meta-analysis, randomized controlled trials, random allocation, fibrinolytic-agents, thrombolytic-therapy, platelet-aggregation-inhibitors, antilipemic agents.

Objectives
1 To establish permanent collaborative groups of trialists which will maintain continuously updated registries of past and current randomised trials in three key categories of vascular disease treatment and prevention: *antiplatelet therapy, fibrinolytic therapy* and *cholesterol-lowering therapy.*
2 To conduct collaborative systematic overviews of these randomised trials; to arrange meetings of collaborators in order to discuss the overview analyses and their interpretation; to agree on further analyses; and to establish priorities for future research.
3 To publish and disseminate the results of these overviews in the names of all collaborators, thus providing up-to-date formal statistical summaries of all randomised evidence for the effects of antiplatelet therapy, fibrinolytic therapy and cholesterol-lowering therapy in vascular disease.

Brief description
The purpose of this Concerted Action is to conduct collaborative systematic overviews of randomised trials in three key categories of vascular disease treatment and prevention: antiplatelet therapy, fibrinolytic therapy and cholesterol-lowering therapy.
The Antiplatelet Trialists' Collaboration is already established, and in the present proposal will:
i update existing reviews;
ii review randomised trials of antiplatelet therapy in new areas (especially acute stroke and pulmonary embolism); and
iii review randomised trials relating to new antiplatelet agents.

The Fibrinolytic Therapy Trialists' Collaboration is also well established and plans similarly to:
i update existing reviews;
ii review randomised trials of fibrinolytic therapy in new areas (e.g. pulmonary embolism and other occlusive vascular disorders); and
iii review randomised trials relating to new fibrinolytic agents.

Cholesterol-Lowering Trialists' Collaboration: at a meeting last year preliminary agreement was reached on setting up a collaborative group of trialists who are currently conducting large randomised trials of cholesterol-lowering therapy. The objectives of this group would be:
i to publish an overview of completed trials using intention-to-treat data (which until now has remained unpublished due to lack of resources); and
ii to plan a prospective overview of current studies which would be published in the name of the Collaborative Group, and would provide (i) a reliable assessment of the effects of lipid lowering on total and cause-specific mortality in primary and secondary

prevention, and (ii) information on the effects of lipid lowering in particular patient groups of special interest (e.g. the elderly and women), which may not be addressed in sufficiently large numbers within individual trials.

The project will help to achieve harmonisation of prescribing policy across Europe, leading to approprately wide use of effective drugs and avoidance of ineffective ones in the treatment and prevention of vascular disease.

Project leader:
Dr. Rory COLLINS
Clinical Trial Services Unit,
Radcliffe Infirmary,
Woodstock Road
UK Oxford OX2 6HE
Phone: +44 86 55 72 41
Fax: +44 86 55 88 17
Contract number: CT931552

Participants:

Prof. R. SCHRODER (DE)
Dr. J.R. O'BRIEN (UK)
Dr. B. MAGNANI (IT)
Ass. Prof. SAMUELSSON (SE)
Dr. A. BASELLINI (IT)
Dr. A. FORESTI (IT)
Dr. A. KEECH (UK)
Dr. A. LEIZOROVICZ (FR)
Dr. A. MAGGIONI (IT)
Dr. A. ORIOL (ES)
Dr. A. SKENE (UK)
Dr. A. VICARI (IT)
Dr. A. Van den BELT (NL)
Dr. A.E. GENT (UK)
Dr. A.E.R. ARNOLD (NL)
Dr. A.H. GERSHLICK (UK)
Dr. A. FUNKE-KUPPER (NL)
Dr. B. BALKAU (FR)
Dr. B. HARTUNG (DE)
Dr. B. KNUDSEN (DK)
Dr. B. MEIER (CH)
Dr. B. NORRVING (SE)
Dr. C.E. ELWIN (SE)
Dr. C. BALGENT (UK)
Dr. C. BLOMSTRAND (SE)
Dr. C. BRUNELLI (IT)
Dr. C. FIESCHI (IT)
Dr. C. FISKERSTRAND (UK)
Dr. C. GRAY (UK)
Dr. C. PATRONO (IT)
Dr. Dirk LAMMERTS (DE)
Dr. D. ARDISSINO (IT)
Dr. D. BONADUCE (IT)
Dr. D. COLLEN (BE)
Dr. D. DUNBABIN (UK)
Dr. D. GRAY (UK)
Dr. D. MENDELOW (UK)

Dr. D. CHAMBERLAIN (UK)
Dr. D.H. COVE (UK)
Dr. D.L. PATTERSON (UK)
Dr. E. ESCHWEGE (FR)
Dr. E. ESMATJES (ES)
Dr. E. JOHANSSON (SE)
LAVENNE-PARDONGE (BE)
Dr. E. LESAFFRE (BE)
Dr. E. ROCHA (ES)
Dr. E. THAULOW (NO)
Dr. E. WYN-JONES (UK)
Dr. E.D. COOKE (UK)
Dr. E.J. ACHESON (UK)
Dr. F. BALSANO (IT)
Dr. F. VERMEER (NL)
Dr. F. VIOLI (IT)
F.J. ESPINA GAYUBO (ES)
Dr. F.W. ALBERT (DE)
Dr. F.W. BÄR (NL)
De la GALA SANCHEZ (ES)
Dr. G. ARAPAKIS (GR)
Dr. G. AVELLONE (IT)
Dr. G. BOYSEN (DK)
Dr. G. CIUFETTI (IT)
Dr. G. DAVL (IT)
Dr. G. LANDINI (IT)
Dr. G. LOWE (UK)
Dr. G. RASMANIS (SE)
Dr. G. SANZ (ES)
Dr. G. STANZ (ES)
Dr. G. VETH (NL)
Dr. DEN OTTOLANDER (NL)
Dr. G.K. MORRIS (UK)
Dr. G.P. SIGNORINI (IT)
Dr. H. ADDRIAENSEN (BE)
Dr. H. Ch. HART (NL)
Dr. H. MULEC (SE)

Dr. H. STIEGLER (DE)
Dr. H. TINDALL (UK)
Dr. H. VINAZZER (AT)
Dr. H.R. BAUR (CH)
Dr. I. CHALMERS (UK)
Dr. Jan-Erik KARLSSON (SE)
Dr. J.E. OLSSON (SE)
Dr. BERTRAND-HARDY (BE)
Dr. J. DALE (NO)
Dr. J. DYCKMANS (DE)
Dr. J. FIGUERAS (ES)
Dr. J. HELKKILA (FI)
Dr. J. HERLITZ (SE)
Dr. J. KAPPELLE (NL)
Dr. J. KELLETT (UK)
Dr. J. LASIERRA (ES)
Dr. J. LODDER (NL)
Dr. J. LOPEZ-SENDON (ES)
Dr. J. MIROUZE (FR)
Dr. J. SANCHO-RIEGER (ES)
Dr. J. SOREFF (SE)
Dr. J. Van der MEER (NL)
Dr. J.L. DAVID (BE)
Dr. DOMENICH-AZNAR (ES)
Dr. J.R. LOUDON (UK)
Dr. KADEL (DE)
Dr. K.A. JOHANNESSEN (NO)
Dr. K.M. FOX (UK)
Dr. K.M. SHAW (UK)
Dr. K.R. KARSCH (DE)
Dr. LOPEZ-TRIGO (ES)
Dr. Lars GRIP (SE)
Dr. Lars WILHELMSEN (SE)
Dr. L. CANDELLSE (IT)

Dr. L. JANZON (SE)
Dr. L. PEDRINI (IT)
Dr. L. REVOL (FR)
Dr. L. VISANI (IT)
Dr. Marcus FLATHER (UK)
Dr. M. BEEN (UK)
Dr. M. BOBERG (SE)
Dr. M. BOSCH (ES)
Dr. M. CARMALT (UK)
Dr. M. CATALANO (IT)
Dr. M. CLOAREC (FR)
Dr. M. DECHAVANNE (FR)
Dr. M. GOLDMAN (UK)
Dr. M. HOMMEL (FR)
Dr. M. MORIAU (BE)
Dr. M. OLDENDORF (DE)
Dr. M. PANNEBAKKER (NL)
Dr. M. PFISTERER (CH)
Dr. M. PINI (IT)
Dr. M. SCHEPPING (DE)
Dr. M. WEBER (DE)
Dr. M.BRAN (BE)
Dr. M.BRITTON (SE)
Dr. M.C. TORKA (DE)
Dr. M.G. FRANZOSI (IT)
Dr. N. BOUSSARD (FR)
Dr. N. BROOKS (UK)
Dr. N. CLAVERELLA (IT)
Dr. N. PFLUGER (CH)
Dr. N. QIZILBASH (UK)
Dr. N. THIBULT (FR)
Dr. N. WAHLGREN (SE)
Dr. N.B. KARATZAS (GR)
Dr. O. FAERGEMAN (DK)
Dr. PASTEYER (FR)
Dr. P. DROUIN (FR)
Dr. P. ELWOOD (UK)
Dr. P. FRANKS (UK)
Dr. P. GRESELE (IT)
Dr. P. GUITERAS (ES)
Dr. P. KOUDSTAAL (NL)
Dr. P. LIJNEN (BE)
Dr. P. MONNIER (CH)
Dr. P. PETERSEN (DK)
Dr. P. POZZILLI (UK)
Dr. P. PRANDONI (IT)
Dr. P. PUTZ (BE)
Dr. P. SANDERCOCK (UK)
Dr. SCHANZENBACHER (DE)
Dr. P.C. ADAMS (UK)
Dr. P.LIEVRE (FR)
Dr. P.S. SORENSEN (DK)
Dr. P.T. HARJOLA (FI)
Dr. P.W. SERRUYS (NL)
Dr. R. CAPILDEO (UK)
Dr. R. COLLINS (UK)
Dr. R. De CATERINA (IT)
Dr. R. GENTILE (IT)

Dr. R. HUGONOT (FR)
Dr. R. LORENZ (DE)
Dr. R. SEABRA-GOMES (PT)
Dr. R.C. KESTER (UK)
Dr. R.G. WILCOX (UK)
Dr. R.G. ZENNARO (IT)
Dr. R. ROSS-RUSSELL (UK)
Dr. STARKMAN (FR)
Dr. S. BALA (UK)
Dr. S. COCCHERI (IT)
Dr. S. ELL (UK)
Dr. S. HEPTI (UK)
Dr. S. PARISH (UK)
Dr. S. PERSSON (SE)
Dr. S.M. RAJAH (UK)
Dr. T. BRÜGGEMAN (DE)
Dr. T. CURTI (IT)
Dr. T. FOLEY (UK)
Dr. T. FOULDS (UK)
Dr. T. LEMMENS (NL)
Dr. T.W. MEADE (UK)
Dr. U. SIGWART (UK)
Dr. U.L.F. BERGLUND (SE)
Dr. CUTHERBERTSON (UK)
Dr. W.S. HILLIS (UK)
Mrs. R. ECKEL (DE)
Mr. A. AUKLAND (UK)
Mr. A. RAHMAN (UK)
Mr. A.D.B. CHANT (UK)
Mr. A.E. CARTER (UK)
Mr. C.A.C. CLYNE (UK)
Mr. C.V. RUCKLEY (UK)
Mr. E.H. WOOD (UK)
Mr. J.A. DORMANDY (UK)
Mr. M.A. WALKER (UK)
Mr. M.D.M. SHAW (UK)
Mr. N.A.G. JONES (UK)
Mr. P.M. SWEETNAM (UK)
Mr. T. GARDECKI (UK)
Ms. C. DICKERSON (UK)
Ms. Daniela GUIDUCCI (IT)
Ms. M.G. WALKER (UK)
Prof. A. Encke (DE)
Prof. UBERLA (DE)
Prof. A. APOLLONIO (IT)
Prof. A. BOLLINGER (CH)
Prof. A. LIBRETTI (IT)
Prof. A. LOWENTHAL (BE)
Prof. A. RASCOL (FR)
Prof. BONEU (FR)
GULRAUD-CHAUMELL (FR)
Prof. C. CERNIGLIARO (IT)
Prof. C.N. McCOLLUM (UK)
Prof. C.P. WARLOW (UK)
Prof. Dr. B. HOFLING (DE)
Prof. Dr. G. SCHETTLER (DE)
Prof. Dr. K. ANDRASSY (DE)
Prof. Dr. R. von ESSEN (DE)

Prof. Dr. W. SCHOOP (DE)
Prof. D. JULIAN (UK)
Prof. D. LOEW (DE)
Prof. D. RAITHEL (DE)
Prof. D. de BONO (UK)
Prof. E. Zeitler (DE)
Prof. F. ROVELLI (IT)
Prof. F. Van de WERF (BE)
Prof. F. ZEKERT (AT)
Prof. F. VERHEUGT (NL)
Prof. G. CRIBLER (FR)
Prof. G. Mattioli (IT)
Prof. G. NENCI (IT)
Prof. G. PAGANO (IT)
Prof. G. SLAMA (FR)
Prof. G. TOGNONI (IT)
Prof. G. VOGEL (DE)
Prof. G.A. FITZGERALD (IE)
Prof. G.V.R BORN (UK)
Prof. H. HESS (DE)
Prof. H. LINKE (DE)
Prof. H.K. TONNESEN (DK)
Prof. H.W. HEISS (DE)
Prof. J.P. BASSAND (FR)
Prof. J. MEYER (DE)
Prof. J. van GIJN (NL)
Prof. J.B. BOISSEL (FR)
Prof. K.L. NEUHAUS (DE)
Prof. K. BREDDIN (DE)
Prof. K.A.A. FOX (UK)
Prof. Lars WALLENTIN (SE)
Prof. L. GREGORATTI (IT)
Prof. L. POMAR (ES)
Prof. M. BROCHLER (FR)
Prof. M. CORTELLARO (IT)
Prof. M. NOBLE (UK)
Prof. M. SIMOONS (NL)
Prof. M. VERSTRAETE (BE)
Prof. M.B. BOUSSER (FR)
Prof. M.J. BROWN (UK)
Prof. M.J.G. HARRISON (UK)
Prof. M.P. VESSEY (UK)
Prof. NOVAK (DE)
Prof. O. KRAUSE (DE)
Prof. P. SLEIGHT (UK)
Prof. P.C. RUBIN (UK)
Prof. R. LIMET (BE)
Prof. R. PETO (UK)
Prof. S. POCOCK (UK)
Prof. S.M. COBBE (UK)
Prof. T. DIPERRI (IT)
Prof. V. COTO (IT)
Prof. V.C. ROBERTS (UK)
Prof. W. KASPER (DE)

COMMUNITY LEARNING ACTION FOR CORONARY RISK ABATEMENT 'CLARA PROJECT'

Key words
Coronary risk factors, cultural model, European code.

Brief description
The Community Learning Action for coronary Risk Abatement project CLARA project has the following main objectives:

A To develop a cultural-model such as a European Code for Cardiovascular Healt containing clear indications on the methodologies to improve the community's knowledge at two levels:
- the lifestyle-related coronay risk factors, in order to reduce them;
- the awarenss of heart attack's symptoms and of coronary facilities, to decrease the time of acute coronary care delivery;

B To review the existing body-of knowledge, paying particular attention to the relevant European experiences, to shape a tôol tailored to European people and easily transferable into local projects;

C To set up two pilot programs to verify the implementation of the cultural model in two different European communities, Friuli-Italy and Bremèn-Germany, where a common monitoring system of cardiovascular diseases has been operational since 1984, according to the who monica project;

D To analyse the results of the pilot phase in order to adapt and integrate the cultural model and support the feasibility of similar activities in other European countries.

The first action of the Clara Project will be that of convening a multidisciplinary workshop of European and international experts in community cardiovascular health communication. Their task will be that of developing the European cultural model and an ad hoc questionnaire to evaluate the baseline and final levels of community knowledge.

The second actiòn of the clara Project will be the establissment of the two pilot programmes in Friuli and Bremen, where, after an initial telephone poll, an active intervention plan will be carried out, for ten months. Eventually a final telephone call will be performed, to evaluate the results. Other indicators will be drawn by the ongoing MONICA project in the two areas.

The third action of the CLARA Project will be a joint analysis and evaluation of the pilot projects.

Project leader:
Professor Giorgio Antonio FERUGLIO
Istituto di Cardiologia,
Ospedale S.M. Misericordia
IT 33100 Udine
Phone: +39 43 255 24 55
Fax: +39 43 255 24 52
Contract number: CT931485

Participant:
Prof. E. GREISER
Bremen Institut für Präventionsforschung
and Sozialmedizin (BIPS)
Grunenstrasse 120
DE Bremen
Phone: +49 421 59 59 60
Fax: +49 421 59 59 665

DIAGNOSIS AND THERAPY OF CORONARY AND CEREBRAL VASCULAR DYSFUNCTION

Key words

Vascular dysfunction, lipid mediators, nitric oxide, endothelin, free radicals.

Brief description

The contribution of vascular dysfunction to clinical syndromes of vascular occlusion, such as myocardial infarction and stroke, has become increasingly appreciated.

This may reflect the generation of biochemical mediators by vascular tissues alone, or in concert with adjacent cells, including platelets and leukocytes.

There is also evidence that the clinical presentation of such diseases may differ between men and women.

Although the mechanisms underlying this observation are poorly understood, they may involve differential generation of and/or response to vascular autacoids.

The present programme is focused upon clarifying the role of three classes of autacoids generated by and acting on the vasculature (lipid mediators, nitric oxide and endothelin-I in clinical syndromes of coronary and cerebral artery instability.

Biochemical methods and animal models will be developed respectively to characterise and assess the biological role of lipid mediators:

i generated by the interaction of platelets, leukocytes and endothelial cells; and

ii by free radical catalysed transformation of arachidonic acid in the cerebral and coronary circulations.

Initial investment will be in physicochemical methodology with later translation to more facile methods, such as enzyme immunoassay.

Identification of biologically appropriate analytical targets will permit study of their biosynthesis in vascular occlusive syndromes in men and women and will aid assessment of the effects of physiological and pharmacological interventions on their biosynthesis.

This will assist the rational design of clinical trials designed to assess the safety and efficacy of therapeutic approaches to the modification of vascular instability in humans.

Project leader:
Professor G. FITZGERALD
Centre for Cardiovascular
Science, Dept. of Medicine &
Experimental Therapeutics
Eccles Street 7
IE Dublin 7
Phone: +353 1 830 74 19
Fax: +353 1 830 70 74
Contract number: CT931533

Participants:
Dr. Jacques MACLOUF
Inserm Unite 348,
Hopital Lariboisiere
6 rue Guy Patin
FR 75475 Paris
Phone: +33 1 42829473
Fax: +33 1 49958579

Prof. Carlo PATRONO
Cardiovascular Pharmacology
Universita G d'Annunzio
Via dei Vestini
IT 66013 Chieti
Phone: +39 871 355775
Fax: +39 871 355718

Prof. Giancarlo FOLCO
Research Centre for Experi-
mental Cadiopulmonary
Pharmacology
9 Via Balzaretti
IT 20133 Milan
Phone: +39 2 20488308
Fax: +39 2 29404961

Prof. Peter KOUDSTAAL
Univ Hospital Rotterdam
Dijkzigt, Dept. of Neurology
Dr. Molewaterplein 40
NL Rotterdam
Phone: +31 10 4639222
Fax: +33 10 4633208

Prof. Raffaele LANDOLFI
Laboratory of Haemostasis,
Universita Cattolica
8 Largo A Gemelli
IT 00168 Roma
Phone: +39 6 3957968
Fax: +39 6 3057968

EUROSTROKE: INCIDENCE AND RISK FACTORS OF ISCHAEMIC AND HAEMORRHAGIC STROKE IN EUROPEAN SUBJECTS

Key words
Ischaemic stroke, haemorrhagic stroke, incidence, mortality, risk factors, haemostatic factors, elderly, dietary factors.

Objectives
1 To study the variation in incidence of fatal and non-fatal ischaemic and haemorrhagic stroke across various European countries.
2 To assess whether the difference in stroke incidence across European countries can be explained by differences in prevalence of established cardiovascular risk factors (risk factor profile) in the populations.
3 To assess the relative importance of selected dietary factors (potassium intake, alcohol consumption), haemostatic disturbances (fibrinogen) and co-morbidity (rheumatic heart disease) compared to established risk factors as determinants of the occurrence of ischaemic and haemorrhagic stroke.

Brief description
In medical, social, and economic terms, cerebrovascular disease has a major impact on society, and the search for possibilities of prevention of cerebrovascular diseases is a clear priority for scientific research.
Mortality from stroke consistently differs across countries. Within Europe a four fold difference in stroke mortality is found across various European countries.
At present, data to explain this variation in stroke mortality is scarce. The difference in stroke mortality, however, strongly suggests a potential for prevention.
An effective, targeted and international approach to prevent cerebrovascular disease is hampered, however, by lack of knowledge.
The proposed collaborative study will mainly focus on a limited number of preventable factors, for which there is sufficient scientific evidence to foster additional research, and that may explain the wide difference in stroke mortality across countries.
To rapidly meet the objectives, a pooled case control approach is proposed based on nine European population-based prospective follow-up studies (cohorts) on the incidence of haemorrhagic and thromboembolic stroke. The ultimate objective is to arrive at guidelines for preventive action.

Project leader:
Professor Diederick GROBBEE
Consultation Centre for Clinical Research
Departement of Epidemiology & Biostatistics
Erasmus University Medical School
PO Box 1738
NL 3000 DR Rotterdam
Phone: +31 10 40 87 489
Fax: +31 10 40 87 494
Contract number: CT931786

Participants:

Dr. A. TRICHOPOULOU
Prof. of Nutrition and
Biochemistry,
Athens School of Public
Health L. Alexandres
GR 196 Athens
Phone: +30 1 642 86 77
Fax: +30 1 643 65 36

Dr. Peter C. ELWOOD
MRC Epidemiology Unit,
Llandough Hospital
UK Penarth South Glamorgan
CF6 1XX
Phone: +44 222 711 404
Fax: +44 222 705 028

Dr. Pierre DUCIMETIERE
INSERM U 258,
Hospital Brussais
96 Rue Didot
FR 75674 Paris Cedex 14
Phone: +33 1 43 959 571
Fax: +33 1 45 434 269

Jukka SALONEN
Research Inst. of Community
Health and General Practice
Univ of Kuopio
P.O. Box 1627
FI 70211 Kuopio
Phone: +358 71 162 910
Fax: +358 71 162 936

Prof. Luigi A. AMADUCCI
Italian National Research
Council, Targeted Project
on Ageieng
Via il Prato 58-62
IT 50123 Firenze
Phone: +39 55 416 9069
Fax: +39 55 414 603

Prof. Dag THELLE
Nordic School of
Public Health
P.O. Box 12133
SE 402 42 Gothenburg
Phone: +46 31 693 948
Fax: +46 31 691 777

Prof. D. GONCALVES
Neurologia 3, Hospital da
Universidade de Coimbra Av
Bissaya Barreto e Praceta
Prof. Mota Pinto
PT 3049 Coimbra CEDEX
Phone: +351 39 722 115
Fax: +351 39 23907

Prof. Dr. med. E. NÜSSEL
Dept. of Clinical Social
Medicine,
Univ of Heidelberg
DE 6900 Heidelberg
Phone: +49 6221 568 751
Fax: +49 6221 565 584

Prof. José FERRO
Dept. of Neurology,
Hospital de Santa Maria
PT 1600 Lisboa
Phone: +351 1 79 34 480
Fax: +351 1 79 34 480

Prof. Peter J. KOUDSTAAL
Dept. of Neurology,
Dijkzigt Hospital,
Erasmus Univ Med. School
P.O. Box 1738
NL 3000 DR Rotterdam
Phone: +31 10 463 37 89
Fax: +31 10 463 32 08

THE ROLE OF ADHESION RECEPTORS IN REGULATION OF THROMBOSIS AND THE DEVELOPMENT OF ANTI-ADHESIVE PEPTIDES

Key words
Thrombosis, B3 integrins, receptor-mediated signalling, cytoskeleton, anti-adhesive peptides.

Brief description
A major challenge in the field of cardiovascular research is (a) the understanding of the molecular mechanisms underlying blood cell interactions with the vasculature and (b) the development of antagonists to prevent uncontrolled cell adhesion events leading to cardiovascular diseases.

Platelet-platelet or platelet-endothelial cell interactions in hemostasis and thrombosis as well as platelet-leukocyte or leukocyte-endothelial cell interactions in inflammatory processes are mediated through a family of cell adhesion receptors called integrins, which require specific receptor-ligand interactions common to a variety of adhesion phenomena involved in celVmatrix interactions.

A key adhesion mechanism in integrin-ligand binding involves the recognition of amino-acid motifs, such as Arg-Gly-Asp (RGD).

In this regard, a major breakthrough has been the discovery of a family of small, RGD containing proteins isolated from viper venoms, potent inhibitors of integrin-ligand interactions and thus termed 'disintegrins'.

In the present proposal, we bring together 5 EEC research teams with established expertise in integrin research to focus on two closely related members of the integrin B3 subfamily, platelet GPIIb-IIIa (integrin aIIbB3) and the endothelial cell vitronectin receptor (integrin avB3) in order to elucidate their functional implications in cardiovascular processes.

Specific aims are:

1 comparative structure/function analysis of native or mutant B3 integrins with emphasis on postranslational regulation of receptor specificity and affinity; generation of B3 integrin mutants by stable cDNA expression in heterologous cells in order;

2 to identify novel extracellular structural domains involved in receptor-ligand interaction as well as;

3 to identify cytoplasmic domains involved in receptor function modulation, cytoskeleton interaction and intracellular signalling;

4 to develop an determine the importance of shear stress on B3 integrin-mediated cell adhesion to the extracellular matrix protein von Willebrand factor, identify functional domains of von Willebrand factor involved in this interaction and evaluate the inhibitory effect of various B3 integrin antagonists; and finally

5 (a) to use native and mutant disintegrins to define the specificity of B3 integrin receptor interactions in adhesion,

(b) develop disintegrins with novel anti-adhesive characteristics to examine non-RGD dependent adhesion events,

(c) examine the potential of disintegrins as prototype antagonists of thrombosis

Conclusion:
The objective of our collaborations is to examine adhesive interactions, by combining structural and functional approaches: from the biochemistry of the isolated receptor and its ligands, through structural analysis by NMR spectroscopy to cell biological models. This objective can only be achieved if the studies are performed at a European level since, unlike the USA, the expertise does not exist in each member state.

Project leader:
Dr. Nelly KIEFFER
Laboratoire Franco-Luxembourgeois de Rercherche Biomédicale
Avenue de la Faiencerie 162 A
LU 1511 Luxembourg
Phone: +352 48 31 98
Fax: +352 40 85 45
Contract number: CT931685

Participants:
Dr. Dominique BARUCH
INSERM U 143, Hôpital de Bicêtre
Rue du Général-Leclerc 78
FR 94275 Le Kremlin-Bicêtre
Phone: +33 1 46 581544
Fax: +33 1 46 719472

Dr. Janice WILLIAMS
National Heart and Lung Inst.
Dovehouse St
UK London SW3 6LR
Phone: +44 71 3518177
Fax: +44 71 3518270

Dr. GONZALEZ-RODRIQUEZ
Unidad de Biophisica,
Inst.o de Quimica Fisica
Serrano 119
ES 28006 Madrid
Phone: +34 15 644564
Fax: +34 15 627518

Dr. Roberto PARRILLA
Fisiologica Endocrina,
Centro de Invewstigaciones Biologicas
Velazques 114
ES 28006 Madrid
Phone: +34 15 644564
Fax: +34 15 627518

STRUCTURE-FUNCTION RELATIONSHIPS OF THE APOA-I PROTEIN: A MULTIDISCIPLINARY APPROACH TO THE MOLECULAR BASIS OF ATHEROSCLEROSIS

Key words

ApoA-I protein, lecithin cholesterol acyltransferase (LCAT), atherosclerosis, X-ray crystallography, NMR spectroscopy, molecular dynamics, CD spectroscopy, differential scanning calorimetry, interactive molecular graphics.

Objectives

The objective of the project is to develop a comprehensive knowledge of the structure-function relationships of human apoA-I. Emphasis is placed on the identification of domains/residues which participate in lecithin cholesterol acyltransferase (LCAT) activation and in the analysis of their contributions to protein stability, dynamics and energetics. The specific aims are:

1 to mutagenize the human apoA-I protein by altering eight repeated amphipathic alphahelices which have been implicated in LCAT activation and in lipid/cell surfaces binding; to isolate apoA-I variants in mg quantities; to produce synthetic peptides corresponding to functional domains;

2 to study the properties of wildtype/mutant apoA-I forms/synthetic peptides by X-ray crystallography, NMR, CD spectroscopy and differential scanning calorimetry;

3 to study the functional properties of apoA-I mutants/synthetic peptides under particular emphasis to LCAT activation and phospholipid cholesterol vesicles/model lipid emulsions/HDL binding;

4 to develop a data base which will correlate structural, dynamic, stability and sequence data with functional properties of the apoA-I protein.

Brief description

In order to approach the molecular basis of diseases, fundamental aspects of biomolecular 3-D structure must be well understood. Apolipoprotein A-I (apoA-I), the main protein component of high density lipoprotein, provides a striking example of benefits resulting from the knowledge of its 3D-structure, both in the understanding at a molecular level of the conditions that predispose 5-10% of humans to atherosclerosis and in the treatment of the disease. Our goal is to analyze in a multidisciplinary approach the structural, dynamic, energetic and functional properties of human apoA-I in order to develop a detailed and comprehensive knowledge its structure-function relationships. The organization of the apoA-I amino acid sequence, highly suggestive of an α-helical bundle folding, makes it possible to address structural aspects in a systematic way. Our strategy is to combine the broad expertise of the collaborating laboratories in the study of a) wild type apoA-I, b) mutant forms of apoA-I which probe either its folding or the roles of functional domains/residues and c)synthetic peptides corresponding to specific structural-functional units apoA-I. Each molecular construction (mutant or synthetic peptide) will be taken through cycles of computer-aided design/modelling, mutagenesis, protein expression and large scale production in bioreactors or chemical peptide synthesis, purification and functional assays; wild type apoA-I and the most interesting constructions will be taken through cycles of structural and physicochemical characterization. The techniques to be used include: X-ray crystallography. NMR spectroscopy, molecular dynamics calculations, CD spectroscopy, differential scanning calorimetry and interactive molecular graphics. Structure-function relationships will be developed from the results obtained from different molecular constructions. One important aspect of the collaboration is the combination of experimental and computational techniques of complementary nature: structural information is complemented by dynamic, energetic, stability and functional data. This creates the basis for an understanding at an atomic level of conditions which predispose humans to atherosclerosis and furthermore, provides an excellent starting point for rational approaches (e.g. drug design) to treat the disease.

Project leader:
Dr. M. KOKKINIDIS
Institute of Molecular Biology & Biotechnology (IMBB)
P.O. Box 1527
GR 711 10 Heraklion, Crete
Phone: +30 81 210091 ext 177
Fax: +30 81 230469
Contract number: CT931454

Participants:
Dr. Paul Rösch
Universität Bayreuth, Lehrstuhl für Struktur
und Chemie der Biopolymere
DE Bayreuth

Dr. P. MATEO ALARCON
Univ of Granada,
Dept. Physical Sciences
ES Granada

Dr. Sandor PONGOR
International Centre for Genetic Engineering
and Biotechnology Laboratory of Protein
Structure and Function
IT Trieste

Dr. Vassilis ZANNIS
Inst. of Molecular Biology and Biotechnology
Foundation for Research and Technology Hellas
P.O. Box 1527
GR 711 10 Heraklion (Crete)

MOLECULAR MECHANISMS OF THE PATHOGENESIS
OF ATHEROSCLEROSIS

Oxidative Modification of Low Density Lipoproteins and its Implication in Atherogenesis

Key words
Atherosclerosis, low density lipoproteins, oxidative modification, lipid peroxidation, lipoxygenase.

Objectives
The aim of this Concerted Action is to investigate the mechanism of oxidative modification of LDL and its impact on atherogenesis. Oxidative modification of LDL will be studied in enzymatic and non-enzymatic subcellular model systems (lipoxygenases, copper ions) as well by mammalian cells relevant to atherogenesis (human monocytes, vascular endothelial cells, vascular smooth muscle cells). Furthermore, the metabolic fate of native and oxidized LDL will be examined. Atherosclerotic lesions of animal atherosclerosis models and man will be investigated for the occurrence of oxygenated lipids and for the expression of lipid peroxidizing enzymes.

Brief description
Atherosclerosis is a multifactorial disease of great socio-economic impact the pathogenesis of which has not been fully understood. Since oxidative modification of low density lipoproteins has been suggested to be a major event in early atherogenesis the aim of this concerted action is to throw light on the mechanism of oxidative modification of LDL in vivo and its impact in atherogenesis. Modification of LDL will be studied in test systems of various integration levels (molecular level, cellular level, whole animals and man). The metabolic fate of native and modified LDL in various cellular systems and the regulatory effects of modified LDL on cell metabolism will also be investigated. A search for inhibitors of LDL oxidation and for cytoprotective substances preventing cell toxicity caused by oxidized LDL is included.

On the molecular level the oxidation of LDL will be studied in various enzymatic and non-enzymatic systems (lipoxygenases, transition metals, uv-irradiation). Analysis of the oxidation products and inhibitor studies ma y lead to the characterization of metabolic pathways involved in cellular oxidative modification of LDL. Furthermore, the metabolism of oxidized LDL by macrophages, the regulatory effects of oxidized LDL on the expression of cytokines, growth factors and heat shock proteins and the impact of LDL metabolism on eicosanoid synthesis will be investigated. Modified lipoproteins extracted from atherosclerotic lesions of animal atherosclerosis models and man will be characterized with respect to its chemical composition. Structure elucidation of oxygenated lipids isolated from atherosclerotic lesions and a comparison with the products formed in the in vitro studies may provide evidence for the mechanism of oxidation reactions in atherosclerotic lesions.

Project leader:
Dr. Hartmut KÜHN
Humboldt University,
Institute of Biochemistry
Hessische Strasse 3-4
DE 10115 Berlin
Phone: +49 30 284 68 538
Fax: +49 30 284 68 600
Contract number: CT931790

Participants:
Dr. Alberico CATAPANO
Univ of Milan,
Inst. of Pharmacological Sciences
Via Balzaretti 9
IT 20133 Milano
Phone: +39 2 29404961

Dr. Andreas HABENICHT
Medizinischse Klinik,
Abt Innere Medizin I, Ruprecht-Karls-
Universität Heidelberg
Bergheimer Str. 58
DE 69115 Heidelberg 1
Phone: +49 6221 565226

Dr. Hermann ESTERBAUER
Insitut für Biochemie, Universität Graz
Schubertstrasse 1
AT 8010 Graz
Phone: +43 316 384092

Dr. Jacky LARRUE
Universite de Bordeaux II,
Inserm U8 Cardiologie
Avenue du Haut-Leveque
FR 33600 Pessac
Phone: +33 563 68979

Dr. Karl Ludwig SCHULTE
Abt für Angiologie, Medizinische Klinik1
Schumannstr. 20-21
DE 10098 Berlin
Phone: +49 30 286 8482

Dr. M. John CHAPMAN
Hospital de la Pitie,
Inserm Unite 231
FR 75651 Paris CEDEX
Phone: +33 1 458 28 198

Dr. Robert SALVAYRE
Universite Paul Sabatier, Labaratoire
de Biochimie Medicale CHU Rangueil
FR 31054 Toulouse CEDEX
Phone: +33 613 22953

Dr. Ulf DICZFALUSY
Huddinge Univ Hospital,
Dept. of Clinical Chemistry CL62
SE 14186 Huddinge
Phone: +46 8 77 48393

MOLECULAR EVENTS INFLUENCING CELLULAR BEHAVIOUR IN AN ESTABLISHED MODEL OF ATHEROSCLEROSIS

Key words
Atherosclerosis, smooth muscle cell proliferation, gene expression, hypoxia, adventitia.

Objectives
1 To study the induction of platelet-derived growth factor (PDGF) and the early growth-response genes c-fos, c-myc, MCP-1 and PCNA in the rabbit carotid artery after adventitial manipulation, following hypoxic cell culture of the BC3H1 myogenic cell line and primary rabbit aortic smooth muscle cells (SMC). Gene transfer techniques will be used.
2 To analyze expression of genes involved in monocyte/macrophage function and lipoprotein metabolism using gene transfer technology. To analyze induction of vascular endothelial growth factor (VEGF) and VEGF receptors in the rabbit carotid artery after adventitial stripping and to clone the rabbit VEGF gene. Subsequently, to transfer this gene into the carotid artery in order to study its effect on lesion initiation and progression.
3 To study the effect of the vastatins on the above genes in cultures of SMCs and also in the collar model in rabbits.

Brief description
An intimal hyperplastic lesion, created by the application of a biologically inert silastic collar to the rabbit carotid, has been postulated to cause intimal SMC proliferation due to occlusion of the adventitial vasa vasorum.
Further development of this model by surgical excision of the adventitia to leave a naked media gives a highly reproducible lesion containing only SMCs on a normal diet but also containing foam cells on a high cholesterol diet. This model allows a controlled proliferative response to take place.
It is hypothesised that these models of adventitial manipulation create a zone of outer medial hypoxia in the artery wall and that hypoxia acts as the stimulus for SMC proliferation and migration to form an intimal lesion. It is further hypothesised that hypoxia in the media caused by thrombotic occlusion of the vasa vasorum may be an initiating factor in human atherogenesis. In London we will test this hypothesis by looking for the induction of PDGF and the early growth-regulated genes c-fos, c-myc, MCP-1 and PCNA in cells cultured under hypoxic conditions and in the rabbit carotid after adventitial stripping by pluronic gel-mediated gene transfer. We will analyse the role of these molecules on lesion progression using the same animal model. In Finland, we will carry out expression analysis of genes involved in monocyte/macrophage function and lipoprotein metabolism. Many of these genes have been cloned and will be used to carry out catheter-mediated retroviral gene transfer into the rabbit carotid following adventitial stripping. In Germany, we will look at the induction of VEGF and VEGF receptors in the rabbit carotid after adventitial stripping. We will also clone the rabbit VEGF gene and, using the catheter-mediated technique developed in Finland, we will transfer this gene into the carotid artery to study its effect on lesion initiation and progression. In Italy, we will study the effect of the vastatins on gene expression in cultured SMCs and also in the collar model. In rabbits we will study the effect of these agents on retroviral - mediated gene expression using the genes cloned by our fellow proposers.

Project leader:
Professor John MARTIN
Department of Medicine,
King's College School of Medicine and Dentistry
Denmark Hill
UK London SE5 9PJ
Phone: +44 81 658 22 11 ext 5391
Fax: +44 81 663 13 25
Contract number: CT931391

Participants:
Dr. Werner RISAU
Max-Planck-Inst. für
Psychiatrie
Am Klopferspitz 18A
DE 8033 Planegg-Martinsried

Prof. Rodolfo PAOLETTI
Universita di Milano
Via Balzaretti 9
IT 20133 Milano

Prof. S. YLA-HERTTUALA
Dept. of Biomedical
Sciences, Univ of Tampere
P.O. Box 607
FI 33101 Tampere

DETERMINATION OF GENETIC ALTERATIONS IN HYPER-TROPHIC CARDIOMYOPATHY AND ASSESSMENT OF THEIR RELATION TO THE CLINICAL EXPRESSION OF THE DISEASE

Key words
Hypertrophic cardiomyopathy, myosin mutations, phenotype.

Brief description
Four multi-disciplinary European groups have been working independently with the goal of:
1 identifying other loci and genes responsible for familial hypertrophic cardiomyopathy;
2 determining the frequency of myosin mutations and thus the feasibility of a DNA diagnostic test for these mutations;
3 determining the relationship between myosin mutations, other gene abnormalities and the HCM phenotype, particularly, in relation to the most difficult management problem, sudden cardiac death.

These four groups include clinicians of recognised expertise and scientists who have made major contributions to the understanding of contractile proteins and the identification of the described myosin mutations. The work of each of the groups, however, is limited by the number and size of pedigrees available for linkage analysis and by sufficient patient numbers in any single centre to determine the frequency of myosin or other mutations. In addition, interpretation of results is limited by different clinical criteria for diagnosis and methods for identifying high risk patients and by differing laboratory methods, particularly in relation to screening the myosin gene for mutations. This concerted action proposes to supply the administrative, secretarial, and databasing infrastructure to facilitate a multi-disciplinary collaboration with the goals listed above. Clinical and scientific exchanges are proposed. The particular resources and skills of the individual centres will be made accessible to the entire group with sharing of families for linkage analysis, standardisation and validation of methods so that myosin mutation data can be pooled and standardisation of clinical protocols so that the entire data set can be utilised to examine the relation of genotype and phenotype. This will also permit examination of the feasability of a molecular diagnosis for myosin mutations. In addition to the clinical benefit to patients and the scientific insight gained into the mechanisms of myocardial hypertrophy, this collaboration will also establish a multi-disciplinary European group for the evaluation of the molecular genetics of cardiovascular disease.

Project leader:
Dr. William McKENNA
St. George's Hospital Medical School, Cranmer Terrace
UK London SW17 ORE
Phone: +44 81 672 99 44
Fax: +44 81 682 09 44
Contract number: CT931788

Participants:
Dr. D. COVIELLO
Laboratory of Molecular Genetics, Univ of
Genova, Inst. of Molecular Genetics
Viale Benedetto XV 6
IT 16132 Genova
Phone: +39 10 353 8980
Fax: +39 10 353 8978

Dr. Ketty SCHWARTZ
Developement, Pathologie, Regeneration
du Systeme Neuromusculaire
INSERM Unite 153
Rue du Fer a Moulin 17
FR Paris
Phone: +33 1 43 364631
Fax: +33 1 43 378522

Prof. Carlo VECCHIO
Div. e de Cardiologia Ente Ospedaliero
Ospedali Galleria
Via Volta 8
IT 16128 Genoa
Phone: +39 10 563 2440
Fax: +39 10 563 2605

Prof. Hans-Peter VOSBERG
Max Planck Inst. WG Kerckhoff Inst.
Benekerstrasse 2
DE 6350 Bad Nauheim
Phone: +49 603 234 5455
Fax: +49 603 234 5419

Prof. Michel KOMAJDA
Service de Cardiologie CHU Pitie-Salpetriere
83 Boulevard de l'Hopital
FR 75351 Paris Cedex 13
Phone: +33 1 45 702426
Fax: +33 1 45 706296

EUROPEAN RANDOMISED CONTROLLED TRIAL OF HORMONE REPLACEMENT THERAPY FOR THE PREVENTION OF CARDIOVASCULAR DISEASE: A FEASIBILITY STUDY

Key words
Cardiovascular, ischaemic heart disease, stroke, oestrogen, progestogen, hormone replacement therapy, menopause, lipids, breast cancer.

Objectives
To establish the feasibility of a European trial to determine the long term balance of risks and benefits of HRT for the prevention of cardiovascular disease in post-menopausal women.

Brief description
Cardiovascular disease is the commonest cause of death and disability in post-menopausal women in Europe. The relationship between oestrogen deficiency and cardiovascular disease is not clear but observational studies suggest that unopposed oestrogen therapy confers worthwhile protection against ischaemic heart disease (IHD) and, to a lesser extent, against stroke. For women with a uterus, however, recommended practice in most European countries is combined oestrogen and progestogen to avoid the increased risk of endometrial cancer associated with oestrogen only treatment. The protective effect of combined, or opposed, therapy on IHD is not clear. Progestogen itself was reported to have adverse effects on blood lipids and blood pressure but recent observational studies suggest that combined HRT may be at least as cardioprotective as oestrogen-only HRT and may afford more protection.

The decision to take or prescribe long-term hormone replacement therapy, HRT, must take account of the overall balance of risks and benefits on metabolic and neoplastic, as well as on vascular disease. This is not clear. On the benefit side, it is generally accepted that oestrogen helps to prevent osteoporosis and progestogen itself has also been reported to confer a small independent benefit against bone mineral loss. On the negative side, the risk of developing breast cancer may also be affected by HRT. A slightly increased risk of breast cancer after 10 years of treatment has been reported in women receiving oestrogen; progestogen is reported, on the one hand, to protect against this oestrogen effects and, on the other, to produce an additional increased risk.

Despite the uncertainty surrounding the long-term consequences of its use ,in some EC countries more than 10% of post-menopausal women are taking HRT. The costs and cost-benefit implications are already large in these countries and, if current trends continue, all member states will soon be affected. An accurate picture of the balance of risks and benefits for HRT and the associated health economic consequences can only be determined by experimental rather than observational studies. Randomised controlled end-point trials should be started as soon as possible so that the estimated 30% of post-menopausal women who will wish to take HRT in Europe in the next decade may make a fully informed decision based on knowledge of long-term effects.

An end-point trial with sufficient power to address the cardiovascular and breast cancer issues requires tens of thousands of women and recruitment might best be achieved in a multi-centre European trial rather than in a single country.

Before a definitive European trial can be undertaken it is essential to show feasibility in countries with different primary care settings, different urban/rural population mixes and different access to health care. This study aims to develop common European trial procedures and documentation, and to estimate eligibility, acceptability, recruitment and early withdrawal rates in different setting in these European countries, the UK, the Netherlands and Ireland.

Outcomes

Year 1   Common trial procedures and documentation.

Year 2   An estimate of the numbers of eligible women in each country and the reasons for ineligibility. The recruitment rate to the trial in a defined number of centres.

Year 3   The withdrawal rates from the trial at 6 months and the reasons for withdrawal. The feasibility of blood sampling and testing for cholesterol, triglycerides, antithrombin III, factor VIIc, fibrinogen. Preliminary results on biochemical changes at 6 months. Preliminary results on blood pressure changes at 6 months. The feasibility of bone densitometry. An informed estimate of the costs of mounting a definitive European trial. The systems and procedures required for a definitive European trial.

Expected impact

The feasibility study will inform the design of a main trial with primary end-points fatal and non-fatal IHD and stroke plus cancer incidence and mortality. Secondary end-points would include blood pressure, blood lipids and clotting factors, osteoporosis and fracture rates. It is expected that, in addition to the three countries participating in the feasibility study other European countries (EC and non-EC) would be involved in a main trial. Upon completion of a main trial benefits would include authoritative information for physicians, patients and service planners on the risks, benefits and costs of different forms of HRT. Physicians could then devise common European clinical guidelines, patients could make informed choices and health care administrators could ensure that appropriate services were provided.

Project leader:
Professor Thomas MEADE
MRC Epidemiology and Medical Care Unit,
Wolfson Institute of Preventive Medicine,
Medical College of St. Bartholomew's Hospital
Charterhouse Square
UK London EC1M 6BQ
Phone: +44 71 982 62 51
Fax: +44 71 982 62 53
Contract number: CT931015

Participants:

Prof. C.C. KELLEHER	Prof. D.E. GROBBEE	Prof. W. SHANNON
Dept. of Health Promotion,	Dept. of Epidemiology and	Royal College of Surgeons
Clinical Service Inst. Univ	Biostatistics Erasmus Univ	in Ireland, Mercers Health
College	Medical School	Centre
IE Galway	P.O. Box 1738	Stephen StreetLower
Phone: +353 91 24411	NL Rotterdam	IE Stephen
Fax: +353 91 22514	Phone: +31 10 408 7489	Phone: +353 14 783544
	Fax: +31 10 408 7494	Fax: +353 14 780797

EUROPEAN CAROTID SURGERY TRIAL

Key words
Random allocation, carotid endarterectomy, perioperative stroke, carotid stenosis, cerebral infarction.

Objectives
Continuation and extension of an existing European wide randomised controlled trial to evaluate the role of carotid endarterectomy for selected patients with transient ischaemic attacks or minor ischaemic stroke in the carotid artery distribution associated with a moderate degree (30-69%) of ipsilateral stenosis at the origin of the internal carotid artery.

Brief description
Continuation and extension of an existing European wide randomised controlled clinical trial which has already recruited over 2,800 patients. It is planned to recruit a total of 3,000 patients. The study will:

1 Evaluate the balance of risk and benefit from carotid endarterectomy for patients with moderate (30-69%) stenosis of the ipsilateral carotid artery.

2 Patients from the first phase of the ECST will continue to be followed up. Analyses will be undertaken to determine whether, in patients with different degrees of stenosis, the short term effects of surgery are maintained in the long term.

3 Evaluation of differences in clinical practise and operative risk across Europe:

a evaluation of the risk of perioperative stroke in different categories of patients in different centres across Europe and the exploration of the reasons for any variation between centres and countries;

b multivariate analyses to identify the profile of patients most likely to benefit from surgery, and most likely to suffer perioperative stroke, in different centres;

c examination of the extent to which proven methods of secondary prevention are applied in different European countries (blood pressure reduction, cholesterol reduction and antithrombotic therapy).

4 Pan-European harmonisation of the method to measure carotid stenosis on X-ray films. Three principal methods have been proposed (ECST, NASCET and Ratio method) and these methods will be applied to the databank of over 2,800 carotid angiogram X-ray films to determine which of these methods is optimum with least observer error and greatest simplicity for use in routine clinical practise in non-specialist departments of radiology.

Project leader:
Professor Charles WARLOW
Department of Clinical
Neurosciences,
Westen General Hospital
Crewe Road
UK Edinburgh EH4 2XU
Phone: +44 31 343 66 39
Fax: +44 31 332 51 50
Contract number: CT931736

Participants:
Dr. C. PRATESI (IT)
Dr. G. Van HOONACKER (BE)
Dr. P. ANZOLA (IT)

Dr. R. DOSSETOR (UK)
Dr. S. BORNHOV (SE)
Mr. W. MORRIS JONES (UK)
Mr. D.T. HOPE (UK)
Prof. L. PROVINCIALI (IT)
Dr. E. HURSKAINEN (FI)
Dr. L. VANHOVE (BE)
Dr. S. KIHLSTRAND (SE)
Dr. ARRUGA (ES)
Dr. A. BARBOD (ES)
Dr. A. FRANK (ES)
Dr. A. GILL-PERALTA (ES)
Dr. A. GIMINEZ-GAIBAR (ES)
Dr. A. MAYOL (ES)

Dr. A. PONCE DE LEON (ES)
Dr. A. VEGA (ES)
Dr. GARCIA-LA TORRE (ES)
Dr. A.G. ALFAGEME (ES)
Dr. B. GUILLAUMET (ES)
Dr. B. STENBURG (SE)
Dr. C. BLOMSTRAND (SE)
Dr. C. COMEZ (ES)
Dr. C. HELMERS (SE)
Dr. C. JIMINEZ-ORTIZ (ES)
Dr. C. OLIVERAS (ES)
Dr. C. RICART (ES)
Dr. C.C. ROURA (ES)
Dr. C.E. SODERSTROM (SE)

Dr. E. DIEZ-TEJEDOR (ES)
Dr. E. LATORRE (ES)
Dr. F. LUNDGREN (SE)
Dr. F. RUBIO (ES)
Dr. G. AMER (ES)
Dr. G. PLATE (SE)
Dr. H.G. Hardemark (SE)
Dr. H. ESPINET (ES)
Dr. H. HOLM (SE)
Dr. I. JOHANSSON (SE)
Dr. J. DIAZ (ES)
Dr. J. ELFSTROM (SE)
Dr. J. LARRACOECHEA (ES)
Dr. J. MUNOZ (ES)
Dr. J. PERES SERRA (ES)
Dr. J. RADBERG (SE)
Dr. J. SWEDENBORG (SE)
Dr. J.G. URIA (ES)
Dr. J.H. LAZARUS (UK)
Dr GARCIA-RODRIGUEZ (ES)
Dr. J.M. CAPDEVILLA (ES)
Dr GONZALEZ-MARCOS (ES)
Dr. K. LUNDHOLM (SE)
Dr. K. SAMUELSSON (SE)
Dr. K. SVENHAMN (SE)
Dr. L.G. HJERNE (SE)
Dr. L. BERGSTEN (SE)
Dr. D'OLHABERRIAGUE (ES)
Dr. L. HAGSTROM (SE)
Dr. L. HJELMAEUS (SE)
Dr. L. HOLM (SE)
Dr. L. KJALLMAN (SE)
Dr. L. SAEZ (ES)
Dr. L. SIKEN (SE)
Dr. L. SKOGLUND (SE)
Dr. L.BRATTSTROM (SE)
Dr. M. CAIROLS (ES)
Dr. M. CALOPA (ES)
Dr. M. GONZALEZ (ES)
Dr. M. LINDQVIST (SE)
Dr. M. MIRALLES (ES)
Dr. M. PALOMAR (ES)
Dr. M. VON ARBIN (SE)
Dr. M.G. MARTINEZ (ES)
Dr. M.SAMUELSSON (SE)
Dr. N. RUDBACK (SE)
Dr. N.G. WAHLGREN (SE)
Dr. O. OLSSON (SE)
Dr. P. BARREIRO (ES)
Dr. P. KONRAD (SE)
Dr. P. MAGALLON (ES)
Dr. P. OLOFSSEN (SE)
Dr. P. QVARFORDT (SE)
Dr. P.L. VILARDELLL (ES)
Dr. R. ALBERCA (ES)
Dr. R. MARES (ES)
Dr. R. MASSOT PUNYET (ES)
R. SEGURA IGLESIAS (ES)
Dr. R. TAKOLANDER (SE)
Dr. R. VILA (ES)
Dr. SIMEON (ES)
Dr. S. ANTON (ES)
Dr. S. KALLERO (SE)
Dr. T. JOHANSSON (SE)
Dr. T. LUNDH (SE)
Dr. T. RANLUND (SE)
Dr. V. KOSTULAS (SE)
V. MARTIN-PARDERO (ES)
Dr. V. ZBORNIKOVA (SE)
Prof. A. ALM (SE)
Prof. J.E. OLSSON (SE)
Dr. Y. ROLLAND (FR)
Ass. Prof. J. SIVENIUS (FI)
Dr. A. ANDREOLI (IT)
Dr. A. CARDON (FR)

Dr. A. DAMIAO (PT)
Dr. A. DAVIES JONES (UK)
Dr. A. GINNANNESCHI (IT)
Dr. A. KEYSER (NL)
Dr. A. KROESE (NO)
Dr. A. LECLUYSE (BE)
Dr. A. LUCAS (FR)
Dr. A. MAMOLI (IT)
Dr. A. MULLIE (BE)
Dr. A. RISSANEN (FI)
Dr. A. ROCHER (BE)
Dr. A. WHITELY (UK)
Dr. A. OP DE COUL (NL)
Dr. A.C. DE VRIES (NL)
Dr. A.C.M. LEYTEN (NL)
Dr. A.J. VERMEY (NL)
Dr. A.M. NEHEN (DK)
Dr. A.P. MOORE (UK)
Dr. A. WATTENDORFF (NL)
Dr. BIHEL-SCHLEICH (FR)
Dr. B. GEORGE (FR)
Dr. B. HOIVIK (NO)
Dr. B. KENDALL (UK)
Dr. B. MJASET (NO)
Dr. B. TETTENBORN (DE)
Dr. B.J. MEEMS (NL)
Dr. B.N. McLEAN (UK)
Dr. B.R.F. LECKY (UK)
Dr. B.S. JENSEN (DK)
Dr. Carlo BUFFA (IT)
Dr. C. BARUFFI (IT)
Dr. C. BJERKELUND (NO)
Dr. C. BURNS-COX (UK)
Dr. C. ELLIS (UK)
C. GARDNER-THORPE (UK)
Dr. C. HORNIG (DE)
Dr. C. PETIT-JEAN (FR)
Dr. C. PORTA (IT)
Dr. C. RABBIA (IT)
Dr. C. RAVETTI (IT)
Dr. C.C. TIJSSEN (NL)
Dr. C.L. FRANKE (NL)
Dr. C.R. BAYLISS (UK)
Dr. DEFER (FR)
Dr. D. BATES (UK)
Dr. D. DECOO (BE)
Dr. D. INZITARI (IT)
Dr. D. JEFFERSON (UK)
Dr. D. LAM (BE)
Dr. D. MAIZA (FR)
Dr. D. ROUGEMONT (FR)
Dr. D. SHEPHERD (UK)
Dr. D. THOMAS (UK)
Dr. D. THRUSH (UK)
Dr. VAN BERGHE-
HENEGOUWEN (NL)
Dr. D.L.W. DAVIDSON (UK)
Dr. E. BIASINI (IT)
Dr. E. BOSCHETTI (IT)
Dr. E. CELLA (IT)
Dr. E. FERRARI (IT)
Dr. E. POZZATI (IT)
Dr. E. SCHELSTRAETE (BE)
Dr. E. SIGNORINI (IT)
Dr. E. TEASDALE (UK)
Dr. Van BRUGGENHOUT (BE)
Dr. E.B. LUND (DK)
Dr. E.C.M. BOLLEN (NL)
Dr. E.N.H. JANSEN (NL)
Dr. FLORIANI (IT)
Dr. Fabio Chiodo GRANDI (IT)
Dr. F. CHEDRU (FR)
Dr. F. GIGOU (FR)
Dr. F. PEINETTI (IT)
Dr. F. PONZIO (IT)

Dr. F. SI MONCINI (IT)
Dr. F. VIADER (FR)
Dr. F. WOIMANT (FR)
Dr. F.G. ROOZENBOOM (NL)
Dr. G. BONALDI (IT)
Dr. G. BOTTINI (IT)
Dr. G. BOYSEN (DK)
Dr. G. BUTH (NL)
Dr. G. DERIU (IT)
Dr. G. D'ALESSANDRO (IT)
Dr. G. JAMIESON (UK)
Dr. G. KRAMER (DE)
Dr. G. LANDI (IT)
Dr. G. MASE (IT)
Dr. G. NEUMANN (DE)
Dr. G. PERKIN (UK)
Dr. G. PISTOLLATO (IT)
Dr. G. ROTHACHER (DE)
Dr. G. TJAN (NL)
Dr. G. VENABLES (UK)
Dr. VAN HELLEMONDT (NL)
Dr. G.J. LAMMERS (NL)
Dr. HETZEL (DE)
Dr. H. GRIESE (DE)
Dr. H. HINGE (DK)
Dr. H. LOBACH (NL)
Dr. H. SPEELMAN (NL)
Dr. H. VAN HOUTTE (NL)
Dr. H.J. TROELSTRA (NL)
Dr. VAN DER LEEUW (NL)
Dr. H.L. DE SMET (NL)
Dr. H.O. LINCKE (DE)
Dr. I. DEHAENE (BE)
Dr. I. ENGE (NO)
Dr. I. MAGNUSSEN (DK)
Dr. I. OKSALA (FI)
Dr. I.F. PYE (UK)
Dr. J. BAMFORD (UK)
Dr. J. CHRISTENSEN (DK)
Dr. J. DE JONGE (NL)
Dr. J. DRIESSENS (BE)
Dr. J. FASTREZ (BE)
Dr. J. GIBSON (UK)
Dr. J. HERN (UK)
Dr. J. HOOGENDAM (NL)
Dr. J. LODDER (NL)
Dr. J. MAGNE (FR)
Dr. J. OLNEY (UK)
Dr. J. PENNINCKX (BE)
Dr. J. REES (UK)
Dr. J. THORBUM (UK)
Dr. J. WADE (UK)
Dr. J.C. SIER (NL)
Dr. J.E. LORENTZEN (DK)
Dr. J.F. PINEL (FR)
Dr. J.H. NEHEN (DK)
Dr. J.J. DE REUCK (BE)
Dr. J.L. MAS (FR)
Dr. J.P.M. CLILESSEN (NL)
Dr. J.R. DRIESSEN (NL)
Dr. J.T.J. TANS (NL)
Dr. J.W. BERENDES (NL)
Dr. KROMHOUT (NL)
Dr. K. FULLERTON (UK)
Dr. K. KAYED (NO)
Dr. K. KOIVISTO (FI)
Dr. K. VAN DEN VELDE (BE)
Dr. L. ANTONUTTI (IT)
Dr. L. CARENINI (IT)
Dr. L. CASTO (IT)
Dr. L. FINDLEY (UK)
Dr. L. INDRIO (IT)
Dr. L. LOIZOU (UK)
Dr. L. PONS (ES)
Dr. L.J. KAPPELLE (NL)

Dr. M. BOSIERS (BE)
Dr. M. BOURGEOIS (BE)
Dr. M. BROWN (UK)
Dr. M. CAMERLINGO (IT)
Dr. M. CAMPBELL (UK)
Dr. M. COLLICE (IT)
Dr. M. CONFORTI (IT)
Dr. M. CRESPO (PT)
Dr. M. DEL PESCE (IT)
Dr. M. DENNIS (UK)
Dr. M. HAEFELE (IT)
Dr. M. HOMMEL (FR)
Dr. M. LANCKNEUS (BE)
Dr. M. LIMBURG (NL)
Dr. M. LUNDT (UK)
Dr. M. PASQUA (IT)
Dr. M. RICE-OXLEY (UK)
Dr. M. TWOHIG (UK)
Dr. M. VAN GEMERT (NL)
Dr. M. VAN ZANDIJCKE (BE)
Dr. M. ZORZON (IT)
Dr. M. D'HOOGHE (BE)
Dr. M.G. CELANI (IT)
Dr. M.G.M. BARWEGEN (NL)
Dr. M.M.B. NARCHAU (BE)
Dr. N. CAPUTO (IT)
Dr. N. CARRARO (IT)
Dr. N. CARTLIDDGE (UK)
Dr. N. MAEDER (DE)
Dr. N. Milligan (UK)
Dr. N.A.J.J. DU BOIS (NL)
Dr. O. ROSJO (NO)
Dr. O. SORTLAND (NO)
Dr. PROVENSOL (FR)
Dr. P.J. TOUBOUL (FR)
Dr. P. ARLIEN-SOBORG (DK)
Dr. P. CANT (BE)
Dr. P. CAO (IT)
Dr. P. CLELAND (UK)
Dr. P. GIANFERRARI (IT)
Dr. P. HARTIKAINEN (FI)
Dr. P. HUMPHREY (UK)
Dr. P. INDEKEU (BE)
Dr. P. KOUDSTAAL (NL)
Dr. P. LAMOTE (BE)
Dr. P. LERMUSIAUX (FR)
Dr. P. LIMONI (IT) ·
Dr. P. LUST (BE)
Dr. P. MARINI (IT)
Dr. P. MARTENS (BE)
Dr. P. MARX (DE)
Dr. P. MILLAC (UK)
Dr. P. NENCINI (IT)
Dr. P. OVBARY (FR)
Dr. P. O'NEILL (UK)
Dr. P. SMITH (UK)
Dr Van GINDERACHTER (BE)
Dr. P. VERCRUYSSE (BE)
Dr. P. VERDRU (BE)
Dr. P. SANDERCOCK (UK)
Dr. P.J. VARHAGEN (NL)
Dr. P.J.B. TILLEY (UK)
Dr. P.K. NEWMAN (UK)
Dr. P.M. SANDSET (NO)
Dr. P.S. SORENSEN (DK)
Dr. R. ADOVASIO (IT)
Dr. R. BULLOCK (UK)
Dr R. CLIFFORD-JONES (UK)
Dr. R. COLEMAN (UK)
Dr. R. CULL (UK)
Dr. R. FOGELHOLM (FI)
Dr. R. GREENHALL (UK)
Dr. R. HARDIE (UK)
Dr. R. JELNES (DK)

Dr. R. ROBERTS (UK)
Dr. R. SCHELLENS (NL)
Dr. R. SELLAR (UK)
Dr. R. SHAKIR (UK)
Dr. R. STERZI (IT)
Dr. R. SUY (BE)
Dr. R. WINTER (DE)
Dr. R. ZONI (IT)
Dr. R.E.M. HEKSTER (NL)
Dr. R.S.G. KNIGHT (UK)
Dr. SETTI (IT)
Dr. S. BLECIC (BE)
Dr. S. CAPPA (IT)
Dr. S. CREMASSCOLI (IT)
Dr. S. CRUIKSHANK (UK)
Dr. S. GIULINI (IT)
Dr. S. NURICK (UK)
Dr. S. RICCI (IT)
Dr. S. VOSTRUP (DK)
Dr. S.P. MOFFETT (UK)
Dr. T. BEISKE (NO)
Dr. T. BROYN (NO)
Dr. T. DAHL (NO)
Dr. T. POWELL (UK)
Dr. T. SCHROEDER (DK)
Dr. T. TROOST (NL)
Dr. VAN WOERKOM (NL)
Dr. T.D.McCUBBIN (UK)
Dr. T.G. SEGEREN (NL)
Dr. T.P.E. MELO (PT)
Dr. T.S. JENSEN (DK)
Dr. U. PASQUINI (IT)
Dr. V. LARRUE (FR)
Dr. V. VAN KAETELL (NL)
Dr. V. De la SAYETTE (FR)
Dr. W. GROENEVELD (NL)
Dr. W. HELDERWEIRT (BE)
Dr. W. McLEOD (UK)
Dr. W. PAASKE (DK)
Dr. W. SCHMIDT (DE)
Dr. Y. GLOCK (FR)
Frau C. LUX (DE)
Miss. A. MANSFIELD (UK)
Mrs. R. CARTER (UK)
Mr. A. BAKER (UK)
Mr. A.D. MENDELOW (UK)
Mr. A.Mc.L. JENKINS (UK)
Mr. A.N. NICOLAIDES (UK)
Mr. B. BLISS (UK)
Mr. C. STRACHAN (UK)
Mr. C.L. WELSH (UK)
D. CHARLESWORTH (UK)
Mr. D. GILMOUR (UK)
Mr. G.J.A. BROWN (UK)
Mr. J. BEARD (UK)
Mr. J. ENGESET (UK)
Mr. J.H.N. WOLFE (UK)
Mr. K.C. CALLUM (UK)
Mr. M. ADISESHIAH (UK)
Mr. M. CALVERT (UK)
Mr. M. CAMERON (UK)
Mr. P. HARRIS (UK)
Mr. P. LEIBERMAN (UK)
Mr. R. KESTER (UK)
Mr. R. NELSON (UK)
Mr. R. QUIN (UK)
Mr. R. SENGUPTA (UK)
Mr. S. DARKE (UK)
Mr. S. PARVIN (UK)
Mr. S.R.S. TAYLOR (UK)
Mr. T.R.K. VARMA (UK)
Mr. V. D'ANGELO (IT)
Prof. A. ALAGUI (IT)
Prof. A. AUTRET (FR)

Prof. A. BES (FR)
Prof. A. DEL FAVERO (IT)
Prof. BECQUEMIN (FR)
Prof. B. MIHOUT (FR)
Prof. B.C. EIKELBOOM (NL)
Prof. C. RAVENNA (IT)
Prof. C.H. LUCKING (DE)
Prof. C.KENNARD (UK)
Prof. DEGOS (FR)
Prof. Dr. P. KITSLAAR (NL)
Prof. D. BERTINI (IT)
Prof. D. CHADWICK (UK)
Prof. D. PALOMBO (IT)
Prof. D.F. DEROM (BE)
Prof. E. KIEFFER (FR)
Prof. F. ALO (IT)
Prof. G. CAZZATO (IT)
Prof. G. Gilles GERAUD (FR)
Prof. G. NENCI (IT)
Prof. G. SPILLNER (DE)
Prof. G. TIBERIO (IT)
Prof. H. CARTON (BE)
Prof. H. GUIDICELLI (FR)
Prof. H. VAN CREVEL (NL)
Prof. H. VAN URK (NL)
Prof. H.C. HOPF (DE)
Prof. I. BONE (UK)
Prof. J. FERNANDES (PT)
Prof. J. HILDEBRAND (BE)
Prof. J. M. ORGOGOZO (FR)
Prof. J. VAN GIJN (NL)
Prof. J. WATTELET (FR)
Prof. J.M. BLARD (FR)
Prof. J.M. DERLON (FR)
Prof. J.P. DEREUME (BE)
Prof. J.R. ALLENBERG (DE)
Prof. K. MATHIAS (DE)
Prof. LOSAPIO (IT)
Prof. L. CASTELLANI (FR)
Prof. L. MOGGI (IT)
Prof. L.A. VIGNOLO (IT)
Prof. J. GRONNIGER (DE)
Prof. O. BUSSE (DE)
Prof. M.J. POLONIUS (DE)
Prof. M. HAGUENAU (FR)
Prof. M. VERMEULEN (NL)
Prof. M.G. BOUSSER (FR)
Prof. M.J.G. HARRISON (UK)
Prof. P. CESARO (FR)
Prof. P. RIEKKINEN (FI)
Prof. P.R.F. BELL (UK)
Prof. R. GREENHALGH (UK)
Prof. R. REUTHER (DE)
Prof Van VROONHOVEN (NL)
Prof. Ulf BERGVALL (UK)
Prof. U. ABILDGAARD (NO)
Prof. U. SENIN (IT)
Prof. V. RUCKLEY (UK)
Prof. V. SCHLOSSER (DE)
Prof. Y. KERDILES (FR)
Dr. J. CAMPOS (PT)
Dr. V. OLIVEIRA (PT)
Dr. J.M. FERRO (PT)
Dr. J.T. HOLTER (NL)
Dr. O.E. HANSEN (DK)

CORONARY ARTERY DISEASE: WHAT ARE THE GENETIC RISK FACTORS?

Key words
Coronary artery disease, genetic risk factors, genetic loci, lipoprotein (a), apolipoprotein E polymorphism.

Brief description
The major risk factors for premature coronary artery disease (CAD) defined as ischaemic symptoms arising before the age of 55 years are hypertension, hyperlipidaemia, cigarette smoking and diabetes mellitus. However studies of concordance rates in monozygotic twins have emphasised the importance of Family History and this implies that genetic risk factors may contribute to susceptibility to the disease. Several genetic loci have already been implicated in the development of the common forms of premature CAD. These include genes coding for lipoprotein (a), Lp(a); the apolipoprotein E polymorphism; apolipoproteins AI and CIII involved in HDL and VLDL-triglyceride transport; and lipoprotein lipase.

The present project aims to compare the relative incidence of each of these variant loci for the development of coronary artery disease in North and South Europe. The apolipoprotein E polymorphism is produced by amino-acid variation at positions 112 and 158 producing E variants termed E2 and E4 respectively (E3 containing cys. and arg. at these positions is considered as the ancestral protein). Different E apolipoprotein variants (e.g. E-4) are associated with increased levels of plasma cholesterol in some populations and the effects are also seen on the prevalence of CAD. The apo AI/CIII/AIV gene cluster on chromosome llq 23 codes for proteins in HDL (involved in reverse cholesterol transport) and VLDL (involved in plasma triglycerid transport). The gene cluster appears very polymorphic with more than twelve restriction site variants in its vicinity. Finally the gene coding for lipoprotein lipase on chromosome 8p 22 involved in the clearance of triglyceride-rich lipoproteins from plasma has recenty been shown to contain a common mutation (frequency in healthy populations of 0.13) in exon 9 that converts serine 447 to a termination codon. In three disease-association studies, this mutation (or linkage markers Within 650 b.pof it) have shown significant associations with dyslipidaemia and/ or premature CAD. All the above loci will be studied in the proposed project.

Project leader:
Professor David J. GALTON
Dept. of Medicine,
St. Bartholomew's Hospital
West Smithfield
UK London EC1A 7BE
Phone: +44 71 601 84 31
Fax: +44 71 601 80 42
Contract number: CT941211

Participants:
Prof. W. KRONE
Policlinic II, Univ. of Koln
Joseph-Stelzmannstrasse
DE 5000 Koln
Phone: +49 221 4780
Fax: +49 221 8907 2489

Dr. M. BARONI
II Clinica Medica,
University La Sapienza
IT 00161 Rome
Phone: +39 6 4423 1139
Fax: +39 6 4423 1141

Prof. L. MASANA
Dept. of Medicine
C/St Llorenc 21
ES 43201 Reus
Phone: +34 977 318 922
Fax: +34 977 310 654

Dr. K. RASLOVA
Dept. of Medicine,
Vojenska nemocnica
Cest mladeze 1
SK 83303 Bratislava

HOMEOCYSTEINE AND VASCULAR DISEASE:
FROM NATURAL HISTORY TO THERAPY

Key words

Homocysteine, red cell folate, vitamin B12, pyridoxine, cardiovascular disease, blood levels, prognosis.

Brief description

Raised blood levels of homocysteine are known to be associated with the development of premature vascular disease. A recently completed EC concerted action has confirmed these findings in the largest case-control study of its kind to date. It is not known however if homocysteine levels relate to prognosis in those with established vascular disease. Blood levels of folic acid, vitamin B12, and pyridoxine are inversely related to homocysteine levels, and treatment with any of these substances should reduce the level of homocysteine in the blood. Further research on these aspects of homocysteine metabolism is required to determine if patients with vascular disease could benefit from such therapy.

There are three objectives for this proposal:

- The first objective is to relate blood homocysteine levels to prognosis in patients with vascular disease. Over 600 patients with cerebrovascular, cardiovascular or peripheral vascular disease were studied for the previous EC project and blood levels of homocysteine are available in all of these. The 18 centres who recruited these patients in 1991 and 1992 for the original case-control study will conduct a follow-up study on these patients to relate mortality and morbidity to the initial homocysteine levels.
- The second objective of this proposal is to examine the interrelations between homocysteine, red cell folate, vitamin B12 and pyridoxine levels in the 600 cases and 600 controls from the previous EC study. Serum/plasma levels of these factors are available but their interrelationships have not been examined. The existing database will be subjected to extensive statistical analysis.
- The objective of this third phase of the proposal is to establish the doses of folic acid, vitamin B12 and/or pyridoxine which will achieve maximal reduction in fasting homocysteine levels. Patients from a number of centres will be entered into clinical trials to examine this question.

Project leader:
Professor Ian M. GRAHAM
Dept. of Cardiology,
Adelaide Hospital
Peter Street
IE Dublin 8
Phone: +353 1 758 971
Fax: +353 1 751 114
Contract number: CT941708

Participants:

Prof. Stephen WHITEHEAD
Dept. of Genetics,
Trinity College
IE Dublin 2
Phone: +353 1 702 1289
Fax: +353 1 679 8558

Prof. Geoffrey BOURKE &
dr. Leslie DALY
Dept. of Public Health
Medicine, University
College Dublin
Earlsfort Terrace
IE Dublin 2
Phone: +353 1 7067 345
Fax: +353 1 7067 407

Dr. Lars BRATTSTROM
Dept. of Neurology,
University Hospital
SE 22185 Lund
Phone: +46 48 048 208
Fax: +46 40 881 998

Dr. Paolo RUBBA
Institute of Disease of
Metabolism & Internal
Medicine, 2nd Medical
School, University of Naples
IT 80131 Naples
Phone: +39 74 62011
Fax: +39 54 66152

Prof. Per URELAND &
prof. Helga REFSUM
Institute Pharmocology &
Toxicology,
University of Bergen
NO Bergen
Phone: +47 240 503
Fax: +47 597 31 15

Prof. Frans J. KOK
Wageningen Agricultural
University, Dept. of Public
Health & Epidemiology
NL Wageningen
Phone: +31 8370 82880
Fax: +31 8370 82782

Dr. Godfried BOERS
Dept. of Endocrinology,
Katholieke Univ. Nijmegen
Postbus 9101
NL 6500 HB Nijmegen
Phone: +31 80 515 599
Fax: +31 80 541 484

Prof. H. DE VALK
Dept. of Internal Medicine,
Utrecht University Hospital
NL Utrecht
Phone: +31 30 506 328
Fax: +31 30 518 238

Prof. A. SALES LUIS
Dept. Cardiology, Hospital
de S. Francisco Xavier
PT 1400 Lisbon
Phone: +351 6173509
Fax: +351 113017533

Dr. Roberto REIS
R. Gregorio Lopes Lt.
1515-80
PT 1400 Lisbon

Prof. Alun EVANS
Belfast Monica Project,
Dept. of Community Medi-
cine & Medical Statistics,
Queens University
Grosvenor Road
UK Belfast BT12 6BJ
Phone: +44 240503
Fax: +44 232236298

Prof. J.C. WAUTRECHT
University Libre de
Bruxelles, Hospital Erasme
BE 1200 Brussels
Phone: +31 2 526 4395
Fax: +32 2 526 4405

Mme. Francois
PARROT-ROULAND
Laboratoire de Biochimie,
Dept. Chromatographie,
Hopital Pellegrin
Place Amelie-Raba-Leon
FR 33076 Bordeaux Cedex
Phone: +33 5679 5679
Fax: +33 5679 5593

Prof. BATT
Hopital St. Rock
Rue Pierre des Volys
FR 06000 Nice
Phone: +33 9203 7730

Prof. MORAND
Hopital Pasteur
30 Av. de la Voie-Romaine,
BP 069
FR 06002 Nice Cedex
Phone: +33 9203 7730

Dr. Daniele GARCON
Laboratoire de Biochimie,
Faculte de Pharmacie
27 Bd Jean Moulin
FR 13005 Marseille
Phone: +33 9178 3658
Fax: +33 9180 2612

Prof. CHANTEL
Hopital Pasteur;
30 Av. de la Voie-Romaine,
BP 069
FR 06002 Nice Cedex
Phone: +33 9203 7730

Mme M. CANDITO
Laboratoire de Biochimie,
Hopital Pasteur
30 Av. de la Voie-Romaine,
BP 069
FR 06002 Nice Cedex
Phone: +33 9203 7730

EUROLIP: CONCERTED ACTION ON THE IMPAIRMENT OF ADIPOSE TISSUE METABOLIC REGULATION AS A GENERATOR OF RISK FACTORS FOR CARDIOVASCULAR DISEASE

Key words
Non-insulin-dependent diabetes mellitus, cardiovascular diseases, metabolic changes, free fatty acids, insulin resistance.

Brief description
Obesity and non-insulin-dependent diabetes mellitus are always associated with an increased prevalence of cardiovascular risk. These diseases have in common certain metabolic abberations and share the same risk factors such as insulin resistance, modifications of blood lipid profile and accumulation of intra-abdominal adipose tissue.

EUROLIP will enable a concerted evaluation of currently separate strands of the accumulating evidence that metabolic changes in adipose tissue underlie the link between insulin resistance, increased circulating non-esterified fatty acid level and cardiovascular disease.

The Concerted Action will facilitate an interdisciplinary approach to the understanding of these metabolic regulation mechanisms and their implications for propen sity to cardiovascular disease. The six proposer in EUROLIP have been examining different facets of the research on adipose tissue metabolic regulation independently under national programs. EUROLIP will focus on the central role of free fatty acids and insulin resistance in the appearance of risk factors for cardiovascular disease. EUROLIP will combine expertise from the molecular to the clinical level on the different components of the lipolytic cascade. EUROLIP should contribute to the solution of technical goals concerning in vivo explorations of metabolic disorders and development of the application of molecular biology techniques to the determination of multiple fat cell markers in human adipose tissue samples.

New in-sights in the pahogenic mechanisms of adipose tissue metabolic regulation are also planned:
- lipid metabolism of normal, obese and insulin-resistant subjects;
- characterization of the highly active human intra-abdominal fat depots;
- study of a physiological state of insulin resistance: pregnancy;
- molecular characterization and study of gene expression regulation of the key components of the adipocyte plasma membrane and triglyceride metabolism in white and brown adipose tissue.

The partners: Lafontan (Toulouse), Belfrage (Lund), Herrera (Madrid), Cannon (stockholm), Frayn (Oxford), Arner (Huddinge) and Stich (Prague). EUROLIP will allow a combination of methodologies otherwise used independently by the different partners and regular exchange of results. By combining techniques, a balanced proportion of clinical and fundamental centres.

Project leader:
Dr. Max LAFONTAN
Unité INSERM 317,
Institut Louis Bugnard CHU Rangueil
Avenue Jean Poulhès 1
FR 31054 Toulouse
Phone: +33 62 17 29 50
Fax: +33 61 33 17 21
Contract number: CT941584

Participants:
Prof. Emilio HERRERA
Departamento de Investigation,
Hospital Universitario Ramon y Cajal,
Universitad de Alcala de Henares
Ctra de Colmenar km. 9
ES 28034 Madrid
Phone: +34 1 336 8077
Fax: +34 1 336 9016

Dr. Keith FRAYN
Oxford Lipid Metabolism Group,
Nuffield Dept. of Clinical Medicine,
Oxford University, Sheikh Rashid Diabetes Unit,
Radcliff Infirmary
UK Oxford OX2 6HE
Phone: +44 865 224 180
Fax: +44 865 224 652

Prof. Per BELFRAGE
Institutionen för Medicinsk och Fysiologisk
Kemi, Molekylär Endokrinologi,
Lunds Universitet
P.O. Box 94
SE 22100 Lund
Phone: +46 46 108 575
Fax: +46 46 110 437

Prof. Barbara CANNON
Institutionene för Metabolisk Forskning,
Wenner-Grens Institutet, The Arrhenius
Laboratories F3, Stockholms Universitet
SE 10691 Stockholm
Phone: +46 8 162000
Fax: +46 8 156756

Prof. Peter ARNER
Lipid Laboratory at the Karolinska Institute,
Dept. of Medicine,
Huddinge University Hospital
SE 14186 Huddinge
Phone: +46 8 746 4113
Fax: +46 8 711 7684

Dr. Vladimir STICH
Unit of Endocrinilogy and Obesity,
Dept. of Internal Medicine IV,
University Hospital
U - Nemocnice 2
CZ Praha 2

IN VIVO NON INVASIVE ASSESSMENT OF ARTERIAL WALL PROPERTIES IN CARDIOVASCULAR DRUG THERAPY

Key words
Arterial hypertension, non-invasive techniques, structure function, arteries, pathophysiology, antihypertensive agents.

Brief description
The major health problems associated with arterial hypertension are due to damage to the vascular system of major target organs: brain, heart and kidneys. Experimental and clinical studies suggest that alterations of arteries are important to evaluate in the cardiovascular morbidity and mortality of patients treated for hypertension. Whereas the heart and the small resistance arteries have been extensively investigated in clinical and experimental models of hypertension there has been no systematic study of the *in vivo* structure and function of large arteries, mainly due to the lack of appropriate techniques, especially non-invasive.

Our objectives are three fold:
1 Evaluation of new devices. The objective is to non-invasively determine the phasic diameter and thickness of large peripheral arteries in animals and patients. Changes in diameter and thickness will be measured as a function of time using new devices with high resolution based on ultrasound (echo-tracking and Doppler-tracking techniques). Simultaneous non invasive measurement of blood pressure will permit to determine the phasic pressure diameter relationships in various experimental conditions.
2 Pathophysiological changes of large arteries. Using the same techniques we will determine the arterial compliance and distensibility as well as tangential wall tension and wall stress. Ultrasound techniques have also become available to determine wall shear rate in large arteries *in vivo*. The study will be performed in normal normotensive animals and humans as a function of age and sex, then applied to several pathological states: hypertension and atherosclerosis.
3 Pharmacological and therapeutic approach. A principal objective will be to investigate the effects of anti-hypertensive agents on the large arteries, mainly those not directly dependent on the decrease in blood pressure, including the counter regulatory neurohumoral mechanisms, the associated mechanical changes such as those related to flow dependent dilation, and changes in endothelial functions. Both acute and long term studies will be performed to investigate in parallel the arterial changes in function (compliance, distensibility, wall tension, wall stress, shear stress) and structure (thickness, collagen and elastin contents, smooth muscle cell.

Project leader:
Dr. Bernard LEVY
INSERM Unit 141,
Dynamique Cardiocirculatoire Biologie
de la Paroi Vasculaire
Bd. de la Chapelle 41
FR 75010 Paris
Phone: +33 1 4285 8672
Fax: +33 1 4281 3128
Contract number: CT941121

Participants:

M. SAFAR
INSERM Unit 337
15 rue de l'Ecole de Médecine
FR 75006 Paris
Phone: +33 1 4329 2961
Fax: +33 1 4539 1193

H. STRUYKER BOUDIER
Dept. of Pharmacology
P.O. Box 616
NL 6200 MD Maastricht
Phone: +31 43 88 14 20
Fax: +31 43 67 09 40

A. HOEKS
Dept. Biophysics
P.O. Box 616
NL 6200 MD Maastricht
Phone: +31 43 88 16 59
Fax: +31 43 67 09 16

G. MANCIA
Centro di Fisiologia,
Clinica e Ipertensione,
Universita di Milano,
Ospedale Policlinico
Via F. Sforza
IT 20122 Milano
Phone: +39 2 5518 4606
Fax: +39 2 5457 666

K.H. RAHN
Dept. of Medicine D,
University of Munster
Albert Schweitzer Strasse 33
DE 4400 Munster
Phone: +49 251 83 75 17
Fax: +49 251 83 69 79

THE ROLE OF FACTOR VII-TISSUE FACTOR PATHWAY IN ISCHAEMIC CARDIOVASCULAR DISEASE

Key words
Cardiocascular diseases, FVII-TF pathway, clotting, standardization, epidemiology, genetic markers.

Brief description
This proposal concerns a Concerted Action whose final goal is to throw light on the role of the FVII-TF pathway, with regard to the pathogenesis of Ischaemic Cardiovascular Disease and its relationship with environmental and dietary habits as well as genetic determinants.

The scientific background for this proposal consists of:

1 epidemiological studies demonstrating that FVII is a risk factor for cardiovascular disease;
2 studies demonstrating the close relationship between cholesterol and the Tissue Factor pathway Inhibitor as well as between triglycerides and FVII;
3 the fact that gene mutations play a role in the plasma levels of FVII, and;
4 that high levels of FVII increase thrombin formation exponentially.

There are, however, unsolved problems:

a there is a lack of basic knowledge on the FVII-TF pathway as a system for initiating clotting;
b there is no agreement on the methods used to measure the haemostatic variables;
c understanding of the factors regulating the expression of FVII, TF and TFPI genes is limited;
d the influence of ethnicity - as studied by gene polymorphisms - on the activation of the pathway is little known, as is;
e the influence of the different lipid fractions on the level of activation of the pathway.

As a consequence, the tasks for this proposal will be:

1 the standardization of available methods for the evaluation of the haemostatic variables;
2 the development of new methods;
3 the evaluation and validation of the haemostatic risk factors through multicentre, multiethnic epidemiological studies;
4 the development and standardization of genetic markers for factors VII, X, TF and TFPI.

The seven Proposers of this CA have a great area of common scientific interest and have complementary scientific experiences, which may, indeed, create a European
action will be managed through a Steering Committee and Task Oriented Groups who will be responsible for and develop the intermediate targets. This CA has an important added scientific value for the Community, since only through the implementation of multicentre programmes is it possible to define the diagnostic value of laboratory data, the influence of the genetic and environmental determinants as well as their relationship to the various clinical pictures of ischaemia.

Project leader:
Professor Guglielmo MARIANI
Hematology Dept. Human Biopathol.,
Thrombosis Research Centre,
University of Rome
Via Chieti 7
IT 00161 Rome
Phone: +39 6 440 37 52
Fax: +39 6 440 37 84
Contract number: CT941202

Participants:
Prof. Francesco BERNARDI
Centro di Studi Biochimici sulle
patologie del genoma umano,
Istituto di Chimica Biologica,
Università di Ferrara
IT Ferrara
Phone: +39 532 210 232
Fax: +39 532 202 723

Prof. Rogier M. BERTONA
Hemostasis and Thrombosis Research Centre,
Leiden University, University Hospital
NL Leiden
Phone: +31 71 262 261
Fax: +31 71 225 555

Prof. Vicente GARCIA
Hematology Unit, Hospital General
Universitario, University of Murcia
ES Murcia
Phone: +34 68 256900
Fax: +34 68 261914

Prof. MEYER SAMANA
Laboratoire Central d'Hématologie,
Hotel Dieu, Laboratoire de Thrombose
Expérimental, Faculté Broussais-Hotel-Dieu
FR Paris
Phone: +33 1 42348266
Fax: +33 1 42348061

Prof. Hans PRYDZ
The Buitechnology Centre of Oslo,
University of Oslo
NO Oslo
Phone: +47 22 958755
Fax: +47 22 694130

Dr. Per Morten SANDSET
Hematological Laboratory, Medical Clinic,
Ullevaal Hospital, University of Oslo
NO Oslo
Phone: +47 22 119247
Fax: +47 22 119181

SOCIO-ECONOMIC VARIATIONS IN CARDIOVASCULAR DISEASE IN EUROPE: THE IMPACT OF THE WORK ENVIRONMENT AND LIFESTYLE

Key words
Cardiovascular diseases, psychosocial and biological risk factors, work environment, family life stressors.

Brief description
Cardiovascular diseases are the main causes of death in Europe and lead to a great social burden of morbidity.

Genetic factors are clearly important in setting individual risks; but genetic factors cannot explain the substantial variations in occurrence of coronary heart disease (CHD) throughout Europe, the dramatic recent declines in CHD in some, but not all, countries of Western Europe and the equally dramatic increases in countries of Central and Eastern Europe. There is strong evidence that variations within and between European countries are related to socio-cultural factors which determine health-related lifestyles (including diet, smoking, weight control, physical activity, alcohol use) and exposure to socio-environment stressors.

A major unsolved problem is the social class gradient in the occurrence of CHD.

People in low status jobs have higher risk of CHD: the lower the job status, the higher the risk.

Thus, the differences spread across all social classes. Over the last decade a substantial body of research has pointed to the importance of adverse environmental and psychosocial conditions at the work site in the aetiology of CHD.

Part of the social class gradient in CHD risk may be due to differences in working conditions among social classes.

This proposal brings together experienced researchers from six European countries: England, Germany, Greece, Italy, the Netherlands and Sweden all of who have active research programs in the field of psycho-social and bio-medical determinants of health.

The main objectives of the proposal are to:

1 distinguish among competing explanations for socioeconomic differences in CHD: in particular to examine the interactions between psychosocial and biological risk factors;

2 to test the hypothesis that the psycho-social work environment and family life stressors are importantly related to risk of CHD and may be a major contributor to generating socio-economic differences in CHD rates, and;

3 to make it possible to study psycho-social factors cross culturally and, therefore, for the first time to be able to address the question of the extent to which international differences in CHD rates may be related to international differences in psycho-social factors.

Project leader:
Professor M. MARMOT
Dept. of Epidemiology & Public Health, University College London
66-72 Gower Street
UK London WC1E 6EA
Phone: +44 71 380 76 02
Fax: +44 71 380 76 08
Contract number: CT941065

Participants:
Prof. Ad APPELS
Rijksuniversiteit Limburg,
Vakgroep Medische Psychologie
Postbus 616
NL 6200 MD Maastricht
Phone: +31 43 881 484
Fax: +31 43 670 952

Prof. Gian Carlo CESANA
Centro Studi Patologia Cronico-Degenerativa,
Ospedale S. Gerardo dei Tintori-Villa Serena
Via Donizetti 106
IT 20052 Monza
Phone: +39 39 3633097/8
Fax: +39 39 365378

Prof. Johannes SIEGRIST
Institute of Medical Sociology, Medical Faculty,
University of Dusseldorf
Moorenstrasse 5
DE 4000 Dusseldorf 1
Phone: +49 211 311 4360/4361
Fax: +49 211 311 2390

Dr. Anna KALANDIDI
Dept. of Hygiene and Epidemiology,
University of Athens Medical School
GR Athens
Phone: +30 1 770 8877
Fax: +30 1 770 4225

Prof. Tores THEORELL
National Institute for Psychosocial
Factors and Health
P.O. Box 60210
SE 10401 Stockholm
Phone: +46 8 7286 400/950
Fax: +46 8 344 143

EFFECTS OF DISEASE AND AGEING ON THE VASCULATURE: FOCUS ON INTRACELLULAR CALCIUM HANDLING

Key words
Ageing vascular disease, smooth muscle cell, calcium handling, humoral factors, neurotransmitters.

Brief description
In an aging population, as throughout the EC, a major cause of heart failure is vascular disease either of the coronary vessels or of the pulmonary and/or systemic vessels. Clearly, susceptibility to vascular disease changes throughout the life cycle, yet previous studies of changing vascular responsiveness with age have been characterised by conflicting or incomplete results.

An obvious common point at which vascular responsiveness can be altered by factors such as vascular aging is at the level of smooth muscle cell calcium handling, yet this hypothesis remains to be tested. The major goal of this project is, therefore, to throw light on the pathogenic mechanisms of aging-related cardiovascular disease by studying the effects of age on the role of calcium in the interplay of cellular and humoral factors.

We aim to investigate changes in vascular responsiveness to humoral factors and neurotransmitters associated with age and age-related cardiovascular diseases such as hypertension, atherosclerosis and chronic heart failure.

We will study resistance vessels from appropriate animal models to identify the risk factors associated with aging and age-related cardiovascular disease. We will do this by combining pharmacological, biochemical and molecular techniques for studying calcium handling. The ultimate aim is to pave the way to the development of new measures to reduce the incidence of cardiovascular disease associated with age.

Project leader:
Professor John McGRATH
Institute of Physiology,
University of Glasgow
UK Glasgow G12 8QQ
Phone: +44 41 330 4483
Fax: +44 41 330 4100
Contract number: CT941375

Participants:
Prof. E. VILA CALSINA
Universitat Autonoma de
Barcelona, Dept. de
Farmacologia i Psiquiatria
Bellaterra
ES 08193 Barcelona
Phone: +34 3 581 1952
Fax: +34 3 581 2004

Prof. Theo GODFRAIND
Universite Catholique de
Louvain, Laboratoire de
Pharmacodynamic Generale
et de Pharmacologie
BE 1200 Brussels
Phone: +32 2 764 7350
Fax: +32 2 764 7308

Prof. James R. DOCHERTY
Royal Collge of Surgeons in
Ireland, Dept. of Physiology
St. Stephen's Green
IE Dublin
Phone: +353 1 780 200
Fax: +353 1 4 780018

Prof. Klaus STARKE
Albert Ludwigs Universitat
Freiburg, Institut für Pharma-
kologie und Toxikologie
Hermann-Herder Strasse 5
DE 7800 Freiburg
Phone: +49 761 203 5313
Fax: +49 761 203 5318

Prof. Jesus MARIN
Universidad Autonoma de
Madrid, Dpto. de
Farmacologia y Terapeutica,
Facultad de Medicina
C/ Arzobispo Morcillo 4
ES 28029 Madrid
Phone: +34 1 397 5380
Fax: +34 1 315 0075

LIPASES AND RECEPTORS AS DETERMINANTS OF LIPOPROTEIN METABOLISM

Key words
Atherosclerosis, cardiovascular diseases, lipoprotein, metabolism, lipoprotein lipase, hepatic receptors.

Brief description
A major cause of heart and circulatory disease in the European countries is atherosclerosis, which is closely linked to derangement of lipoprotein metabolism. A number of epidemiological factors which seem to promote atherogenesis through lipoproteins are known, but there are wide gaps in understanding of how these epidemiological factors act at a mechanistic level.

Rational approaches to improved prevention and treatment requires insight at a mechanistic level.

Lipoproteins are secreted into plasma from the intestine as chylomicrons carrying dietary lipids, and from the liver carrying endogenous lipids. The first step in metabolism of these lipoproteins is mediated by lipoprotein lipase at vascular surfaces in many peripheral tissues. Through the hydrolytic action of this enzyme, fatty acids are liberated from lipoprotein triglycerides for use in cellular metabolic reactions. The lipoproteins become degraded to triglyceride-poor remnant particles, which are either cleared rapidly from blood by receptor-mediated pathways, primarily in the liver, or are remodelled into the slowly metabolized cholesterol-rich lipoproteins, LDL and HDL.

Epidemiological correlations to disease processes have focused mainly on the levels of LDL and HDL in fasting plasma. This creates a paradox since the epidemiological studies have indicated that major factors are the amount and type of dietary triglycerides, as well as exercise. Indeed, a "metabolic syndrome" has recently been suggested as a common denominator. Yet there are few if any direct mechanistic links between energy metabolism and turnover of cholesterol-rich lipoproteins. In contrast, there are ample connections between metabolic regulation and the lipases. For instance, large and rapid changes occur in lipase activity in response to meals to exercise.

The focal point for this proposal is the recent demonstration from Dr. Beisiegel's laboratory (in collaboration with the Umeå group) that lipoprotein lipase may act as a decisive ligand for the interaction of remnant particles with hepatic receptors. This suggests that the lipases may in fact have a dual role in lipoprotein metabolism, by degrading the primary triglyceride-rich lipoproteins to remnants and mediating interaction of remnants with receptors. This opens new perspectives on the coupling between risk factors and lipoproteins. In view of the enormous impact of atherosclerosis on health in the European countries, it is urgent that these new perspectives are pursued vigorously.

Neither of the proposed collaborating laboratories can do this effectively alone, but together we would form a strong team.

Project leader:
Professor T. OLIVERCRONA
Department of Medical Biochemistry & Biophysics
University of Umeå
SE 901 87 Umeå
Phone: +46 90 165234
Fax: +46 90 167840
Contract number: CT941244

Participants:
Johan AUWERX
Département d'Arthérosclérose, Laboratoire de
Biologie des Régulations ches les Eucaryotes
1 Rue Calmette
FR 59019 Lille
Phone: +33 20 87 77 88
Fax: +33 20 87 77 88

Ulrike BEISIEGEL
Medizinische Klinik,
Universitätskrankenhaus Eppendorf
Martinistrasse 52
DE 20246 Hamburg
Phone: +49 40 468 3917
Fax: +49 40 468 4592

Jorgen GLIEMANN
Institute of Medical Biochemistry,
University of Aarhus
DK 8000 Aarhus C
Phone: +45 86 12 93 99
Fax: +45 86 13 11 60

Sabine GRIGLIO
INSERM Unité 321, Lipoprotéines et
Athérogénèse, Hôpital de la Pitié,
Pavillon Benjamin Delessert
83 Boulevard de l'Hôpital
FR 75651 Paris Cedex 13
Phone: +33 1 42 17 78 59
Fax: +33 1 42 82 81 98

Miquel LLOBERA
Unitat de Biochemia Biologica
Molecular, Universitat de Barcelona
Avda. diagonal 647
ES 08028 Barcelona
Phone: +34 3 402 1525
Fax: +34 3 402 1559

Senén VILARO
Unitat de Biologia Cellular,
Universitat de Barcelona
Avinguda Diagonal 645
ES 08071 Barcelona
Phone: +34 3 402 1536
Fax: +34 3 411 2967

Hans WILL
Heinrich-Pette-Institut für Experimentelle
Virologie und Immunologie an der
Universität Hamburg
Martinistrasse 52
DE 20251 Hamburg
Phone: +49 40 4805 1221/1223
Fax: +49 40 464709

EUROPEAN CONCERTED ACTION ON ANTICOAGULATION

Key words
Anticoagulants, standardisation, prothrombin time, heparin, computerised system.

Brief description
European Concerted Action on Anticoagulation Anticoagulants are widely administered in EC member states for prevention and treatment of occlusive vascular disorders. The purpose is to develop a uniform strategy to make the treatment safer and more effective on an EC basis.

Oral Anticoagulants
The lack of standardisation of the prothrombin time (PT) test used for control has led to great differences in dosage between centreà. A WHO scheme for PT standardisation based on International Normalised Ratios (INR) was launched in 1983. The INR system should have greatly benefited EC member states but so far has only had limited application because:

1 INR are based on the manual PT technique now superseded in most EC hospital laboratories by automated methods. Automation reduces the reliability of INR, producing variable effects even between instruments of the same commercial brand of coagulometer.
2 The present INR calibration procedure is imprecise and complex.
3 INR are also unfamiliar to many clinicians who base dosage on direct PT ratios or percentage activities.

The aims of the study involving participants in ten EC member states with a minimum of 10 sub-participant centres in each will be:

a to improve reliability of Inrs using a new simplified system of PT calibration performed locally based on lyophilised calibrated plasmas;
b to standardise clinical dosage by computerised programmes of INR based oral anticoagulant dosage to improve clinical efficacy.

Heparin
Similar problems affect heparin administration, the dose varying between centres because of differing control methods and from variations in clinical dose regimens. A current international study including laboratories from EC member states shows considerable differences in target ranges based on the control test, the activated partial thromboplastin time (APTT). A multi-centre study will be undertaken to develop:

1 a consensus approach to therapeutic ranges;
2 a computerised system for heparin dosage.

Project leader:
Professor Leon POLLER
Dept. of Pathological Sciences,
Medical School
Oxford Road
UK Manchester M13 9PT
Phone: +44 61 275 5300
Fax: +44 61 275 5289
Contract number: CT941349

Participants:

Dr. J. ARNOUT
Thrombosis & Vascular
Research,
Campus Gasthuisberg
Herestraat 49
BE 3000 Leuven
Phone: +32 16 21 57 75
Fax: +32 16 34 59 90

Porf. H. BEESER
Medicine & Coagulation,
Dept. of Transfusion,
Universität Freiburg
DE Freiburg
Phone: +49 761 270 3480
Fax: +49 761 270 3245

Prof. M. SAMAMA
Service d'Hematologie,
Hotel Dieu de Paris
FR 75181 Paris Cedex 04
Fax: +33 1 42 34 80 61

Prof. J.A. IRIARTE
Hospital Civil de Basurto
Avenida Montevideo 18
ES 48013 Bilbao
Phone: +34 4 315 388
Fax: +34 4 441 4362

Prof. Jorgen JESPERSEN
Dept. of Clinical Chemistry,
Ribe County Hospital
DK Esbjerg
Phone: +45 75 181 900
Fax: +45 75 139 603

Dr. KONTOPOULOU-
GRIVA
Haematologist, 1st Regioonal
Transfusion Center,
Anticoagulant Unit,
Hippocration Hospital
GR Athens
Fax: +30 1 7702 959

Prof. P.M. MANNUCCI
Centro Emofilia e Trombosi,
Ospedale Maggiore di Milano
Via Pace 9
IT Milan
Fax: +39 2 55 16093

Dr. VAN DEN BESSELAAR
Haemostasis & Thrombosis
Research Center,
Academisch Ziekenhuis
NL Leiden
Phone: +31 71 261 893
Fax: +31 71 225 555

Dr. Brian OTRIDGE
Consultant Haematologist,
Mater Misericordiae Hospital
IE Dublin 7
Phone: +353 1 384 444/188
Fax: +353 1 874 8975

Prof. J. PINA CABRAL
Centro de Fisiologia da
Hemostase,
Universidade do Porto,
Faculdade de Medicina
Hospital de S joao
PT 4200 Porto
Fax: +351 2 510 1462

Prof. Klaus LECHNER
Medizinische Klinik der
Universität Wien
Zarettgasse 14
AT 1040 Wien
Phone: +43 1 404 0020
Fax: +43 1 402 6930

Prof. Nils EGBERG
Dept. of Clinical Chemistry,
Karolinska Hospital
SE 17176 Stockholm
Phone: +46 8 729 2212
Fax: +46 8 30 34 61

Prof. Ulrich ABILDGAARD
Medical Dept. A,
Aker Sykehus
NO 0514 Oslo
Phone: +47 22 894 000
Fax: +47 22 894 008

Dr. Martti SYRJALA
Laboratory Department,
Helsinki University
Central Hospital,
Meilahti Hospital
FI 00290 Helsinki
Phone: +358 0 4714308
Fax: +358 0 4714001

Prof. LAMMLE
Central Haematology
Laboratory,
University Hospital Bern
CH 3010 Bern
Phone: +41 31 632 3301
Fax: +41 31 632 9366

REGRESSION OF CORONARY ATHEROSCLEROSIS ASSESSED WITH INTRACORONARY ULTRASOUND

Key words

Coronary atherosclerosis, coronary angiography, intracoronary ultrasound, randomized study, evaluation.

Brief description

Background: Prevention is the key strategy in the approach to coronary atherosclerosis, the most important cause of morbidity and mortality in the European Community. The methods used to assess the efficacy of the interventions available to avoid progression and facilitate regression of coronary atherosclerosis are inadequate because they are unable to directly visualize the atherosclerotic plaque.

Objectives: Aim of this study is the use of intracoronary ultrasound in patients with symptomatic coronary artery disease to assess regression of atherosclerosis after 2 years of treatment with HMG-CoA reductase inhibitors.

Patient population: Two hundred fifty patients undergoing coronary angiography or angioplasty with the presence of angiographically and echocardiographically visible atherosclerotic changes suitable for quantification are enroled in a prospective, randomized, placebo-controlled study.

Methods: Progression/regression of the atherosclerotic lesion is assessed using quantitative coronary angiography and quantitative intracoronary ultrasound. Three-dimensional reconstruction of the acquired ultrasonic cross-sections using a motorized pull-back and automated contour detection are used to increase accuracy and reproducibility of the lumen-plaque volume measurements.

Follow-up: Angiography and intravascular ultrasound are repeated after 6 months and 2 years of treatment with placebo or active medication.

Project leader:
Dr. J.R.T.C. ROELANDT
Thorax Centre,
Div. Cardiology, University
Hospital Rotterdam
Dijkzigt Bd. 408
NL 3000 DR Rotterdam
Phone: +31 10 463 53 12
Fax: +31 10 436 30 96
Contract number: CT941626

Participants:
Dr. P. HANRATH
I Medizinischer Klinik,
RWTH Aachen
Pauwelstrasse 30
DE 5100 Aachen
Phone: +49 241 808 93 00
Fax: +49 241 888 84 14

Dr. R. ERBEL
University GBS-Essen
Hufelandstrasse 55
DE 4300 Essen 1
Phone: +49 201 723 24 93
Fax: +49 201 723 59 51

Dr. I. DE SCHEERDER
U.Z. Gasthuisberg
49 Herestraat
BE 3000 Leuven
Phone: +32 16 332 211
Fax: +32 16 343 449

Dr. S. CHIERCHIA
Ospedale San Raffaele
Via Olgettina 60
IT 20132 Milano
Phone: +39 2 226 431
Fax: +39 2 264 373 98

Dr. P. MARZILLI
Istituto di Fisiologia Clinica,
C.N.R.
via P. Savi 8
IT 56100 Pisa
Phone: +39 50 583 111
Fax: +39 50 553 461

EUROPEAN PROSPECTIVE COHORT
ON THROMBOPHILIA (EPCOT)

Key words
Thrombosis risk factor, protein C, protein S, antithrombin III, hereditary deficiencies.

Brief description
The aim of this project is to establish the risk of thrombosis in individuals who are deficient of natural coagulation inhibitors (protein C, protein S or antithrombin III).
The ultimate goal is to obtain reliable risk estimates that will allow the formulation of balanced guidelines for the clinical management of these individuals.
Hereditary deficiencies of protein C, protein S or antithrombin III are associated with an increased risk of thrombosis. The extent of this risk is unknown.
This poses a dilemma in the treatment of these individuals, of whom many still are asymptomatic, because the treatment with anticoagulants, which is highly efficient in the prevention of thrombosis, has a substantial risk of bleeding complications, as well as teratogenic side-effects. At present, no data are available to weigh the risks pro and contra anticoagulant treatment in these individuals.
This has ethical and social implications, since many individuals are detected as deficient because of a symptomatic relative in the family, whereas they are without any symptoms themselves.
The project will be conducted as a multicentre controlled prospective follow-up study. The study will include 900 individuals with one of the coagulation inhibitor protein deficiencies, and 900 healthy control subjects. Total follow-up will be approximately 6,000 person-years. Major endpoints are venous thrombosis and death.
The large size of the study will yield accurate risk estimates. The project brings together the leading European centres in thrombosis research, with the highest standards of laboratory and clinical experience. The expected results of the project will relate to the risk of thrombosis in deficient individuals versus healthy controls, in symptomatic versus asymptomatic carriers, in specific circumstances (pregnancy, oral contraceptive use, puerperium, hospital stay), in the presence or absence of anticoagulation, and in the various types and subtypes of the coagulation inhibitor protein deficiencies.
An important sub-aim will be to investigate the risk of miscarriage in women with these deficiencies.
A laboratory quality control system will be part of the study. Therefore, this project will lead to much needed harmonisation in laboratory methods, diagnostic criteria and clinical management. Thrombosis is a major cause of morbidity and mortality throughout the community. The losses in human lives, quality of life and in capital due to thrombosis can only be minimized by a uniform approach, which requires cost-benefit-analyses based on reliable information, as will be supplied by this study.

Project leader:
Dr. Frits ROSENDAAL
Haemostasis Thrombosis Research Centre, Department of Haematology, University Hospital
Building 1, C2-R
P.O. Box 9600
NL 2300 RC Leiden
Phone: +31 71 26 22 17
Fax: +31 71 21 28 32
Contract number: CT941565

Participants:

Prof. E. BRIET
Hematologie, Building 1 C2-R
University Hospital Leiden
P.O. Box 9600
NL 2300 RC Leiden
Phone: +31 71 262 261
Fax: +31 71 225 555

Dr. J. CONARD
Service d'HematologieImmunologie,
Hotel-Dieu de Paris
1 Place du Parvis Notre-Dame
FR 75181 Paris Cedex 04
Phone: +33 1 4234 8264
Fax: +33 1 4234 3100

Dr. J. FONTCUBERTA
Hospital de la Santa Creu i Sant Pau,
Servei d'Hematologia
Avgda S. A. M. Claret 167
ES 08025 Barcelona
Phone: +34 3 2919290
Fax: +34 3 2919192

Prof. G. MARIANI
Dept. Human Biopathology,
Hematology Section,
La Sapienza University
Via Benevento 6
IT 00161 Roma
Phone: +39 6 4403752
Fax: +39 6 4403753

Dr. G. PALARETI
Dept. Angiology and
Blood Coagulation,
University Hospital S. Orsola
Via Massarenti 9
IT 40138 Bologna
Phone: +39 51 6363411
Fax: +39 51 341642

Prof. F.E. PRESTON
Royal Hallamshire Hospital
Glossop Road
UK Sheffield S10 2JF
Phone: +44 742 739107
Fax: +44 742 756126

Prof. I. SCHARRER
Klinikum der
J.W. Goethe-Universität,
Abteilung für Angiologie
Theodor-Stern-Kai 7
DE 6000 Frankfurt am Main
Phone: +49 69 6301 5051
Fax: +49 69 6301 6738

Dr. I. WALKER
Thrombosis Research Group,
Dept. of Haematology,
Royal Infirmary
UK Glasgow G4 OSF
Phone: +44 41 5525692
Fax: +44 41 3044919

Dr. E. BERNTORP
Dept. for Coagulation
Disorders,
Dept. of Medicine,
University of Lund,
Malmö General Hospital
SE 21401 Malmö
Phone: +46 40 331000
Fax: +46 40 336255

Dr. I. PABINGER
Klin. Abteilung Hämatologie-
Hämastaseologie,
Allgemeines Krankenhaus
der Stadt Wien
Währinger Gürtel 18-20
AT 1090 Wien
Phone: +43 1 40400
Fax: +43 222 4026930

MULTI-LEVEL EPIDEMIOLOGICAL STUDY OF CORONARY HEART DISEASE IN EUROPEAN WOMEN

Key words
Coronary heart diseases women, risk factors, epidemiology.

Brief description
This is a collaborative research project between six well established centers in the field of cardiovascular epidemiology in France, UK, Finland and Spain. The aim is to describe the main features of the epidemiology of coronary heart disease among women aged 25-64 and to improve the understanding of the gender differences in the mortality, incidence and medical management of this disease.

The project will describe:

a mortality, attack and case fatality population rates of acute myocardial infarction for women over a 5-year period;

b the distribution and 5-year trends of risk factors;

c compare gender case-fatality rates and gender differences in medical management for the acute phase of myocardial infarction;

d study the associations between fatality from CHD and medical management during the acute phase of myocardial infarction at the individual level by pooling data from all centres and at aggregate level (population) taken into account the effect of socio-economic, health services variables and other confounders.

The project will use data from general population surveys, existing myocardial infarction registers and vital statistics, corresponding to the resident population of eight geographical defined areas. All the centres involved have been using the same highly standardized methods to collect the data.

Special emphasis will be put into the development and use of appropiate statistical methods to pool data and to study the ecological associations. The study will be run by a coordinating centre, a project management group, and a data centre will carry out the central analysis.

At the end of this project it is expected to improve the knowledge about chd in european women by quantifying the problem, thus helping in the planning and organization of health services by having information on the provision of medical care to women during the acute phase of myocardial infarction in different parts of europe, and by knowing the trends in the main coronary risk factors in current middle-aged women and therefore identifying needs for prevention of a major cause of disability in elder women.

Project leader:
Dr. Susana SANS
Chronic Diseases Prevention and Control Programme
Sant Antoni Claret 167
Pavello Convent, 2nd floor
ES 08025 Barcelona
Phone: +34 34 56 79 02
Fax: +34 34 33 15 72
Contract number: CT941779

Participants:
Prof. Pekka PUSKA
National Public Health Institute
Mannerheimintie 166
FI 00300 Helsinki
Phone: +358 0 47441
Fax: +358 0 1462185

Prof. Jaakko TUOMILEHTO
National Public Health Institute,
Dept. of Epidemiology and Health Promotion
Mannerheimintie 166
FI 00300 Helsinki
Phone: +358 0 47441
Fax: +358 0 1462185

Prof. Alun EVANS
The Queen's University of Belfast, Dept. of
Epidemiology and Public Health, Mulhouse
Building, Institute of Clinical Science
Grosvenor Road
UK Belfast BT12 6BJ
Phone: +44 2322 40503
Fax: +44 2322 36298

Prof. Hugh TUNSTALL-PEDOE
University of Dundee,
Cardiovascular Epidemiology Unit,
Ninewells Hospital & Medical School
UK Dundee DD1 9SY
Phone: +44 38264 4255
Fax: +44 38264 1095

Dr. Jean-Pierre CAMBOU
INSERM, Unité 326,
Hôpital Purpan
Place du Dr Baylac
FR 31059 Toulouse Cedex
Phone: +33 6149 1853
Fax: +33 6149 6749

Dr. Dominique ARVEILER
Université Louis Pasteur, Laboratoire
d'Epidémiologie et de Santé Publique,
Faculté de Medécine
4 Rue Kirschleger
FR 67085 Strasbourg Cedex
Phone: +33 88 368 597
Fax: +33 88 240 131

MOLECULAR GENETICS OF HUMAN HYPERTENSION

Key words
Hypertension, blood pressure, molecular mechanisme, environmental factors.

Brief description
Elevation of blood pressure in human essential hypertension is a major risk factor in western countries and is present in approximately 15% of the adult population. The hereditary and the environmental components of high blood pressure (BP), both very well documented, define hypertension as a multifactorial disease, with complex non-mendelian inheritance. Polymorphic variation of the structure of genes regulating BP are likely to be responsible for the hereditary part of BP, but the genes involved have not been identified. Only recently, the angiotensinogen gene was shown to have a role in human hypertension (cell 71, 169, 1992). The search for genes involved in BP hypertension is now made possible by the molecular cloning of several candidate genes, the possible development of linkage and genetic epidemiology methods. A complete exploitation of these methods in hypertension research requires multiple expertise in clinical medicine, genetics, epidemiology and molecular biology.

The purpose of this project is to facilitate the exchange of expertise between complementary groups in europe, involved in the various fields concerned by hypertension research. The project will favour continuation of collaborations already started. These exchanges will:

1 Encourage this research;
2 Improve its performance, and;
3 Allow large-scale studies required to confirm epidemiological and genetic results. Funds from ec will allow regular working sessions associating the different groups, the exchange of materials and human ressources between groups and the rapid exchange of results.

The final goal is to understand:
a The molecular basis of hypertension and its major related end-organ damages;
b How these molecular mechanisms interact with environmental factors.

This will allow an improved and comprehensive prevention, the design of drugs targeted to the molecular mechanisms of the disease and ultimately reduce the cost of this disease in western countries and its morbidity and mortality.

Project leader:
Dr. Florent SOUBRIER
INSERM Unit 36,
College de France
Rue d'Ulm 3
FR 75005 Paris
Phone: +33 1 44 27 16 73
Fax: +33 1 44 2716 91
Contract number: CT941353

Participants:
Prof. D. GANTEN
Max Delbrück Center for Molecular Medicine
Robert Rössle-Strasse
DE 01115 Berlin Buch
Fax: +49 30 949 7008

Dr. STAESSEN
Hypertension and Cardiovascular
Rehabilitation Unit, U.Z. Gasthuisberg
Herestraat 49
BE 3000 Leuven
Fax: +32 16 34 57 63

Prof. E. RITZ
University of Heidelberg, Dept. of Internal
Medicine and German Institute for
High Blood Pressure Research
Bergheimer Strasse 56a
DE 6900 Heidelberg
Fax: +49 6221 402 485

Dr. CONNOR
Glasgow Duncan Guthrie Institute of Medical
Genetics, MRC Blood Pressure Unit,
University of Glasgow, Dept. of Public Health
Yorkhill
UK Glasgow G3 8SJ
Fax: +44 41 357 4277

Dr. J. CONNELL
MRC Blood Pressure Unit, Western Infirmary
UK Glasgow G11 6NT
Fax: +44 41 357 4277

Dr. G. WATT
Dept. of Public Health, University of Glasgow
2 Lilybank Gardens
UK Glasgow G12 8RZ
Fax: +44 41 357 4277

Dr. D.E. GROBBEE
Dept. of Epidemiology and Biostatistics,
Erasmus University Medical School
P.O. Box 1738
NL 3000 Rotterdam
Fax: +31 10 408 7494

Prof. G. BIANCHI
Cattedra di Nefrologia, Divisione di Nefrologia
Dialisi e Ipertensione, Ospedale San Raffaele
Via Olgettina 60
IT 20132 Milano
Fax: +39 2 33500408

Dr. MARTINEZ-AMENOS
Unitat Hipertensio Arterial,
Servei de Nefrologia,
Hospital Princeps d'Espanya
c/Freixa Larga s/n
ES 08097 LHospitalet de Llobregat,
Barcelona
Fax: +34 3 263 1561

Dr. F. CANBIEN
SC7 INSERM
17 rue du Fer-à-Moulin
FR 75005 Paris
Fax: +33 1 4707 1741

Dr. M. LATHROP
INSERM U358, Hôpital Saint Louis
1 avenue Claude Vellefaux
FR 75010 Paris
Fax: +33 1 4240 1016

DEVELOPMENT OF A NEW NON-INVASIVE APPROACH TO THE EARLY IDENTIFICATION OF ALTERATION IN NEURAL CONTROL OF CIRCULATION IN CARDIOVASCULAR DISEASE

Key words
Cardiovascular diseases, blood pressure, non-invasive technique, computer analysis, diagnosis.

Objectives
The main objective of the proposed concerted action is the development of a diagnostic tool, based on computer analysis of blood pressure and heart rate fluctuations, for the early identification of alterations in autonomic cardiovascular control. These alterations characterize cardiovascular complications of a number of important diseases, such as diabetes and hypertension, and are associated with the ageing processes.

The diagnostic procedure will include two different phases. Firstly blood pressure and heart rate changes will be continuously measured over prolonged time periods in subjects under different behavioral conditions. Data collected will be further be analyzed by computerized procedures.

The main objective of the project will be achieved by two intermediate targets:

1 creation of guidelines to standardize the procedures for non-invasive continuous blood pressure monitoring by existing devices (finapres) and validation of a new device for continuous non-invasive 24 hour finger blood pressure recording in ambulant subjects (portapres);

2 development of innovative computerized procedures for the analysis of long-term blood pressure recordings, focusing on the various components of blood pressure and heart rate variability.

Brief description
The benefit from this project will be the development and validation of a simple approach to early diagnosis of cardiovascular complications through the computer analysis of beat-by-beat blood pressure and heart rate recordings. This non-invasive approach will reduce the need of invasive procedures in diagnosing autonomic dysfunction and, by extending such an evaluation to daily life conditions out of the artificial laboratory environment, will greatly increase the accuracy of our diagnostic approach to these pathologic conditions. It will also allow to assess the impact of treatment on these alterations.

Project leader:
Professor A. ZANCHETTI
Istituto di Clinica Medica Generale e Terapia Medica
Università degli Studi di Milano
Ospedale Maggiore
Via F. Sforza 35
IT 20122 Milano
Phone: +39 2 55 01 12 95
Fax: +39 2 55 18 75 06
Contract number: CT941455

Participants:

Dr. Gianfranco PARATI
Divisione di Malattie Cardiovascolari
e Riabilitazione Cardiologia,
Centro Auxologico Italiano
Via Spagnoletto 3
IT 20149 Milano
Phone: +39 2 48041
Fax: +39 2 48047 4127

Ing. Marco DI RIENZO
Centro di Bioingegneria,
Fondazione Pro-Juventute Don Gnochhi
Via Gozzadini 7
IT 20148 Milano
Phone: +39 2 4870 5848
Fax: +39 2 2686 1144

Dr. Karel H. WESSELING
TNO Biomedical Instrumentation,
Academisch Medisch Centrum, Room LO-002
Meibergdreef 15
NL 1105 AZ Amsterdam
Phone: +31 20 566 5844
Fax: +31 20 697 6424

Dr. Thomas SCHMIDT
Praventiv- und Verhaltensmedizin,
Abteilung Epidemiologie und Sozialmedizin,
Medizinische Hochschule Hannover
Postfach 610180
DE 3000 Hannover 61
Phone: +49 511 532 4422
Fax: +49 511 532 5347

Prof. R.I. KITNEY
Biomedical Systems Group,
Dept. of Electrical Engineering,
Imperial College of Science/
Technology and Medicine
Exhibition Road
UK London SW7 2BT
Phone: +44 71 581 3128
Fax: +44 71 823 8125

Prof. Ein O'BRIEN
The Blood Pressure Unit,
Beaumont Hospital
POB 1297, Beaumont Road
IE Dublin 9
Phone: +353 1 2803 865
Fax: +353 1 2803 688

Dr. Jan STAESSEN
Inwendige Geneeskunde-Cardiologie,
U.Z. Gasthuisberg
Herestraat 49
BE 3000 Leuven
Phone: +32 16 347 104
Fax: +32 16 345 763

Prof. Jean-Luc ELGHOZI
Nephrologie/Hypertension,
Laboratoire de Pharmacologie,
Faculté de Medecine Necker
156 Rue de Vaugirard
FR 75015 Paris
Phone: +33 1 4566 5585
Fax: +33 1 4061 5584

Prof. Giuseppe MANCIA
Cattedra di Medicina Interne,
1a Divisione di Medicina,
Universita degli Studi di Milano,
Ospedale S. Gerardo dei Tintori
Via Donizetti 106
IT 20052 Monza
Phone: +39 39 3633 357
Fax: +39 39 3222 74

II.4 RESEARCH ON MENTAL ILLNESS
AND NEUROLOGICAL DISEASES

Introduction

The understanding of the nervous system and in particular of the functions of the brain is one of the greatest scientific challenges of today and a unique theme of interest to society in general. The applications in medicine are far-reaching and may contribute to an improvement in the situation of persons suffering from major neurological and psychosocial disorders.

Neuroscience has made astonishing progress in the last few decades, based upon the new capabilities created by molecular biology and genetics, novel instrumentation and information technology. Thus, multi-disciplinary research has to be promoted if we want to accelerate the pace of unraveling the basic mechanisms underlying mental and neurological diseases, with the aim of promoting appropriate and effective treatment and prevention. This is the ultimate goal of this part of the BIOMED 1 Programme.

As such, a global approach to the study of etiopathogenic mechanisms, control disease and prevention and effects of prophylactic and therapeutic measures was undertaken.

Three ongoing actions dealing with epidemiological, neuropathological and basic approaches to prior diseases research illustrate how European neuroscience knowledge can benefit from inter- and multidisciplinary collaboration.

Another successful example is the creation of the first European Brain Bank for neurobiological studies in neurological and psychiatric disorders, aimed to serve as a bridge between clinicians, neuropathologists and neuroscientists investigating the various mental and neurological disorders.

From 1991 to 1994, financial support for the coordination of 532 research teams involved in 45 different projects has been committed. These activities have set the scene for a further structured and developed brain research area which will be implemented under BIOMED 2 of the Fourth Framework Programme (1994-1998).

Maria Vidal, MD

GENETIC ANALYSIS OF EPILEPSY

Key words
Epilepsy, genetics brain, gene mapping.

Objectives
The main objective of the Concerted Action is to promote and facilitate a collaborative European research programme on the molecular genetic analysis of epilepsy. The ultimate aim of this programme is to identify genes predisposing to the common familial epilepsies and to characterise the genetic contribution to its aetiology at a molecular level.

Brief description
Epilepsy is the most common serious neurological disorder. It is a heterogenous group of disorders with a genetic cause in about 20% of patients. The molecular genetic basis of these familial epilepsies is entirely common. Methods now exist, using positional cloning or candidate gene analysis, which should allow epilepsy genes to be identified. The task is more difficult than that of identifying genes for mendelian disorders. It is first necessary to assemble a large resource of families in which full clinical information is available on affected individuals. An extensive laboratory effort is then required in the analysis of DNA from family members. These tasks can only be achieved by the collaborative effort of several groups.
The Concerted Action is designed to allow the many European groups working on the genetic analysis of epilepsy to work together.

Project leader:
Professor R.M. GARDINER
Department of Paediatrics,
University College London Medical School,
The Rayne Institute
5 University Street
UK London WC1E 6JJ
Phone: +44 71 380 99 17
Fax: +44 71 380 96 81
Contract number: CT920456

Participants:
Dr. K. JOHNSON
Dept. of Anatomy, Charing Cross and
Westminster Medical School,
St. Dunstan's Road
UK London W6 8RP
Phone: +44 81 846 7038
Fax: +44 81 846 7025

Dr. S.D. SHORVON
National Hospital for
Nervous Diseases
Queen Square
UK London WC1N 3BG
Phone: +44 2407 71927
Fax: +44 2407 3991

Prof. O. DULAC
Hopital St. Vincent de Paul
74 Avenue Denfert Rochereau
FR 75674 Paris
Phone: +33 1 4048 8055
Fax: +33 1 4634 1656

Dr. A. MALAFOSSE
Institut de Biologie,
Lab.de Med. Experimentale
Boulevard Henri IV
FR 34060 Montpellier Cedex
Phone: +33 6760 9474
Fax: +33 6760 9478

Dr. M. LATHROP CEPH
27 Rue Juliette Dodu
FR 75010 Paris
Phone: +33 1 4249 9870
Fax: +33 1 4018 0155

Dr. M. DARLISON
Universitats-Krankenhaus Eppendorf
Martinistrasse 52
DE 2000 Hamburg 20
Phone: +49 40 468 4551
Fax: +49 40 468 4541

Dr. A. BIANCHI
UO Neurofisipatologia,
Presidio Ospedasiovi USL 23
Via Fonte Veneziana 17
IT 52100 Arezzo
Phone: +39 575 305 222
Fax: +39 575 305 257

Dr. L. FERRER-VIDAL
Spanish League Against Epilepsy
Escuelas Pias 89
ES 08017 Barcelona
Phone: +34 3 417 9716
Fax: +34 3 201 4324

Dr. F. ALVAREZ
Hospital Sant Joan de Deu
Carrefera d'Esplugues
ES 08034 Barcelona
Phone: +34 3 203 4000
Fax: +34 3 203 3959

Dr. KASTELEIJN-NOLST TRENITE
Instituut voor Epilepsiebestrijding
Meer en Bosch - De Cruquiushoeve
Achterweg 5
NL 2103 SW Heemstede
Phone: +31 23 294 323

Prof. Jose KEATING
Portugese League Against Epilepsy,
University of Coimbra
Rua Boavista 713
PT 4000 Porto
Phone: +351 2 302 525

Dr. M. SANTIAGO
Hosp. da Univ. de Coimbra
PT 3000 Coimbra
Phone: +351 39722115

Dr. A. COVANIS
Dept.of Neurology
Neurophysiology,
Aghia Sophia
Children's Hospital
GR 11527 Athens
Phone: +30 1 7771 811

Prof. EEG-OLOFSSON,
dr. WADELIUS &
prof. GUSTAVSON
Dept. of Paediatrics,
University Hospital
SE 75185 Uppsala
Phone: +46 18 663 000
Fax: +46 18 665 853

Prof. D. LINDHOUT
Faculteit der Geneeskunde en
Gezondheidswetenschappen,
Erasmus Universiteit
NL 3000 DR Rotterdam
Phone: +31 10 408 7215
Fax: +31 10 436 7133

Dr. M. FRIIS
Dept. of Neurology,
Odense University Hospital
DK 5000 Odense C
Phone: +45 66 11 33 33
Fax: +45 66 13 28 54

Prof. DE LA CHAPELLE &
dr. A.E. LEHESJOKI
Dept. of Medical Genetics,
University of Helsinki
Haartmaninkatu 3
FI 00290 Helsinki
Phone: +358 0 434 61
Fax: +358 0 434 6677

Dr. A. SUNDQVIST
Soder Hospital
SE 11883 Stockholm
Phone: +46 86 161 000
Fax: +46 86 162 957

RISK FACTORS FOR DEMENTING DISEASES

Key words
Dementia, Alzheimer's disease, vascular dementia, neurologic diseases, epidemiology, cognitive function, elderly populations, epidemiologic methods, incidence, risk factors.

Objectives
The general objective of the proposed Concerted Action is to detect preventable causes of the dementing diseases. The specific objectives are:
1 to study the variation in the incidence of dementia in the European community;
2 to study risk factors for dementia specifically for Alzheimer's disease and vascular dementia.

Brief description
Dementing diseases are a major public health problem. They include a wide range of debilitating pathological conditions, the most common of which are Alzheimer's disease and vascular dementia in Europe, the prevalence of dementia among those aged 65 years and older is at least 5%. The prevalence increases exponentially with age, affecting more than 25% of those 80 years and older. There are major gaps in our knowledge about the etiology of these age-associated diseases, and it is generally agreed that follow up epidemiologic studies of risk factors can assist in broadening and deepening our understanding in this field.

General design
This Concerted Action is based on European prospective follow-up studies on the incidence of dementing diseases which follow the same protocol. It is designed as a collaborative cohort study of risk factors for dementia and its sub-types Alzheimer's disease and vascular dementia.

Incidence studies
These incidence studies include community and institutional residents who are surveyed at baseline and followed up two to three years later. At baseline risk factors are measured and prevalent cases of dementia are detected and excluded from the cohort. The same case-finding procedures are repeated at the follow-up examination to enumerate the incident cases that occurred during the interval. Procedures have been developed to track all those who withdraw or die so that all new cases are identified.

Collaborative cohort study
The relation will be investigated between dementia and various risk factors. The risk factors for Alzheimer's disease and vascular dementia will be studied separately. The centres cover a cohort of approximately 43,000 individuals 65 years of age and older that will accumulate an anticipated 95,000 person-years. Based on the most recent estimates of the incidence of dementia we expect approximately 1,000 incident cases of dementia including 600 Alzheimer's disease patients and 250 vascular dementia patients. This would comprise the largest ever incident case series of Alzheimer disease and vascular dementia patients.

Selection of cases
This study will focus on moderate to severe cases of dementia identified through the two stage case-finding procedure outlined in the Eurodem protocol. In this procedure, the whole cohort is screened on cognitive functioning and on that basis a sub-sample is

selected to undergo a more extensive examination to diagnose dementia and its sub-types (ie., Alzheimer's disease, vascular dementia other dementia). A panel will review each case according to criteria that conform to internationally accepted diagnostic guidelines for dementia and its sub-types.

Risk factors

A set of core risk factors is measured at baseline by all participating centres. We will study the following putative risk factors for Alzheimer's disease, family history of dementia, epilepsy, Parkinson's disease, and Down's syndrome, history of thyroid disease, epilepsy, Parkinson's disease, head trauma and depression, and use of tobacco, alcohol and psychotropic medication. Information on socio-economic status and education will also be available. For vascular dementia the following putative risk factors will be examined: family history of dementia and stroke; history of hypertension obesity, diabetes mellitus, age of menopause, cardiac and cerebra-vascular events, use of tobacco and alcohol, as well as socio-economic status and education.

Data analysis

Each centre will enter data into a uniform data base. The data management and data analysis will be coordinated by the Department of Epidemiology & Biostatistics, Erasmus University Medical School, the Netherlands. The overall analytical strategy will be developed in concert with the MRC Biostatistics Unit, Cambridge, United Kingdom. Each centre will use this approach to analyze and write-up for publication at least one set of risk factors. These analyses will yield estimates of the absolute risk for Alzheimer's disease and vascular dementia, the relative risk associated with the putative risk factors, and the attributable risks for the preventable causes of dementia.

Project leader:
Professor A. HOFMAN
Dept. of Epidemiology &
Biostatistics, Erasmus
University, Medical School
P.O. Box 1738
NL 3000 DR Rotterdam
Phone: +31 10 408 74 88
Fax: +31 10 408 74 94
Contract number: CT920653

Participants:
Prof. J.F. DARTIGUES
FR 33076 Bordeaux-Cedex

Prof. L.A. AMADUCCI
IT 50123 Firenze

Prof. A. HOFMAN &
dr. L.J. LAUNER
NL 3000 DR Rotterdam

Dr. A. DROUX
PT 4420 Gondomar

Prof. A. LOBO
ES 50009 Zaragoza

Prof. J.M.R. COPELAND &
mr. M. DEWEY
UK Liverpool L69 3BX

Prof. N.E. DAY
UK Cambridge CB2 2BW

Ms. C. CHADWICK
UK Liverpool L69 3BX

Prof. T.H.D. ARIE &
dr. K. MORGAN
UK Nottingham NG7 2UH

Prof. J. GRIMLEY EVANS
UK Oxford LX2 68E

Prof. E. PAYKEL &
dr. C. BRAYNE
Prof. D.W.K.KAY

Drs. M. ROELANDS

Prof P. KRAGH-SORENSEN
& dr. A. LOLK
DK 5000 Odense C

Dr. A. ALPEROVITCH
FR 94807 Villejuif-Cedex

Prof. O. HAGNELL
SE 220 06 Lund

Prof. B. WINBLAD
SE 144186 Huddinge

Dr. C. JAGGER
UK Leicester LE2 7LX

Prof. A. MANN
UK London SE5 8AF

EUROPEAN COLLABORATIVE STUDY ON AFFECTIVE DISORDERS: INTERACTION BETWEEN GENETIC AND PSYCHOLOGICAL VULNERABILITY FACTORS

Key words
Genetic, affective disorders, psychosocial factors.

Objectives
1 To study the genetics of manic depressive illness (MDI) at the molecular level using the candidate gene strategy (molecular genetics and linkage techniques).
2 To explore the quantitative effect of psychosocial factors on gene expression for MDI in large population samples and in large affected pedigrees.
3 To study the interaction between genetic and psychosocial factors.

Brief description
There is now cumulative evidence (family, twins and adoption studies) that genetic factors are involved in the vulnerability and expression of Major Affective disorders such as manic-depressive illness (MDI) and recurrent unipolar depressive disorder.

Although these findings strongly support an important role of heredity, they do not elucidate the underlying genetic mechanisms.

Furthermore, non genetic (environmental, psychosocial) factors may also be operational, but their quantitative effect on gene(s) expression can not be predicted. Recent progress in molecular genetics and chromosomal markers studies constitute a powerful strategy for demonstrating gene effects regarding the etiology of major psychiatric disorders.

Linkage studies with classical genetic markers (such as colour blindness and glucose-6-phosphate dehydrogenase) were conducted and provided evidence for the presence in MDI of a Major single gene located in the distal end of the long arm of the X chromosome. The localisation of a gene situated on the distal part of the short arm of chromosome It has also been reported in one family originating of the Amish community but this result was not confirmed in other pedigrees.

These different findings (X and non X-linked forms of the illness) suggest the genetic heterogeneity of MDI which is one of the major problem to cope with in linkage studies of affective disorders. Indeed, these linkage analyses only function optimally for diseases caused by a single gene with specified genetic parameters (gene penetrance, allele frequency, mode of inheritance).

Several others factors limit the interpretation of linkage studies such as diagnostic uncertainties, assortative mating and cohort effect.

It is then of interest to apply other methods that do not require specification of penetrance and mode of inheritance (non parametric analysis such as marker association segregation chi-quare method and affected sib-pair method). These methods require a large number of subjects.

Beside genetic factors, psychosocial variables have been shown to affect the onset and the course of MDI and depression. Social adjustment, family functioning, level of expressed emotion and self-esteem are some of the most relevant psychosocial vulnerability factors and predictors of relapses. However, the interaction between genetic and psychosocial factors has not been properly studied yet.

The research tasks of this Program are to study the molecular genetics of manic depressive illness and the interactions with psychosocial factors in a large scale interdisciplinary and multicentric European project.

Modern molecular genetic techniques using the candidate gene approach, detected by Polymerase Chain Reactions (PCR) will be applied to marker association, sib-pair and linkage studies. Special attention will be given to candidate genes (i.e. the GABA receptor alpha 3 gene (GABRA3) and tyrosine hydroxylase (TH) and in candidate regions (i.e. XQ 27-28; 11 P 15). Simultaneously, the random genome search approach will be applied for available markers chosen for their high polymorphic information content. (SSR: highly polymorphic simple sequence repeats).

These analyses will be performed in large samples of patients, normal controls and families. The issues of diagnostic uncertainties and disease variation (problem of phenocopies) will be addressed and new concepts of diagnostic management will be applied (probability of being a true case rather than a phenocopy).

Analysis of interactions between genetic and psychosocial factors will focus on the above mentioned factors, most relevant for the onset and course of affective illnesses. For psychosocial factors, logistic regressions and weight factors approach will be used to appreciate their quantitative effects in relation to genetic determinants of affective disorders.

Project leader:
Professor J. MENDLEWICZ
Dept. of Psychiatry,
Erasmus Hospital
route de Lennik 808
BE 1070 Brussels
Phone: +32 2 555 44 09
Fax: +32 2 555 45 15
Contract number: CT921217

Participants:
Dr. D. BLACKWOOD
UK Edinburgh EH 10 5HF

Prof. G. TACAGNI &
dr. N. BRUNELLO
IT 20133 Milano

Dr. S.Z. LANGER
FR 92225 Bagneux Cedex

Dr. L. ORUC
Paula Goranina GR 16
71000 Sarajevo

Prof. C. PULL
LU 1210 Luxembourg

Prof. B. SALETU
AT 1090 Vienna

Dr. T. MELLERUP
DK 2100 Copenhagen

Dr. F. MACCIARDI
IT 20122

Prof. E. SMERALDI
IT 20147 Milano

Prof. B. LERER
IL 91120 Jerusalem

Prof. N. MATUSSEK &
prof. M. ACKENHEIL
DE 8000 Munchen 2

Prof. L. WETTERBERG
SE 11281 Stockholm

Prof. C. STEFANIS &
prof. G. PAPADIMITRIOU
GR 11528 Athens

Dr. PINTO DE AZEVEDO
PT 3049 Coimbra

Prof. P. COSYNS
BE 2650 Edegem

Prof. J.J. LOPEZ-IBOR
ES 28035 Madrid

Prof. J. ANGST
CH Zurich

Prof. VAN DE WETERING
NL Rotterdam

Dr. O. DEBRAY
FR 75730 Paris Cédex 15

Dr. PELTONEN-PALOTIE
FI 00300 Helsinki

Dr. VAN BROECKHOVEN
BE 2610 Antwerpen

Dr. L.A. SANDKUIJL
NL 2611 Delft

Prof. J. MENDLEWICZ
BE 1070 Brussels

CLINICAL AND MOLECULAR GENETIC STUDY OF CYTOGENETIC ABNORMALITIES ASSOCIATED WITH SCHIZOPHRENIA AND AFFECTIVE PSYCHOSIS

Key words
Schizophrenia, affective disorders, psychotic, chromosome abnormalities, cloning, molecular.

Objectives
A search will be made linking clinical psychiatric and cytogenetic centres in Scotland and Denmark for abnormalities of karyotype that co-segregate or significantly associate with schizophrenia and affective psychosis. Families showing the co-inheritance of mental illness, mental retardation and/or physical dysmorphic features will also be examined for chromosomal abnormalities. Once identified such abnormalities define candidate regions containing genes for these mental illnesses. Microdissection and microcloning of DNA from these areas will involve molecular genetic centres in Austria and Scotland and a joint approach will be made to isolate the genes and develop new and novel methods of microdissection and cloning to improve the rapidity and efficiency of gene isolation.

Brief description
The MRC Human Genetics Unit in Edinburgh has maintained and expanded a registry for cytogenetic abnormalities defined for large population groups for several years. Detailed karyotyping and genealogical tracing has identified a large series of families with inherited constitutional abnormalities and yearly clinical follow up on all carriers and controls in such pedigrees allows the identification of abnormalities that associate with mental illness. Denmark also has extensive cytogenetic information on individuals collected over many years and databases exist for all persons in Denmark who have had treatment for psychiatric disorders. Dr. Mors is cross-linking these two data sets to find subjects who have psychiatric illness and abnormality of karyotype. Our aim is to combine the Edinburgh and Aarhus data to increase the power to detect significant associations. In addition families in which psychotic disorders, mental retardation and physical dysmorphisms appear to run together are being identified in Scotland. Such multiple handicaps increase the likelihood of a microscopically visible chromosomal rearrangement or one that can be rendered visible by chromosome 'painting' methods, and both these approaches will be studied.

Abnormalities that are found to significantly co-associate with schizophrenia or affective psychosis will form the base for molecular studies. Dr. Weith in Vienna has already developed powerful chromosomal microdissection techniques that can be used to generate region specific DNA libraries. The chromosomes are dissected unstained and the average insert size of the libraries is several kilobases, and thus ideally suited to be used as probes in their own right, to screen genomic cosmid and YAC libraries for contig mapping purposes, to identify new dinucleotide and trinucleotide repeat polymorphisms useful in genetic mapping, and to screen brain cDNA expression libraries for genes of interest. The methodology will be further developed with the aim of reducing the number of chromosomes that need to be cut to generate a library improving the specificity of the technique. The eventual aim is to obtain representative libraries from a single cut using PCR based methodology.

Microdissection will be applied in combination with other cloning techniques to examine chromosomal re-arrangements that are found linked to psychiatric disorders with the aim of identifying genes in these particular regions that may be causal for psychiatric disorder in the particular patients with abnormal karyo-type, and form candidate genes for schizophrenia and affective psychosis in general.

Project leader:
Dr. W.J. MUIR
University Department of Psychiatry,
Royal Edinburgh Hospital,
Kennedy Tower
Morningside Park
UK Edinburgh EH10 5HF
Phone: +44 31 447 20 11
Fax: +44 31 447 68 60
Contract number: CT921560

Participants:

Dr. D.H.R. BLACKWOOD
Univ. Dept. of Psychiatry,
Kennedy Tower,
Royal Edinburgh Hospital
Morningside Park
UK Edinburgh EH10 5HF
Phone: +44 31 447 2011
Fax: +44 31 447 6860

Prof. Christine M. GOSDEN
Medical Research Coucil
Human Genetics Unit, Western General Hospital
Crewe Road
UK Edinburgh EH4 2XU
Phone: +44 31 332 2471
Fax: +44 31 343 2620

Dr. David M. St. CLAIR
Univ. Dept. of Psychiatry,
Kennedy Tower,
Royal Edinburgh Hospital
Morningside Park
UK Edinburgh EH10 5HF
Phone: +44 31 447 2011
Fax: +44 31 447 6860

Dr. Andreas WEITH
Forschungsinstitut für
Molekulare Pathologie
Dr. Bohr-Gasse 7
AT 1030 Vienna
Phone: +43 222 797 30 625
Fax: +43 222 798 71 53

Dr. Ursala FRIEDRICH
Psychiatric Hospital
Skovagervej 2
DK 8240 Risskow
Phone: +45 86 177777
Fax: +45 86 175977

Dr. Ole MORS
Inst. Psychiatric Demograp.,
Psychiatric Hospital
Skovagervej 2
DK 8240 Risskow
Phone: +45 86 177777
Fax: +45 86 175977

INCIDENCE AND RISK FACTORS FOR PARKINSON'S DISEASE: A EUROPEAN COLLABORATIVE STUDY

Key words
Parkinson's disease, epidemiology, incidence, risk factors.

Objectives
The specific objectives of the Concerted Action are:
- To compare the incidence of PD, as measured through repeated population surveys, in 5 cohort studies from 4 European countries, and investigate the distribution of PD by age, sex, occupation, education, and other personal characteristics.
- To investigate environmental and genetic risk factors for PD through a case-control study nested within 5 European cohort studies of ageing populations. To estimate the degree of risk (relative risk) associated to occupations, toxic exposures, smoking, head trauma, family history, and other putative risk factors.

Brief description
The Concerted Action is a collaborative comparison of incidence data on Parkinson's disease obtained with similar case-finding strategies and common diagnostic criteria. Five cohort studies conducted France (1), Italy (1), Spain (2) and the Netherlands (1) on both community and institutional residents of well-defined populations are included in the collaborative project. The combined sample of the 5 cohorts comprised approximately 24,000 individuals yielding to an expected number of 120 incident cases of Parkinson's disease.

The general structure of the incidence study is common across centres:
1 initial assessment of disease status and collection of risk factor information through a direct personal contact (initial door-to-door survey);
2 follow-up for 2 or 3 years (according to the centre), with or without interim assessment of disease status;
3 final assessment of disease status on the entire cohort at end of study (final door-to-door survey); and
4 retrospective reconstruction of medical events occurring in the time elapsed between contacts.

The principal risk factors to be investigated are: occupation, use of herbicides and pesticides, exposure to industrial chemicals, farming practices, residences during life, migrations, well-water drinking, smoking, head trauma, age at viral infections, previous diseases, family history of PD, family history of Alzheimer's disease, personality, education, and other psychosocial factors. These factors will be assessed using routine questionnaire during the survey Conducted at the beginning of the study.

A two-phase design will be used for case-finding. During phase 1, a brief screening instrument is administered to each subject; in phase 2, the presence of PD is confirmed or excluded by a neurologist only in those subjects who screened positive. A common protocol is used by neurologists for the clinical diagnosis of PD and for the differential diagnosis with other types of parkinsonism.

Geographic differences in the incidence of PD will be investigated by comparing age-specific rates calculated in each of the 5 cohorts for men and women separately. In addition, the incidence pattern by occupation, education, and other variables will be described. For the various risk factors to be investigated, relative risk will be estimated through the calculation of odds ratio.

Project leader:
Dr. A. ALPEROVITCH
INSERM U360
16, Av. Paul Vaillant Couturier
FR 94807 Villejuif Cédex
Phone: +33 1 45 59 51 86
Fax: +33 1 45 59 51 70
Contract number: CT921101

Participants:
Dr. Monique M.B. BRETELER
Dept. of Epidemiology and Biostatistics,
Erasmus University Medical School
PO Box 1738
NL 3000 DR Rotterdam
Phone: +31 10 408 7393
Fax: +31 10 408 7494

Dr. Jean Francois DARTIGUES
INSERM Unité 330, Département d'Informatique Médicale, Université de Bordeaux II
146 Rue Léo-Saignat
FR 33076 Bordeaux Cedex
Phone: +33 5757 1010/1393
Fax: +33 5699 1360

Dr. Secundino LOPEZ-POUSA
Grupo de Estudio de Epidemiologia en Girona
(GRESEPGI), Hospital Sta. Caterina
Placa Hospital 5
ES 17001 Gironaerdam
Phone: +34 7220 1450
Fax: +34 7222 6205

Dr. José Maria MANUBENS BERTRAN
Dpto. Neurologia y Neurocirugia,
Unidad de Alzheimer, Clinica Universitaria,
Facultad de Medicina Universidad de Navarra
ES 31080 Pamplona
Phone: +34 4810 9469/9319
Fax: +34 4817 0515

Dr. Walter A. ROCCA
CNR - Progetto Finalizzato Invecchiamento and
Institute of Neurology, Centro SMID,
University of Verona
Via il Prato 58
IT 50143 Firenze
Phone: +39 55 230 2920/48/49
Fax: +39 55 230 2919

ROLE OF THE DOPAMINE D₃ RECEPTOR IN PHYSIOLOGY, SCHIZOPHRENIA AND AS A TARGET FOR ANTIPSYCHOTIC DRUGS

Key words
Dopamine receptor, neurotransmission, antipsychotics, schizophrenia, behaviour, molecular genetics.

Objectives
The major aim is to understand the physiological roles of the dopamine D_3-receptor (D3R) in cerebral neurotransmission, to assess its involvement in schizophrenia and other mental disorders and to develop a new generation of antipsychotic agents.

Brief description
The recently identified D_3R has been shown to be recognized by antipsychotic drugs and to be selectively expressed in rodents in the limbic brain areas, suggesting that its blockade may play an important role in the treatment of schizophrenia. We plan to further investigate its role by an interdisciplinary approach.

The pharmacological subprogram will be to design selective compounds, for which chemical leads have already been identified, by a classical structure-activity study as well as by a three-dimensional D_3R model based on its amino acid sequence. The localization subprogram will establish the dopamine pathways in CNS using the D_3R by a combination of autoradiography with a selective radioligand and in situ hybridization performed in sections of rodent and human brains. Biological effects of D_3R activation and intracellular pathways involved in D_3R-mediated responses will be studied by classical biochemical and electrophysiological approaches, using either identified neurons bearing this receptor or cultured transfected cells. Behavioral responses will be characterized in rodents among stereotyped manifestations and locomotor behaviours, using selected specific agonists and antagonists identified in the pharmacological subprogram. Monitoring in vivo DA neurotransmission using microdialysis, correlated with measurement of Fos expression will provide information on the role of D_3R in specific brain areas.

Finally, the molecular genetic subprogram will assess the possible role of the D_3R in the aetiology of schizophrenia by performing linkage and association studies, using DNA polymorphisms that have already been identified in the D_3-receptor gene.

Project leader:
Professor P. SOKOLOFF
INSERM, Unité 109, Centre Paul Broca
2 ter, Rue d'Alésia
FR 75014 Paris
Phone: +33 1 40 78 92 41
Fax: +33 1 45 80 72 93
Contract number: CT921086

Participants:

Prof. J.C. SCHWARTZ
Unité de Neurobiologie et Pharmocologie (U.
109) de l'INSERM, Centre Paul Broca
2ter rue d'Alésia
FR 75014 Paris
Phone: +33 1 4589 8907
Fax: +33 1 4580 7293

Dr. C.G. WERMUTH
Laboratoire de Pharmacochimie Moléculaire,
ERA 393 CNRS
5 rue Blaise Pascal
FR 67000 Strasbourg
Phone: +33 88 66 90 77
Fax: +33 88 67 47 94

Dr. P.F. SPANO
Dipartimento di Scienze Biomediche e
Biotecnologie, Facolta di Medicina e Chirurgia,
Università degli Studi di Brescia
Via Valsabbina 19
IT 25124 Brescia
Phone: +39 30 3996 286
Fax: +39 30 3701 157

Dr. L. CAZIN
UA 650 CNRS, Faculté des Sciences
B.P. 118
FR 76134 Mont Saint Aignan Cedex
Phone: +33 35 14 66 24
Fax: +33 35 14 69 46

Prof. G. SEDVALL
Dept. of Psychiatry and Psychology,
Karolinska Hospital
SE 104 01 Stockholm
Phone: +46 8 729 4445
Fax: +46 8 346 563

Dr. M.A. CROCQ
Centre Hospitalier Spécialisé
FR 68250 Rouffach
Phone: +33 89 78 70 67
Fax: +33 89 78 51 24

Dr. A. MAYER
Institut Humangenetik und Anthropologie
Breisacherstrasse 33
DE 7800 Freiburg
Phone: +49 761 270 7051
Fax: +49 761 270 7041

Prof. J. CESTENTIN
UER de Médecine et Pharmacie, Laboratoire de
Pharmacodynamie et Physiologie
Avenue de l'Université, B.P. 97
FR 76800 Saint Etienne du Rouvray
Phone: +33 35 66 08 21
Fax: +33 35 66 08 21

Prof. G. DI CHIARA
Institute of Experimental Pharmacology and
Toxicology, University of Cagliari
Via Porcell 4
IT 09124 Cagliari
Phone: +39 70 303 819
Fax: +39 70 300 740

SURVEILLANCE OF CREUTZFELDT-JAKOB DISEASE IN THE EUROPEAN COMMUNITY

Key words
Creutzfeldt-Jakob disease, epidemiology, case-control study, neuropathology, molecular biology.

Objectives
The objectives on the European Collaborative Study on CJD are firstly to study the frequency of human spongiform encephalopathies in Europe in relation to animal spongiform encephalopathies and secondly to assess the risk of CJD and other human spongiform encephalopathies in relation to genetic, occupational and nutritional factors with particular emphasis on animal spongiform encephalopathies.

Brief description
Registries of Creutzfeldt-Jakob disease have been set up in a number of European countries in order to monitor the frequency of CJD and to serve as a basis for further epidemiological and molecular genetic studies. Detailed diagnostic criteria have been agreed by all participants and cases are ascertained by direct referral from neurologists, neuropathologists and others including psychiatrists in some countries. Where possible, death certificates are used as a safety net in order to identify cases not directly referred.

Each identified patient is visited and details of clinical features and investigations are obtained. A standard questionnaire addressing potential risk factors including occupation, past medical history, dietary exposure and contact with animals is used to obtain information from the relatives of each patient. In parallel a case-control study is being carried out using hospital-based age- and sex-matched controls in which the standard questionnaire is again used. Blood is obtained from all possible cases for molecular biological analysis and post mortem is obtained in a high proportion of patients.

The main analysis of this data is to determine whether the incidence of Creutzfeldt-Jakob disease is similar throughout the EC and if there is any major difference between putative risk factors in various countries.

Project leader:
Dr. R.G. WILL
CJD Surveillance Unit, Western General Hospital
UK Edinburgh EH4 2XU
Phone: +44 31 332-2117
Fax: +44 31 3431404
Contract number: CT920988

Participants:
Dr. J. COLLINGE
Dept. of Biochemistry & Molecular Genetics, St.
Mary's Hospital Medical School
Norfolk Place
UK London W2 1PG
Phone: +44 71 723 1252
Fax: +44 71 706 3272

Dr. A. ALPEROVITCH
INSERM U.360
16 Avenue Paul-Vaillant-Couturier
FR 94807 Villejuif Cedex
Phone: +33 1 4559 5186
Fax: +33 1 4559 5170

Prof. L. AMADUCCI
Centro SMID
Via Il Prato 58
IT 50123 Firenze
Phone: +39 55 230 2948
Fax: +39 55 230 2914

Prof. A. LECHI
Clinica Neurologica
Via del Quartiere 4
IT 43100 Parma
Phone: +39 521 28 27 76
Fax: +39 521 23 28 66

Prof. G. MACCHI
Clinica Neurologica, Universita Cattolica Sacro
Cuore
Largo Gemelli 8
IT 00168 Roma
Phone: +39 6 33 05 42 42
Fax: +39 6 30 51 343

Prof. V. BONAVITA
Clinica Neurologica, Nuovo Policlinico
Via Pansini 5
IT 80131 Napoli
Phone: +39 81 54 65 402
Fax: +39 81 54 65 402

Prof. A. HOFMAN
Dept. of Epidemiology & Biostatistics,
Erasmus University Medical School
PO Box 1738
NL 3000 DR Rotterdam
Phone: +31 10 408 7365
Fax: +31 10 408 7494

Prof. S. POSER
Klinik und Poliklinik für Neurologie,
Georg-August-Universität Göttingen
Robert-Koch-Strasse 40
DE 3400 Göttingen
Phone: +49 551 39 6603
Fax: +49 551 39 8405

Dr. T. WEBER
Klinik und Poliklinik für Neurologie,
Georg-August-Universität Göttingen
Robert-Koch-Strasse 40
DE 3400 Göttingen
Phone: +49 551 39 6603
Fax: +49 551 39 8405

Dr. P. BROWN
Laboratory of CNS Studies, NINDS Bld 36
Room 5B21, National Institutes of Health
Bethèsda
US Maryland 20892-0036
Phone: +1 301 496 5292
Fax: +1 301 496 8275

CONCERTED ACTION ON T-CELL AUTOIMMUNITY IN MULTIPLE SCLEROSIS

Key words
Multiple Sclerosis, Pathogenesis, Diagnosis, Immunotherapy, T-Iymphocytes, Lymphokines, Autoimmunity, Immunogenetics.

Objectives
1 Characterization of specific mechanisms of T cell-mediated immune response to the CNS in multiple sclerosis (MS).
2 Identification of associations between MS and immune response genes.
3 Development of rational bases for non-toxic immunotherapies of MS in order to establish successful clinical trials in MS.
4 Identification of markers useful for the monitoring of disease activity and efficacy of immunotherapies in MS.

Brief description
Multiple Sclerosis (MS) is an inflammatory and demyelinating disease of the Central Nervous System (CNS) of unknown etiology, characterized by progressive neurological impairment. In Europe the disease affects 1/1000 individuals and represents, excluding trauma, the most frequent cause of disability in young adults.

Independently considering each European country, public and private investments in MS have not reached the critical mass needed for efficiently developing rational basis of non toxic treatments of MS, but the total European resources dedicated to the study of autoimmune mechanisms in MS are remarkable.

Coordination of MS research currently ongoing in each European country, may:
- promote adequate interdisciplinary cooperation, gathering complementary methodological competences;
- promote a more rational planning and efficient handling of most of human and economical resources currently devoted to international cooperation.

T-cell mediated autoimmunity against myelin antigens is currently considered the major pathogenetic mechanism in MS, but thus far the target antigen(s) and therefore the pathogenetic T-cell clones, have not been identified. Characterization of pathogenetic T-cells and their specific inactivation, allowing development of selective immunosuppressive therapeutic strategies, is therefore the ultimate goal of the research in this field. Recent advances in cellular and molecular immunology allow now to study antigen specific T-cells at clonal level In addition, new more sensitive molecular genetics techniques are now available for identification of possible immune response genes associations to the disease.

The present Concerted Action will coordinate studies of qualified European research centers on:
- characterization of specific mechanisms of T-cell mediated immune response to the CNS in MS; monitoring of disease activity and efficacy of immunosuppressive treatments in MS; identification of association between MS and immune response genes.
- identification of associations between MS and immune response genes;
- development of rational bases for non-toxic immunotherapies of MS in order to establish successful clinical trials in MS;

- identification of markers useful fot the monitoring of disease activity and efficacy of immunotherapies in MS.

Project leader:
Dr. Luca MASSACESI
Dipartimento di Scienze Neurologiche e Psichiatriche
Viale Morgagni 85
IT 50134 Firenze
Phone: +39 55 43 22 24
Fax: +39 55 41 36 03
Contract number: CT931531

Participants:

Dr. Hans LASSMANN
Neurol. Inst. der Universität
Wien (Obersteiner-Institut)
LX Schwarzpanierstr. 17
AT 1090 Wien
Phone: +43 140 480 257
Fax: +43 140 340 77

Dr. Jef RAUS
Dr. L. Willems Institute Uzw
Universitaire Campus
BE 3590 Diepenbeek
Phone: +32 11 226 721
Fax: +32 11 269 312

Dr.Eric. SEBOUN
Genethon
1 Rue de l'International
FR 91000 Every
Phone: +33 1 6947 2959
Fax: +33 1 6077 8698

Dr. Hans Peter HARTUNG
Neurologische Universitäts-
klinik und Poliklinik
Jos. Schneider-Str. 11
DE 8700 Würzburg
Phone: +49 93 1201 2250
Fax: +49 93 1201 2697

Prof. Hartmut WEKERLE
MPI fur Psychiatrie, Abt.
Neuroimmunologie
Am Klopferspitz 18a
DE 8033 Martinsried
Phone: +49 8985 781
Fax: +49 8985 783/790

Prof. Carlo POZZILLI
Dipartimento di Scienze
Neurologiche, III Clinica La
Sapienza
Viale dell'Università
IT 00185 Rome
Phone: +39 6 4991 4716
Fax: +39 6 4457 705

Prof. Bruno TAVOLATO
Università di Padova,
Ospedale Geriatrico
Via Vendramini 7
IT Padua
Phone: +39 498 216 347
Fax: +39 498 216 358

Dr. Tomas OLSSON
Dept. of Neurology,
Huddinge Hospital
SE 14186 Huddinge
Phone: +46 8776 1000
Fax: +46 8774 4822

Dr. Margreet JONKER
TNO Rijswijk,
Radiobiol. and Immunolog.
Lange Kleiweg 151,
P.O. Box 5815
NL 2280 HV Rijswijk
Phone: +31 15 842 842
Fax: +31 15 843 999

Dr. Hans VAN NOORT
TNO Medical Biological
Laboratory
Lange Kleiweg 151,
P.O. Box 5815
NL 2280 HV Rijswijk
Phone: +31 15 842 3106
Fax: +31 15 843 989

Prof. Alastair COMPSTON
Dept. of Medicine University
of Cambridge, Clin. School
Addenbrooke's Hospital
Hills Road
UK Cambridge CN 2 200
Phone: +44 223 245 151
Fax: +44 223 216 926

A MULTICENTRE PROSPECTIVE STUDY OF THE EVERYDAY LIFE RISKS IN PATIENTS WITH EPILEPSY

Key words
Epilepsy, risk, cohort study, morbidity, accident, insurance.

Objectives
1 To deliver proper information to physicians, patients and their caretakers, and employers about the extent of the everyday life risks in patients with epilepsy as compared to a normal, non-epileptic population;
2 To provide reliable data on the everyday life risks which could be utilized by the insurance companies as a reference to assess the terms of insurability of patients with epilepsy.

The following risks will be specifically assessed in patients with epilepsy and controls: (i) risk of morbidity; (ii) risk of accident.
Secondary goals are the assessment of the risk by patient and disease characteristics, in general and within each European country.

Brief description
A review of the literature and the results of a recent workshop on *Epilepsy, Risks and Insurance*, documented a substantial lack of information about the everyday life risks among people with epilepsy.

The present investigation is a cohort study which intends to provide reliable estimates of the everyday life risks (morbidity, accidents, and related events) attributable to epilepsy. The main aim of the study is to estimate the relative risks of morbidity (ie, any event requiring medical attention which is not an accident) and the relative risk of accidents (i.e. any untoward event, which is not a disease, leading to physical damage requiring medical attention or resulting in financial obligation) by comparing patients with epilepsy to a referent non-epileptic population. Secondary targets are assessment of the risks by disease categories, treatment modalities, and country of origin.

In each European country involved in the study the target epileptic population will be selected by reviewing the medical records of patients with epilepsy (i.e. one or more unprovoked epileptic seizures under treatment) firstly diagnosed in that center in the previous five years.

For each eligible patient two matched controls will be randomly selected - from individuals with no epileptic seizures (one of whom is a relative) and matched for sex, age ($\pm$ 5 years), race, current occupation or social class. After informed consent, patients with epilepsy and controls are given monthly diaries to record the number of medical contacts, accidents (type and circumstances), illnesses, hospital admissions, and days off-work. Follow-up visits will be set at 3-month intervals up to 24 months.

Combining these end-points, the relative risks of morbidity and accident will be calculated for the entire study population and for specific subpopulations (according to the patient and disease characteristics and to the country of origin). To pursue the objectives of the study, a minimum sample size of 733 patients with epilepsy and 733 controls is required.

Project leader:
Dr. Ettore BEGHI
Laboratory of Clinical
Pharmacology
Istituto di Ricerche
Farmacologiche
'Mario Negri'
Via Eritrea 62
IT 20157 Milano
Phone: +39 2 39 01 41
Fax: +39 2 33 20 02 31
Contract number: CT931428

Participants:
Dr. Cinzia CAVESTRO
Istituto di Richerche
Farmacologiche Mario Negri
Via Eritrea 62
IT 20157 Milano

Dr. CORNAGGIA,
dr. DAVID &
dr. GIANATTI
Ospedale Maggiore
Via F. Sforza 35
IT 20122 Milano

Dr. Luisa ANTONINI &
dr. Maria Pia PASOLINI
Servizio di Neurofisiopato-
logia, Centro Regionale
Epilessia, Ospedale Civili
P.zza Ospedali Civili
IT 25100 Brescia

Prof. Giuliano AVANZINI &
Sig. ARIENTI
Servizio di Neurofisipato-
logia, Istituto Neurologico
C. Besta
Via Celoria 11
IT 20133 Milano

Dr. BEGHI, dr. BOGLIUN
& dr. FIORDELLI
Divisione di Neurologia,
Ospedale S. Gerardo
IT Monza, Milano

Dr. DEFANTI, dr. BOATI
& dr. PINTO
Neurologia I, Centro
Regionale Epilessia,
Ospedali Riuniti
Largo Barozzi 1
IT 24100 Bergamo

Dr. Francesco PISANI &
dr. Rosa TRIO
Clinica Neurologica I,
Università di Messina
IT 98100 Messina

Prof. Amalia TARTARA &
dr. Raffaele MANNI
Clinica Neurologica,
Centro Regionale Epilessia,
Fondazione C. Mondino
Via Palestro 3
IT 27100 Pavia

Dr. ZACCARA,
dr. COSOTTINI &
dr. BORGORESE
Servizio di Neurofisiopato-
logia, Ospedale San Salvi
Via San Salvi 12
IT 50136 Firenze

Dr. Pierluigi ZAGNONI &
dr. Silvia GIUBERGIA
Ospedale S. Croce
Via Michele Coppino 26
IT 12100 Cuneo

Dr. ZOLO, dr. BIANCHI &
dr. SEVERI
Neurologia, Osp. S. Donato
Via Pietro Nenni
IT 52100 Arezzo

Luigi Maria SPECCHIO
Clinica Neurologica II,
Ospedale Regionale
Policlinico
Via G. Cesare
IT 70124 Bari

Dr. Michelle ZARRELLI
Divisione di Neurologia,
Ospedale Casa Sollievo delle
Sofferenza
IT 71013 S. Giovanni
Rotondo (FG)

Dr. Marc BEAUSSART
Associotion Francaise pour
l'Epilepsie, G.R.I.N.E.
11 Avenue de President
Kennedy
FR 59800 Lille

Dr. Stephen W. BROWN &
dr. Helen COYLE
The David Lewis Centre
for Epilepsy
Mill Lane, Nr. Alderly Edge
UK Cheshire CK9 7UD

Dra. C. DIAZ-OBREGON
c/Berlin 5-4
ES 28020 Madrid

Dr. Luis F.V. OLLER
Liga Espanola contra
la Epilepsia
Escuelas Plass 89, planta
ES 08017 Barcelona

Dr. Birthe PEDERSEN
Neuromedicinsk afdeling,
Aalborg Sygehus Syd
P.O. Box 365
DK 9100 Aalborg

Dr. Arthur E.H. SONNEN
Epilepsiecentrum,
Dr. Hans Berger Kliniek
P.O. Box 90108
NL 4800 RA Breda

Dr. Peter WOLF &
mr. Rupprecht THORBECKE
Epilepsiezentrum Bethel
Maraweg 21
DE 4800 Bielefeld 13

Prof. Aleen W. HAUSER
Gertr. H. Sergievsky Centre,
Columbia University
603 West 168th street
US New York N.Y. 10032

Dr. Joop N. LOEBER
International Bureau
for Epilepsy
P.O. Box 21
NL 2100 AA Heemstede

THE EUROPEAN MULTICENTRE STUDY
ON ATTEMPTED SUICIDE

Key words
Attempted suicide, risk groups, suicidal behaviour, prediction, assessment, comparison, evaluation.

Objectives
1 To collect, coordinate and analyze dat from identical follow-up studies carried out in 14 research centres representing 11 European countries, with the ultimate purpose to work out guidelines and recommendations as to prevention and intervention in the field of suicidal behaviour.
2 Data from each participating centre will be transferred to the centre in Odense, which will be responsible for pooling, processing and analyzing the data.

Brief description
The proposed project is an European multicentre study, involving 14 research centres from 11 European countries. At these centres follow-up studies of parasuicide population, as a special high risk group for further suicidal behaviour, are being carried out with a view to identifying social and personal characteristics predictive of future suicidal behaviour.

Five intermediate targets have been recognized:
a identification of personal and social characteristics predictive of future suicidal behaviour;
b evaluation of existing scales which are designed to predict suicidal behaviour;
c estimation of the social, psychological and economic burden of repeated suicide to the individual, his/her community, and the society as a whole;
d assessment of the utilization of health and social services by the suicide attempters and the effectiveness of the different treatment offered; and
e comparison of differences in personal characteristics (clinical, sociodemographic, psychological, etc.) among suicide attempters from different cultural and economic settings.

Project leader:
Professor Unni BILLE-BRAHE
Unit for Suicidological Research,
Odense Universitet
Tietgens Allé 108
DK 5230 Odense
Phone: +45 66 11 33 33
Fax: +45 65 90 81 74
Contract number: CT931090

Participants:

Dr. Konrad MICHEL
Universitätspoliklinik
Mürtenstrasse 21
CH 3010 Bern
Phone: +41 31 64 88 11
Fax: +41 31 25 13 31

Dr. Paolo Crepet &
dr. L. LO RUSSO
Via della Gensola 38
IT 00153 Roma
Phone: +39 65 80 66 23
Fax: +39 65 83 67 36

Dr. Imanol QUEREJETA
University of the Basque
Country, Hospital de
Guipuzcoa
ES 20014 San Sebastian
Phone: +34 43 45 40 00
Fax: +34 43 46 97 00

Prof. Juoko LONNQVIST
National Public
Health Institute
Mannerheimintie
FI 00300 Helsinki
Phone: +358 47 13 990
Fax: +358 47 15 471

Dr. Christian HARING
Dept. of Psychiatry,
Medical School,
University of Innbruck
AT 6020 Innsbruck

Dr. Ad J.M.F. KERKHOF
Dept. of Clinical & Health
Psychology, Univ. of Leiden
Postbus 9555
NL 2360 RB Leiden
Phone: +31 71 27 37 45
Fax: +31 71 27 36 19

Dr. Diego DE LEO
Instituto di Clinica
Psichiatrica,
Univ. Degli Studi di Padova
Via Vendramini 7
IT 35137 Padova
Phone: +39 49 821 62 62
Fax: +39 49 821 62 64

Dr. Danuta WASSERMAN
Suizidpräventivt Center,
Karolinska Institutet
Tomtebodavägen 11 F
P.O. Box 230
SE 171 77 Stockholm
Phone: +46 872 80 26
Fax: +46 830 64 39

Beata TEMESVARY
Dept. of Neurology and
Psychology,
University of Szeged
Postbox 397
HU 6701 Szeged
Phone: +36 62 10 011
Fax: +36 62 21 752

Prof. Tore BJERKE
Norsk Institut for
Naturforskning
Faberg Gate 106
NO 2600 Lillehammer
Phone: +47 62 60 611
Fax: +47 62 60 007

Dr. SALANDER-RENBERG
& prof. L. JACONSSON
Dept. of Psychiatry,
University of Umea
SE 901 85 Umea
Phone: +46 90 10 10 00
Fax: +46 90 10 22 02

Dr. Armin SCHMIDTKE
Universitäts-Nervenklinik
Füchsleinstrasse 15
DE 8700 Würzburg
Phone: +49 931 203 248
Fax: +49 931 203 365

Dr. H.J. MOLLER
Dept. of Psychiatry,
University of Bonn
Sigmund Freud Strasse 25
DE 5300 Bonn

VIRUS MENINGITIS AND ENCEPHALITIS

Key words
Virus, meningitis, encephalitis, diagnosis, treatment, epidemiology, quality control.

Objectives
The ultimate objective of the Concerted Action is to contribute to a reduction in the mortality and morbidity associated with virus infection of the central nervous system.

Brief description
The purpose of the proposed CA is to develop agreed methods and protocols to achieve rapid and specific diagnosis of viral meningitis and encephalitis. The establishment of such protocols will allow:
1 Improved patient management together with timely and rational use of specific antiviral therapy. The resulting decrease in mortality and morbidity and the requirement for long term institutionalised care of neurologically damaged patients will impact on costs of Health Care.
2 The establishment of defined diagnostic parameters which will result from the CA will allow meaningful studies and trials to evaluate new antiviral drugs.
3 The proposed management structure of the CA together with agreed standards for use of the new diagnostic procedures will, for the first time, allow the collection and collation of epidemiological data related to:
i The true incidence of viral meningitis and encephalitis.
ii The incidence of viral involvement in unusual presentations of CNS disease.

This will be the first time that such pan European data will have been assembled and without doubt it will have significance for future planning of diagnostic, treatment, and immunisation strategies.

Project leader:
Dr. G.M. CLEATOR
Division of Virology,
Dept. of Pathological Sciences,
The Medical School,
University of Manchester
Oxford Road
UK Manchester M13 9PT
Phone: +44 61 274 42 00
Fax: +44 61 275 54 31
Contract number: CT931716

Participants:
Dr. Peter MUIR
Dept. of Virology,
United Medical and Dental
Schools of Guys &
St. Thomas' Hospitals
Lambeth Palace Road
UK London SE1 7EH
Phone: +44 71 928 0730
Fax: +44 71 928 0730

Prof. Volker TER MEULEN
Institut fur Virologie und
Immunobiologie,
Universitat Wurzburg
Verbacherstrasse 7
DE 8700 Wurzburg
Fax: +49 931 201 3934

Dr. PUCHHAMMER-
STOCKL
Institute of Virology,
University of Vienna
Kinderspitalgasse 15
AT 1095 Vienna
Phone: +43 1 222 40490
Fax: +43 1 222 432161

Dr. Clive TAYLOR &
dr. Malik PIERIS
Dept. of Virology,
The Royal Victoria Infirmary
Queen Victoria Road
UK Newcastle-upon-Tyne
NE1 4LP
Phone: +44 91 232 5131
Fax: +44 91 201 0155

Dr FABER VESTERGAARD
Dept. of Virology,
Statens Seruminstitut
5 Artillerivej
DK 2300 Copenhagen S
Phone: +45 326 83453
Fax: +45 326 83148

Dr. Jose M. ECHEVARRIA
Centro Nacionale
Microbiologia,
Inst. de Salud Carlos III
Cart, Majadahonda-Pozuelo
ES 28220 Majadahonda
(Madrid)

Dr. Marianne FORSGREN
Central Microbiological
Laboratory,
Stockholm County Council
PO Box 70470
SE 10726 Stockholm

Prof. Giuseppe GERNA &
dr. Fausto BALDANTI
Institute of Infectious Disease, University of Pavia
6 Taranelli
IT Pavia 27100

Dr. Anton M. VAN LOON
Laboratory of Virology,
National Institute of Public
Health and Environmental
Protection
A. van Leeuwenhoeklaan 9,
P.O. Box 1
NL 3729 BA Bilthoven

Dr. Paul KLAPPER
North Manchester Virus
Laboratory, Booth Hall
Childrens Hospital
Charlestown Road
UK Manchester M9 2AA

Dr. M. KOSKINIEMI
Dept. of Virology,
University of Helsinki
Haartmaninkatu 3
FI 00290 Helsinki

Prof. Pierre LEBON
Service de Bacteriologie,
Virologie et Hygiene,
Lab. de Recherche sur les
Infections Virales,
Hospital St Vincent de Paul
82 Avenue Denfert-Rocherau
FR 75674 Paris cedex 14

Prof. Christian J.M. SINDIC
& dr Philippe MONTEYNE
Laboratoire de Neurochimie,
Universite Catholoque de
Louvaine
Avenue Mounier 5359
BE 1200 Brussels

Dr. Maria CIARDI
Instituto di Malattie Infettive,
Universita La Sapienza
Viale Regina Elen 3307
IT 00161 Rome

Dr. Paola CINQUE
Centro Ricera e Cura
Patologie HIV-Correlate,
Division di Malattie Infettive,
Ospedale San Raffaele
Via Stamina d'Ancona
IT 20127 Milan

Prof. Monica GRANDIEN &
dr. Annika LINDE
National Bacteriological
Laboratory
SE 105 21 Stockholm
Phone: +46 8 7351000
Fax: +46 8 7303248

Prof. Tapani HOVI
Enterovirus Laboratory,
National Public Health
Institute
Mannerheiminte 166
FI 00300 Helsinki

ESTABLISHMENT AND USE OF EDMUS AS A DATABASE SYSTEM FOR MULTIPLE SCLEROSIS RESEARCH IN EUROPE

Key words
Multiple Sclerose, database, epidemiology, predictive factors, clinical trials, genetic, usceptibility.

Brief description
Establishment of *EDMUS: a European database for multiple sclerosis* has been one of the main themes of the 1990-1992 European Concerted Action for Basic Research and Treatment in Multiple Sclerosis. The concertation has taken place since January 1989 through an EDMUS Steering Committee composed of members from the various countries of the EEC. The conceptual and technical design of the EDMUS system has been published (J Neurol Neurosurg Psychiat 1992;55:671-676).

The system is user-friendly, fast and easy to complete and runs on Apple and IBM-PC personal microcomputers. It is agreed by the French Commission Nationale 'Informatique et Libertés' (CNIL). It has been made available since October 1992. On August 31, 1993, it was implemented in 57 European and 1 US centres.

Several collaborative international multi-centre actions are organized:
- EVALUED (EVALUation of the EDmus system) is a methodological project aimed at validating the impairment scale and the whole system within and among European centres. By the end of the experiment, sharing of results and analysis of potential sources of inter-observer inconsistencies/disagreements in the use of the EDMUS form will result in a finalization of thew whole system.
- PRIMS (PRegnancy In Multiple Sclerosis) is an epidemiological project aimed to ascertain in a prospective manner the effect of pregnancy and the post partum period on the course of multiple sclerosis (MS).
- PRESTIMUS (PRedictive ESTImates in Multiple Sclerosis) is aimed to identify clinical and paraclinical parameters which may reliably and early predict disease course and severity.
- ERAZMUS (EaRly AZathioprine in Multiple Sclerosis) is a therapeutic trial aimed at assessing the possible benefit of treating with azathioprine in the early phase of the disease.
- GAMES (Genetic Analysis of Multiple sclerosis in the European Society) is aimed at identifying the number and location of genes conferring susceptibility to MS with the differences, if any, between various European populations.

There are other areas, including genetic analysis of twins and multiplex families and epidemiological analysis and various ethnical and geographical settings.

The Lyon Clinique de Neurologie as coordinating centre and the EDMUS Steering Committee as advisory board are interacting for the improvement, development and diffusion of the system, the organization of collaborative actions, the setting of an EDMUS central database and the connection with biological material banking facilities. It is hoped that the European Economic Community will contribute to setting up and maintaining this central coordinating facility which could be pivotal in all future research in MS throughout Europe.

Project leader:
Prof. C. CONFAVREUX
Service de Neurologie,
Hopital de L'Antiquaille
1 rue de L'Antiquaille
FR 69321 Lyon
Phone: +33 72 38 51 82
Fax: +33 72 38 51 43
Contract number: CT931529

Participants:
Mr. Albert BIRON
Service de Neurologie,
Hôpital de l'Antiquaille
1 rue de l'Antiquaille
FR 69001 Lyon
Phone: +33 72 38 51 82
Fax: +33 72 38 51 43

Prof. Patrice ADELEINE
Laboratoire de Statistiques
Médicales
162 avenue Lacassagne
FR 69424 Lyon Cedex 03
Phone: +33 72 11 51 37/36
Fax: +33 72 11 51 41

Dr M.P. AMATO,
dr L. MASASCESI &
prof L. AMADUCCI
Clinica Neurologica I,
Ospedale di Careggi
Viale Morgagni 85
IT 50134 Firenze
Phone: +39 55
416969/432224
Fax: +39 55 413603

Prof. Jean-Pierre BOISSEL
Unité de Pharmacologie
Clinique
162 avanue Lacassagne
FR 69242 Lyon Cedex 03
Phone: +33 72 11 52 32
Fax: +33 78 53 10 30

Prof. Bruno BROCHET &
Prof. ORGOGOZO
Département de Neurologie,
Groupe Hospitalier Pellegrin
Tripode, Centre Hospitalier
et Universitaire de Bordeaux
Palce Amélie Raba-Léon
FR 33076 Bordeaux Cedex
Phone: +33 56 79 55 20
Fax: +33 56 79 55 93

Prof. Giancarlo COMI
Associazione Amici Del
Centro Sclerosi Multipla,
HSR, Istituto Scientifico
H. San Raffaele
Via Olgettina 60
IT 20132 Milan
Phone: +39 2 26 43 23 39
Fax: +39 2 26 43 23 35

Prof. Alastair COMPSTON
Neurology Department,
Addenbrooke's Hospital
Hills Road
UK Cambridge CB2 2QQ
Phone: +44 223 217091
Fax: +44 223 216926

Prof. Gilles EDAN
Service de Neurologie,
Hôpital de Pontchaillou
Rue Henri le Guilloux
FR 35033 Rennes Cedex
Phone: +33 99 284293
Fax: +33 99 284132

Dr. Oscar FERNANDEZ
Servicio de Neurologia,
Hospital Regional de Malaga
Carlos Haya
Avda Carlos Haya s/n
ES 29010 Malaga
Phone: +34 9 52 39 04 00
Fax: +34 9 52 28 83 49

Dr. Richard GONSETTE
Centre National de la
Sclérose en Plaques
Vanheylenstraat 16
BE 1820 Melsbroek
Phone: +32 27 51 80 30
Fax: +32 27 51 52 45

Prof. Hans-Peter HARTUNG
Neurologischer Klinik
Josef-Schneider-Strasse 1
DE 8700 Wurzburg
Phone: +49 931 201 2502
Fax: +49 931 201 2697

Prof. Otto HOMMES
Dept. of Neurology,
Radboud University Hospital
P.O. Box 9101
NL 6500 HB Nijmegen

Dr. Michael HUTCHINSON
Dept. of Neurology,
St. Vincent's Hospital
Elm Park
IE Dublin 4

Dr. Ludwig KAPPOS
Neurologische
Universitätspoliklinik,
Kantonsspital Basel
Petergraben 4
CH 4031 Basel

Dr. KOCH-HENRIKSEN
Dept. of Neurology,
Aalborg Hospital
DK 9000 Aalborg

Prof. Paolo LIVREA
Clinica Neurologica del
l'Universita
Piazza G. Cesare
IT 70124 Bari

Prof. Antonio MAGALHAES
Servico de Neurologica,
Hospital Universitario
de Santa Maria
Av. Egas Moniz
PT 1600 Lisboa

Prof. Chris POLMAN
Dept. of Neurology, University Hospital Free University
De Boelelaan 1117,
P.O. Box 7057
NL 1007 MB Amsterdam

Dr. A. THOMPSON,
dr. D. MILLER &
prof. W. MCDONALD
Institute of Neurology,
The National Hospital
Queen Square
UK London WC1N 3BG

DEPRESSION OF OLDER AGE: DETECTION, TREATMENT AND GEOGRAPHICAL VARIATION

A Collaborative Study among Research Centres in the European Community

Key words
Depression, elderly, epidemiology, community.

Objectives
A To quantify the variation in prevalence of depression in people aged 65 and over living in Europe.
B To quantify the profile of depressive symptoms in each centre studied, and to compare these profiles across centres.
C To use other social and economic variables collected at an individual level to explain differences found in (A, B).
D To establish the equivalence of other social and economic variables available at an ecological level, to relate them to differences found in (A, B), and to generate hypotheses to be tested in later individual studies.
E To measure the rate of treatment of persons identified as depressed, to quantify the differences between centres, and to relate these to differences in social conditions and health service practices.
F To measure the social networks of study respondents, to relate these to levels of depression, and to compare them with networks of other people.
G To quantify the life events and social stresses suffered by respondents, and to relate those to differences found in (A, B, F).

Brief description
It is estimated that approximately eight million European community citizens aged 65 and over suffer from potentially treatable forms of depression yet only 4% of community depressions receive specific treatment. This concerted action aims to compare the prevalence of old age depression in the European Community, identify reasons for geographical variation and to investigate the causes of the failure to treat.
Several European groups are already using standardised methods of case-finding and diagnosis developed by the coordinating centre for studies in the Comparative Epidemiology of the mental disorders of older age. It is proposed to capitalise on these studies. Nine participating centres are already undertaking or planning locally funded population based studies:
- Liverpool (coordinating centre) and London (UK), Porto (Portugal), Rotterdam, Amsterdam and Maastricht (Netherlands), Zaragoza (Spain), Dublin (Ireland), Verona (Italy).

The aims of the Concerted Action will be pursued through the extension of common measures, exchange of study data between centres and central analysis.

Project leader:
Professor J.R.M. COPELAND
The University of Liverpool,
Department of Psychiatry, Royal Liverpool University Hospital
P.O. Box 147
UK Liverpool L69 3BX
Phone: +44 51 706 41 41
Fax: +44 51 709 37 65
Contract number: CT931781

Participants:
Prof. DE VRIES
IPSER
P.O. Box 214
NL 6200 AE Maastricht
Phone: +31 43 299 774
Fax: +31 43 299 708

Prof. Arnaldo DROUX
Unidade de Saude Mental de
Gondomar do Hospital do
Conde de Ferreira
Av. General Humberto
Delgado 1275
PT 4420 Gondomar
Phone: +351 2 6183589
Fax: +351 2 6183589

Prof. A. HOFMAN
Dept. of Epidemiology,
Erasmus University
Postbus 1738
NL 3000 DR Rotterdam
Phone: +31 10 408 7365
Fax: +31 10 408 7494

Dr. Chris HOOIJER
Vakgroep Psychiatrie VU,
Secr. AMSTREL Project
Valeriusplein 9
NL 1075 BG Amsterdam
Phone: +31 20 673 3535
Fax: +31 20 662 3677

Prof. A. LOBO
Hospital Clinico Universitario
Avda San Juan Bosco
ES 50009 Zaragoza
Phone: +34 76 55 97 95
Fax: +34 76 35 79 63

Prof. A. MANN
Institute of Psychiatry
Decrespigny Park,
Denmark Hill
UK London SE5 8AF
Phone: +44 71 703 5411
Fax: +44 71 277 0283

Dr. Cesare TURRINA
Instituto di Psichiatria,
Universita di Brescia
3o CPS via Manara 7
IT 25126 Brescia
Phone: +39 30 2410 774
Fax: +39 30 2411 246

Dr. M. WRIGLEY
Consultant Psychiatrist in the
Psychiatry of Old Age,
James C. Memorial Hosp.
Blanchardstown
IE Dublin 15
Phone: +353 1821 3844
Fax: +353 1820 3564

EUROPEAN BRAIN BANK NETWORK (EBBN) FOR NEUROBIOLOGICAL STUDIES IN NEUROLOGICAL AND PSYCHIATRIC DISORDERS

Key words
Brain bank, neurological disorders, neuropathology, molecular biology, Alzheimer's disease, Parkinson's disease, Multiple Sclerosis, Amgotrophic Lateral Sclerosis, sudden infant death syndrome, schizophrenia, brain tumours.

Brief description
The European Brain Bank Network (EBBN) consists of groups operating in several European countries and can make optimal use of the existing and well-functioning brain bank facilities providing tissues for various other Concerted Actions.

Relevance to the work-programme:
A To establish an efficient network of European Brain Banks as a bridge between scientists, disorders according to Area II.4 of the summary work programme.
B To collaborate with various Concerted actions providing brain tissue from patients with neurological and psychiatric disorders as well as with control non-demented patiens.

Objectives
1 Standardization and registration of data.
2 Standardization of protocols (clinical diagnosis, criteria for neuropathological diagnosis, protocols for collecting material).
3 Multi-center European concordance studies to study a variety of diseases including: AD, Parkinson's disease (PD), Hungtinton disease, Diffuse Lewvy body disease, multiple sclerosis (MS), AIDS, amyotrophic lateral sclerosis (ALS) and several other conditions.
4 Multi-center studies on risk factors in various diseases to investigate molecular, genetic and environmental factors wich may play a role in the various diseases.
5 To meet scientists of different countries in plenary meetings or limited workshops to establish strategies directed to improving knowledge of neurological and psychiatric disorders.

The scientific output will no doubt exceed the total output and results of the local brain banks and will make it possible to have a large amount of material for research (also for other CA), many patients data for reliable statistical analysis.
In addition, the CA matches the objetives by allowing the necessary infrastructure which will connect various Europeans Brain Banks.

Project leader:
Dr. Felix F. CRUZ-SÁNCHEZ
Banco de Tejidos Neurológicos, Universidad de Barcelona, Hospital Clínico y provincial
Villarroel 170
ES 08036 Barcelona
Phone: +34 34 54 70 00 ext 2212
Fax: +34 34 51 52 72
Contract number: CT931359

Participants:

Dr. R. RAVID
The Netherlands Brain Bank
Meibergdreef 33
NL 1103 Amsterdam ZO

Prof. W. POEWE
Depart. of Neurology,
Universitätsklinikum
Rudolph Virchows
Augestenburger Platz 1
DE 13353 Berlin

Dr. A.J. LEES &
dr. S.E. DANIEL
Parkinson's disease
Society Brain Bank
1 Wakefield Street
UK London WC1N 1PJ

Dr. M.L. ROSSI
Scientifica Fondazione Istituto
Neurologico Casimiro
Mondino, Universita di Pavia
Via Palestro 3
IT 27100 Pavia

Prof. N. KNOPP
Faculté de Medicine
Alexis Carrel
Rue Guillaume Paradin
FR 69006 Lyon Cedex 8

Porf. D. SWAAB
Netherlands Institute
for Brain Research
Meibergdreef 33
NL 1105 Amsterdam ZO

Dr. E. TOLOSA
Servico de Neurologia, Hospital Clínico y Provincial
c/Villarroel 170
ES 08036 Barcelona

Prof. CERVOS-NAVARRO
Institute für Neuropathologie,
Freie Universität Berlin
Hindenburgdam 30
DE 12200 Berlin

Prof. J.J. HAUW
Laboratoire de
Neuropathologie Raymond
Escourolle,
Hôpital de la Salpêtrière
47 Bd de l'Hôpital
FR 75651 Paris Cedex 13

Dr. N. MAHY
Facultad de Medicina,
Unidad de Bioquímica
Av. Diagonal 643
ES 08028 Barcelona

Prof. D. GRAHAM
Dept. of Neuropathology,
Institute of Neurological
Sciences,
Southern General Hospital
1345 Govan Road
UK Glasgow G51 4TF

Dr. T. SKLAVIADIS
Dept. of Pharmaceutical
Sciences,
Laboratory of Pharmacology
University Campus Aristotle
GR 54006 Tsaloniki (TK)

Dr. F. JAVOY-AGID
Laboratoire de Medicine
Experimentale,
Hôpital de la Salpêtrière
47 Bd de l'Hôpital
FR 75651 Paris

Prof. P. LANTOS &
dr. N. CAIRNS
Dept. of Neuropathology,
Institute of Psychiatry
De Crespigny Park
UK London SE5 8AF

Dr. M.L. CUZNER
Multiple Sclerosis Laboratory, Institute of Neurology
1 Wakefield Street
UK London WC1N 1PJ

Prof. P. RIEDERER &
dr. W. GSELL
Klinische Neurochemie,
Psychiatrische Klinik
und Poliklinik,
Universitätsnervenklinik
Füchsleinstrasse 15
DE 97080 Würzburg

Dr. G.P. REYNOLDS
University of Sheffield
Western Bank
UK Sheffield S10 2TN
Phone: +44 742 824 662
Fax: +44 742 765 413

Dr. J. LUCENA
Instituto Anatómico Forense
c/Villarroel 170
ES 08036 Barcelona
Phone: +34 3 453 4271
Fax: +34 3 453 4248

Dr. ESCALONA-ZAPATA
Dept. of Pathology,
Hospital Gregorio Maranon
Dr. Esquerdo 46
ES 28007 Madrid
Phone: +34 1 568 8162
Fax: +34 1 586 8018

Prof. H. BUDKA
Klinisches Institut für
Neurologie der Universität
Wien, Neues Allgmeines
Krankenhaus 04J
Währinger Gürtel 18-20
AT 1090 Wien
Phone: +43 1 40400 5501
Fax: +43 1 40400 5511

Prof. K. JELLINGER
L. Boltzmann Institute of
Clinical Neurobiology,
Lainz Hospital
AT 1130 Wien
Phone: +43 1 22280 110
Fax: +43 1 22280 45401

Prof. B. WINBLAD &
dr. N. BOGDANOVIC
Dept. of Geriatric Medicine,
Huddinge University Hospital
SE 14186 Huddinge
Phone: +46 8746 3613
Fax: +46 8711 1751

Prof. W. JANISCH
Institut für Pathologische
Anatomie
Charite Universität 20/21
DE 10117 Berlin
Phone: +49 30 798 2339

CYTOKINES IN THE BRAIN

Key words
Neurosciences, Cytokines, Neuroimmunomodulation, Neural degeneration, Sickness, Fever, Neural plasticity.

Objectives
1 Establish a centralized facility to produce rat recombinant proinflammatory cytokines and antibodies to these cytokines and distribute these standardized reagents to participating European laboratories.
2 Intensify contact and coordination within the European Community by harmonising experimental protocols between laboratories for investigating different neuronal endpoints of cytokine action.
3 Organize workshops enabling exchange of information and expertise between neurobiologists and immunologists.
4 Improve training of European scientists in methodological and technical aspects of research into the neurobiology of cytokines.

Brief description
Cytokines have been identified as primary mediators of cellular communication within the immune system but it is now evident that they exert potent physiological actions in the brain and function as important communication signals between the immune system and the brain. Neurotropic activities of cytokines include fever, activation of the pituitary-adrenal axis and induction of sickness behaviour. These responses play an important role in the host response to infection and inflammation. Moreover, cytokines and their receptors are expressed in the brain and are directly involved in neural degeneration (e.g., brain ischemia and trauma) and neuropathology (e.g., Alzheimer's disease and neurological symptoms of infection by neurotropic viruses, including HIV).

Understanding the mechanisms of the neural effects of cytokines is a multidisciplinary task which is critically dependent on: (1) the availability of species specific recombinant cytokines and appropriate immunopharmacological tools and, (2) an effective cooperation between immunologists and neurobiologists.

In terms of project methodology, the project has two core elements: (1) the establishment of a centralized facility to produce high quality reagents; and (2) a network of leading immunologic and neurobiologic laboratories to provide support services for the research.

Establishment and functioning of the centralized facility
The centralized facility is responsible for (a) the production of recombinant rat interleukin-1 α, interleukin-1 ß, interleukin-6 and tumour necrosis factor α; (b) the production of polyclonal and affinity-purified antibodies to these recombinant preparation; (c) the quality control and distribution of these reagents to the participating laboratories.

Coordination and cooperation between the participating laboratories is carried out by means of the commonly used modalities (workshops, expert meetings, site and contact visits, exchange of personnel, exchange of data).

The time schedule of 'Cytokines in the brain' comprises 36 months of research.

Project leader:
Dr. Robert DANTZER
INSERM U. 176
rue Camille Saint-Saens
FR 33077 Bordeaux Cedex
Phone: +33 56 00 02 50
Fax: +33 56 98 90 29
Contract number: CT931450

Participants:
Dr. A.M. GUERIN
U282 INSERM, Hormones et
différenciation cellulaire,
Hôpital Henry Mondor
FR 94010 Créteil

Dr. Marcienne TARDY
U282 INSERM, Hormones et
différenciation cellulaire,
Hôpital Henry Mondor
FR 94010 Créteil

Dr. Flora ZAVALA
U25 INSERM, Maladies
auto-immunes,
Hôpital Necker
161 Rue de Sèvres
FR 75743 Paris Cedex 15

Dr. J. MARIANI
Institut des Neurosciences
CNRS URA 1488,
Laboratoire de Neurobiologie
du Développement Université
Pierre et Marie Curie
9 Quai Saint-Bernard
FR 75005 Paris

Dr. B. CALVINO
INSERM CJF 91.02,
Faculté de Médecine
8 Rue de Général Sarrail
FR 94010 Créteil Cedex

Dr. P. GIRAUDON
CJF 90-10 INSERM,
Laboratoire d'Anatomie
pathologique, Faculté de
Médecine Alexis Carrel
Rue Guillaume Paradin
FR 69372 Lyon Cedex 08
Phone: +33 78 01 00 95
Fax: +33 78 77 86 12

Dr. E. WOLLMAN
U283 INSERM,
Rue du Faubourg St. Jacques
FR 75674 Paris Cedex

Dr. F. HAOUR
28 Rue du Docteur Roux
FR 75724 Paris Cedex 15

Prof. Eugen ZEISBERGER
Physiologisches Institut
Aulweg 129
DE 35392 Giessen

Prof. H.E. BESEDOVSKY
Fachbereich Humanmedizin,
Institut für Normal und
Pathologische Physiologie,
Philipps-Universität Marburg
Deutschhausstrasse 2
DE 35037 Marburg

Prof. Gennaro SCHETTINI
Facolta di Medicina
Farmacologia cellulare et
moleculare, Universita degli
Studi di Napoli Frederico II
Via Sergio Pansini 5
IT 80131 Napoli

Dr. C. GUAZA
Instituto Cajal CSIC
Avda Dr. Arce 34
ES 28002 Madrid

Prof. F. TILDERS
Dept. of Pharmacology,
School of Medicine, Free
University of Amsterdam
Van der Boechorstraat 7
NL 1081 BT Amsterdam

Dr. A. HERMUS
Vakgroep Endocriene
Ziekten, Faculteit det
Medische Wetenschappen,
Katholieke Universiteit
Nijmegen
Postbus 9101
NL 6500 HB Nijmegen

Dr. C.D. DIJKSTRA
Vrije Universiteit
Van der Boechorstraat 7
NL 1081 BT Amsterdam

Prof. E. RON DE KLOET
University of Leiden
P.O. Box 9503
2300 AA Leiden

Dr. N.J. ROTHWELL
University of Manchester,
Stopford Building
Oxford Road
UK Manchester M13 9PT

Dr. S.P. BUTCHER
Fujisawa Institute
of Neuroscience,
The University of Edinburgh
1 George Square
UK Edinburgh EH8 9JZ

Dr. V. Hugh PERRY
University of Oxford
Mansfield Road
UK Oxford OX1 3QT

Dr. M. WOODROOFE
1 Wakefield Straat
UK London WC1N 1PJ

Porf. I.V. ALLEN
Institute of Pathology, The
Queen's University of Belfast
Grosvenor Road
UK Belfast BT12 6 BL

Dr. s. LIGHTMAN
Dept. of Medicine,
University of Bristol,
Bristol Royal Infirmary
Marlborough Straat
UK Bristol BS2 8HW
Phone: +44 272 282 871
Fax: +44 272 282 212

Dr. A.B. GROSSMAN
Dept. of Endocrinology,
St. Bartholomew's Hospital
UK London EC1A 7BE
Phone: +44 71 601 8343
Fax: +44 71 601 8505

Dr. S. POOLE
NIBSC, Division of
Endocrinology
Blanche Lane, South Mimms,
Potters Bar
UK Hertfordshire EN6 3QG
Phone: +44 707 654 753
Fax: +44 707 646 730

MOLECULAR STUDIES OF PLASMA MEMBRANE
AND VESICULAR NEURONAL TRANSPORTERS

Key words
Neurotransmitter transporters, neurotransmitter uptake, synaptic vesicles, antidepressants, Parkinson's disease, MPTP neurotoxicity, serotonin, glycine, choline.

Objectives
The Programme will develop our knowledge on four different transporters: the vesicular monoamine transporter and the plasma membrane transporters of serotonin, choline and glycine.
Four different levels will be investigated: cloning of the genes, protein purification, structure-function analysis and physiology (regulation) of the transporters.

Brief description
The proposal is aimed to the study of four different neuronal transporters: the monoamine vesicular one and the serotonin, glycine and choline plasma membrane transporters. These proteins play an important role in neurotransmission, either during the biogenesis of synaptic vesicles or in terminating the neurotransmitter effect. They are important pharmacological targets (5-HT transporter/tricyclic antidepressants) or markers (vesicular monoamine transporter/parkinson's disease). Their physiological role is not fully appreciated (the glycine transporter might modulate NMDA receptors) and their regulations have to be studied. Moreover, their pharmacology is either unsatisfactory (reserpine/vesicular transporter) or poor (glycine transporter).
Finally these transporters might be involved in various pathologies and disorders: migraine, chronic depression, compulsive disorders (5-HT), Alzheimer's disease (choline), epilepsy (glycine), MPTP neurotoxicity and parkinson's disease (monoamine vesicular).

1 The molecular genetics of the four transporters will be developed, starting from current knowledge, to clarify the possibility of isoforms (with different biochemical or pharmacological properties), expressed or regulated in different ways (for the choline, glycine or monoamine transporters).

2 Wild type and mutated serotonin transporter will be overexpress and purified for structural studies, including Fourier transform IR spectroscopy and 2D and 3D crystallization trials. Rapid kinetics of that transporter expressed in well defined E. Coli vesicles will be initiated.

3 All four transporters will be analyzed for topological and structure-function relationship, using:

i site directed mutagenesis and expression of the cloned genes in eucaryotic heterologous cells or:

ii selection of randomly mutated genes expressed in stable cell lines.

4 Regulations will be analyzed at:

i the level of the activity of the transporters, by following the effects of *in vivo* and *in vitro* phosphrylation, and:

ii at the level of their synthesis, by following the level of mRNA after stimulation of the cells.

Project leader:
Dr. Jean-Pierre HENRY
URA 1112, CNRS, IBPC
Rue Pierre et Marie Curie 13
FR 75005 Paris
Phone: +33 1 43 25 26 09
Fax: +33 1 40 46 83 31
Contract number: CT931110

Participants:
Dr. Carmen ARAGON
Universidad Autonoma de Madrid,
Centro de Biologia Molecular,
Dept. de Biologia Molecular Cantoblanco
ES 28049 Madrid
Phone: +34 1 397 4855
Fax: +34 1 397 4799

Dr. Heinrich BETZ
Abteilung Neurochemie,
Mac Planck Institut für Hirnforschung
Deutschordenstrasse 46
DE 60496 Frankfurt
Phone: +49 69 96 76 92 60
Fax: +49 69 96 76 94 41

Dr. George ROBILLARD
Groningen Biomolecular Sciences &
Biotechnology Institute
Nijenborgh 4
NL 9747 AG Groningen
Phone: +31 50 634 321
Fax: +31 50 634 165

Dr. Clive WILLIAMS
Dept. of Biochemistry,
Trinity College
IE Dublin 2
Phone: +353 1 702 21 51
Fax: +353 1 671 51 98

A SCREENING INSTRUMENT FOR THE DETECTION
OF PSYCHOSOCIAL RISK FACTORS IN PATIENTS
ADMITTED TO GENERAL HOSPITAL WARDS

Key words
General hospital, psychiatry, co-morbidity, risk factors, instrument, screening, cost-effectiveness.

Objectives
The main objectives of this Concerted Action are:
a to enhance the awareness and appropriate treatment by medical doctors and nurses of patients with physical illnesses and mental health problems admitted to general hospital wards; and
b when needed referral to mental health consultation-liaison services.

Brief description
Background: Although a series of psychosocial factors have demonstrated to have a negative effect on the outcome on physical illness and its costs for treatment, doctors and nurses are not trained in its systematic assessment, nor do they have instruments feasible in the clinical practice to apply this available knowledge. As mental health intervention studies have demonstrated its positive mental and cost effects in several sub-populations, the development of such a risk screening instrument is most needed. An European effort will by-pass all kinds of local ideosyncratic and redundant instrument development.

Resources for the CA: An earlier COMAC-HSR CA action (MR*-340-NL) has resulted in a research network and an extensive database (n=15.000) on mental health service delivery in 57 general hospitals in 12 European countries. Recently 2.500 pertinent articles describing this specific mental health field have been documented in a database. This network and these two databases will be an important source for the development of the screening instrument in this CA.

Procedures and outcome of the CA: The developed network in the COMAC-HSR CA will be used for the data analyses, instrument building, and field testing, including feasibility and validity studies. The study will among others result in a series of protocols which can be submitted for national funding to:
a further assess the instrument validity; and
b use the instrument as a screener for much needed specific prevalence/incidence studies, and clinical trials assessing the (cost)effectiveness of mental health interventions in the medically ill.

European effects: As in the first CA action, the CA will be a second impulse on the growth of research; its results will provided health care policy makers with much needed currently lacking information.

Project leader:
Dr. Frits HUYSE
General Hospital Psychiatry and Psychosomatics,
Free University Hospital Amsterdam
De Boelelaan 1117
NL 1007 MB Amsterdam
Phone: +31 20 548 59 48
Fax: +31 20 548 59 49
Contract number: CT931180

Participants:
Graca M.P. CARDOSA
Servico Psiquiatria, Hosp. Santa Maria
Av. Egas Moniz 7
PT 1699 Lisboa Codex
Fax: +351 1 388 5736

Trevor FRIEDMAN
Dept. of Psychiatrym Leicester General Hospital
Gwendolen Road
UK Leicester LE5 4PW
Phone: +44 533 490 490
Fax: +44 533 584 745

Dr. T. HERZOG
Psychother. und Psychosom. Med.,
Klin. Albert Ludwigs Un. Psych. un. kl.
Hauptstrasse 8
DE 7800 Freibrug
Phone: +49 761 270 6878
Fax: +49 761 270 6885

Prof. A. LOBO
Dept. of Psychiatry,
Universidad de Zaragoza
ES 50009 Zaragoza
Fax: +34 76 56 58 52

Prof. A.F. MALT
Psychosomatik avd., Rikshospitalet
Pilestredet 32
NO 0027 Oslo 1
Phone: +47 22 868 140
Fax: +47 22 868 149

Prof. M. RIGATELLI
Clinica Psichiatrica,
Policlinico Universita di Modena
Via del Pozzo
IT 41100 Modena
Phone: +39 360 386
Fax: +39 593 725 40

HEALTH SERVICES RESEARCH RELATED TO REHABILITATION FOR PERSONS WITH MULTIPLE SCLEROSIS

Key words
Multiple Sclerosis, rehabilitation, health services, long-term-management.

Objectives
Quality improvement of care and designing more cost effectiveness means of providing rehabilitation programs for MS patients and their caregivers in the different Member States:
1 Identification of the needs and priorities.
2 Identification of appropriate scales for assessment of Disability and Handicap.
3 Identification of the Health Care Systems related to rehabilitation.
4 Identification of Rehabilitation programs adapted to MS.
5 Identification of cost-efficiency of different Health Care Systems.

Brief description
Multiple sclerosis (MS) is the most common progressive neurologic disease of young Europeans. With a prevalence of 30 to 200 in 100.000 inhabitants, MS affects over 250.000 persons in Europe.

MS can drastically decrease quality of life. Somatic symptoms may reduce social interaction and may have an impact on educational or vocational attainment over time. Family life may deteriorate or disintegrate. The impact of MS on the individual and society goes far beyond direct medical consequences. (As the EEC treaty of Maastricht (title X, art.129) points out community action shall be directed towards major health scources and will be aimed at the promotion of economic and social progress.) Most of the persons with MS have a relatively normal life span and will live with the disease for decades. They will develop some permanent neurologic disability as a consequence of their disease. The patients and their families will face a variety of health care needs. The health care services and complementary resources differ substantially in the different member states. The full economic cost of MS to society and individuals with the disease is uncertain, but is most likely considerable.

The proposed concerted action would concist in a workpackage of 5 tasks:
1 Definition of health care needs of the MS patients and their caregivers.
2 Research to accurate assessment instruments to evaluate impairment, disability and handicap in MS 3. Evaluation of the different health care services available in the different member states.
4 Definition of accurate rehabilitation programs for MS patients.
5 Research related to cost-effectiveness, cost-efficiency and cost-utility in MS.

The proposal is managed by rehabilitation in MS (R.I.M.S.) with involvement and supervision of members of the European MS platform (E.M.S.P.) and hospital committee of the European Community (H.C.E.C.).

Project leader:
Dr. Pierre KETELAER
National Schiftings- en
Readaptie-Centrum voor
Multiple Sclerose
Vanheylenstraat 16
BE 1820 Melsbroek
Phone: +32 2 751 80 30
Fax: +32 2 751 52 45
Contract number: CT931453

Participants:
Dr. J. BAGUNYA
Institut Guttmann
ES 08027 Barcelona

Prof. M. BATTAGLIA
Associazione Italiana de
Sclerosi Multipla
IT 16128 Genova

Mrs. R. BENCIVENGA
Associazione Italiana de
Sclerosi Multipla
IT 16128 Genova

Dr. C. BENETON
Centre Médical
Germaine Revel
FR 69440 Mornant

Dr. F. BORGEL
Clinique Neurologique,
rééducation et réadaptation
fonctionnelle, C.H.R.U. de
Grenoble, Hôpital Nord
FR 38043 Grenoble

Dr. D. CASTRO
25 de Julio 54
ES 38004 Santa Cruz de
Tenerife

Dr. M. CHARLIER
National MS Centre
Vanheylenstraat 16
BE 1820 Melsbroek

Dr. CHRISTIDIS
ELEA
Kerkyras 140
GR 11363 Athens

Mrs. M. CRENESSE
FR 75013 Paris

Dr. G. CRIMI
IT 45100 Rovigo

Prof. W. DEWEERDT
BE 3000 Leuven

Mrs. M. DUPORTAIL
BE 1820 Melsbroek

Mrs. A. FAGERBERG
Humlegarden, Box 109
SE 193 23 Sigtuna

Mrs. E. FISCHBACHER
CH 8003 Zürich

Dr. K. FROHRIEP
CH 8881 Knoblisbühl

Dr. A. GUSEO
Seregelyesi UT 3
HU 8001 Szekesfehervar

Mr. B. INGOLDSBY
IE Dublin 4

Dr. R. JONES
Horfield Road
UK Bristol BS2 8ED

Mrs. JONSSON
RINGSTEDVEJ 106
DK 4690 hASLEV

Dr. N. KONIG
DE 82335 Berg 1

Mr. B. LANDSTEDT
Humlegarden, box 109
SE 193 23 Sigtuna

Prof. G. LANKHORST
NL 1007 MB Amsterdam

Prof. L. MCLELLAN
UK Southampton 509 4XY

Dr. J. MERTIN
DE 8873 Ichenhaüsen

Dr. M.F. MILLET
FR 69440 Mornant

Mrs. C. MOLLEMAN
BE 3000 Leuven

Mr. VAN NUIJSENBURG
NL 3961 AV Wijk bij
Duurstede

Prof. J. PACOLET
BE 3000 Leuven

Prof. VAN DER PLOEG
NL 1081 BT Amsterdam

Dr. P. POHL
AT 6020 Innsbruck

Dr. C. POLAMN
NL 1007 MB Amsterdam

Dr. M. PROSIEGEL
DE 80804 München

Dr. M. RAVNBORG
DK 2100 Copenhagen

Dr. J. RUUTIAINEN
FI 21251 Masku

Prof. K. SCHUTYSER
BE 3000 Leuven

Dr. A.J. THOMPSON
UK London WC1N 3BG

Mr. L. VLEUGELS
BE 1820 Melsbroek

Dr. B. VRACKO-KONCAN
SI 61000 Ljunljana

Prof. K. WRIGHT
Centre for Health Economics,
University of York
UK York YO1 5DD

IDENTIFICATION OF GENE SUSCEPTIBILITY FACTORS IN MANIAC-DEPRESSIVE ILLNESS USING NON-PARAMETRIC METHODS

(i.e. Association and Sib-Pair Studies)

Key words
Manic-depressive illness (MDI).

Objectives
Identification of gene susceptibility factors in manic-depressive illness using non-parametric methods (i.e. Association and Sib-Pair Studies).

Brief description
Manic-depressive illness (MDI) is a severe and common psychiatric syndrome affecting 1% of the general population. The etiology of MDI is not known; an ascertained fact is that it presents an hereditary component.

Previous attempts to identify genetic risk factors implicated in the etiopathogenesis of MDI, using parametric methods of analysis, have given contradictory results, because of the complexity of MDI, which is a genetically heterogeneous disease. Moreover, MDI is not a clinically homogeneous disease. In order to avoid the pitfalls of parametric linkage analysis, this study envisages the utilization of non parametric methods (sib-pair and association analysis) for the systematic study of the whole genome of a very large sample of families and individuals collected by a collaborative international effort. This international collaboration allows for similar standardised diagnostic procedures in the gathering of a great number of familial and sporadic cases, a result unattainable by a single centre or a single country.

Our analysis will be based on the sib-pair method using the collected families (n=200 to 300 families in total). In parallel, a sample of unrelated patients (n=100 per centre) and unaffected controls of the same geographic origin will be collected in each country to perform association studies with candidate genes (genes which code for proteins relevant to neurotransmission).

Three hundred markers of the microsatellite type which can be exploited by PCR (polymerase chain reaction), evenly spaced on the genome, will be used to identify regions of vulnerability by using the sib-pair method. This study will take place at Généthon, which has the technical competence to handle large numbers of samples simultaneously.

The participating laboratories will carry out:
1 association analysis studies with markers close to candidate genes, and;
2 search for mutations in candidate genes utilising the PCR-SSCP (Polymerase Chain Reaction Single Strand Conformation Polymorphism) technique.

The identification of genetic factors conferring susceptibility to MDI will:
- improve our understanding of the disease for its diagnosis and treatment;
- help in the designing of new and more effective drugs;
- elucidate the role of environmental factors and open a completely new field of prevention of MDI.

These results will yield a reduction of the economic burden of the public health structures in caring for a chronic disease such as MDI. Moreover, with better care, better drugs and prevention the patients will be better integrated into society thus reducing the strain on themselves and their families. Finally, a better understanding of the neurophysiology of the brain in normal and pathological conditions will give new insights in the study of higher mental functions.

Project leader:
Dr. Jacques MALLET
Lab. de Génétique
moléculaire de la
Neurotransmission
Av. de la Terrasse 1
C.N.R.S. bâtiment 32
FR 91198 Gif-sur-Yvette
Phone: +33 1 69 82 36 46
Fax: +33 1 69 82 35 80
Contract number: CT931508

Participants:
Dr. T. HERZOG
Klinikum Albert Ludwigs
Universität
Haupstrasse 8
DE 79104 Freiburg
Phone: +49 761 270 68 42
Fax: +49 761 270 68 85

Prof. F. CREED
Manchester Royal Infirmary,
Dept. of Psychiatry
Rawnsley Bldg.
Oxford Road
UK Manchester M13 9WL
Phone: +44 61 276 53 31
Fax: +44 61 273 21 35

Prof. A. LOBO
Dept. de Psiquiatriá, Hospital
Clinico Universitario
Planta 11
ES 50009 Zaragoza
Phone: +34 76 55 97 95
Fax: +34 76 53 18 15

Prof. M. RIGATELLI
Clinica Psichiatrica
Via del Pozzo 71
IT 41100 Modena
Phone: +39 59 37 94 36
Fax: +39 59 37 25 40

Prof. U. MALT
Rikshospitalet,
Psykosomatik Avd.
Pilestredet 32
NO 0027 Oslo
Phone: +47 2 86 81 40
Fax: +47 2 36 04 59

Dr. G.CARDOSO
Hospital Santa Maria,
Servico Psiquiatria
Av. Egas Moniz 7
PT 1699 Lisbon
Phone: +351 1 80 21 31
Fax: +351 1 797 88 21

Dr. P. McKEON
Dept. of Medical Genetics,
Trinity College
Lincoln Place
IE Dublin 2
Phone: +353 1 677 54 23
Fax: +353 1 679 88 65

Prof. S. SORBI
Dip. di Scienze Neurologiche
e Psichiatriche, Univ. Degli
Studi di Firenze
Viale G. Morgagni 85
IT 50134 Firenze
Phone: +39 55 41 26 34
Fax: +39 55 41 87 18

Dr. O. MORS
Institute of Basic Psychiatric
Research, Dept. of Psychiat-
ric Demography, Psychiatric
Hospital in Aarhus
Skovagervej 2
DK 8240 Risskov
Phone: +45 86 17 77 77
Fax: +45 86 17 59 77

Mr. M. BURKE
University of Wales,
College of Medicine
Heath Park
UK Cardiff CF4 4XN
Phone: +44 222 74 77 47
Fax: +44 222 74 29 14

Prof. P. McGUFFIN
University of Wales,
College of Medicine
Heath Park
UK Cardiff CF4 4XN
Phone: +44 222 74 32 41
Fax: +44 222 74 78 39

Dr. W. MAIER
Dept. of Psychiatry,
University of Mainz
Untere Zahlbacher Strasse 8
DE 55101 Mainz
Phone: +49 6131 17 24 74
Fax: +49 6131 17 66 90

Mr. A. INGLE
Institute of Psychiatry
De Crespigny Park
Denmark Hill
UK London SE5 8AF
Phone: +44 71 703 54 11
Fax: +44 71 701 90 44

Dr. M. GILL
Dept. of Psychological Medi-
cine, Institute of Psychiatry
De Crespigny Park
Denmark Hill
UK London SE5 8AF
Phone: +44 71 703 60 91
Fax: +44 71 701 90 44

Dr. J.F. FONCIN
Lab. de Neurohistologie,
Ecole Pratique des
Hautes Etudes
Boulevard de l'Hopital 47
FR 75651 Paris Cedex 13
Phone: +33 1 45 70 28 20
Fax: +33 1 45 70 99 90

Dr. J. BECKMANN
Centre d'Etude du
Polymorphisme Humain
Juliette Dodu 27
FR 75010 Paris
Phone: +33 1 42 49 98 67
Fax: +33 1 40 18 01 55

Prof. M. ACKENHEIL
Neurochemistry Dept.,
Psychiatric Hospital,
University of Munich
Nussbaumstrasse 7
DE 80336 Munich
Phone: +49 89 5160 27 30
Fax: +49 89 5160 47 41

MULTIGENERATIONAL STUDIES OF FUNCTIONAL PSYCHOSES IN A FOUNDED POPULATION

Key words
Functional psychoses, molecular genetics, founder population.

Objectives
The aim of this study is to locate genes which contribute to the aetiology of psychiatric disorders in a large multigenerational founder population.

Brief description
Psychiatric disorders cause considerable human suffering. They are often severely disabling and socially stigmatising and inflict immense personal, family and economic cost. There is considerable evidence for a genetic contribution to the aetiology of major psychiatric disorders such as schizophrenia. Recent advances in molecular genetic techniques provide us with the capability to locate genes which may play a role in the development of psychiatric disease.

We will study the pattern of psychiatric disorders and genetic marker transmissions through several generations of a founder population. We have used as a starting point some striking accounts of insanity, deviant and suicidal behaviour in three progenitors living in a genetically isolated population in Norway, during the 17th and 18th Centuries. A variety of genealogical paths have been traced from these progenitors to the present day population of geographically delimited area of rural Norway. A family cohort of 2000 have been identified of which 120 are patients, 60% of which have been traced back to the three progenitors. We will employ comprehensive assessments of phenotypes relying on continuous and multidimensional clinical measurements as well as categorical diagnoses.

We believe that this study in genetic epidemiology creates a unique background for us to carry out linkage and association studies in large multigenerational families, small families, sib-pairs and unrelated individuals. A systematic search for genetic linkage will be performed using microsatellite markers based at 10cM intervals. Furthermore, a Representational Difference Analysis (RDA) will be carried out to isolate DNA similarities between affected family members and a common founder, compared to a control group. The statistical analysis will also take account of shared chromosome segments in patients using a method developed by Dr. Sandkuijl.

Project leader:
Professor Peter McGUFFIN
Dept. of Psychological Medicine,
University of Wales, College of Medicine
Heath Park
UK Cardiff CF4 4XN
Phone: +44 22 274 77 47
Fax: +44 22 274 78 39
Contract number: CT931759

Participants:
Dr. M. OWEN
Dept. of Psychological Medicine,
University of Wales College of Medicine
Heath Park
UK Cardiff CF4 4 XN
Phone: +44 222 743 058
Fax: +44 222 747 839

Prof. U.F. MALT
Dept. of Psychosomatic and Behavioural
Medicine, University of Oslo,
The National Hospital
NO 0027 Oslo 1
Phone: +47 22 86 81 40
Fax: +47 22 86 81 49

Dr. Torfinn HYNNEKLEIV
Psykosomatisk Avdeling,
Universitetsklinikk, Rikshospitalet
Pilestredet 32
NO 0027 Oslo 1
Phone: +47 22 86 81 40
Fax: +47 22 86 81 49

Dr. J.E. ANDERSEN
Psykosomatisk Avdeling,
Universitetsklinikk, Rikshospitalet
Pilestredet 32
NO 0027 Oslo 1
Phone: +47 22 86 81 40
Fax: +47 22 86 81 49

Dr. Lodewijk SANDKUIJL
Voorstraat 27a
NL 2611 Delft
Phone: +31 15 12 36 38
Fax: +31 15 14 39 25

Dr. Julie WILLIAMS
Dept. of Psychological Medicine,
University of Wales, College of Medicine
Heath Park
UK Cardiff CF4 4XN
Phone: +44 222 743 058
Fax: +44 222 747 839

Dr. Anne FARMER
Dept. of Psychological Medicine,
University of Wales, College of Medicine
Heath Park
UK Cardiff CF4 4XN
Phone: +44 222 743 228
Fax: +44 222 747 839

EUROPEAN NETWORK FOR STRIATAL TRANSPLANTATION IN HUNTINGTON'S DISEASE (NEST-HD): PRECLINICAL DEVELOPMENT AND CLINICAL TRIAL METHODOLOGY

Key words
Striatal transplantation, Huntington's disease, animal models, methodology.

Objectives
The aim of the NEST-HD project is to establish the experimental ground work and clinical methodology essential for undertaking the first multicentre trials of striatal transplantation in Huntington's disease.

Brief description
Much of the pioneering experimental and clinical work on reversal of CNS dysfunction by intracerebral neuronal grafting has been undertaken in Europe. NECTAR, the European Network of European CNS Transplantation and Restoration, was established in 1991 to coordinate basic and animal experimental and clinical research in this field. Attention was first directed to Parkinsons disease (PD). A number of PD patients have so far been operated with promising results, and this area is now to be supported by a BIOMED Concerted Action. These trials involve the implantation of fetal nigral cells from the midbrain, which is diseased in PD, into the striatum, which is healthy, but deprived of its normal input from nigra (i.e. heterotopic grafting).

Huntington's disease (HD) is a dominantly inherited degenerative neurological disorder, most commonly starting in the fourth and fifth decades. It causes a progressive decline of motor function, behaviour, personality and intellect leading to death after a mean of 17 years. Neurons die prematurely in a number of different brain areas, but especially in the striatum. Symptomatic treatment is of limited benefit, and no treatment influences the course of the disease. The responsible gene was identified in March 1993, but how it causes cell loss is not known. In the coming years, a number of candidate therapies may emerge. One of these is transplantation of fetal striatal cells into diseased striatum (i.e. orthotopic).

Requirements
Before human trials of striatal transplantation can begin, the ground work must be laid, and this is the purpose of the NEST-HD Concerted Action. The key elements are:
1 the basic and animal experimental work underpinning striatal transplantation will be coordinated and developed;
2 an appropriate clinical methodology incorporating repeated neurological, neuropsychological, psychiatric and neurophysiological measures, and functional (PET, SPECT) and anatomical (MRI) imaging will be developed and;
3 cohorts of HD patients will be prospectively and longitudinally followed in order to establish data on the natural history of the disease.

Project leader:
Dr. Niall QUINN
Institute of Neurology
Queen Square
UK London WC1N 3BG
Phone: +44 71 837 36 11
Fax: +44 71 278 56 16
Contract number: CT931621

Participants:
Prof. Anders BJORKLUND
SE 223 62 Lund

Dr. Stephen DUNNETT
UK Cambridge CB2 3EB

Prof. Peter HARPER
UK Cardiff CF4 4XW

Dr. Marc LEVIVIER
NY New York 10032

Prof. Olle LINDVALL
SE 221 85 Lund

Dr. Marc PESCHANSKI
FR Creteil Cedex

Dr. Cornelis VARKEVISSER
NL 2403 HD
Alphen aan de Rijn

Dr. Alfredo BERARDELLI
30IT Rome

Dr. Richard BROWN
UK London WC1N 3BG

Dr. David CRAUFORD
UK Manchester

Dr. Serge GOLDMAN
BE 1070 Bruxelles

Dr. Philippe HENTRAYE
FR Orsay 91406

Dr. John HODGES
UK Cambridge CB2 2QQ

Dr. Juan J LOPEZ-LOZANO
ES Madrid

Prof. Johannes NOTH
DE 5100 Aachen

Dr. Karen OSTERGAARD
DK 5000 Odense C

Dr. Raymund ROOS
NL 2300 RC Leiden

Prof. David BROOKS (replacing
Dr. G. V. SAWLE)
UK LONDON W12 0HS

Dr. Vincenzo SILANI
IT 201 22 Milano

Dr. Christian SPENGER
CH 3010 Bern

Dr. Karl KIEBURTZ
US Rochester NY 14642

Dr. Rene DOM
BE 3000 Leuvern

Dr. J Garcia DE YEBENES
ES Madrid

Dr. Berry KREMER
NL 65 HB Nijmegen

Dr. Anders LUNDIN
SE 171 76 Stockholm

Dr. Hartmut MEIERKORD
DE 10117 Berlin

Dr. Patrick MORRISON
UK Belfast

Dr. Wolfgang OERTEL
DE 8000 Munich 70

Prof. W POEWE
DE Berlin

Prof. Horst PRZUNTEK
DE Bochum
Dr. Sheila SIMPSON

UK Aberdeen AB9 2ZB

Dr. Alfredo BERARDELLI
IT 00185 Rome

Dr. Christian SPENGER
CH 3010 Bern

Dr. Cornelis VARKEVISSER
NL 2403 HD

Dr. David CRAUFORD
UK Manchester

Dr. Guy SAWLE
UK London W12 0HS

Dr. John HODGES
UK Cambridge CB2 2QQ

Dr. J.L. LOPEZ-LOZANO
ES 28035 Madrid

Dr. Karen STERGAARD
DK 8000 Aarhus C

Dr. Karl KIEBURTZ
US Rochester NY 14642

Dr. Marc LEVIVIER
US New York NY 10032

Dr. Marc PESCHANSKI
FR 94010 Creteil Cedex

Dr. Philippe HENTRAYE
FR 91406 Orsay

Dr. Raymund ROOS
NL 2300 RC Leiden

Dr. Richard BROWN
UK London WC1N 3BG

Dr. Serge GOLDMAN
BE 1070 Bruxelles

Dr. Vincenzo SILANI
IT 201 22 Milano

Dr. Wolfgang OERTEL
DE 8000 Munich 70

Prof. Anders BJORKLUND
SE 223 62 Lund

Prof. Johannes NOTH
DE 5100 Aachen

Prof. Olle LINDVALL
SE 221 85 Lund

Prof. Peter HARPER
UK Cardiff CF4 4XW

Dr. Stephen DUNNETT
UK Cambridge CB2 3EB

MONOCLONAL ANTIBODIES FOR UNDERSTANDING MYASTHENIA GRAVIS AND ACETYLCHOLINE RECEPTOR

Key words

Monoclonal antibodies, myasthenia gravis, acetylcholine receptor, autoimmunity, autoantibodies, rembuant proteins, protein function.

Brief description

This proposal aims at the coordination of the best possible use, by 12 competent European laboratories, of a unique library of 150 monoclonal antibodies (mabs) against the acetylcholine receptor (Achr) in multidisciplinary studies on Achr and myasthenia gravis (MG). MG is a neuroimmune disease caused by the destructive activity of anti-Achr autoantibodies at the neuromuscular junction. Antibody-mediated Achr loss, or blockage, severely affects the skeletal muscles of the patients. Current treatments of MG (200,000 patients) are non-specific and unsatisfactory.

The coordinators extensive anti-Achr mab library has been proved valuable in numerous Achr and MG studies by the participants and other investigators. This is largely due to the continuous discovery of novel properties of these mabs as their characterization advances. The library will be further expanded, characterized and organized. mabs and corresponding data will be widely available for use as tools and as model autoantibodies towards understanding the molecular mechanisms of MG and Achr (muscle and neuronal) and treating the disease.

Tasks and expected achievements of the proposal are as follows:

1 Anti-Achr mab production, maintenance and fine characterization: continuous maintenance of mab stocks, quality control and recloning; expression of recombinant animal and human mabs (Fv) and mutants; mab characterization and epitope mapping (by molecular genetics, peptide chemistry, crystallography, NMR.

2 Establishment of a comprehensive mab data bank and dissemination of information, mabs and related material.

3 Coordination of the use of the mabs for the study of Achr and MG:

a characterization of recombinant human Achr domains, subunits, intact molecules and mutants;

b imaging Achr by scanning tunnelling microscopy;

c Achr phosphorylation-function relationship;

d differences between slowly and rapidly degrading Achr;

e fine specificities of human MG antibodies;

f thymoma proteins with Achr epitopes;

g immunotherapeutic approaches (anti-idiotypes and recombinant mab Eragments as protective drugs) for MG;

h localization, structure and function of neuronal Achr.

European collaboration is indispensable to the project. It will accomplish the maximum exploitation of a valuable set of tools towards.

Project leader:
Dr. Socrates J. TZARTOS
Hellenic Pasteur Institute,
Biochemistry Dept,
Vas. Sofias Avenue 127
GR 115 21 Athens
Phone: +30 16 43 00 44
Fax: +30 16 42 34 98
Contract number: CT931100

Participants:
Dr. K.R. ACHARYA
Dept. of Biochemistry, University of Bath
Claverton Down
UK Bath BA2 7AY
Phone: +44 225 826 134
Fax: +44 225 826 449

Dr. Sonia BERRIH-AKNIN
Dept. de Physiologie Humaine, Lab. d'Immuno-
logie Cellulaire, Hopital Marie Lannelongue
133 av. de la Resistance
FR 92350 Le Plessis-Robinson
Phone: +33 1 4537 1551
Fax: +33 1 4630 4564

Dr. M.T. CUNG & dr. M. MARRAUD
Lab. Chimie-Physique Macromoleculaire,
C.N.R.S.-U.A. 494, ENSIC-INPL
1 rue Grandville
FR 54041 Nancy
Phone: +33 8330 2248
Fax: +33 8337 9977

Prof. F. CLEMENTI & dr. G. FUMAGALLI
Dept. of Medical Pharmacology,
University of Milan
Via Vanvitelli 32 '
IT 20132 Milan
Phone: +39 2 7014 6254
Fax: +39 2 7490 937

Prof. F. CORNELIO &
dr. R. MANTEGAZZE
Dept. of Neuromuscular Diseases,
Istituto Nationale Neurologico Carlo Besta
Via Celoria N. 11
IT 20133 Milan
Phone: +39 2 23941
Fax: +39 2 70638217

Dr. M. DE BAETS
Dept. Immunology, Faculty of Medicine,
University of Limburg
P.O. Box 616
NL 6200 MD Maastricht
Phone: +31 43 888 586
Fax: +31 43 436 080

Prof.MULLER-HERMELINK &
prof. T. KIRCHNER
Pathologisches Institut, Lultpoldkrankenhaus,
Universitat Wurzburg
DE 8700 Wurzburg
Phone: +49 931 2013 793
Fax: +49 931 2013 440

Prof. J. NEWSOM-DAVIS & dr. A. VINCENT
Neurosciences Group, Inst. Molecular Medicine,
John Radcliffe Hospital
Headington
UK Oxford OX3 9DU
Phone: +44 865 222 322
Fax: +44 865 222 402

Dr. N. OIKONOMAKOS
Dept. of Biology,
Nat. Hellenic Research Foundation
48 Vas. Constantinou Ave.
GR Athens
Phone: +30 1 723 9965
Fax: +30 1 722 9811

Prof. C. SAKARELLOS
Dept. of Chemistry, University of Ioannina
GR Ioannina
Phone: +30 651 98390
Fax: +30 651 45840

Dr. V. WITZEMANN
Abteilung Zellphysiologie, Max-Planck Institute
für Medizinische Forschung
Jahnstrasse 29
DE 6900 Heidelberg 1
Phone: +49 6221 486 475
Fax: +49 6221 486 351

BASIC APPROACHES TO RESTORE
NEURONAL FUNCTIONS (BARNEF)

Key words
Neurodegenerative disorders, neuronal function, excitatory amino acids, immunocompetent cells, developmental genes, surface molecules, neuromodulators.

Brief description
Despite the explosive growth and development of new knowledge in neuroscience, preventive and restorative medicine of neurodegenerative disorders is less advanced with respect to other systemic and local diseases. One of the major disadvantages of the Central Nervous System of humans and other mammalian forms is its intrinsic inhability to restore impaired nerve connections.

The aim of the proposed project is to carry out multidisciplinary approaches which combine knowledge from many areas such as molecular biology, embryology, neurochemistry, neuropharmacology, neuroanatomy and physiology.

The participants to the project have well established experience in these areas. The responsible scientists belong to nine laboratories from five different State Members. A possible concerted management of their work will make possible this close-knit group of researchers and investigators working both individually and in combination. The research tasks of the present project include molecular genetics and developmental neurobiology aimed to investigate the role of early developmental genes and factors modulating cell growth, plasticy and differentiation of neurons. This knowledge will help to define basic mechanisms underlying mental and neurological disorders in order to provide some experimental cues for therapeutic approaches aimed to prevent/restore neuronal degeneration and to promote repair of nerve cell connections.

To this aim, experimental models and protocols are defined to the following specific and strictly interconnected objectives:

1 To determine the role of excitatory amino acid receptors in neuronal degeneration and synapse elimination.Increased knowledge of the molecular mechanisms underlying toxic effects of excitatory amino acids can help to prevent/restore nerve cell degeneration;

2 To determine the role of intracerebral immunocompetent cells (IC) in recognizing and destroying degenerating neurons. This knowledge can help to interfere with IC in order to prevent/restore neuronal degeneration;

3 To determine the role of early developmental genes in neuronal specification. Increased knowledge of molecular genetics of the developing brain can help the use of embryonal grafts to restore neuronal function;

4 To determine the role of transiently expressed surface molecules in neuronal development and regeneration. This knowledge may be of crucial importance for promoting restorative nerve cell growth and repairing nerve connections;

5 To determine the role of neuromodulators/neurotrophins in neuronal morphogenesis and trophism. Increased knowledge in this field can help the use of peptides in neurodegenerative disorders.

The final goal of this proposal is to provide some experimental cues to be disseminated to the industrial environment which in turn will integrate the basic achievements of the present project.

Project leader:
Professor P. BAGNOLI
Dept of Environmental Sciences,
University of Tuscia
Via S. Camillo de Lellis
IT 01100 Viterbo
Phone: +39 761357113
Fax: +39 761357114
Contract number: CT941378

Participants:
Dr. B. BERGER
Batiment de Pedriatrie,
INSERM Hopital Salpetriere
47 Bld. de l'Hopital
FR 75651 Paris 13
Phone: +33 1 4582 61 00
Fax: +33 1 4570 99 90

Dr. L. DOMENICI
Institute of Neurophysiology,
Italian Research Council
Via S. Zeno 51
IT 56127 Pisa
Phone: +39 50 559 706
Fax: +39 50 559 725

Dr. D. KARAGOGEOS
Institute of Molecular Biology
and Biotechnology
P.O. Box 1527
GR Heraklion, Crete
Phone: +30 81 261 975
Fax: +30 81 230 469

Dr. E.D. KOUVELAS
Department of Physiology, Medical School,
University of Patras '
Panepistimioupolis
GR 26500 Patras
Phone: +30 61 992 389
Fax: +30 61 997 215

Dr. J. MARIANI
Lab. de Neurobiologie du Developpement,
Université P&M Curie
9 Quai Saint Bernard
FR 75003 Paris
Phone: +33 1 4427 32 36
Fax: +33 1 4407 15 85

Dr. E. PATSAVOUDI
Hellenic Pasteur Institute
127 Vassilis Sofias Avenue
GR 11521 Athens
Phone: +30 1 646 22 82
Fax: +30 1 642 34 98

Dr. L. PUELLES
Department of Morphol. Pathol. Anat. and
Psychobiol., University of Murcia
Campus de Espinardo
ES Murcia
Phone: +34 68 83 30 00
Fax: +34 68 36 39 55

Dr. S. THANOS
Abteilung Physikalische Biologie,
Max-Planck Institute für Entwicklungsbiologie
Spemannstrasse 35/1
DE 7400 Tubingen 1
Phone: +49 7071 294 796
Fax: +49 7071 293 730

STUDY ON PHYSIOLOGICAL ROLES OF TWO NEUROTROPHIC FACTORS NAMED MIDKINE (MK) AND HEPARIN AFFIN REGULATORY PEPTIDE (HARP) AND THEIR POTENTIAL USE IN NEURONAL DYSFUNCTIONS AND REPAIR

Key words

Neurotrophic growth factors, neuronal survival, differentiation, neurodegenerative disorders, brain damage, repair.

Brief description

This proposal describes how five European teams, by combining complementary expertises in biochemistry, molecular biology, cell biology, neuroanatomy, neurophysiology and cell transplants, address key questions on the mechanisms of action of two neurotrophic growth factors, named Midkine (MK) and Heparin Affin Regulatory Peptide (HARP), their role in neuronal cell survival, differentiation and their implication in brain damage repair and in neurodegenerative diseases.

The necessary biochemical, immunological and molecular tools allowing the identification, the localization, the quantification of these factors and the gene message for their production are now becoming available from group 1 and group 2 and can be therefore used to study the mechanisms of action and identify functional receptors, as well as to study the biological role of these factors on various cells of neuronal origin in tissue culture. Organotypic cultures of brain slices provide unique opportunities for studies of neuron-glial interactions, cell differentiation and electrophysiology, as well as the cellular localisation of HARP and MK at all stages of development by in situ hybridizations.

In vivo studies on the role of these factors in brain damage repair will be performed, using local injections of excitotoxic drugs as a model for some neuro-degenerative diseases or mechanical lesions as a model of wound healing.

Furthermore, transplantations of homotypic fetal neurons have demonstrated that regeneration of synaptic contacts with afferent responsible axons can be maintained if continuous supply of neurotrophic factors is provided. Groups 2 and 4 will also assess MK and HARP in cellular transplantation models.

The last approach to be proposed concerns the use of transgenic mice to evaluate the effects of over-expression of these molecules in the developing and adult mice.

It must be stressed that group 1 has succeeded in producing recombinant HARP which has three aminoacids more at the N-terminal than previously described forms and which is 10 to 100-fold more active than previously described HARP.

This molecule is patent pending.

Project leader:
Professor D. BARRITAULT
Laboratoire CRRET, Université Paris XII-Val de Marne
Av. du Général de Gaulle
FR 94000 Creteil
Phone: +33 1 48 99 60 98
Fax: +33 1 48 99 60 98
Contract number: CT941168

EUROPEAN NETWORK FOR THE DEVELOPMENT OF A NEURAL TRANSPLANTATION THERAPY IN PARKINSON'S DISEASE: METHODOLOGICAL DEVELOPMENT AND CLINICAL TRIALS

Key words
Transplantation, Parkinson's disease, methodology, clinical trials.

Brief description
The goal of the program is to develop efficient, reliable, safe and ethically acceptable transplantation therapies for patients with Parkinson's disease (PD) through a Concerted Action among all European clinical and experimental research groups active in this field. From the results obtained so far this goal seems feasible. However, it is clear that efficient progress can only be made through joint forces between several centres. Brain transplantation is still in its infancy and a wide range of issues related to, for example, immunology, implantation surgery, trophic mechanisms, cell preparation, scaling-up from experimental animals to humans, functional assessment, and techniques for in vivo monitoring of graft survival and function, need to be addressed in an efficient, goal-directed manner.

The network program will comprise the following four parts:

1 A registry coupled to a data bank and an assessment program to coordinate clinical trials with neural transplantation in PD patients, carried out in different centres in Europe. The purpose of the registry is to facilitate planning, evaluation, coordination and data sharing between different European centres.

2 Coordinated and collaborative experimental research for technical and methodological development as a basis for future clinical trials. The purpose of this program is (i) to solve critical methodological and immunological problems raised by the ongoing clinical trials; (ii) to develop improved techniques for the assessment of graft viability and function; (iii) to improve the efficacy of current transplantation procedures; an (iv) to develop new alternative sources of cells for transplantation in PD patients which will reduce or eliminate the need to use fetal tissue.

3 Annual Network conferences supplemented by small group meetings as a basis for planning, data sharing and follow-up of the clinical and experimental research programs carried out by the participating groups.

4 A Network secretariat for the coordination and administration of the joint network programs and planning of the annual conferences. In addition, the secretariat will provide service for the member institutions on legal and ethical issues and follow developments in different European countries with respect to legislation and regulations in the field of brain transplantation.

The secretariat will also publish a regular a fax-based newsletter for rapid dissemination of information among the member institutions.

Project leader:
Professor A. BJÖRKLUND
Department of Medical Cell Research
Biskopsgatan 5
SE 223 62 Lund
Phone: +46 46 10 79 05
Fax: +46 46 10 79 27
Contract number: CT941316

Participants:

Dr. Gerard J. BOER
Netherlands Institute for Brain Research
Meibergdreef 33
NL 1105 AZ Amsterdam
Phone: +31 20 566 5509
Fax: +31 20 691 8466

Dr. Stephen B. DUNNETT
Dept. of Experimental Psychological
Downing Street
UK Cambridge CB2 3EB
Phone: +44 223 333 567
Fax: +44 223 333 564

Prof. Olle LINDVALL
Dept. of Neurology, University Hospital
SE 22185 Lund
Phone: +46 46 171 292
Fax: +46 46 188 150

Prof. Wolfgang OERTEL
Ludwig Maximilian's University,
Dept. of Neurology,
Klinikum Grosshadern
DE 8000 Munchen 70
Phone: +49 89 7095 3678
Fax: +49 89 7095 8839

Dr. Marc PESCHANSKI
Centre Hospital-Universitaire Henri Modor,
Dept. Neurosciences Medicales
FR 94010 Creteil
Phone: +33 1 4981 3682
Fax: +33 1 4981 2326

THE HUMAN PRION DISEASES: FROM NEUROPATHOLOGY TO PATHOBIOLOGY AND MOLECULAR GENETICS

Key words
Human prion diseases, neuropathology, pathobiology, data bases, tissue bank.

Objectives
Establishment of the European Neuropathological Data Base on Prion Diseases (ENDA-PRID). Since definite diagnosis of human prion diseases is made by neuropathology, the incidence of biopsy- or autopsy-proven Creutzfeldt-Jakob disease (CJD), Gerstmann-Sträussler-Scheinker disease (GSS) and fatal familial insomnia (FFI) throughout Europe will be determined both retrospectively and prospectively, to analyze eventual secular or geographic clustering or shifts.
Establishment of the European Neuropathological Tissue Bank of Prion Diseases (ENTI-PRID). Tissues and body fluids from biopsy- or autopsy-proven prion disease will be collected from retrospective and prospective cases in the appropriate way, for information of and distribution to interested researchers.
Definition of neuropathological diagnostic criteria for prion diseases, including standardized immunocytochemistry for the prion protein (PrP).
Definition of a standardized tissue handling protocol for prion diseases which is both safe and practical.
Establishment of the Neuropathological Clearing House for Prion Diseases (ENCLEAP-RID) for special evaluation of difficult, atypical or insufficiently diagnoses cases, including application of immunolabeling for the prion protein (PrP) and, if necessary in selected cases, immunochemical, molecular biologic (PRNP gene) and experimental transmission studies. Diagnostic neuropathology support can be provided to laboratories with limited experience in these rare diseases or lack of appropriate methodology.
Clinico-neuropathological investigations into the relation between clinical phenotype and the distribution of pathology, including the pattern of PrP deposition and of synaptic pathology. Better insight into the mechanism of neuronal degeneration by study of apoptosis/DNA fragmentation.
Molecular biologic investigations of familial and iatrogenic human prion diseases with differing phenotypes, examining mutations and polymorphisms (especially at codon 129) of the PRNP gene.
Infectivity and in vitro studies for clarification of the nature of the yet enigmatic infectious agent and its effect upon the biomolecular machinery of neural cells.
Support of local research subprojects in the field by sharing of materials and special techniques.
Improving neuropathological experience and application of modern diagnostic and research techniques in prion diseases by exchange of scientific/laboratory personnel on a Europe-wide scale.

Brief description
Dissemination of information on all parts of this project by a regularly distributed newsletter and yearly meetings. This is of special importance for information on ENTIPRID materials available to interested researchers for local subprojects and for further European expansion of this CA to additional groups with potentially useful contribution.
ENDAPRID: central storage and processing of prion disease patient data (identification

number, sex, age, length of disease, clinical phenotype, neuropathology report), evaluation and storage of confirmatory histological slides (minimum one each of cerebrum and cerebellum). Data will be collected both prospectively and retrospectively for the last 10 years. Problem cases and cases to be confirmed will enter ENCLEAPRID.

Project leader:
Professor H. BUDKA
Klinisches Institut für Neurologie der Universität Wien
Klinische Abteilung für Neuropathologie und Neurochemie
Neues Allgemeines Krankenhaus 04
Währinger Gürtel 18-20
AT 1090 Wien
Phone: +43 1 40400 5501
Fax: +43 1 40400 5511
Contract number: CT941484

Participants:

Prof. F. SEITELBERGER (AT)

Prof. K. JELLINGER (AT)

Dr. R. KLEINERT (AT)

Dr. H. MAIER (AT)

Dr. P. PILZ (AT)

Prof. J.M. BRUCHER (BE)

Prof. J.J. MARTIN &
Dr. P. CRAS (BE)

Prof. C.J.M. SINDIC (BE)

Dr. E. MITROVA (SK)

Prof. H. LAURSON (DK)

Dr. P.S. TEGLBJAERG (DK)

Prof. M. HALTIA (FI)

Dr. H. KALIMO (FI)

Dr. J. KOVANEN (FI)

Dr. M.B. DELISLE (FR)

Mme. J. DOERR-SCHOTT (FR)

Dr. D. DORMONT (FR)

Prof. F. DUBAS (FR)

Prof. F. GRAY (FR)

Prof. J.J. HAUW (FR)

Dr. N. HELDT (FR)

Prof. J. MIKOL (FR)

Prof. Cl. VITAL (FR)

Dr. J.W. BOELLAARD (DE)

Prof. J. CERVOS-NAVARRO
& Dr. S. PATT (DE)

Prof. E. DAHME (DE)

Dr. H. DIRINGER (DE)

Prof. H.H. GOEBEL &
Dr. J. BOHL (DE)

Prof. F. GULLOTTA (DE)

Prof. M. KIESSLING (DE)

Dr. H. KLEIN (DE)

Prof. H.A. KRETSCHMAR
(DE)

Prof. P. MEHRAEIN (DE)

Prof. W. POEWE &
Dr. K. JENDROSKA (DE)

Prof. W. SCHACHENMAYR
(DE)

Prof. W. SCHLOTE (DE)

Prof. J.M. SCHRODER (DE)

Prof. R. SCHRODER

Prof. D. STAVROU &
Dr. R. LAAS (DE)

Prof. B. VOLK (DE)

Prof. G.F. WALTER &
Dr. A. HORI (DE)

Prof. O.D. WIESTLER

Dr. K. MAJTENYI (HU)

Dr. G. GEORGSSON (IS)

Prof. S.J. BALLOYANNIS
(GR)

Prof. P. DAVAKI

Prof. E. PATSOURIS (GR)

Dr. C. KEOHANE (IE)

Dr. W. KAMPHORST (NL)

Prof. D. SCHIFFER (IT)

Prof. O. BUGIANI (IT)

Prof. A. LECHI &
Prof. G.R. TRABATTONI (IT)

Prof. G. MACCHI &
Prof. C. MASULLO (IT)

Dr. M. POCCHIARI (IT)

Prof. S.J. MORK (NO)

Dr. P.P. LIBERSKI (PL)

Dr. C. COSTA &
Dr. J. PIMENTEL (PT)

Dr. C. LIMA (PT)

Dr. A. PETRESCU (RO)

Prof. M. POPOVIC (SI)

Dr. F.F. CRUZ-SANCHEZ
(ES)

Dr. J.A. BERCIANO (ES)

Dr. F.J. FIGOLS (ES)

Prof. M. GUTIERREZ-
MOLINA & Dr. C. MORALES-
BASTOS (ES)

Prof A. BRUN (SE)

Prof. K. KRISTENSSON (SE)

Prof. Y. OLSSON (SE)

Dr. E.C. GESSAGA (CH)

Prof. R.C. JANZER (CH)

Prof. P. KLEIHUES (CH)

Dr. B. OESCH (CH)

Dr. G. PIZZOLATO &
Dr. A. CAROTA (CH)

Prof. J. ULRICH (CH)

Prof. M. VANDEVELDE (CH)

Prof. Ch. WEISSMANN (CH)

Dr. P.V. BEST (UK)

Prof. L.W. DUCHEN &
Dr. F. SCARAVILLI (UK)

Dr. M.M. ESIRI (UK)

Prof. P.L. LANTOS (UK)

Prof R.O. WELLER (UK)

CONCERTED ACTION TO SUPPORT RESEARCH ON THE MOLECULAR GENETIC BASIS OF THE LATE ONSET AUTOSOMAL DOMINANT CEREBELLAR ATAXIAS

Key words
Neurodegenerative disorders, autosomal dominant cerebellar ataxia, SCAI and SCA2 genes, clinical phenotype.

Brief description
Autosomal dominant cerebellar ataxia (ADCA) is a genetically heterogeneous group of autosomal dominant neurodegenerative disorders determining cerebellar ataxia.
The overall goal of this Concerted Action program is to define the molecular genetic basis of the ADCAS:

1 SCAI, the gene on chromosome 6 that determines one of the ADCAS, has been precisely localized to 6P23, between two highly polymorphic microsatellite markers (STRS) in an interval of 3-4CM that contains 3 other Strs in linkage disequilibrium with the disease locus. SCAI will be precisely localized on physical maps of Yacs, cosmids and restriction fragments of uncloned genomic DNA. Precisely mapped fragments from these maps, suspected of carrying SCAI, will be searched for transcripts likely to be the gene. Sequence information from cdnas found with candidate transcripts will be used to test DNA from patients and controls to find mutations involving one or a few base pair changes. CDNA clones will also be used as probes to search for rearrangements in genomic DNA from patients and controls.

2 SCA2 has recently been localized to chromosome 12q22-q24 by linkage mapping, and this ADCA gene will be precisely genetically localized with Strs mapped to this chromosomal region.

3 Other ADCA genes will be identified by linkage mapping with Strs mapped on all the autosomes.

4 We will attempt to define a clinical phenotype for each identified ADCA locus and for specific mutations existing at each locus.

The project is designed to make available DNA and detailed and uniformly collected clinical data from disease families, physical mapping resources, molecular techniques for characterizing ADCA mutations and highly informative already mapped genetic markers to the participants in order to achieve the above described objectives.

Project leader:
Professor Howard M. CANN
Centre d'Etude du Polymorphisme Humain
27, rue Juliette Dodu
FR 75010 Paris
Phone: +33 1 42 49 98 70
Fax: +33 1 40 18 01 55
Contract number: CT941243

Participants:

Dr. A. BRICE
INSERM U 289, Hôpital de la Salpétrière,
Bâtiment Nouvelle Pharmacie
47 bd de l'Hôpital
FR 75651 Paris Cedex 13

Prof. S. DI DONATO
Divisione di Biochimica e Genetica,
Istituto Nazionale Neurologico C. Besta
via Celoria 11
IT 20133 Milano

Prof. M. FRONTALI
Istituto Medicina Sperimentale, CNR
Viale Marx 15
IT 00137 Roma

Prof. A. HARDING
Institute of Neurology
Queen Square
UK London WC1N 3BG

Prof C. MOROCUTTI
Istituto di Clinica delle Malattie Nervose e
Mentali, Universita la Sapienza
Viale Dell'Universita 30
IT 00185 Roma

Prof. L. TERRENATO
Dipartimento Di Biologia,
Il Universita di Roma Tor Vergata
Via E. Carnevale
IT 00173 Roma

Prof A. ZIEGLER
Inst. of Experimental Oncology and
Transplantation Medicine, Universitätsklinikum
Rudolf Virchow, Standort Charlottenburg
Spandauer Damm 130
DE Berlin 19

PSYCHOTHERAPIES IN EUROPE

Key words
Psychotherapeutic intervention.

Brief description
The aim of this research is to confront the psychoterapeutic approaches in different countries.

The research is divided into two phases: the first one (descriptive) will last one year and it is focused on the assessment of the extent and nature of the variability in structure and processes (resources, organisation, training and practice), cost of psychotherapies and counselling in a sample of public Mental Health Services of European countries. Rates and ratio of patients treated with individual and group psychotherapy proportion of clients suffering of different mental disease, cancer, AIDS and other pathology will be estimated too.

In the second phase, the psychological and social outcome of patients (clients) admitted to psychotherapy and counselling in public Mental Health service across Europe will be evaluated and compared (follow up six months and one year after the beginning of treatment).

A set of instruments - questionnaire, standardized tests, etc. - for evaluating the socio-cultural and structural variables and psychotherapeutic aspects of different psychotherapeutic approaches, will be prepared by researches of different countries. We will develop a common set of outcome tools (tacking into account theoretical aspects of different point of view) to be used for the routine planning and evaluation of psychotherapeutic intervention in Europe. We will also be able to define effectiveness levels (criteria and thereshold of outcome) to which the outcome of one's own psychotherapeutic intervention may be compared across countries and psychotherapeutic schools.

Project leader:
Dr. Marcello CESA-BIANCHI
Istituto di Psicologia,
Facoltà di Medicina,
Università degli Studi di Milano
Via Francesco Sforza 23
IT 20122 Milano
Phone: +39 2799082
Fax: +39 2785481
Contract number: CT941445

Participants:

Prof. M.A. REDA
Istituto di Psicologia Generale e Clinica,
Facoltà Medica, Università di Siena
Piano dei Mantellini 35
IT 53100 Siena
Phone: +39 577 29 80 75
Fax: +39 577 29 80 70

Dr. M. CARTA
Istituto di Clinica Psichiatrica,
Facoltà Medica,
Università degli Studi di Cagliari
Viale Liguria 13
IT 09100 Cagliari
Phone: +39 70 48 51 46
Fax: +39 70 49 62 95

Prof. O. PELC
Service di Psychiatrie, Hospital Brugman
Place Athur Van Gehuchten 4
BE 1020 Brussels
Phone: +32 2 477 27 05
Fax: +32 2 478 51 70

Prof. J.M. CALDAS DE ALMEIDA
Clinica Universitària de Saùde Mental e
Psiquiatria, Universitade Nova de Lisbona,
Facultade de Ciencias Medicas
Calçada de Tapada 155
PT 1300 Lisboa
Phone: +351 1 64 46 51
Fax: +351 1 363 12 64

Dr. M. POWER
Royal Halloway,
University of London
UK Egham TW20 0EX Surrey
Phone: +44 784 44 35 26
Fax: +44 784 43 43 47

Prof. C. PERRIS
Department of Psychiatry III,
University of Umea
SE 901 Umea
Phone: +46 90 10 10 00
Fax: +46 90 10 22 02

Prof. H.U. WITTCHEN
Max-Planck Institut für Psychiatrie,
Klinisches Institut
Kräpelinstrasse 10
DE 80804 München
Phone: +49 89 30 62 2/1
Fax: +49 89 30 62 22 00

Prof. V. KOVESS
Institute National Marcel Riviere
Ches la Verriere
FR 78320 Le Mesnil Saint Denis
Phone: +33 1 34 61 18 18
Fax: +33 1 34 61 38 18

NEURONAL ACETYCHOLINE NICOTINIC RECEPTORS IN THE BRAIN: INTERACTIONS WITH DOPAMINERGIC RECEPTORS

Key words
Nicotinic acetylcholine receptors, dopaminergic system interaction, transgenic animals, cell culture.

Brief description
Central nicotinic acetylcholine receptors are increasingly recognized as functional to the function of mammalian central nervous system, in particular in circuits related to reward and higher cognitive functions. Accordingly, nicotinic transmission is thought to be involved in two highly relevant medical problems, cigarette smoke and Alzheimer's dementia. Many studies have shown that nicotine reinforcing effects are mediated through the central dopaminergic system.

The working hypothesis of this project is that the interplay between nicotine and dopamine in meso-cortico-limbic systems is mediated by an interaction between nicotinic and dopaminergic receptors. This interaction will be examined in animal experimental systems *in vivo* (normal and transgenic animals) as well as in cell cultures (primary and transfected cells), in animal models of human pathologies (nicotine dependence, nicotine prenatal exposure, aging), and in human fetal, embryonic and perinatal material.

Methods of molecular biology, biochemistry, chemical neuroanatomy, microdialysis and electrophysiology will be used to assess the presence of a relevant interactions between these two types of receptors at genomic, second messenger, and membrane levels.

Project leader:
Dr. Jean-Pierre CHANGEUX
Institut Pasteur, Molecular Neurobiology Laboratory
rue du Docteur Roux 25
FR Paris 75724 Cédex 15
Phone: +33 1 45 68 88 05
Fax: +33 1 45 68 88 36
Contract number: CT941060

Participants:
Dr. A. FAIRÉN
Consejo Superior de Investigaciones
Cientificas, Instituto Cajal
Av. Doctor Arce 37
ES 28002 Madrid
Phone: +34 1 585 47 05
Fax: +34 1 585 47 54

Dr. A. DE LA CALLE
Universidad de Malaga, Department of Cellular
Biology, Campus Universitario de Teatinos
ES 29071 Malaga
Phone: +34 1 213 19 56
Fax: +34 1 213 20 00

Dr. K. FUXE
Karolinska Institutet, Department of
Neuroscience, Division of Cellular
and Molecular Neurochemistry
Doktorsringen 12
SE 171 77 Solna
Phone: +46 8 728 70 77
Fax: +46 8 33 79 41

NEUROENDOCRINOLOGY OF STRESS AND DEPRESSION: BASIC AND CLINICAL STUDIES

Key words
Chemic stress, depression, neurochemical, neurophysiological mechanisms.

Brief description
The maintenance of homeostasis in response to stressors is under a coordinated control of neural and endocrine (i.e. neuroendocrine) systems. It is believed that if communication within these systems deranges, such as that occuring in depressed subjects, hormone-dependent gene-mediated central mechanisms come into action that may precipitate into mental disorders such as depression, symptoms of which include severe changes in sleep patterns, in eating, sexual and cognitive behavioural patterns.

This project is aimed at gaining better understanding of the neurochemical and neurophysiological mechanisms (at the level of brain, pituitary and adrenals) involved in chronic stress and in the genesis and maintenance of depression.

The proposed project co-ordinates research, which extends from laboratories to clinics, on the neuro-endocrinology of stress and depression at different levels of biological complexity.

The project combines five well-defined research programmes, in six countries, which are aimed at examining the various levels of biological organization involved in the pathophysiology of depression. These programmes are:
1 Handling of stressful information and behaviour;
2 Chemical and molecular markers for behaviour;
3 Pharmacological manipulations of neuronal circuits underlying behavioural adaptation;
4 Cellular and molecular mechanisms of action, and;
5 Clinical studies.

Stress is one of the main causes of pathology, notably for its connection with mental breakdown and cardiovascular diseases, especially in the elderly.

The findings of this project will path the way to the formulation of new drugs (therapeutic purposes in depression.

Project leader:
Professor E.R. DE KLOET
Centre for Drug Research,
University of Leiden
P.O. Box 9503
NL 2300 RA Leiden
Phone: +31 71 27 62 10
Fax: +31 71 27 62 92
Contract number: CT941108

Participants:
Prof. L. ANGELUCCI
Pharmacology 2A, Faculty of
Medicine and Surgery
Piazzale Aldo Moro
IT 00185 Rome
Phone: +39 6 4991 25 96
Fax: +39 6 494 05 88

Prof. S. LIGHTMAN
Department of Medicine,
Bristol Royal Infirmary
UK Bristol BS2 8HW
Phone: +44 272 28 28 71
Fax: +44 272 28 22 12

Dr. J.A. FUENTES
Dpto. de Farmacologia, Fac.
Farmacia, Universidad
Complutense de Madrid
Ciudad Universitaria
ES 28040 Madrid
Phone: +34 1 394 17 66
Fax: +34 1 394 17 42

Prof. F. HOLSBOER
Max Planck Institute of Psychiatry, Clinical Institute
Kraepelinstrasse 2
DE 80804 Munich 40
Phone: +49 89 3062 22 20
Fax: +49 89 3062 24 83

Prof. W. ROSTENE
INSERM, Research Centre
Paris Saint Antoine
184 rue du Faubourg Saint
Antoine
FR 75571 Paris Cedex 11
Phone: +33 1 4928 46 00
Fax: +33 1 4343 32 34

A STUDY OF SKEW AND TORSIONAL EYE MOVEMENTS, VISUAL IMPAIRMENT AND SPATIAL DISORIENTATION IN NORMAL SUBJECTS AND PATIENTS WITH OPHTHALMOLO-GICAL, OTOLOGICAL AND NEUROLOGICAL DISEASE

Key words
Eye disorders, head movement, perception, neurophysiological techniques, patho-physiology.

Objectives
We are lacking in our understanding of the various mechanisms of these disorders, in appropriate diagnostic techniques and how the disorders relate to associated problems of posture and balance. Accordingly, the specific targets of the study are:

A What are the control mechanisms and respective dynamics of cyclovertical eye movements and head movement responses to tilt? What does the subject perceive with skew and torsion of the eyes and body tilt? How do the eyes move vertically and skew and tort under normal Circumstances in response to head movements and structure of the visual field and how well is cyclovertical tropia is maintained by the brain in the absence of bin- or monocular vision?

B How do vestibular signals of head motion (i.e in roll eardown-to shoulder) and tilt influence cyclovertical eye movement and head posture and interact with visual cues to fusion and motion.

C How do eye position and vestibular signals combine to give perception of verticality and cues to orthostatic posture in the roll plane. How this may become disordered in ophthalmic, neurological and otological disease and its interrelationship with postural instability.

D To determine what derangements of visual, vestibular or tropic mechanisms are involved in patients with central neurological disease involving cyclovertical eye movement, deranged head posture and perceptual disorders of verticality.

E The inputs to vertical coordination are vision, vestibular signals of head roll and tilt and central mechanisms of orthotropic alignment. The areas of the nervous system where lesion affects roll coordination are notably the cerebellum, brainstem and midbrain, the peripheral vestibular apparatus and visual and oculomotor pathways. Hence, what are the relationships between these functions in perceiving the earth-vertical? and what are the differential effects of individual derangements? Via imaging of pathological processes affecting these structures together with clinical neurophysiological techniques we aim to determine the functional anatomy of the organisation of head-eyeperceptual verticality.

Brief description
Ophthalmological, otological and neurological disease may cause disorders of eye and head movement and perception which affect patients upright orientation. The consequences of such disorientation may be abnormal postural tilt, imbalance, ataxia, latero-pulsion and susceptibility to falling. Cyclovertical heterotropias of the eyes may provoke diplopia and torsional and skewing nystagmus. The patient may also experience poor localisation of the direction of verticality and postural instability.

The mechanisms controlling vertical orientation of the eyes head and body and how they become disordered by disease are poorly understood. The purpose of this concerted action is to investigate these mechanisms.

Eye movement disorders affecting vertical orientation are referred to as the 'cyclovertical disorders' and include abnormal torsion (rotation about the optical axis) and skew (differential movement in vertical directions) which give rise to diplopia (caused by 'heterotropic' positions of the eyes) and are associated with false perception of orientation and disorders of postural control. These disorders are poorly understood, impart disabling symptoms to patients and are difficult to treat. Skew and torsional disorders may arise from dysfunction of the extraocular muscles, imbalance of peripheral and central nervous vestibular signals controlling reflex eye movements and lesions of the central nervous system affecting the motor mechanisms responsible for aligning the eyes in orthotropia but understanding the principles of how to interpret a particular case, especially involving neurological pathology, are lacking.

Disorders of head posture and movement with respect to earth vertical correspond to problems with eye movement and include abnormal head tilts (associated with postural abnormalities of the whole body) and torticollis. Mechanisms governing head movement are even less well understood than those for eyes but a significant contribution is thought to be derived from the vestibular system, some neck dystonias, for example may be profoundly modulated by altered position of the head with respect to gravity.

Complementary to motor disturbances are perceptual derangements of orientation and relative motion of the self (body and head axes) and the external world which are equally implicated in diseases affecting eye-head coordination.

In many instances it is not known whether a disorder of balance is a consequence of disordered perception of orientation or an independent derangement caused by common underlying pathophysiological mechanisms.

This proposal is for a concerted interdisciplinary study of cyclovertical eye movements, head posture and tilt, associated perceptual consequences and relationship to diseases of the nervous system and of the eyes and ears.

Project leader:
Dr. M. GRESTY
MRC, Human Movement and Balance Unit,
Institut of Neurology
8-11 Queen Square
UK London WC1N 3BG
Phone: +44 71 837 36 11
Fax: +44 71 837 72 81
Contract number: CT941179

Participants:

Prof. Eberhard KOENIG
Neurologische Universitatsklinik,
Abteilung Allgemeine Neurologie
Hoppe-Seyler-Strasse 3
DE 7400 Tubingen
Phone: +49 7071 292 057
Fax: +49 7071 352 136

Prof. Thomas BRANDT
Dept. of Neurology, Klinikum Grossharden,
University of Munich
Marchionistrasse 15
DE 8000 Munchen
Phone: +49 8970 952 571
Fax: 649 8970 958 883

EUROTAURINE: REGULATION AND FUNCTION OF TAURINE IN THE MAMMALIAN CENTRAL NERVOUS SYSTEM

Key words
Taurine, synthesis, metabolism, pharmacological actions, neuroprotectim, central nervous system.

Brief description
Taurine (2-aminoethanesulphonic acid) is present in relatively high concentrations in the brain.

Despite quite extensive studies of its synthesis, release in response to nerve stimulation and possible neuronal or extraneuronal uptake, there still is no consensus regarding its function(s).

It has variously been designated as a neurotransmitter, neuromodulator, osmo-regulator or an antioxidant.

It is also reported to have anticonvulsant and, perhaps, actions.

This project concerns the assessment of the modes of action of taurine by a combined chemical, enzymological, neurochemical, neuroanatomical, pharmacological and toxicological approach.

The synthesis of novel taurine analogues will be used to define the behaviour of the system in more detail and in attempts to manipulate taurine levels in the CNS.

These compounds will also be assessed for their potential as therapeutic agents, either as a result of their direct mimetic actions or their effects on central taurine levels.

The specific and interrelated objectives are summarised below:

a Synthesis of novel taurine derivatives and analogues for assessing the roles and metabolism of taurine and their pharmaceutical potential. These compounds will also be used in studies of the catabolism of taurine under different physiological conditions.

b Investigations of the release, uptake and binding of taurine in the basal ganglia and the effects of the synthetic analogues on these processes.

c Studies on the pharmacological actions of taurine with particular stress on its possible actions as a modulator of calcium-ion mediated processes and anticonvulsant behaviour.

d Investigation of the neuroprotective effects of taurine using tissue slices and in vivo systems exposed to oxidative, osmotic and neurotoxic insult.

These studies will also involve biochemical and neuroanatomical investigations of the distribution and redistribution of taurine in stressed systems and an investigation of the effects on the respiratory burst in reactive glial cells, which can represent a source of toxic oxygen radicals. Alterations of the levels of taurine and its metabolites will also be determined in postmortem human brain samples as a function of age and neurodegenerative disease status.

Project leader:
Professor Laura DELLA CORTE
Università degli Studi di Firenze, Dip. Farmacologia Preclinia e Clinica, 'Mario Alazzi-Mancini'
Viale Morgagni 65
IT 50134 Firenze
Phone: +39 55 41 11 33
Fax: +39 55 43 16 13
Contract number: CT941402

Participants:

Prof. K.F. TIPTON
Department of Biochemistry,
University of Dublin,
Trinity College
IE Dublin 2
Phone: +353 1 702 16 08
Fax: +353 1 677 24 00

Dr. H.B.F. DIXON
Department of Biochemistry,
University of Cambridge
Tennis Court Road
UK Cambridge CB2 1QW
Phone: +44 223 33 36 72
Fax: +44 223 33 33 45

Dr. M. PALMI
Istituto Policattedra di Scienze Farmacologiche,
Università di Siena
via E. Piccolomini 170
IT 53100 Siena
Phone: +39 577 22 12 55
Fax: +39 577 28 19 28

Dr. P. BOLAM
Department of Pharmacology,
University of Oxford
Mansfield Road
UK Oxford OX1 3TH
Phone: +44 865 27 18 69
Fax: +44 865 27 16 47

QUALITY ASSURANCE (QA) IN CONSULTATION LIAISON PSYCHIATRY AND PSYCHOSOMATICS (CL). DEVELOPMENT AND IMPLEMENTATION OF A EUROPEAN QA SYSTEM

Key words
Psychiatry, psychomatics, Quality Assurance programme.

Brief description
10 to 15% of non-psychiatric general hospital (GH) in patients need special assessment or treatment of mental health disorders and problems to be provided by consultation liaisonu services (CL). CL can significantly improve diagnosis and treatment and reduce costs. Across Europe, approaches to the integration of physical, mental and social health care in the GH through CL and the relative importance given to it (e.g. training, allocation of resources) differ Widely. There are no agreed standards for the adequacy of such care and no reliable, valid and feasible system for it's routine documentation (process, outcome) in a clinically relevant Way. Moreover, there are virtually no European quality assurance (QA) programs sensu strictu in mental health generally.
The proposed study addresses these issues. It will build on experiences, research instruments and a large data-base of an earlier Concerted Action. It will develop and field-test a set of simple, reliable and valid instruments for QA (questionnaires re hospital and CL service characteristics, course and outcome of case-episodes, documentation of audit cycles) and formulate European and local standards for CL (consensus meetings). Based on these it will initiate and QA using a quasi-experimental design. At leas one pair of matched services each from Norway, United Kingdom, the Netherlands, Germany, Italy, Spain and potugal will participate with consecutive CL episodes, to be split into the QA-group and the NO-QA-group. After baseline assessment regular feedback will be provided to the QA group only (9 month) as basis for an audit cycle. Implementation of QA programs will be monitored and evaluated. Feedback to both groups and review at the end of data collection will be used for readjustment of standards and instruments.
The study will provide a feasible European instrument for documentation of strucural, process and outcome quality in CL and initiate a European process of the continuing development and evaluation of practices and standards. It will help to improve professional training and other structural standards of mental health care for GH patients on European and national levels. It should provide a paradigm for QA research and implementation in mental health care delivery generally.

Project leader:
Dr. Thomas HERZOG
Abt. Psychotherapie und Psychosomatische Medizin,
Psychiatrische Universitätsklinik
Hauptstrasse 8
DE 7800 Freiburg
Phone: +49 761 2706866
Fax: +49 761 2706885
Contract number: CT941706

Participants:
Dr. F.J. HUYSE
Free University Hospital,
Department of CL Psychiatry
De Boelelaan 1117
P.O. Box 7057
NL 1007 MB Amsterdam

Dr. G. CARDOSO
Hospital de Santa Maria,
Departamento de Psiquiatria de Ligacao,
Servicio de Psiquiatria
Av. Egas Moniz
PT 1699 Lisboa Codex

Prof. F. CREED
University of Manchester, Department of
Psychiatry, Manchester Royal Infirmary,
Rawnsley Building
Oxford Road
UK Manchester M13 9WL

Prof. U.F. MALT
The National Hospital, Department of
Psychosomatic and Behavioral Medicine
Pilestredet 32
NO 0027 Oslo

Prof. M. RIGATELLI
Clinica Psichiatrica,
Modena School of Medicine
Via del Pozzo 71
IT 41100 Modena

Prof. A. LOBO
Hospital Clinico Universitario,
Department of Psychiatry
Planta 11
ES 50009 Zaragoza

MECHANISMS OF CHRONIC PAIN IN RELATIONSHIP TO CHRONIC PAIN DISORDERS OF GREAT SOCIO-ECONOMIC IMPACT

Key words
Chronic pain, glutamate, serotin, substance P, CGRP, excitotoxic lesion, hyperalgesia.

Brief description
Disorders with pain as the main disabling symptom (for example low back pain and fibromyalgia) are a major health problem in the industrialized countries. Since they are one of the main causes for longlasting sick leave and disability pensions these diseases are of great socio-economic impact.
The aim of this project is through concerted actions to improve the understanding of the causes and mechanisms of these illnesses related to neurologic and mental disorders. This knowledge may be the basis for new strategies for development of novel neuropharmacological therapeutic agents as well as for preventive measures for reducing the incidence of occupation-related disease. To achieve this goal the four research groups propose to join forces to study mechanisms of pain regulation in the spinal cord, particularly focused on the dorsal horn. The role of several transmitter substances (glutamate, serotonin, substance P, CGRP), of subgroups of receptors for these substances, and functionally important interactions, as well as mechanisms of plasticity and long term changes, will be studied. It has been hypothesized that longlasting and strong pain may induce excitotoxic lesions of small inhibitory gaba-ergic dorsal horn neurons, due to a great release of excitatory amino acids and possibly an enhancement of this effect by substance P. This may result in increased pain and hyperalgesia. If the experiments show this hypothesis to be correct, this makes possible new strategies for treatment as well as for prevention.
The possibility that chronic pain may develop due to mechanisms in the spinal cord similar to long term potentiation and learning also will be investigated. The role of changes in gene expression in this type of neuronal plasticity will be studied. Electrophysiological, neurochemical and neuroanatomical methods, as well as several behavioural tests of nociception, will be employed.
We expect that after one year and a half we may know whether or not noxious stimulation may result in excitotoxic damage in the dorsal horn, and after three years understand the major mechanisms involved, how to prevent such damage, and suggest how to proceed with clinical investigations.

Project leader:
Dr. Kjell HOLE
Laboratory of
Neurophysiology,
Dept. of Physiology,
University of Bergen
Aarstadveien 19
NO 5009 Bergen
Phone: +47 52 06 412
Fax: +47 52 06 410
Contract number: CT941758

Participants:
Dr. A.H. DICKENSON
Dept. of Pharmacology,
University College London
UK London WC1E 6BT
Phone: +44 71 387 70 50
Fax: +44 71 380 72 98

Prof. E. BRODIN
Department of Pharmacology,
Karolinska Institutet
P.O. Box 60400
SE 104 01 Stockholm
Phone: +46 8 728 79 49
Fax: +46 8 31 71 35

Prof. O.G. BERGE
Astra Pain Control,
Preclinical Research
SE 151 85 Södertälje
Phone: +46 855 32 80 63
Fax: +46 855 32 89 05

HORMONAL AND GENETIC DISORDERS GENDER SPECIFIC BRAIN DIFFERENTIATION

Key words
Brain development, genetic factors, hormonal factors, genetic models.

Brief description
The human brain undergoes sexual differentiation during early development. As in many mammalian species sex hormones such as steroids are believed to have organizing effects on human hypothalamic neurones. Certain relevant conditions such as Turner Klinefelter and the androgen insensitivity syndromes also affect development suggestlng a role for hormones. Abnormalities in steroid condition of the human fetus or in the sensitivity of target cells in the brain caused by lack of steroid receptors disrupt the direction of neuroanatomical sex differentiation and behavioural sex orientation.

We shall study genetic and epigenetic (hormonal) factors which influence brain development with special reference to the sexual differentiation of hypothalamic neurones in areas related to behaviour.

The work will focus on steroid hormones, androgen, oestrogens and corticosteroids, which are known to be key agents in brain differentiation and neural plasticity both during fetal and in early postnatal development. Normal brain differentiation will be studied and the effects of certain abnormal endocrine conditions both in development and ageing, on sex differentiation of the human brain. Particular emphasis will be placed on enzymes forming neuroactive steroids in hypothalamic areas and the receptors required for their actions. The conversion of androgen to oestrogen by aromatase within hypothalamic cells is a key regulatory proces in brain differentiation. Specific imaging methods for measuring human hypothalamic nuclei are available for this project to allow immunocytochemical localisation of aromatase and oestrogen receptors within cells of the developing brain.

Concurrent experimental work using animal models will define developmental changes in formation of neuroactive steroid metabolites and their receptors. Primary cell culture will be used to study steroid effects on hypothalamic neurone development. Genetic models (e.g. the TFM mouse model for androgen insensitivity) will be used to study androgen receptor deficits in the brain. In addition, gene cloning and sequencing techniques will be employed to prepare CDNA probes for steroid-metabolising enzymes (notably aromatase) and steroid receptors to localize gene expression at critical developmental phases of steroid.

Project leader:
Dr. John HUTCHISON
MRC Neuroendocrine Development and Behaviour Group,
Institute of Animal,
Physiology and Genetics Research
Babraham
UK Cambridge CB2 4AT
Phone: +44 223 832312
Fax: +44 223 836122
Contract number: CT941536

Participants:

Dr. J. KOOLHAAS
Dept. of Animal Physiology, Biologisch
Centrum, University of Groningen
P.O. Box 14
NL 9750 AA Haren
Phone: +31 50 63 23 40
Fax: +31 50 63 52 05

Dr. SWAAB
Netherlands Institute for Brain Research
Meibergdreef 33
NL 1105 AZ Amsterdam
Phone: +31 20 566 55 00
Fax: +31 20 691 84 66

Dr. REISERT
Abteilung Anatomie und Zellbiologie,
Universität Ulm (Medical Faculty)
Albert-Einstein-Allee
DE 7900 Ulm
Phone: +49 731 502 32 20
Fax: +49 731 502 32 17

Dr. PILGRIM
Abteilung Anatomie und Zellbiologie,
Universität Ulm (Medical Faculty)
Albert-Einstein-Allee
DE 7900 Ulm
Phone: +49 731 502 32 20
Fax: +49 731 502 32 17

Dr. VAZQUEZ
Departamento de Anatomia e Histologia
Humanas, Facultad de Medicina,
Universidad de Salamanca
Avda. del Campo Charro
ES 37007 Salamanca
Phone: +34 23 29 45 46
Fax: +34 23 29 45 59

Dr. STEIMER
Division of Psychopharmacology, Institut
Universitaire Psychiatrie de Geneve
8 Chemin du Petit-bel-Air
CH 1225 Chene Bourg Geneva
Phone: +41 22 48 33 11 Ext. 226
Fax: +41 22 305 53 98

PHYSIOLOGY AND PHARMACOLOGY OF BRAIN ADENOSINE RECEPTORS. IMPLICATIONS FOR THE RATIONAL DESIGN OF NEUROACTIVE DRUGS (ADEURO)

Key words
Brain, adenosine receptors physiopathology, synthesis, design, molecules.

Brief description
The envisaged research in this Concerted Action 'ADEURO' addresses research tasks under the headings 2d and 2e in the work-programme, viz. molecular neuro-biological, neuro-psychopharmacological, and neuro-endocrinological aspects of adenosine receptor function in the brain. Particular emphasis is on age-related diseases. Our integrated approach uniting 13 teams in 7 member states, will allow a truly transnational collaboration of multiple disciplines. Our strategy may prove useful for other brain receptors as well, and could serve as a pilot case for a general strategy in drug research.

The goals of the proposed CA are two fold:
- a better understanding of the function and role of adenosine receptors in the brain, particularly with respect to (patho)physiological conditions in the elderly (e.g., vascular and senile dementia, stroke, sleep, and dopamine-related diseases)
- the rational design and synthesis of key molecules (lead compounds), from which future drugs will be derived.

Project leader:
Dr. A.P. IJZERMAN
Centre for Bio-Pharmaceutical Sciences,
Div. of Medicinal Chemistry
P.O. Box 9502
NL 2300 RA Leiden
Phone: +31 71 274651
Fax: +31 71 274277
Contract number: CT941153

Participants:
Dr. M.P. ABBRACCHIO
University of Milan,
Department of Pharmacology
Via Balzaretti 9
IT 20133 Milan
Phone: +39 2 2048 83 74
Fax: +39 2 2940 49 61

Prof. F. CATTABENI
University of Milan,
Dept. of Pharmacology
Via Balzaretti 9
IT 20133 Milan
Phone: +39 2 2048 83 74

Prof. G. CRISTALLI
University of Camerino,
Dip. di Scienze Chimiche
Via S. Agostino 1
IT 62032 Camerino (MC)
Phone: +39 737 403 55
Fax: +39 737 373 45

Dr. M. DANHOF
LACDR, Div. of Pharmacology
P.O. Box 9503
NL 2300 RA Leiden
Phone: +31 71 27 26 22
Fax: +31 71 27 62 14

Prof. B.B. FREDHOLM
Karolinska Institute,
Dept. of Pharmacology
P.O. Box 60400
SE 104 01 Stockholm
Phone: +46 8 32 29 04
Fax: +46 8 33 16 53

Dr. M. FREISSMUTH
University Wien,
Inst. of Pharmacology
Wahringer Strasse 13a
AT 1090 Vienna
Phone: +43 1 404 80 Ext. 298
Fax: +43 1 402 48 33

Prof. K. FUXE
Karolinska Institute,
Inst. for Histology and Neurobiology
P.O. Box 60400
SE 10401 Stockholm
Phone: +46 8 34 05 60
Fax: +46 8 33 79 41

Prof. U. HACKSELL
Biomed. Center Uppsala,
Dept. of Org. Pharm. Chemistry
SE 75123 Uppsala
Phone: +46 855 32 74 39
Fax: +46 855 284 50

Prof. P. HERDEWIJN
Rega Instituut, Kath. Universiteit Leuven
Minderbroedersstraat 10
BE 3000 Leuven
Phone: +32 163 373 41
Fax: +32 163 33 73

Dr. M. LOHSE
Universität München,
Lab. für Molekulare Biologie,
Max Planck Inst. für Biochemie
DE 85152 Martinsried
Phone: +49 89 8578 39 41
Fax: +49 89 8578 37 95

Prof. G. PEPEU
Univ. degli Studi di Firenze,
Dip. di Farmacologia
Viale G.B. Morgagni
IT 50134 Florence
Phone: +39 5 541 11 33
Fax: +39 5 436 16 13

Prof. J.A. RIBEIRO
Inst. Gulbenkian de Ciencia,
Dept. of Pharmacology
Rua da Quinta Grande
PT 2781 Oeiras
Phone: +351 1443 07 07
Fax: +351 1443 16 31

Prof. U. SCHWABE
Universität Heidelberg,
Dept. of Pharmacology
Im Neuenheimer feld 366
DE 6900 Heidelberg
Phone: +49 6221 56 39 03
Fax: +49 6221 56 39 44

BORNA DISEASE VIRUS INFECTION AS ETIOLOGICAL FACTOR OF NEUROLOGICAL DISEASES IN MEN AND ANIMALS

Key words
Borna Disease Virus, BDV-specific antibodies, human, animals.

Brief description
The goal of this common project is to study the relationship of borna disease virus (BDV) or a BDV-like agent to neurological disorders in man. Such a combined approach, involving different scientific groups throughout Europe is justified since BDV infection as an animal disease has been studied in great detail. BDV is known to cause a non-purulent mening oencephalomyelitis in horses and sheep.

Furthermore it could successfully be transmitted to a variety of experimental animals. Most recently the clinical neurological picture of a cat disease could also be shown to be related to an at least BDV-like agent.

Over the last five years different research groups contributed to the assumption that a BDV infection exists in man. Our group has been able to demonstrate that the prevalence of BDV-specific antibodies in patients is associated with a certain pattern of disease symptoms. Furthermore by using BDV-specific monoclonal antibodies we have been able to demonstrate the existence of BDV antigen in such patients.

The available data so far suggests that BDV or BDV-like infections occur in man as well as in animals and are spread worldwide involving different patient groups. Based on previous studies of our and th operating groups in Italy, Sweden, and Spain this common project provides the unique chance to illucidate a well characterized animal virus infection and its relationship to similar infections in man. Each of the four groups contributes from its great scientific experience and potention. The Berlin group with its longtime knowledge on such animal and human infections will contribute to this project with its know-how and provide the organisatorical background for the total project.

Project leader:
Professor Hans LUDWIG
Institut für Virologie
Nordufer 20
DE 1000 Berlin 65
Phone: +49 30 4503 301
Fax: +49 30 4503 328
Contract number: CT941791

Participants:

Dr. M. CARAMELLI
Istituto Zooprofilattico
Sperimentale del Piemonte,
Liguria e Valle d'Aosta
Via Bologna 148
IT 10154 Torino
Phone: +39 11 268 62 51
Fax: +39 11 24 87 70

Dr. F. CRUZ-SANCHEZ
Banco de Tejidos
Neurologicos,
Universidad de Barcelona,
Hospital Clinico y Provincial
Villarroel 170
ES 08036 Barcelona
Phone: +34 34 54 70 00
Fax: +34 34 51 52 72

Dr. A.L. LUNDGREN
Dept. of Pathology, Swedish
University of Agric. Sciences
P.O. Box 7028
SE 75007 Uppsala
Phone: +46 18 67 21 77
Fax: +46 18 67 35 32

THE FAMILY OF THE SCHIZOPHRENIC PATIENT: OBJECTIVE AND SUBJECTIVE BURDEN AND COPING STRATEGIES

Key words
Schizophrenia, relative, burden, coping strategies.

Brief description
The proposed study aims to explore the objective and subjective burden on the relatives of schizophrenic patients, and the coping strategies of these relatives, in different geographic contexts and in relation to different patterns of psychiatric care.

Recruitment will be performed, within each centre, in an outpatient unit. Every consecutive patient attending the unit during a 12-month period will be asked to participate, If meeting the following criteria:

a age between 18 and 50 years;

b diagnosls of schizophrenia according to ICD-10, verified by present State Examination (PSE-10);

c presence of at least one adult relative living with the patient and having contacts with him/her at least five days/week during the last year;

d no hospitalization during the last month;

e absence of disabling physical or psychiatric diseases or drug abuse in the relatives living with the patient.

Patient will provide their informed consent by signing an appropriate form, whose content will be fully explained to them. For each patient recruited in the study, the key-relative will be contacted and asked to participate in the project. In each enrolled patient, the psycho-patological status will be assessed by means of the PSE-10, and the degree of social disability will be evaluated by administering the Disability Assessment Schedule to the key-relative. In each key-relative, the psycho-pathological status will be also evaluated by the PSE-10 and the global physical status by the Health Status Index. Moreover, each key-relatives will compile the Questionnaire on Family Problems and the Family Coping Questioñnaire. A socio-demographic schedule will also be compiled for each patient and each key-relative. The pattern of care available in each centre will be characterized by means of an ad-hoc schedule, based on the World Health Organlzation Quality Assurance Criteria for Mental Health Services.

Project leader:
Professor Mario MAJ
Dept of Psychiatry, First Medical School,
University of Naples
Largo Madonna delle Grazie
IT 80138 Napels
Phone: +39 81 566 65 02
Fax: +39 81 449 938
Contract number: CT941615

Participants:
Dr. G. FADDEN
Aylesbury Valle Community Healthcare,
NHS Trust, The Tindal Centre
Bierton Road
UK Aylsebury Bucks HP20 1HU
Phone: +44 29 63 93 363
Fax: +44 29 63 99 332

Prof. J.M. CALDAS DE ALMEIDA
Clinica Univ. de Saude Mental e Psiquiatria,
Fac. de Ciencias Medicas,
Univ. Nova de Lisboa
Calcada da Tapada 155
PT 1300 Lisboa
Phone: +351 11 36 44 651
Fax: +351 11 36 31 264

Dr. M. MICHAEL
Community Mental Health Center,
Faculty of Medicine, University of Athens
14 Delou Street Kessariani
GR 16121 Athens
Phone: +30 17 64 01 11
Fax: +30 17 66 28 29

Dr. T. HELD
Landschaftsverband Rheinland,
Rheinische Landesklinik Bonn
Postfach 170169
DE 53027 Bonn
Phone: +49 228 551 21 00
Fax: +49 228 551 24 84

A MULTI-CENTRE ASSOCIATION STUDY OF THE
MOLECULAR GENETICS OF SCHIZOPHRENIA

Key words
Schizophrenia, molecular genetics, multi-centre association study.

Brief description
A powerful, multi-centre association study of schizophrenia is proposed using a candidate gene approach. The sample will comprise 1,500 schizophrenics (DSM-III-R) and 1,500 controls. Detailed phenotypic information will be collected on each patient using standard diagnostic techniques. Patients and controls will be comprehensively matched. The Haplotype Relative Risk method will be utilised to further control for the possible effects of population stratification. Fifteen candidate genes will be examined with an initial emphasis on genes involved in the dopamine system.

Recent research strongly suggests that genes of moderate to minor effect play a significant role in the aetiology of schizophrenia. It is suggested that using the association paradigm in combination with a very powerful sample, provides the only viable means of detecting genes of minor effect.

Project leader:
Professor Peter McGUFFIN
Institute of Psychological
Medicine,
College of Medicine,
University of Wales
Heath Park
UK Cardiff CF4 4XN
Phone: +44 222 74 77 47
Fax: +44 222 74 78 39
Contract number: CT941556

Participants:
Dr. WIILLIAMS, dr. OWEN
& dr. FARMER
Institute of Psychological
Medicine,
College of Medicine,
University of Wales
Heath Park
UK Cardiff CF4 4XN
Phone: +44 222 747 747
Fax: +44 222 747 839

Dr. MACCIARDI,
dr. CAVALLINI,
dr. CAULI & dr VERGA
Dip. Science Neuropsichich,
Univ degli Studi di Milan
Via Prinetti 29
IT 20147 Milan
Phone: +39 2 2643 1000
Fax: +39 2 2643 3265

Prof. PROPPING,
dr NOTHEN, dr KORNER
& dr RIETSCHEL
Institute of Human Genetics,
University of Bonn
Wilhelmstrasse 31
DE 5300 Bonn 1
Phone: +49 22 8287 2346
Fax: +49 22 8287 2380

Dr. Harald ASCHAUER
Psychiatrische
Universitatsklinik,
Universitat Wien
Wahringer Gurtel 18-20
AT 1090 Wien
Phone: +43 40 400 3560
Fax: +43 40 400 3560

Dr. Ole MORS
Inst. Psychiatric Demograp.,
Aarhus Psychiatric Hosp.
Skovagervej 2
DK 8240 Risskov
Phone: +45 86 17 7777
Fax: +45 86 17 5977

Dr. Jacques MALLET
Lab de Genetique
Moleculaire de la
Neurotransmission, CNRS
1 Ave de la Tewrrasse
FR 91198 Gif Sur Yvette
Phone: +33 1 6982 3646
Fax: +33 1 6982 3580

Prof. Costas STEFANIS
Dept. of Psychiatry,
Athens Univ Medical School
72 Vas. Sophia
GR 11528 Athens
Phone: +30 1 721 7763
Fax: +30 1 724 9902

Dr. PATO, dr. COEHLO
dr. AZEVEDO
Dept. of Psychiatry,
Faculdade de Medicina,
Universidad de Coimbra
PT 3049 Coimbra Cedex
Phone: +351 39 28 121
Fax: +351 39 23 236

Dr. Mike GILL
Genetics Section, Institute of
Psychiatry, De Crespigny
Park, Denmark Hill
UK London SE5 8AF
Phone: +44 71 703 5411
Fax: +44 71 703 5796

PSYCHIATRIC REHABILITATION-STANDARDIZATION OF PROCEDURES FOR THE ASSESSMENT OF ACTIVITIES AND COSTS/BENEFITS

Key words
Psychiatric rehabilitation, activities assessment, cost, benefits.

Brief description
With the transfer of psychiatric assistance from the mental hospital to community-based care, psychiatric rehabilitation has gained considerable theoretical and economic relevance.

The principle objectives of our project are the following:

A   to determine,in a measurable and comparable form, what specific psychiatric rehabilitation activities are being carried out in European facilities working in this sphere;

B   to define a methodology for the multiaxial evalutation(socio-economic, individual and familial) of the cost and benefits of the various psychiatric rehabilitation programs currently being implemented within the EEC.

Reaching these goals requires the designing, testing and validation in the five participating countries of two ad hoc instruments, as appropriate means of assessment are currently unavailable.

Project leader:
Dr. Carmine MUNIZZA
Centro Studi e Ricerche in Psichiatria,
Servizio Sanitario Nazionale,
Regione Piemonte USSL Torino VI
Piazza Donatori del Sangue 3
IT 10155 Torino
Phone: +39 11 201044
Fax: +39 11 2426846
Contract number: CT941304

Participants:

Dr. P. DE JONG
Dept. of Social Psychiatry,
Faculty of Medicine,
University of Groningen
Oostersingel 59
P.O. Box 30.001
NL 9700 RB Groningen
Phone: +31 50 61 20 79
Fax: +31 50 69 67 27

Prof. C. PERRIS
University of Umea,
Dept. of psychiatry III
SE 901 85 Umea
Phone: +46 9010 10 00
Fax: +46 9010 22 02

Prof. L. SALVADOR
CIM-PROM/Universidad de
Cadiz, Edif. CYCAS 7°D
Urb. El Bosque
ES 11405 Jerez de la Fra
Phone: +34 56 30 02 17
Fax: +34 56 22 31 39

Dr. G. THORNICROFT
PRISM, Institute of
Psychiatry
De Crespigny Park
Denmark Hill
UK London DE5 8AF
Phone: +44 71 703 54 11
Fax: +44 71 277 14 62

Dr. M. VON CRANACH
Bezirkskrankenhaus
Kaufbeuren, Fachkranken-
haus für Psychiatrie
und Neurologie
Keumnater Str. 16
Postfach 1143
DE 8950 Kaufbeuren
Phone: +49 834 17 21
Fax: +49 834 172 12 00

Dr. M. KNAPP
PSSRU, The University
Cornwallis Building
UK Kent CT2 7NF
Phone: +44 227 47 54 67
Fax: +44 227 76 43 27

THE ROLE OF LIMBIC TELENCEPHALIC REGIONSIN THE PATHOGENESIS OF PSYCHIATRIC DISEASES OF NEURO-DEVELOPMENTAL AND NEURODEGENERATIVE ORIGIN

Key words
Limbic telencephalic regim, psychiatric diseases, neurodevelopment, neurodegeneration, neurotransmitter.

Brief description
Recent results in physiological, hodological, and behavioural brain research of non-primates and primates including man point to a highly elaborated parallel processing of external or internal sensory stimuli within cortical as well as subcortical structures. To understand the function of the normal and the diseased human brain, it is indispensable to concentrate on a generally excepted psychopathology, to investigate neuropathologically complete hemispheres, to exclude confounding agonal factors, and to focus interdisciplinary research on regions of interest.

Alzheimer's disease, a neurodegenerative disease, and schizophrenia, as neurodevelopmental disease, both afflict limbic as well as paralimbic cortical and subcortical structures. Both diseases occur with a relatively high frequency. They have detrimental effects and are associated with immense care costs. Both diseases represent natural experiments with primary disturbances of limbic neuronal circuits.

The contribution of morphological changes, imbalancies or decreases of neurotransmitters, changes in peptide concentrations or disturbances of neurotrophic factors and the aetio-pathogenic role of trace elements can be only assessed in a multi-disciplinary concerted action on rare human CNS tissue. By means of neuropathological, neuroanatomical, morphological as well as autoradiographic, immunocytochemical, biochemical, pharmacological and molecularbiological methodology this concerted EC-project is aimed at investigating the particular role of the regions of interest (see above) to facilitate psychotic symptoms in a neurodevelopmental (schizophrenia) and neurodegenerative (Alzheimer dementia) disease.

Attention is made' to the dopamine-glutamate, dopamine-GABA and dopamine-neuropeptide interaction. Studies desianed to characterize the molecular biology of dopaminergi D4-receptors in limbic areas are in line with the aforementioned hypotheses. EC-harmonization of post-mortem methodology and clinical prerequisits is highlightened in this Concerted Action. The project cannot be performed on a national basis.

Project leader:
Professor Peter F. RIEDERER
Department of Psychiatry,
Clinical Neurochemistry,
University of Würzburg
Füchsleinstrasse 15
DE 8700 Würzburg
Phone: +49 941 203318
Fax: +49 941 203425
Contract number: CT941563

Participants:

Dr. T. HÖKFELT
Dept. of Histology,
Karolinska Institute
P.O. Box 60500
SE 104 01 Stockholm
Phone: +46 8 728 70 70
Fax: +46 8 33 16 92

Dr. P. EMSON
Medical Research Council
Group, Dept. of
Neurobiology,
Inst. of Animal Physiology
and Genetics Research
Babraham
UK Cambridge CB2 4AT
Phone: +44 223 83 23 12
Fax: +44 223 83 66 14

Dr. G.P. REYNOLDS
School of Biological
Sciences, Dept. of
Biomedical Sciences,
The University of Sheffield
UK Sheffield S10 2TN
Phone: +44 742 76 85 55
Fax: +44 742 76 54 13

Dr. F.F. CRUZ-SANCHEZ
Banco de Tejidos
Neurologicos, Servicio de
Neurologia, Hospital Clinic i
Provincial
Villarroel 170
ES 08036 Barcelona
Phone: +34 3 454 60 00
Fax: +34 3 451 95 54

Prof. KOPP
Université Lyon 1, Fac. de
Medecine Alexis Carrel
Rue Guillaume Paradin
FR 69372 Lyon Cedex 08
Phone: +33 7 874 85 89
Fax: +33 7 877 86 12

Prof. K.F. TIPTON
Biochemistry Department,
Trinity College
IE Dublin 2
Phone: +353 1 77 29 41
Fax: +353 1 77 24 00

Prof. L. CALCZA
Lab. di Fisiopatologia
del Sistema Nervoso,
Hesperia Hospital
Via Arqua 80/A
IT 41100 Modena
Phone: +39 59 39 27 88
Fax: +39 59 39 48 40

Prof. G.L. GESSA
Universita di Cagliari,
Dip. di Neuroscienze
Bernard B. Brodie
Via Procell 4
IT 09124 Cagliari
Phone: +39 70 66 94 70
Fax: +39 70 65 72 37

prof. G.U. CORSINI
Università degli Studie di
Pisa, Cattedra di
Neuropsicofarmacologia
Via Roma 55
IT 56100 Pisa
Phone: +39 50 56 01 09
Fax: +39 50 55 14 34

Prof. K. JELLINGER
LBI for Clinical
Neurobiologie, Lainz hospital
Wolkersbergenstr. 1
AT 1130 Vienna
Phone: +43 1 801 103 431
Fax: +43 1 804 54 01

Prof. D.K. TEHERANI
Österreichisches
Forschungszentrum
Seibersdorf Ges. m.b.H.
AT 2444 Seibersdorf
Phone: +43 2254 780 3509
Fax: +43 2254 780 74060

Prof. F. GERSTENBRAND
Department of Neurology,
University of Innsburck
Anichstr. 35
AT 6020 Innsbruck
Phone: +43 512 504 38 50
Fax: +43 512 58 23 39

Dr. J. LESZEK
Lower Silesian Alzheimer
Association,
Family Support Program
90/4 St. Olszewskiego
PL 51-646 Wroclaw
Phone: +48 71 48 61 78
Fax: +48 71 22 54 15

Dr. Z. SOUSTEK
Department of Pathology
CZ 334 41 Dobrany
Phone: +42 19 97401
Fax: +42 19 97520

THE RELATION BETWEEN STRUCTURE AND FUNCTION IN THE INNER EAR SENSORY ORGANS. A CONFOCAL MICROSCOPY STUDY ON LIVING TISSUE

Key words
Inner ear, structure, function, receptors, confocal microscopy.

Brief description
The sensory structures of the inner ear are highly specialised in the transduction of the mechanical stimuli of sound and of head movements into sensory information directly available to the central nervous system. This information is vital for appropriate adaptation of our behaviour to any changes of the external world.

In spite of their fundamental importance, our knowledge regarding to the specialized functions of the different components of inner ear sensory organs is at present largely based on hypothesis.

This limited present knowledge must be expanded in order to understand the etiology of hearing and equilibrium disorders, to develop more accurate clinical tests and to find better ways of prevention and medical treatment.

An investigative tool is needed that would permit high-resolution functional imaging of intact living preparations of these sensory receptors.

The objective of this project is to develop such a tool and to apply it to the correlative study of structure and function in the cochlea and vestibular sensory receptors from healthy animals. It will then be possible to address problems such as the cellular origins of pathological disorders of hearing and equilibrium.

The BIOMED I program will permit the rapprochement of techniques that are necessary to the realisation of this project. These techniques are presently implemented in different laboratories:
- Image acquisition will use laser scanning confocal microscopy, a new imaging technique that combines optical sectioning properties with high resolution imaging.
  Although the applications of this technique to living tissue have, so far, been sparse, they have revealed an extraordinary potential. This set up is installed in Montpellier:
- Tissue preparations specific to the vestibular organ as well as vital fluorescent staining of cellular structures and metabolism are done in Aarhus.
- Physiological investigations of inner ear sensory receptors involving the implementation of sensory cells mechanical microstimulation and the design of experimental chambers are done in Stockholm.
- Animal models for inner ear dysfunctions involving exposure to sustained changes of the apparent acceleration of gravity are done in Amsterdam.

This proposal expresses the desire of these four participants to bring together their specialized expertise, their equipment and their interest in inner ear sensory functions.

Project leader:
Dr. E. SCARFONE
INSERM, Unité 254,
Laboratoire de Neurophysiiologie Sensorielle,
Univ. de Montpellier II
Place Eugène Bataillon
FR 34095 Montpellier Cedex 05
Phone: +33 67 14 32 77
Fax: +33 67 14 36 96
Contract number: CT941793

Participants:
Prof. A. SANS
Lab. de Neurophysiologie Sensorielle,
UMII-CP 089
Place Eugéne Batallon
FR 34095 Montpellier Cedex 05
Phone: +33 671 432 77
Fax: +33 671 436 96

Prof. J.M. JORGENSEN
Department of Zoophysiology,
University of Aarhus, Institute
of Biological Sciences, Bldg. 131
Universitetsparken
DK 8000 Aarhus C
Phone: +45 8620 27 11
Fax: +45 8619 41 86

Prof. W.J. OOSTERVELD
Vestibular Department, ENT Clinic,
Academic Medical Centre,
University of Amsterdam
Meibergdreef 9
NL 1105 AZ Amsterdam
Phone: +31 20 566 35 21
Fax: +31 20 566 39 16

Dr. J. VAN MARLE
Academic Medical Centre,
University of Amsterdam
Meibergdreef 9
NL 1105 AZ Amsterdam
Phone: +31 20 205 663 521
Fax: +31 20 205 663 916

Prof. A. FLOCK
Department of Physiology and Pharmacology,
Division of Physiology II,
Karolinska Institutet
SE 17177 Stockholm
Phone: +46 8 728 72 51
Fax: +46 8 32 70 26

Prof. M. ULFENDAHL
Department of Physiology and Pharmacology,
Division of Physiology II,
Karolinska Institutet
SE 17177 Stockholm
Phone: +46 8 728 72 56
Fax: +46 8 32 70 26

Dr. M. GROSS
Medizinische Poliklinik
Pettenkoferstrasse 8a
DE 8000 München 2
Phone: +49 89 5160 3546
Fax: +49 89 5160 4480

METABOLISM AND TRANSPORT OF GLUTAMATE: IMPLICATIONS FOR MENTAL HEALTH

Key words
Mental disorders, neurodegeneration, glutamate, metabolism, transport, neuron, glial cells.

Brief description
Major neurological and psychiatric disorders (such as epilepsy, dementia, depression, Parkinson's, schizophrenia and stroke) are poorly understood; treatment is currently at best ameliorative rather than curative. With the increase in life-span, urbanization, mobility and the breakdown of integrated family life in developed countries, such problems will escalate in the coming decades in Europe and intense research is taking place in Universities and industries.

A wide variety of techniques is being employed in attempts to unravel the underlying principals, and a considerable amount of knowledge is accumulating from studies at cellular and subcellular levels on brain cell cultures and whole cell tissue preparations of the brain, to the extent that applications to studies in the brain in vivo, and in the conscious human brain, are now becoming feasible.

Yet underlying mechanisms for the degeneration and/or dysfunction of selected neurons in these disorders remain unknown.

Current hypotheses on the pathophysiological basis for the disorders noted above focus on the amino acid glutamate.

Glutamate is now regarded as the major mediator (transmitter) of excitatory signals in the brain, and several types of glutamate receptors have recently been identified and cloned.

This mediator is probably involved in most aspects of brain function. In particular it is implicated in plasticity, such as in processes of memory and learning, and ontogenetic development.

However, glutamate is also potentially toxic if it accumulates in the extracellular space, such as is believed to occur during deranged cerebral activity in several brain disorders.

An important aspect in this area is the metabolic relationship between neurons and glial cells in thei uptake and handling of glutamate and of related compounds such as lactate, glutamine, or tricarboxylic acid cycle intermediates.

Investigation of the role of glutamate and related metabolites in these disorders requires an array of techniques, in which the consortium of participating laboratories involved in the proposed collaborative research have extensive experience and expertise.

The emphasis will be on the use of a variety of model systems (cultured cells liposomes, superfused tissue, cell preparations and *in vivo* studies) and molecular modeling, with extensive exploitation of the expertise of our participants in NMR spectroscopy and imaging, electron microscopic immunocytochemistry, in situ hybridization, HPLC mass spectroscopy and microdialysis.

Project leader:
Dr. Ursula SONNEWALD
MR-Center SINTEF UNIMED
NO 7034 Trondheim
Phone: +47 7 99 77 00
Fax: +47 7 99 77 08
Contract number: CT941248

Participants:
S.B. PETERSEN
MR-Center SINTEF/UNIMED
NO 7034 Trondheim
Phone: +47 73 9977 00/03
Fax: +47 73 997708/944145

A. SCHOUSBOE & N. WESTERGAARD
Pharma Biotech Res. Center,
Dept. of Biological Scinces,
Royal Danish School of Pharmacy
DK 2100 Copenhagen
Phone: +45 35 370 850
Fax: +45 35 375 744

H. BACHELARD
MR-Centre, University Park Nottingham,
Dept. of Physics
UK Nottingham NG7 2RD
Phone: +44 602 514 752
Fax: +44 602 515 166

D. LEIBFRITZ
University Bremen, FB 2-Chemistry
Leobener Strasse/NW 2
DE 2800 Bremen 33
Phone: +49 421 218 2818
Fax: +49 421 218 4264

H. SANTOS & M. CARRONDO
CTQB
Rua da Quinta Grande 6, Apartado 127
PT 2780 Oeiras
Phone: +351 1 4426146
Fax: +351 1 4428766

F. FONNUM
Defence Research Institute,
Division for Environmental Toxicology
P.O. Box 25
NO 2007 Kjeller
Phone: +47 63807800/22854601
Fax: +47 63807811

J. STORM-MATHISEN
Dept. of Anatomy, University of Oslo
P.O. Box 1105 - Blindern
NO 0317 Oslo
Phone: +47 22 851 258
Fax: +47 22 851 278

STUDY OF PREVALENCE, PATHOPHYSILIOLOGY, AND MOLECULAR DEFECT OF ADENYLOSUCCINASE DEFICIENCY, AND USE OF THIS ENZYME AS A TARGET FOR CHEMIOTHERAPY

Key words
Adenylosuccinase, mental retardation, pathophysiology, neurotransmitters, asase gene.

Brief description
Adenylosuccinase (adenylosuccinate lyase, EC 4.3.2.2., Asase) catalyses two reactions in purine metabolism:

1 conversion of succinylaminoimidazole carboxamide ribotide (SAICAR) into aminoimidazole carboxamide ribotide (AICAR), the 8th step of the de novo synthesis of purine nucleotides;
2 conversion of adenylosuccinate (S-AMP) into AMP, the 2nd step of the conversion of IMP into AMP.

Asase deficiency is the first deficiency of an enzyme of the de novo synthesis of purines dlscovered in man. It is revealed by the presence of succinyl-aminoimidazole carboxamide riboside (SAICAR-riboside) and succinyladenosine (S-Ado) in body fluids. These succinylpurines are the products of the dephosphorylation of the two substrates of Asase. The enzyme deficiency is manifested clinically by variable degrees of psychomotor delay, often autistic features and/or convulsions, sometimes growth retardation and muscular dystrophy. Its inheritance is autosomal recessive. Asase defiency is not that rare, since in a few years at least 13 cases have been diagnosed.
The project includes:

1 Screening of a large population of patients with unexplained mental retardation, in order to establish the prevalence of Asase deficiency in Europe and its spectrum of clinical presentation.
2 Studies of the pathophysiological mechanism(s) underlying the psycho-motor retardation in Asase deficiency, centered on the possibilities that the succinylpurines may interfere with receptors for neurotransmitters, compromise G-protein activity, and/or cerebral glucose metabolism.
3 Characterisation of normal and mutant Asase, and of its gene(s), particularly with respect to the existence of isozymes.
4 Investigations of the susceptibility of Asase and of its isozymes to modulators of their activity and synthesis.

It is expected that the project will lead to a better understanding of Asase deficiency, and perhaps of other neurological, psychiatric and muscular disorders. The studies should also allow prenatal prevention and possibly therapeutic approaches of the enzyme defect. Finally, owing to the dual role of Asase in purine biosynthesis, new insights into its function, and the synthesis of inhibitory analogues of its substrates.

Project leader:
Dr. Georges VAN DEN BERGHE
UCL, ICP 75.39, International Institute
of Cellular and Molecular Pathology
Av. Hippocrate 75
BE 1200 Brussels
Phone: +32 2 764 75 39
Fax: +32 2 764 75 73
Contract number: CT941384

Participants:

Dr. M. GROSS
Medizinische Poliklinik
Pettenkoferstrasse 8a
DE 8000 München 2
Phone: +49 89 5160 3546
Fax: +49 89 5160 4480

Prof. C. SALERNO
Sezione Biochimica Clinica,
Dipartimento di Biopatologia Umana,
Universita degli Studi di Roma La Sapienza
Viale Regina Elena 324
IT 00161 Roma
Phone: +39 6 44 63 776
Fax: +39 6 44 64 698

Dr. R.A. DE ABREU
Kindergeneeskunde,
Academisch Ziekenhuis Nijmegen
Geert Grooteplein 20
Postbus 9101
NL 6500 HB Nijmegen
Phone: +31 80 61 69 33
Fax: +31 80 54 05 76

Dr. J.A. DULEY
Purine Research Laboratory, Floor 18,
Guy's Tower, Guy's Hospital
London Bridge
UK London SE1 9RT
Phone: +44 71 955 40 24
Fax: +44 71 407 66 89

Prof. T.W. STONE
Department of Pharmacology,
University of Glasgow
UK Glasgow G12 8QQ
Phone: +44 41 330 44 81
Fax: +44 41 330 41 00

Dr. R.T. SMOLENSKI
Department of Biochemistry,
Academic Medical School
PL Gdansk

Dr. I. SEBESTA
Center for Inborn Errors of Metabolism,
Charles University
CZ Praha

ACTIVATION STUDIES WITH POSITRON EMISSION TOMOGRAPHY (PET) ON RECOVERY FROM APHASIA

Key words
Aphasia, Positron Emission Tomography assessment, recovery logopedic, pharmacologic therapy.

Brief description
Aphasia after stroke is a disabling disorder and comprises a major socio-economic health problem.

Information on the functional reorganisation of the language system after stroke is of paramount interest for the improvement of rehabilitation of aphasic patients.

Recovery of function after stroke is often observed, although the morphological lesion that has caused the deficit persists. Changes in the organisation of the brain, corresponding to sprouting of new synapses, increase in efficiency of existing connections and others have been seen as possible mechanisms in animal experiments. Today, Positron Emission Tomography (PET) is the only technique available to address this question directly in man.

Activation studies with PET looking at changes in regional cerebral blood flow as a marker of synaptic funtion have shown that widespread functional reorganisational changes may take place in the motor system after stroke. These studies have broadened our view on the organisation of the motor system of the normal human brain.

It is the aim of this project to assess in a similar way the changes in the language system after stroke.

At the second stage the reorganisational changes elicited by PET are used to assess the influence of logopedic or pharmacological therapy. Intersubject averaging will be used to increase sensitivity in the assessment of the systemic components of functional reorganisation. Highly selected groups of patients in terms of linguistic characteristics and lesion site have to be formed.

Large data bases of centers with longstanding interest in aphasia have to be screened.

Linguistic paradigms have to be developed, adapted to different languages and tested.

Intensive logopedic therapy and pharmacological experience must be available on site for the second part of the study.

High quality PET scanning for sophisticated activation studies is only available at a number of limited centers in Europe.

Thus, an interdisciplinary multi-center approach, merging neurological, linguistic, and PET experience is required.

This necessitates the transfer of data and centralised data analysis as well as bringing together suitable patients.

Five centers with a longstanding interest in aphasia and language therapy (Toulouse, Brescia, Milano, Aachen, Lisboa) will design appropriate linguistic paradigms, select and train groups of patients with defined aphasia syndromes and guarantee a standardised logopedic therapy. PET scanning with MRI corregistration will be performed at Essen and Milano, with centralised data analysis at Essen.

Because of major relocation wirk the London center will have a consultant role in the beginning only.

Drugs suitable to influence the process of functional reorganisation will be tested at the Essen center.

Project leader:
Dr. C. WEILLER
Neurologische Klinik und Poliklinik
der Universität - GHS - Essen
Hufelandstrasse 55
DE 4300 Essen
Phone: +49 201 723 24 67
Fax: +49 201 723 5901
Contract number: CT941261

Participants:
Dr. F. CHOLLET
Service de Neurologie, Hôpital Purpan
Place du Docteur Baylac
FR 31059 Toulouse Cedex
Phone: +33 61 77 76 40
Fax: +33 61 15 01 93

Dr. S.F. CAPPA
Clinica Neurologica, Universita degli
Studi di Brescia Spedali Civili
Piazzale Ospedale
IT 25125 Brescia
Phone: +39 30 399 54 89
Fax: +39 30 39 43 13

Dr. D. PERANI
Instituto di Neuroscienze e Bioimmagni,
Hospitale San Raffaele
Via Olgettina 60
IT 20132 Milano
Phone: +39 2 264 13431
Fax: +39 2 264 15202

Dr. W. HUBER
Neurologische Klinik und
Poliklinik der RWTH Aachen
Pauwelsstr. 30
DE 52057 Aachen
Phone: +49 241 808 96 09
Fax: +49 241 808 96 05

Dr. A. CASTRO-CALDAS
Laboratorio de Estudos de Linguagem,
Centro de Estudos Egas Moniz
PT 1600 Lisboa
Phone: +351 1 793 44 80

Dr. R.S.J. FRACKOWIAK
MRC Cyclotron Unit,
Hammersmith Hospital
Ducane Road
UK London W12 0HS
Phone: +44 81 740 31 72
Fax: +44 81 743 39 87

Dr. M. INGVAR
Karolinska Hospital,
Dept. of Clinical Neuroscience
SE 171 76 Stockholm
Phone: +46 8 729 51 34
Fax: +46 8 33 99 53

Dr. R. BINIEK
Neurologische Klinik der
Rheinischen Landesklinik Bonn
Kaiser-Karl Ring 20
DE 53111 Bonn

II.5 THE AGEING PROCESS, AND AGE-RELATED HEALTH PROBLEMS AND HANDICAPS

Introduction

The area of *The ageing Process, and age-related problems and handicaps* covers, by definition multidisciplinary research on illness and affections of, at one end of the scale infants and children at birth, and at the other end, research to maintain optimal quality of life for the aged.

As such this multidisciplinary approach, covers fields such as prevention, screening, epidemiology, basic research, treatment and clinical trials and health care organisation and health services research.

These disciplines form together with the numerous specific diseases which are represented such as diabetes, arthritis, osteoporosis, blindness, asthma, bladder dysfunction, toxoplasmosis etc., an appropriate matrix in which the networks built for the concerted actions can promote the scientific collaboration in the EC.

Without going into details for each concerted action some examples of selected research projects can be given in the different fields. As basic research, cellular and molecular research on diabetic nephropathy and glomerular diseases, retinitis pigmentosa, and the role of modification of glial cells in ageing can be mentioned.

Other studies such as on genetic counselling or prenatal diagnosis of Alport Syndrome, mosaicism, chrondrodystrofy, intrauterine growth retardation, on screening of blindness and paediatric visual defects, on quality control of screening practices and finally on organisational aspects of care delivery, in particular perinatal care, are directly or indirectly oriented towards prevention. Better understanding of the health status in the EC will also be provided by studies on childhood diabetes, congenital toxoplasmosis, and osteoporosis etc.

As clinical oriented research, projects in the field of treatment of arthritis through immunotherapy, the therapeutic approach of cystic fibrosis, a nicotinamide diabetes intervention trial, the transplantation of islet pancreatic cells in diabetes, and treatment of inherited polycystic renal disease can be mentioned.

Finally, a series of projects deal specifically with bone marrow and organ transplantation, in particular on the genetic diversity of HLA, the matching criteria, and on donor organ storage techniques.

It is felt the results of this broad spectrum of research will be able to promote appropriate new insights for the orientation of future health policy initiatives related to diseases with an important social impact.

Dr. Alain Vanvossel

GENETIC DIVERSITY OF HLA IN EUROPE: IMPACT ON TRANSPLANTATION AND PREVENTIVE MEDICINE

Key words
HLA, genes, diversity, transplantation, autoimmunity.

Brief description
Knowledge of the genetics of the HLA region is a scientific prerequisite to understand the biology of antigen presentation and T cell activation; it will also provide new markers for use in organ and bone marrow transplantation and in predictive medicine. EThe aims of the proposed Concerted Action are to:

1 Obtain definitive genetic information, including the polymorphism of new genes, at the DNA sequence level, for HLA region genes from the multi-ethnic European population.

2 Develop, standardise and apply to the study of the HLA diversity, DNA technologies in a network of European laboratories.

3 Study the impact of these DNA based polymorphisms on organ transplantation, bone marrow transplantation and disease susceptibility.

4 Organise and coordinate research projects using the genetic material and information described above. These will include studies of the repertoire of HLA and associated peptides in cells from normal and diseased individuals and the diversity of expression of T cell receptors in relation to the HLA haplotypes and diseases will be also determined.

5 Collect the above data and make them available through a permanent Database established in Europe as an interconnected European network of core and satellite centres which will be linked worldwide to US and Asian equivalents.

The work will be organised in a central component (antigens and haplotype societies) and in specific satellite components as follows:
- HLA-peptides interactions;
- Cell immune responses (T cell receptors);
- Transplantation (organ and Bone marrow);
- Disease susceptibility studies (diabetes, HIV-infection, allergy, cancer).

Project leader:
Professor D. CHARRON
Université P. et M. Curie,
Laboratoire d'Immunogénéti-
que Moléculaire, Institut
Biomédical des Cordeliers
r. de l'Ecole de Médecine 15
FR 75006 Paris
Phone: +33 1 40 46 03 58
Fax: +33 1 43 26 76 13
Contract number: CT921699

Participants:
Dr. Michel JEANNET (CH)
Dr A. SANCHEZ-MAZAS (CH)
Dr. Agatha ROSENMAYR (AT)
Prof. R. WOLFGANG (AT)

Dr. Henriqueta BREDA (PT)
Prof. Antero GUIMARAES (PT)
Dr. Filipe INACIO (PT)
Dr. Armando MENDES (PT)
Dr. Francois HENTGES (LU)
Dr. C. PAPASTERIADES (GR)
Dr. C. STAVROPOULOS (GR)
N. CONSTANTINIDOU (GR)
Dr. Niels GRUNNET (DK)
Prof. Lars U. LAMM (DK)
Dr. H. LOWENSTEIN (DK)
Prof. Arne SVEJGAARD (DK)
Dr. Soren BUUS (DK)
Dr. Claire BOUILENNE (BE)

Dr. Marc DE BRUYERE (BE)
Prof. Etienne DUPONT (BE)
Dr. L. MUYLLE (BE)
Dr. Jean Cl. OSSELAER (BE)
Dr. Marie Paul EMONDS (BE)
Dr. Flament JOCELYNE (BE)
Clara ALONSO (ES)
M. R. ALVAREZ-LOPEZ (ES)
Pr. A. ARNAIZ-VILLENA (ES)
Dr. Gonzalez ESCRIBANO (ES)
Prof. Federico GARRIDO (ES)
Dr. J. Miguel KREISLER (ES)
Dr. Carlos LAHOZ (ES)
N. CLERICI LARRADAT (ES)

Dr. C. LOPEZ LARREA (ES)
Pr. M. SANCHEZ-PEREZ (ES)
Dr. Jose L. VICARIO (ES)
Dr. Antonio GAYA (ES)
Dr. Wil ALLEBES (NL)
Dr. Ronald BONTROP (NL)
Dr. Ella VAN DEN (NL)
Dr. Leo Pieter DE WAAL (NL)
Prof. P. C. ENGELFRIET (NL)
Prof. Pavol IVANYI (NL)
Dr. Simon P.M. LEMS (NL)
Dr. Ilias DOXIADIS (NL)
Dr. Ieke SCHREUDER (NL)
Prof. Jon J. VAN ROOD (NL)
Dr. Marcal G.J. TILANUS (NL)
Prof. Domenico ADORNO (IT)
Prof. Francesco BARBONI (IT)
Dr. Elena BENAZZI (IT)
Dr. Sergio BAROCCI (IT)
Prof. Licinio CONTU (IT)
Prof. Emilio S. CURTONI (IT)
Dr. Simonetta TRABACE (IT)
Prof. Giovanni BATTISTA (IT)
Dr. Maria Pia PISTILLO (IT)
Prof. Enrico GANDINI (IT)
Dr. Ciro MANZO (IT)
Dr. Maria C. MAZZILLI (IT)
Dr. Miryam MARTINETTI (IT)
Prof. F. MERCURIALI (IT)
Prof. Pier Luigi MATTIUZ (IT)
Prof. Alberto PIAZZA (IT)
Dr. Giuseppe PELLEGRIS (IT)
Prof. Francesco PUPPO (IT)
Dr. Maria PURPURA (IT)
Prof. Patricia RICHIARDI (IT)
Dr. Luca RICHELDI (IT)
Dr. Anna RUFFILLI (IT)
Prof. Alfredo SALERNO (IT)
Prof. Mario SAVI (IT)
Dr. Raffaella SCORZA (IT)
Prof. Girolamo SIRCHIA (IT)
Dr. Rosa SORRENTINO (IT)
Dr. Roberto TOSI (IT)
Prof. S. ZAPPACOSTA (IT)
Dr. D. ALCALYA (FR)
Dr. Brigitte CAVELIER (FR)
Dr. Herve BETUEL (FR)
Dr. Jean-Denis BIGNON (FR)
Prof. Alain BERNARD (FR)
Prof. Claude BOITARD (FR)
Dr. M.D. BOULANGER (FR)
Dr. C. COUSSEDIERE (FR)

Dr. J.H.M. COHEN (FR)
Dr. Jean Claude BENSA (FR)
Dr. Brigitte COEFFIC (FR)
Dr. P.M. DANZE (FR)
Prof. D. CHARRON (FR)
Dr. Jacques COLOMBANI (FR)
Prof. Jean DAUSSET (FR)
Prof. Laurent DEGOS (FR)
Prof. Jacques HORS (FR)
Prof. Patrice DEBRE (FR)
Dr. DROUET (FR)
Dr. Francoise DUFOSSE (FR)
Dr. Gabriel PELTRE (FR)
Dr. Jean Francois ELIAOU (FR)
Dr. H. FARAHMAND (FR)
Prof. Renee FAUCHET (FR)
Dr. Dominique FIZET (FR)
Dr. Claude FEREC (FR)
Dr. Eliane GLUCKMAN (FR)
Dr. GRIVEAU (FR)
Dr. Fredy GUIGNIER (FR)
Prof. G. HAUTPMANN (FR)
S. CAILLAT-ZUCMAN (FR)
Dr. KANDEL (FR)
Dr. Cecile KAPLAN (FR)
Prof. M.P. LEFRANC (FR)
Dr. Jean C. LE PETIT (FR)
Dr. James LESPINASSE (FR)
Dr. Pierre MERCIER (FR)
Dr. Marie-M. TONGIO (FR)
Dr. Anne CAMBON (FR)
Dr. Pascale PERRIER (FR)
Dr. Gilbert SEMANA (FR)
Dr. D. ZELISZEWSKI (FR)
Dr. Pierre TIBERGHIEN (FR)
Prof. Jean P. CLAUVEL (FR)
Prof. E. D. ALBERT (DE)
Dr. Dagmar BARZ (DE)
Dr. Gregor BEIN (DE)
Dr. Manfred BALLAS (DE)
Dr. Volker LENHARD (DE)
Dr. Harro WALGER (DE)
Dr. Bernhard O. BOEHM (DE)
Prof. Xaver BAUR (DE)
Dr. Hans-Peter RIHS (DE)
Dr. Th. H. EIERMANN (DE)
Dr. S. F. GOLDMANN (DE)
Dr. G. HOLZBERGER (DE)
Dr. J. KUEHR (DE)
Dr. SCHONEMANN (DE)
Prof. Peter KUEHNL (DE)

Dr. C. LOELIGER (DE)
Prof. Bernard LANG (DE)
Prof. Gottfried MAUFF (DE)
Dr. Ch. G. MEYER (DE)
Dr. Claudia MULLER (DE)
Dr. Gertrud MUELLER (DE)
Dr. Marion NAGY (DE)
Dr. Hans NEUMEYER (DE)
Dr. Graham PAWELEC (DE)
Dr. Inga MELCHERS (DE)
Dr. Rainer BLASCZYK (DE)
Prof. Gerd SCHMITZ (DE)
Dr. P. M. SCHNEIDER (DE)
Prof. Walter STANGEL (DE)
Dr. Stephan VOLKER (DE)
Dr. Rudolf WANK (DE)
Dr. Ralf WASSMUTH (DE)
Dr. Sibylle WEGENER (DE)
Dr. Eckhard WESTPHAL (DE)
Prof. Elisabeth WEISS (DE)
Dr. Hovanes AVAKIAN (UK)
Mr. Gary CAVANASH (UK)
Prof. J. BATCHELOR (UK)
Dr. Julia G. BODMER (UK)
Sir Walter F. BODMER (UK)
Prof. G.F. BOTAZZO (UK)
Prof. Benjamin BRADLEY (UK)
Dr. Godfrey J. LAUNDY (UK)
Dr. R.D. CAMPBELL (UK)
Dr. John RAYMOND (UK)
Prof. A.G. DALGLEISH (UK)
Dr. A. DEMAINE (UK)
Dr. Cristopher DARKE (UK)
Dr. Philip A. DYER (UK)
Dr. Nelson FERNANDEZ (UK)
Dr. Keith GELSTHORPE (UK)
Dr. Craig TAYLOR (UK)
Dr. Shirley JOBSON (UK)
Dr. Derek MIDDLETON (UK)
Dr. Mike BUNCE (UK)
Prof. Peter MORRIS (UK)
Dr. Cristina NAVARRETE &
MR. Colin BROWN (UK)
Dr. W.E.R. OLLIER (UK)
Dr. W.M. HOWELL (UK)
Dr. John SMITH (UK)
Dr. Giselle SCHWARZ (UK)
Dr. John TROWSDALE (UK)
Dr. S.J. URBANICK (UK)
Dr. J.S. LANCHBURY (UK)

IMMUNOTHERAPY OF CHRONIC ARTHRITIS: EXPERIMENTAL BASIS

Key words
Immunology, rheumatoid arthritis, immunogenetics, pre-clinical studies, immunotherapy.

Objectives
1 Facilitation and coordination of human immunogenetic studies, more specifically:
- the establishment and distribution of a B cell line repository from multiplex RA families for genetic studies;
- the establishment of a bank of HLA-DR transfectants for functional studies;
- exploring whether elution of peptides from HLA molecules may provide a clue to the triggering antigen(s).
2 To stimulate an optimal use of the experience from animal models for the design of therapeutic experiments in patients.
3 Coordination of, and providing facilities for pre-clinical studies of promising immunotherapy strategies in non-human primates.

Brief description
Rheumatoid Arthritis (RA) and other forms of chronic arthritis are a major cause of disability, particularly in the aged. Therapy is symptomatic, not very effective and/or associated with serious side effects.

In the past 10 years our understanding of the pathogenesis of these diseases has made considerable progress. Several lines of evidence suggest that inappropriate presentation of (a) thus far unknown antigen(s) to disease inducing T cells plays an important role at least in the pathogenesis of RA. In the same period the molecular basis of antigen presentation to T cells has been unravelled, which led to extremely successful immune intervention approaches in experimental animal models of T cell mediated immunopathological and auto-immune diseases. These immune interventions are aimed at either blocking the presentation of antigen to disease inducing T cells or inducing a response against such T cells. Stimulated by these experimental findings, several groups have started or are considering clinical trials of similar immunotherapy modalities in patients with RA.

Mid 1989 a European Concerted Action on *Immunopathogenesis and Immunotherapy of Chronic Arthritis* was started to coordinate the research and clinical activities in this rapidly moving area. Based on the results of this successful Concerted Action and exploiting the established network, a proposal for a new Concerted Actions has been formulated aimed at coordinating studies relating to the experimental basis of the new immunotherapeutic modalities.

Project leader:
Professor R.R.P. DE VRIES
Dept. of Immunohaematology & Blood Bank,
University Hospital, Bldg 1 E3-Q
P.O. Box 9600
NL 2300 RC Leiden
Phone: +31 71 26 38 69
Fax: +31 71 21 67 51
Contract number: CT921038

Participants:

Prof. H.H. PETER &
dr. I. MELCHERS
DE 7800 Freiburg

Prof. G. RIETHMULLER
DE 8000 München 2

Dr. J. ROUDIER
FR 130005 Marseille

Prof. J. SANY
FR 34059 Montpellier

Prof. J. SMOLEN
Wolkesbergenstrasse 1
AT 1130 Vienna

Prof. N.A. STAINES
UK London W8 7AM

Prof. S.W. SERJEANTSON
P.O. Box 334
AU Canberra ACT 2601

Dr. J. TROWSDALE &
dr. J. HEYES
UK London WC2A 3PX

Prof. F.C. BREEDVELD
NL 2300 RC Leiden

Prof. H. WALDMANN
Tennis Court Road
UK Cambridge CB2 1QP

Dr. L. ADORINI ·
IT 20132 Milano

Dr. A.E. BAERT
200 Rue de la Loi
BE 1049 Brussels

Dr. J. BELL
UK Oxford OX3 9DU

Dr. W.B. VAN DEN BERG
& prof. VAN DE PUTTE
NL 6500 HB Nijmegen

Dr. C. BOGDAN
Str. Berceni 12
RO 75622 Bucharest

Dr. G. BURMESTER
Krankenhausstrasse 12
DE 8520 Erlangen

Dr. S. BUUS
Blegdamsvej 3B
DK 2200 Copenhagen N

Prof. D. CHARRON
15 rue de 'Ecole de Médecine
FR 75006 Paris

Prof. J. CLOT &
dr. J.F. ELIAOU
FR Montpellier Cedex

Dr. F. CORNELIS
27 Rue Juliette Dodu
FR 75010 Paris

Dr. W. VAN EDEN
P.O. Box 80150
NL 3508 TD Utrecht

Dr. P. EMMERY
UK Birmingham B15 2TT

Dr. F. EMMRICH
Schwabachanlage 10
DE 8520 Erlangen

Prof. O. FORRE
Akkerbakken 27
NO 0172 Oslo

Dr. C. FOURNIER
FR 75674 Paris Cedex 14

Dr. M. JONKER
P.O. Box 45
NL 2280 AA Rijswijk

Prof. J.R. KALDEN
Krankenhausstrasse 12
DE 8520 Erlangen

Prof. L. KLARESKOG
P.O. Box 575
SE 751 85 Uppsala

Dr. J. LANCHBURY &
Prof. G.S. PANAYI
UK London Bridge SE1 9RT

Dr. B. LANG
P.o.Box 100662
DE 8400 Regensburg

Dr. A.W LOHSE
Langenbeckstrasse 1
DE 6500 Mainz 1

Prof R.N. MAINI &
Dr. M. FELDMANN
6 Bute Gardens
UK London W6 7DW

Dr. MARTVON
Drug Research Institute
Horná 36
CS 90001 Modra

Dr P. MIOSSEC
FR 69437 Lyon Cedex 03

Prof. H. MOUTSOPOULOS
Dept. of Internal Medicine;
School of Medicine
GR 55110 Ioannina

Dr. W.E.R. OLLIER &
Prof. A.J. SILMAN
Univ. of Manchester
Oxford Road
UK Manchester M13 9PT

EUROPEAN NICOTINAMIDE DIABETES
INTERVENTION TRIAL (ENDIT)

Key words
Insulin-dependent diabetes mellitus (IDDM), prevention, clinical trial, nicotinamide.

Objectives
To establish in a prospective, randomized, placebo-controlled trial whether it is possible to prevent or delay the clinical manifestation of IDDM with daily oral administration of nicotinamide in first degree relatives at increased risk of contracting the disease, and more specifically:

1 To establish an organizational structure for management of the study.
2 To complete screening of 22,000 first degree relatives of children with IDDM for islet cell antibodies.
3 To identify a minimum of 525 individuals with confirmed ICA ≥ 20 JDF units and to determine their first phase insulin response (FPIR) prior to entry to the study.
4 To undertake a 5 year prospective study in individuals randomized to nicotinamide ($1.2gm/m^2/day$) or placebo, and to test the null hypothesis that nicotinamide cannot achieve a 40% overall reduction in the rate of progression to IDDM over the study period, or a 25% reduction in the group at greatest risk; the Study should have 90% power to detect such a difference.
5 To establish which subgroups, if any, benefit from nicotinamide and to devise a clinical and research programme for their future investigation and clinical management.
6 To establish a European collaborative network capable of undertaking a programme of prompt, high quality and cost-effective intervention trials in individuals at high risk of progression to IDDM.

Brief description
The European Nicotinamide Diabetes Intervention Trial (ENDIT) is a multinational randomized placebo-controlled intervention study aiming at establishing the utility of nicotinamide in preventing or delaying the clinical presentation of insulin-dependent diabetes mellitus (IDDM) in individuals at increased risk of contracting the disease. Nicotinamide is a water soluble group B vitamin which has been shown to be effective in preventing onset of diabetes in animal models, has produced promising results in uncontrolled trials in non-diabetic relatives with high levels of islet cell antibodies (ICA), and may have some benefit in prolonging beta cell function in recently diagnosed patients with insulin-dependent diabetes. No serious side effects have been reported from its use at the doses proposed in man or other species. The trial will be undertaken on a European multinational basis. Relatives of patients developing diabetes under the age of 21 will be screened for islet cell antibodies. Those with confirmed levels ≥ 20 JDF units and meeting the age criteria will be asked to undergo both oral and intravenous glucose tolerance tests and will be invited to take part in a prospective randomized placebo controlled trial of nicotinamide vs placebo. It is aimed to screen 22,000 first degree relatives in order to identify and recruit 525 eligible individuals, on the assumption that 422 will complete the trial. Up to 5 years of treatment are required to demonstrate or exclude any clinically useful benefit from nicotinamide (i.e. a 90% power to identify an overall 40% reduction in risk of progression to diabetes over the study period, and a 25% risk reduction in the sub-group at highest risk). An interim analysis will be under-

taken after 3 years. This first major European study to attempt intervention in the prodromal phase of childhood diabetes, has already attracted support from well established centres with a sufficiently large screening population to ensure rapid recruitment of the large numbers needed for such an endeavour.

A project management team is responsible for the practical conduct of the trial, under the supervision of an independent review committee. There are annual workshop meetings, and an active laboratory exchange and training programme for those involved in screening, together with data and safety monitoring, and site and contact meetings are foreseen.

Project leader:
Dr. E.A.M. GALE
Diabetes & Metabolism
St. Bartholomew's Hospital
West Smithfield
UK London EC1A 7BE
Phone: +44 71 601 74 46
Fax: +44 71 601 74 49
Contract number: CT920957

Participants:
Dr. Edith SCHOBER
Währinger Gürtel 18-20
AT 1090 Wien

Dr. Frans K. GORUS
Laarbeeklaan 103
BE 1090 Brussels

Dr. John DUPRE
399 Windermere Road
CA London -
Ontario N6A 5A5

Dr. Velimir PROFOZIC
Dugi dol 4a
HR 41000 Zagreb

Dr. Jesper I. REIMERS
DK 2820 Gentofte

Dr. Polly J. BINGLEY
West Smithfield
UK London EC1A 7BE

Dr. Mikael KNIP
Aapiste 3
FI 90220 Oulu

Dr. LEVY-MATCHAL
FR 75019 Paris

Dr. Frank BECKER
Rodthohl 6
DE 6300 Giessen

Dr. Denise KEPPLER
Athens Children's Hospital
GR 11527 Athens

Mrs. Margir GYORKO &
dr. Gyula SOLTESZ
7 Jozsef A. Street
HU 7623 Pecs

Dr. T. MITCHELL
IE Wilton - Cork

Dr. D.J. CARSON
Grosvenor Street
UK Belfast NT12 6B7

Dr. Paolo POZZILLI
Via G. Bagliui 12
IT 00161 Rome

Dr. G.J. BRUINING
PO Box 70029
NL 3000 LL Rotterdam

Prof. Hab Ida KINALSKA
PL 15276 Bialystok

Prof. A.M ROZIKIEWICZ
Dluga 1/2
PL 61848 Poznan

Dr. M.M.A. RUAS
PT 3049 Coimbra Codex

Prof. Eugene I. SCHWARTZ
Litovskaya street 2
RU 194100 St. Petersburg

Dr. Stephen GREEN
Dept. of Child Health,
Ninewells Hospital
UK Dundee DD1 9SY

Dr. Dagmar MICHALKOVA
I Paediatric Dept. Children
University Hospital
Limbova I
SK 833 Bratislava

Dr. Alberto DE LEIVA
Servicio de Endocrinologia,
Hospital de San Pablo
S. Antonio Ma Claret 167
ES 08025 Barcelona

Prof. SERRANO-RIOS
Cea Bermudez 66
ES 28003 Madrid

Prof. Johnny LUDVIGSSON
Dept. of Paediatrics,
Faculty of Health Sciences,
University Hospital
SE 58185 Linkoping

Dr. Eugen J. SCHOENLE
Universitäts-Kinderklinik,
Kinderspital Zürich
Steinwiesstrasse 75
CH 8032 Zürich

Prof. W.J. RILEY
UT Houston Medical School,
Dept. of Paediatrics
6431 Fannin
US Houston 77030

Dr. Hasan ILKOVA
Division of Metabolism &
Diabetes, Istanbul University,
Cerrahpasa Medical Faculty
Aksaray
TR Istanbul

COORDINATION OF CYSTIC FIBROSIS
RESEARCH AND THERAPY

Key words
Cystic fibrosis, networking, data bases, genetic diagnosis, mutations, population screening, new therapies.

Objectives
This Concerted Action on *Cystic Fibrosis Research and Therapy* has the following objectives:
- Development of a patient data base and software to correlate phenotype with genotype within the EC population.
- Development of and training in new testing methods for the identification of novel CF mutations, particularly in Southern Europe.
- Development of central reference labs with appropriate training for each EC country to coordinate quality control, distribution of reagents and training of laboratory personnel.
- Development of a European map of CF mutations.
- Coordinated efforts to design novel and rational approaches to treatment.
- Linking of research laboratories to clinical centres.
- Distribution of common reagents, reference standards, and coded samples for testing.
- Provision of funding for exchanges of staff between EC labs to assist in the achievement of these objectives and provide future networks.
- Establishment of effective population screening programmes.
- Sharing of resources and skills through networking and workshops.

Brief description
A Steering Committee will develop strategies to meet these objectives. It will consist of the following persons: Prof. Michel Goossens, project leader (FR); Prof. Bob Williamson (GB); Prof. J.J. Cassiman (BE); Prof. John Dodge (GB); Dr. Xavier Estivill (ES); Dr. Hans Scheffer (NL); Prof. Dimitris Loukopolous (GR); Prof. Pier-Franco Pignatti (IT); and Dr. Marianne Schwartz (DK). Subcommittees will also be established to organise and coordinate broadly grouped initiatives.

Throughout the three years of the action, steering committee meetings, reference lab meetings and workshops will be held on a regular basis. The venues will be rotated so as to involve as many EC countries as possible. Newsletters will be produced to ensure information exchanges on all the various initiatives proposed for the Concerted Action. Biological materials and personnel will be exchanged on an ongoing basis. These exchanges and workshops will accelerate the development of new testing methods for the identification of mutations, new approaches to treatment and the linking of research laboratories and clinical centres. It will also allow for the identification and discussion of technical, legal and ethical issues arising from new treatments and screening, as well as issues affecting quality control.

Project leader:
Professor M. GOOSSENS
INSERM, U. 91, Hôpital Henri Mondor,
Laboratoire de Biochimie
FR 94010 Créteil Cédex
Phone: +33 1 49 81 28 61
Fax: +33 1 49 81 28 42
Contract number: CT921391

Participants:

Dr. Miguel DE ARCE
IE Dublin 2

Prof. André BOUE
FR 75016 Paris

Prof. D.J.H. BROCK
UK Edinburgh EH42X4

Prof. Antonio CAO
IT 09121 Cagliari

Dr. A. CARBONARA
IT 10126 Turin

Prof. J.J. CASSIMAN
BE 3000 Leuven

Dr. J. CHEADLE &
dr. L. MEREDITH
UK Cardiff CF4 4XN

Dr. Mireille CLASUSTRES
FR 34060 Montpellier

Prof. J.A. DODGE
UK Belfast BT12 6BJ

Dr. Xavier ESTIVILL
ES 06907 Barcelone

Dr. Maurizio FERRARI
IT 20132 Milano

Dr. Claude FEREC
FR 29275 Brest cedex

Dr. Dicky HALLEY
NL 3000 DR Rotterdam

Prof. Jürgen HORST
DE 4400 Münster

Dr. Joao LAVINHA
PT 1699 Lisboa Codex

Dr. W. LISSENS
BE 1001 Brussels

Prof. D. LOUKOPOULOS
GR 11527 Athens

Dr. A. MAGGIO
IT 910146 Palermo

Prof. G. MASTELLA
IT 37126 Verona

Prof. Jean NAVARRO
FR 75019 Paris

Prof. P.F. PIGNATI
IT 37134 Verona

Dr. Edith PUCHELLE
FR 51092 Reims Cedex

Dr. Giovanni ROMEO
IT 16148 Genova

Dr. Hans SCHEFFER
NL 9713 AW Groningen

Dr. J. SCHMIDTKE
DE 30000 Hannover 61

Dr. B. SCHOLTE
NL 3000 DR Rotterdam

Dr. Marianne SCHWARTZ
DK 2100 Copenhagen

Dr. Maurice SUPER
UK Manchester M27 1HA

Dr. B. TUMMLER
DE 30000 Hannover

Dr. D. VALERIO
NL 2280 HV Rijswijk

Prof. R. WILLIAMSON &
mrs. C. WILLIAMS
UK London W2 1 PG

AETIOLOGY OF CHILDHOOD DIABETES ON AN EPIDEMIOLOGICAL BASIS (EURODIAB ACE)

Key words
Type 1 (insulin-dependent) diabetes mellitus, epidemiology, aetiology, genetics, mortality, immunology.

Brief description
EURODIAB ACE was established as Subarea A of the previous Concerted Action EURODIAB (1988-1991). The EURODIAB ACE network is now used to conduct research in order to:
1 Unravel the aetiology and pathogenesis of insulin-dependent diabetes mellitus (IDDM) with the ultimate goal of preparing the way for prevention of the disease;
2 Identify determinants related to clinical presentation and early mortality of IDDM aiming at defining means of reducing the severity and mortality in the early phases of the disease.

The research is performed in five sub-studies as follows:
Study 1 Continued surveillance of IDDM incidence. This study continues the previous EURODIAB Subarea A in the detailed characterisation of the geographical distribution of childhood onset IDDM, incl. time trends in incidence. The study also represents the basic incidence network from which cases and samples for the following studies are drawn. Participation in Substudy 1 is mandatory for full membership of the EURODIAB ACE Research Network.
Study 2 Identification of non-genetic determinants of IDDM. This study includes case-control research on possible non-genetic determinants of IDDM in various European populations.
Study 3 Clinical aspects of IDDM. This study describes clinical and biochemical characteristics of childhood IDDM at onset in various European populations according to background risk level.
Study 4 Investigations of the mortality of childhood IDDM. This study describes factors associated with onset and short-term mortality in childhood onset IDDM in various European populations.
Study 5 Genetic and immune markers of susceptibility to IDDM. This study is based on immune and genetic marker technology in order to describe the genetic and immunologic susceptibility of IDDM in different European populations. Based on this information, combined with epidemiological and clinical data, it will be possible to obtain a model on the aetiology of IDDM.

In terms of project methodology, the project has two core elements: (i) the basic incidence network described above, and (ii) a network of leading genetic and immunologic laboratories to provide support services for the research.
The project will be carried out by means of the commonly used modalities (workshops, expert meetings, site and contact visits). It will be managed by a Project Coordinator, assisted by a Steering Committee and with the input from an Advisory Board.
Progress will be reported by frequent Newsletters, by information at Workshops, and by annual Progress Reports.
The time schedule of EURODIAB ACE comprises 36 months of research.

Project leader:
Dr. A. GREEN
Genetic Epidemiology Research Unit,
Odense University
Winslowparken 15-17
DK 5000 Odense C
Phone: +45 66 15 86 00
Fax: +45 65 90 63 94
Contract number: CT920043

Participants:

Dr. Kirsten Ohm KYVIK (DK)

Dr. Edwin GALE (UK)

Dr. Polly BINGLEY (UK)

Dr. C. LEVY-MARCHAL (FR)

Dr. Raisa LOUNAMAA (UK)

Dr. Gyula SOLTESZ (HU)

Dr. Marco SONGINI (IT)

Dr. Gisela DAHLQUIST (SE)

Dr. Edith SCHOBER (AT)

Dr. Ch. VANDEWALLE (BE)

Dr. J. KREUTZFELDT (DK)

Dr. Arni V. THORSSON (IS)

Dr. Paul CZERNICHOW (FR)

Dr. Christos BARTSÓCAS (GR)

Dr. N. PAPAZOGLOU (GR)

Dr. Maarten REESER (NL)

Dr. G. CHIUMELLO (IT)

Dr. Paolo POZZILLI (IT)

Dr. Francesco PURRELLO (IT)

Prof. LARON (IL)

Dr. Brone URBONAITE (LT)

Dr. Girts BRIGIS (LV)

Dr. Toomas PODAR (EE)

Dr. C. DE BEAUFORT (LU)

Prof. Guido GIANI (DE)

Dr. Geir JONER (NO)

Dr. Silvestre ABREU (PT)

Dr. Casimiro MENEZES (PT)

Dr. Elsa A. PINA (PT)

Dr. Vladimir CHRISTOV (BG)

Dr. C. IONESCU-TIRGEVISTE (RO)

Dr. Alberto GODAY (ES)

Dr. David HADDEN (UK)

Dr. Hannes BOTHA (UK)

Dr. Dorota WOZNICKA (PL)

Dr. Zbigniew SZYBINSKI (PL)

Dr. Ciril KRZISNIK (SI)

Dr. Gojka ROGLIC (HR)

Dr. D. MICHALKOVA (SK)

Dr. Jan VAVRINEC (CZ)

THE PROPHYLACTIC AND THERAPEUTIC EFFECT OF N-3 FATTY ACIDS IN PRETERM BIRTH, PRE-ECLAMPSIA AND INTRAUTERINE GROWTH RETARDATION

Key words
Fatty acids, preterm birth, pre-eclampsia, intervention studies.

Objectives
The primary objectives of the study are to assess the potential usefulness of fish oil supplementation in pregnancy on the prevention of new cases to arise of preterm delivery, fetal growth retardation and pre-eclampsia, and in the therapy of already diagnosed cases of fetal growth retardation and preeclampsia. Subordinate objectives are to assess biochemical effects of fish oil supplementation in pregnancy in order to obtain a better understanding of pathophysiological mechanisms.

Brief description
Clinical and theoretical studies suggest that consumption of n-3 fatty acids prolongs the duration of pregnancy. A possible cardiovascular and metabolic effect of n-3 fatty acids seems to be valuable in the prevention/treatment of pre-eclampsia and intrauterine growth retardation (IURG).

The purpose of the study is - by means of randomised controlled trial - to investigate whether a dietary supplement of n-3 fatty acids (2.8 grammes/day) given from midpregnancy (16th to 24th week of gestation) until birth has a *preventative effect* on:
1 Pre-term birth.
2 Pre-eclampsia.
3 Birth of infants small for gestational age (=SGA).

Furthermore, the purpose of the study is to investigate whether n-3 fatty acids (6.3 grammes/day) have a *therapeutic effect* on the progress of diagnosed cases of intrauterine growth retardation and pre-eclampsia.

Main hypotheses:
1 Supplementation of n-3 fatty acids (2.8 grammes/day) during pregnancy reduces the recurrence risk in woman *who in an earlier pregnancy* have had pre-term delivery.
2 Supplementation of n-3 fatty acids (2.8 grammes/day) during pregnancy reduces the recurrence risk in women *who in earlier pregnancy* have had pre-eclampsia and/or given birth to a growth retarded child.
3 Supplementation of n-3 fatty acids (6.3 grammes/day) has a beneficial effect on the progress of *recognised* pre-eclampsia and intrauterine growth retardation in the child.

Project leader:
Professor N.J. SECHER
Department of Obstetrics & Gynaecology, University Hospital Aarhus
37-39 Norrebrogade
DK 8000 Aarhus C
Phone: +45 86 12 55 55
Fax: +45 86 19 74 13
Contract number: CT921906

Participants:

Dr. J. TROVIK
Kvinneklinikken,
Haukeland Sykehus
NO 5021 Bergen
Phone: +47 55 298 060
Fax: +47 55 974 968

Dr. B. STRAY-PEDERSEN
Dept of Obstetrics and Gynaecology,
Aker Sykehus
NO 0514 Oslo
Phone: +47 22 894 000
Fax: +47 22 894 150

Dr. A. BJORKLUND
Kvinnoklinikken, Danderyds Sjukhus
SE Stockholm
Phone: +46 8655 5000
Fax: +46 8655 6998

Prof. J.G. GRUDZINSKAS
Dept of Obstetrics and Gynaecology,
The London Hospital
UK London E1 1BB
Phone: +44 71 3777 340
Fax: +44 71 3777 294

Dr. P. ROBERTS
Dept of Obstetrics and Gynaecology,
Newham General District Hospital
UK London E13
Phone: +44 71 4761 400
Fax: +44 71 4732 480

Prof. J. WALKER
University Dept of Obst and Genaecology,
Glasgow Royal Infirmary
10 Alexander Parade
UK Glasgow G31 2ER
Phone: +44 4155 23535
Fax: +44 4155 31367

Ass. prof. A. TABOR
Dept of Obstetrics and Gynaecology,
Rigshospitalet
DK 2100 Kopenhagen
Phone: +45 3545 3545
Fax: +45 3545 4285

Ass. prof. T. WEBER
Dept of Obstetrics
and Gynaecology,
Hvidovre Hospital
DK 2650 Hvidovre
Phone: +45 3632 3332
Fax: +45 3632 3361

Dr. B. LJUNGSTROM
Dept of Obstetrics and Gynaecology,
Odense Centralsygehus
1DK 5000 Odense C
Phone: +45 6611 3333
Fax: +45 6541 2322

Dr. K. SOGAARD
Dept of Obstetrics and Gynaecology,
Naestved Centralsygehus
DK 4700 Naestved
Phone: +45 5372 1401
Fax: +45 5372 3926

ALTERATIONS OF EXTRACELLULAR MATRIX COMPONENTS IN DIABETIC NEPHROPATHY AND OTHER GLOMERULAR DISEASES

Key words
Diabetes, genetic marker, glomerulopathy.

Objectives
This CA proposes coordinated studies addressing these issues with 5 basic objectives:
1 The changes in renal basement membrane composition in diabetes and their relation to proteinuria will be assessed by studying: (a) the expression of mRNA for basement membrane components, including perlecan (the major heparan sulphate proteoglycan of basement membranes), in IDDM diabetic models; (b) expression of these components at the protein level in diabetic and non-diabetic basement membranes using semi-quantitative immunohistochemistry; (c) investigating a new rat modes with spontaneous glomerulopathy, establishing the functional parameters and investigating alterations within the basement membranes of these animals, and; (d) examining the synthesis of basement membrane components and heparan sulphate in cell culture of diabetic patients with and without complications, to shed light on the possible mechanisms involved in susceptibility.
2 Identification of cDNA clones encoding previously uncharacterised components of basement membranes, with a focus on: (a) identification of cDNA clones encoding novel basement membrane proteoglycans, and; (b) identification of new variants of basement membrane components and the analysis of these clones in diabetes and congenital renal diseases.
3 Determining the effects of diabetes on the synthesis of the heparan sulphate side chains themselves, by: (a) analysis of the effect of diabetes on the activity of a key enzyme in heparansulphate synthesis, N-deacetylase; (b) isolation of the complete cDNA clones for this enzyme and determination of the gene and promoter structure, and; (c) determination of the influence of diabetes on the domain structure of the heparan sulphate side chains.
4 A search for genetic markers for susceptibility to diabetic complications, determining: (a) genetic polymorphisms in the N-deacetylase gene and; (b) in the genes encoding basement membrane components.
5 Analysis of potential therapeutic agents by: (a) expanding studies on the effectiveness and mechanism of exogenous glycosarninoglycan administration in preventing diabetic complications, and; (b) examining the microstructural domains of heparan sulphate that interact with growth factors and those that have an apparent protective potential.

Brief description
Objective 1
Goal 1: Examination of the effect of diabetes on collagen IV and perlecan in animal models and the relationship of these effects to micro and macroalbuminuria.
Goal 2: Establishment of an animal model with spontaneous glomerulopathy caused by abnormal heparan sulphate biosynthesis.
Goal 3: Examination of glycosaminoglycan metabolism in cell cultures of renal tissues and fibroblasts from diabetic and normal volunteer patients.
Goal 4: Semi-quantitative immunohistochemical studies of the cell types affected in diabetes.

Objective 2
Goal 1: Isolation of cDNA clones encoding unique basement membrane components.
Goal 2: Isolation of variants of basement membrane components and of genes involved in congenital renal diseases.

Objective 3
Goal 1: Characterisation of the reduction of N-deacetylase in diabetes.
Goal 2: Isolation and characterisation of the full length cDNA and characterisation of the mouse and human N-deacetylase genes.
Goal 3: Determination of the influence of diabetes on the domain structure of heparan sulphate.

Objective 4
Goal 1: Determination of genetic polymorphisms of the N-deacetylase enzyme.
Goal 2: Determination of genetic polymorphisms in basement membrane components.

Objective 5
Goal 1: Determination of the effectiveness and mechanisms of glycosarninoglycan administration on preventing diabetic matrix alterations.
Goal 2: Growth factor - heparan sulphate interaction, structural determination and exogenous glycosarninoglycan therapeutic agents.

Project leader:
Dr. D. NOONAN
Istituto Nazionale per la Ricerca sul Cancro
Viale Benedetto XV 10
IT 16132 Genova
Phone: +39 10 353 42 12
Fax: +39 10 35 29 99
Contract number: CT921766

Participants:
Bruno BAGGIO &
Giovanni GAMBARO
IT 35128 Padova

Jo BERDEN &
Jaap VAN DEN BORN
NL 6500 HB Nijmegen

Guido DAVID
BE 3000 Leuven

T. DECKERT &
A KOFOED-ENEVOLDSEN
DK 2820 Gentoft

John GALLAGHER
UK Manchester M20 9BX

L. VAN DEN HEUVEL &
Jacques VEERKAMP
NL 6500 HB Nijmegen

Lena KJELLEN
SE 75123 Uppsala

Erwin SCHLEICHER
DE 8000 München

Karl TRYGGVASON
FI 90570 Oulu

PREVENTION OF BLINDNESS: MOLECULAR RESEARCH AND MEDICAL CARE IN RETINITIS PIGMENTOSA (RP)

Key words
Retinitis pigmentosa, molecular genetics.

Objectives
- To understand the basis of inherited blindness.
- To ascertain patients from specific ethnic groups and geographic clustering.
- To understand the pathogenesis.
- To search for prophylactic measures and eventual therapies.
- To disseminate scientific information throughout the Community.
- To support health-care delivery.
- To share common resources, rare material, expensive technologies in the EC.
- To support advanced training.

Brief description
Molecular genetic studies have resulted in recent and considerable progress, Gene mapping and gene cloning were successful in a number of eye disorders allowing clinical use in some of these. This progress, predominantly from European research, has been achieved by participants in this Concerted Action as exemplified by two recent publications in *Nature* which were based on material collected all over Europe, greatly facilitated by our Concerted Action.

An ascertainment programme for rare informative patient material (blood-DNAs from pedigrees with arRP, Usher Syndrome, dominant cystic macula dystrophy etc.) will be coordinated in participating European centres and this material will be shared with experienced molecular genetics groups. These will perform molecular genetics studies such as linkage analyses, fine mapping, physical mapping and cloning of disease genes. In adRP and arRP, pedigrees will be screened for mutations in the rodtransducin, CRBP I an II and CHMP-PDE genes. The latter are involved in the transport of retinal, or directly, in the visual cascade which involves eight different proteins/subunits of the transducin cycle proper and at least six further regulatory proteins. In Usher syndrome, DNAs will be submitted for mutation analysis of the CHML-gene, a recently isolated choroideremia homologue mapping to the Iq32-42 region.

Concerted Action supported studies on small G proteins will transfer new techniques of utmost importance from the US to Europe and may advance the leading role of one European centre (Nijmegen) in relation to basic research into choroideremia.

The proposed Concerted Action-aided Primer Bank promises an added value for three reasons:

1 European areas where technical skills are still limited may take advantage of the particular strength of leading European centres by receiving primers pretested in experienced labs;
2 clinical use of molecular diagnostics and mutation analyses will be accelerated in participating Member States;
3 *bulk* synthesis and European-wide distribution of pretested industrial products may represent a benefit for industry.

A Concerted Action-aided improvement of hard and software of Humphrey Visual Fields Analyser which is not available on the market seems promising for three reasons:

1 the highest available technical standard in computer-aided perimetry is disseminated in participating European centres;
2 rare patient material (=pedigrees classified by molecular subtypes) will be more intensely exploited on a common basis for phenotype/genotype correlation;
3 experiences with the modified device collected European-wide may be of benefit for industry. *EC Courses for Scientists in Ophthalmology* and *EC Courses for Technicians-Academicians* offer an opportunity of advanced training and some European areas will take advantage of the particular strength of leading centres.

A *Directory of European Services*: (i) will disseminate information on European scientific interests and expertise; (ii) will increase the awareness of clinicians for specific patient material needed in basic research, and; (iii) may advance health care delivery in the EC.

Project leader:
Professor I.H. PAWLOWITZKI
Institute of Human Genetics,
Westfälische Wilhelms-Universität
Vesaliusweg 12-14
DE 48149 Münster
Phone: +49 251 83 69 96
Fax: +49 251 83 69 97
Contract number: CT921789

Participants:
Dr. J. FREZAL (FR)
Dr. M. WARBURG (DK)
F. BRUNSMANN (DE)
Prof. E. ZRENNER (DE)
Prof. H.H. ROPERS (NL)
Prof. J. MARSHALL (UK)
Prof. A. WRIGHT (UK)

EUROPEAN STUDY GROUP ON CONGENITAL TOXOPLASMOSIS

Key words
Toxoplasma, toxoplasmosis, pregnancy, screening, infection, blindness, congenital infections.

Objectives
1 Develop and evaluate new technologies for diagnosis of toxoplasma in pregnancy.
2 Standardisation and quality control of current and emerging diagnostic tests for toxoplasmosis.
3 Establish a clinical and biological case definition and stage classification of congenital toxoplasmosis.
4 Establish a register of children with congenital toxoplasmosis diagnosed after common guidelines.
5 Evaluate current treatment strategies and propose treatment schedules to be evaluated in a European multi-centre study.
6 Develop common guidelines for appropriate advice to pregnant women on how to avoid infection (health promotion).
7 Investigate transmission of Toxoplasma infection to human populations, and between mother and child.

Brief description
Infections with *Toxoplasma gondii* are found all over the European Community. In the EC, 3,5 million children were born in 1989. Of these, it is estimated that 7,700 mothers were infected with toxoplasmosis during pregnancy, and 3,100 children were infected before birth (assuming 40% transmission rate). Two hundred and fifteen children will have severe damage like hydrocephalus and mental retardation, and the remaining will have a high risk of presenting retinochoroiditis within the first 20 years of life.

Objective 1: The network will identify promising novel diagnostic techniques and reference laboratories that wish to evaluate these tests (see below).

Objective 2: Appropriate control and reference specimens, which will compromise serum samples, amniotic fluid and foetal blood samples, will be produced ¨and exchanged between the laboratories.

Objective 3: The concerted action will assemble and combine current knowledge of the clinical, serological and microbiological manifestations of congenital toxoplasmosis.

Objective 4: Pregnant mothers with suspected acute toxoplasmosis and children with suspected congenital toxoplasmosis will be offered registration in a European register of congenital toxoplasmosis. The register will be kept at Division of Prenatal Medicine and Obstetrics, A.Z. V.U.B., Brussels (Belgium) which will be responsible for data analysis and follow up. The establishment of a central register will have to be approved by national ethical committees.

Objective 5: The concerted action will establish a working group to consider the feasibility of conducting a European multicentre trial of treatment of congenital toxoplasmosis.

Objective 6: Informal, qualitative interviews will be conducted with small groups of pregnant women.

Objective 7: The working group will initiate research to identify risk factors associated with exposure to Toxoplasma infection in different countries. Such information can be used to develop better targeted health education programmes.

Project leader:
Dr. E. PETERSEN
Statens Seruminstitut,
Laboratory of Parasitology
Artillerivej 5
DK 2300 Copenhagen S
Phone: +45 32 68 32 23
Fax: +45 32 68 32 28
Contract number: CT921572

Participants:
Prof. P. AMBROISE-THOMAS
FR 38043 Grenoble

Prof. H. ASPÖCK &
Dr. HASSL
AT 1095 Vienna

Dr. A.H. BALFOUR
UK Leeds LS15 7TR

Dr. R. BERGER
CH 4058 Basel

Dr. M.H. BESSIERES
FR 31054 Toulouse Cedex

Prof. J.P. SEGUELA
FR 31054 Toulouse Cedex

Dr. R. BLATZ
DE 7022 Leipzig

Dr. A. DECOSTER ·
FR Lille Cedex

Prof. F. DEROUIN
FR 75475 Paris Cedex 10

Dr. G.N. DUTTON
UK Glasgow G11 6NY

Prof G. ENDERS
DE 7000 Stuttgart

Dr. M. FORSGREN
SE 107 26 Stockholm

Dr. W. FOULON
BE 1090 Brussels

Dr. R. GILBERT
UK London WC1N 1EH

Dr. T. VAN GOOL
NL 1105 AZ Amsterdam

Dr G.B. HASTINGS
UK Glasgow G4 0RQ

Dr. K. HEDMAN
FI 00290 Helsinki

Prof. P. HENGST
DE Berlin

Dr. D.O. HO-YEN
UK Inverness IV2 3UJ

Dr. R.E. HOLLIMAN
UK London SW1T 0QT

Dr. P. JACQUIER
CH 8057 Zürich

Dr. K. JANITSCHKE
DE Berlin 65

Dr. P. JENUM
NO 0462 Oslo

Dr. D.H.M. JOYNSON
UK Swansea SA2 8QA

Dr. T.T. KIEN
FR 6700 Strasbourg

Dr. J. KJELDSEN
DK 6400 Sonderborg

Dr. P.E. KLAPPER
UK Blackley Manchester

Dr. F. VAN KNAPEN
NL 3720 BA Bilthoven

Dr. B. LÉCOLIER
FR 75674 Paris Cedex 14

Dr. E. LINDER
SE 105 21 Stockholm

Dr. V. LUYASU
BE 1340 Ottignies

Dr. K. MELBY
NO 0407 Oslo

Dr. B. MILEWSKA-BOBULA
PL 04 736 Warsawa

Dr. A. NAESSENS
BE 1090 Brussels

Dr. H. PADELT
DE Berlin

Dr. A.PAJOR
HU 1082 Budapest

Prof. J. PHILIP
DK 2100 Copenhagen

Dr. J.M. PINON
FR 51092 Reims

Prof. A. POLLAK
AT 1090 Vienna

Dr. M. RUSSO
IT 80135 Naples

Prof. J.P. SEGUELA
FR 31054 Toulouse

Prof H.M. SEITZ
DE 5300 Bonn 1

Dr. M.A.E. CONYN-
VAN SPAENDONCK
NL 3720 BA Bilthoven

Dr. B. STRAY-PEDERSEN
NO 0514 Oslo

Dr. D.W. TAYLOR
UK Cambridge CB2 1QP

Dr. J.G. THORNTON
UK Leeds LS2 9LN

Dr. P. THULLIEZ
FR 75014 Paris

Dr. B. OVLISEN
DK 3400 Hillerod

TREATMENT OF DIABETES BY ISLET CELL TRANSPLANTATION

Key words
Diabetes, transplantation, ß cells, therapy.

Objectives
1 Production and banking of standardized human ß cell aggregates in sufficient quantity and quality for clinical and investigational use in a European network.
2 Organization of clinical trial on islet cell transplantation in diabetic patients using quality controlled grafts of insulin-producing ß cells.
3 Training of clinical and basic investigators, with a commitment to establish new centres and laboratories in our network.

Brief description
The long-term goal of the project is to develop a cure for diabetes by implantation of insulin-producing ß cells.

The working hypothesis is that successful transplantation of islet ß cells in man requires standardized preparation of purified grafts with selected size, composition and function. The cell biologic properties of the grafts should be adjusted to the metabolic and immunologic status of the recipient. Purified grafts are expected to increase the efficacy of accompanying measures against (auto)immune reactivity.

Human pancreata are procured by 15 European transplantation centres of our network and are shipped, together with blood and donor data, to the central unit in Brussels. Donor organs are processed at the central facility in Brussels, according to international regulations for handling material intended for implantation in man. For each donation, pancreatic and blood samples are taken for morphologic, toxicologic and microbiologic control as well as for storage; genetic, medical and laboratory information of the donor is collected and stored.

Human ß cell isolation proceeds via the methods which have been developed for laboratory animals. The isolated ß cells fulfil all basic requirements of viability and glucose-regulated functions. Each isolated ß cell preparation will be characterized by quality control data which assess the morphologic and functional state of the cells.

A clinical trial is planned to start in 1993. The purpose of this trial is to test the usefulness of purified ß cell grafts which have been composed on the basis of cell biologic parameters. An expert committee will outline protocols for the clinical trial of islet cell grafts, defining patient selection, surgical act, drug treatment, follow-up. This protocol will be submitted to the national and local ethical committees and to the participating centres. Grafts will be distributed from the central unit to the islet cell transplant centres through Eurotransplant/Bio Implant Services. The clinical trial is coordinated by the central unit where data of donors, recipient and grafts are stored.

Project leader:
Professor D. PIPELEERS
Diabetes Research Center, Vrije Universiteit Brussel
Laarbeeklaan 103
BE 1090 Brussels
Phone: +32 2 477 45 59
Fax: +32 2 477 45 45
Contract number: CT920805

Participants:

R. AERTS
Dept. of Surgery,
Katholieke Univ. Leuven
Herestraat 49
BE 3000 Leuven

R. BOUILLON
Dept. of Endocrinology,
Katholieke Universiteit
Leuven
Herestraat 49
BE 3000 Leuven

L. DE PAUW
Dept. of Surgery, Université
Libre de Bruxelles
Route de Lennik 808
BE 1070 Brussels

E. VAN SCHAFTINGEN
Chem. Physiology,
Universite Libre de Bruxelles
Avenue Hippocrate 10
BE 1200 Brussels

P. PATTIJN
Dept. of Surgery,
Rijksuniversiteit Gent
De Pintelaan 185
BE 9000 Gent

R. VAN HEE
Dept. of Surgery,
Universitaire Instelling
Antwerpen
Wilrijkstraat 19
BE 2650 Edegem

M. MEURISSE
Dept of Surgery,
Universite de Liege
Sart Tilman B35
BE 4000 Liege 1

J.P. SQUIFFLET
Avenue Hippocrate 10
BE 1200 Brussels

G. DELVAUX
Laarbeeklaan 101
BE 1090 Brussels

H. MARKHOLST
Niels Steensensvej 6
DK 2820 Gentofte

K. SALMELA
Haartmaninkatu 3A
FI 00290 Helsinki

P. CZERNICHOW
48 bd. Sérurier
FR 75019 Paris

R. LANDGRAF
Ziemssenstrasse 1
DE 80336 München

P. PETERSEN
DE 8000 München

D. ABENDROTH
Steinhövelstrasse 9
DE 7900 Ulm a.d. Donau

G. PAPADOPOULOS
GR 45332 Ioannina

G. TOMKIN
Fitzwilliam Square 1
IE Dublin 2

F. PURRELLO
Dept of Endocrinology,
University of Catania
Piazza s. Maria di Gèsu
IT 95123 Catania

B. ROEP
NL 2333 AA Leiden

T. DE BY
Bio Implant
Services/Eurotransplant
P.O. Box 2304
NL 2301 RC Leiden

C. ERICHSEN
National Hospital
Pilestredet 32
NO 0027 Oslo

J. ANSELMO
Dept of Endocrinology,
Hospital of Lisbon
Rua Nova do Almada 11 4D
PT 1200 Lisbon

C. HELLERSTROM
Dept of Medical Cell
Biology,
University of Uppsala
Husargatan 3
SE 751 23 Uppsala

A. LERNMARK
Dept of Endocrinology,
Karolinska Institute,
University of Stockholm
SE 10401 Stockholm

C. GROTH
Dept of Transplantation
Surgery, Karolinska Institute,
Huddinge Hospital
SE 141 86 Huddinge

N. PERSSON
Dept of Surgery, Malmö
General Hospital,
University of Lund
SE 214 01 Malmö

J. WADSTROM
Dept of Surgery, University
of Uppsale
SE 851 85 Uppsala

DETERMINANTS OF OSTEOPOROTIC HIPFRACTURE AND THEIR IMPLICATIONS FOR PUBLIC HEALTH IN EUROPE: A PROSPECTIVE MULTICENTRE STUDY

Key words

Osteoporis, hip fractures, vertebral fractures, risk factors, bone remodelling, bone densitometry, radiological morphometry, clinical biochemistry, bone histomorphometry.

Objectives

1 To unravel the aetiopathogenesis of fragility fractures of the hip ans spine, to explain the large variation in their incidence across Europe and ultimately to prepare the way for disease prevention and better treatments.

2 To identify the risk factors associated with the development of osteoporotic (fragility) fractures of the hip and spine in the people of Europe, for use in developing public health strategies for their management.

Brief description

The prevalence of spinal fractures in 30 European centres has been described in the COMAC-Epid *EVOS* study. 28 of these centres (including 6 non-EC/COST), with 4 additional EC centres will study prospectively, in these and new subjects drawn from population-based registers, the incidence of hip, spine and other fractures associated with bone fragility. Incident spine fractures will be measured on interval X-rays.

Fractures will be related to diet, lifestyle (including smoking and alcohol), exercise and other risk factors determined from questionnaires (including reproductive history) as well as falls, bone mass measurements, bone loss rates, and biochemical indices of bone turnover. The occurrence of hip fractures is so variable throughout Europe and rates of secular age-specific increase are so different between centres that the study derives great power from its wide geographical spread (> 25,000 subjects).

Power: The sample size will be sufficient to give it a power of 95% with the ability to detect a relative risk of 1,5 or higher for a given exposure.

Ascertainment of outcome (fractures) will be based on: (i) annual questionnaires; (ii) positive radiological and clinical verification of reported fractures and (iii) radiological identification of new vertebral fractures in a sample of 15,000 at an interval of 3-4 years after x-ray.

Specialised Methods: (i) bone densitometry of proximal femur and femoral neck length measurement using Dual X-ray Absorptiometry standardised with the European Spine Phantom (ESP); (ii) measurement of 8 biochemical markers as risk factors for hip fracture (nested case-control design). These are ostcocalcin, uncarboxylated osteocalcin, PTH, 25(OH) vitamin D, deoxypyridinoline, bone specific alkaline phosphatase, albumin and creatinine. (iii) histological evaluation of microstructure and remodelling in biopsies taken from the fracture site (femoral neck fractures, Garden types 3 or 4).

Management: The Project Steering Group will be based on the ERVOS Management Group and continuity with EVOS will be assured. The statistical evaluation will be shared between Manchester and Cambridge (UK). The designated biochemistry centre will be Lyon (FR) with histology shared between UK and FR. Radiology will be Berlin's responsibility (DE).

This study will provide valuable information on the age-specific incidence for spine and hip fractures in defined populations and will identify statistical determinants of fracture risk. It is likely that new risk factors will be identified which will be of practical value in developing Public Health strategies for reducing fracture rates in the future.

Project leader:
Dr. J. REEVE
Institute of Public health,
University Forvie Site
Robinson Way
UK Cambridge CB2 2SR
Phone: +44 223 330344
Fax: +44 223 330399
Contract number: CT920182

Participants:

Prof. Donato AGNUSDEI
IT 53100 Siena

Prof.BENEVOLENSKAYA
RU 115522 Moscow

Prof. Jorge CANNATA
ES 33080 Oviedo

Prof. Guzin DILSEN
TR Istanbul

Prof. Emmanuel DRETAKIS
GR 711 10 Heraklion (Crete)

Prof. Dieter FELSENBERG
DE 1000 Berlin 45

Prof. Dietrich BANZER
DE 1000 Berlin 37

Dr. Ashok BHALLA
UK Bath BA1 1RL

Dr. Juliet COMPSTON
UK Cambridge CB2 2QQ

Dr. Cord DODENHOF
DE 05010 Erfurt

Dr. Jan FALCH
NO 014 Oslo

Prof. Fernando GALAN &
prof. Ramon PEREZ CANO
ES 41009 Sevilla

Prof. Piet GUESENS
BE 3212 Lubbeek

Dr. Krysztow HOSZOWSKI
PL 03737 Warsaw

Dr. Olof JOHNELL
SE 214 01 Malmö

Dr. Heikki KROGER
FI 70201 Kuopio

Dr. Paul LIPS
NL 1007 MB Amsterdam

Prof. Roman LORENC
PL 04 736 Warsaw

Prof. Stanislav HAVELKA
CZ 128 50 Praha 2

Prof. Ivo JAJIC
HR 4100 Zagreb

Prof. Kay-Tee KHAW
UK Cambridge CB2 2QQ

Dr. A. AROSO
PT Porto

Prof. George LYRITIS
GR Kiifisia Athens

Dr. Francois MARCHAND
FR 71300

Dr. Tomasz. MIAZGOWSKI
PL 71 455 Szezecin

Dr. Gyula POOR
HU 1023 Budapest

Prof. W. REISINGER
DE 0 1040 Berlin

Dr. Pavol MASARYK
SK 921 01 Piestany

Dr. Jose ORTEGA
ES 28040 Madrid

Dr. Huibert A.P. POLS
NL 3000 DR Rotterdam

Prof. Heiner RASPE
DE Lübeck

Dr. David M. REID
UK Aberdeen AB9 8AU

Prof. H. SCHATZ
DE 4630 Bochum 1

Dr. C. SCHEIDT-NAVE
DE 6900 Heidelberg 1

Dr. Christopher TODD
UK Cambridge CB2 2SR

Dr. Anthony WOOLF
UK Cornwall TR1 2HZ

Prof. Jan STEPAN
CZ 12621 Prague 2

Dr. Kurt WEBER
AT 8036 Graz

A MULTIDISCIPLINARY APPROACH TO THE PATHOGENICITY OF THE TRANSTHYRETIN RELATED DISORDERS

Key words
Amyloidoses, amyloidogenesis, transthyretin related disorders.

Brief description
Human plasma transthyretin (TTR) is a protein known to transport both thyroxine (T4) and retinol binding protein (RBP). Polychlorinated byphenils (PCBs) also bind specifically to TTR. The three dimensional structure of the protein has been elucidated and its association with diseases constitutes an important tool to investigate the biology of the protein. More than 20 mutations have been described in TTR.

Most of these TTR variants are associated with familial amyloid polyneuropathies (FALP) and familial amyloid cardiomyopathies (FAC), diseases characterized by the extracelluar deposition of fibrilar material composed of TTR. TTR amyloid also occurs in the heart of old people but in these cases non mutated TTR is involved and the condition is denominated senile systemic amyloid (SSA). SSA is a frequent postmortem finding in patients over 80 years of age, retrospectively associated with antemortem congestive heart failure and cardiac arrhythmias. Non amyloidogenic TTR variants have been also reported and among these, two of them affect thyroxine binding. How TTR mutations affect the structure, function and metabolism of TTR has not yet been fully explored. Furthermore, information is lacking, and is needed, about the factors that cause mutant TTR molecules to polymerize into amyloid fibrils.

Several alternative and non-exclusive hypotheses can be considered to try to explain the pathogenic mechanisms underlying the TTR related amyloidoses. Synthetic TTR mutants produced by recombinant DNA techniques have been obtained that can serve to explore the amyloidogenic potential of TTR. Comparative X-Ray crystallography of both amyloid and non-amyloid TTR mutants combined with ligand binding studies will provide information about a possible conformational model for amyloidogenesis. The *in vivo* approaches use animal models to study not only the amyloidogenic potential of TTR, but especially the factors that modulate amyloidogenesis. Such studies might give insights into circulating or tissue factors responsible for the clinical heterogenecity observed among FAP and FAC patients. One possible modulating factor is the proteolytic system that degrades TTR. Analyses of fibrils from some FAP and FAC patients and from patients with SSA showed, along with intact TTR, fragments that always encompass the same region of the TTR monomer. A proteolytic mechanism might represent a common pathway of amyloid formation from both mutant and normal TTR. Whether proteolysis induces a particular conformation, thus triggering polymerization, or is a secondary event in amyloid formation remains to be determined and can be tested in available transgenic mice carrying and expressing a mutant TTR.

Both the *in vitro* and the *in vivo* approaches should help to understand the amyloid formation process and in devising treatment strategies for the TTR related disorders, in particular the cardiomyopathies.

Project Leader:
Professor M.J. SARAIVA
Centro de Estudos de Paramiloidose, Hospital de Santo Antonio
PT 4000 Porto
Phone: +351 2 606 61 49
Fax: +351 2 606 61 06
Contract number: CT921076

Participants:
Dr. Colin BLAKE
Molecular Biophysics, University of Oxford,
The Rex Richards Building
South Parks Road
UK Oxford OX1 3QU
Phone: +44 865 275 373
Fax: +44 865 510 454

Dr. Abraham BROUWER
Dept. of Toxicology,
Wageningen Agricultural University
Biotechnion/De Dreijen 12
NL 6700 EV Wageningen
Phone: +31 8370 839 71
Fax: +31 8370 849 31

Dr. Ana M. DAMAS
Biofysica, Instituto de Ciencias Biomedicas,
Universidade do Porto
PT 4000 Porto
Phone: +351 2 2080 288
Fax: +351 2 2001 918

Dr. Erik LUNDGREN
Dept. of Cellular and Molecular Biology,
Umea University
SE 901 87 Umea
Phone: +46 90 133 536
Fax: +46 90 111 420

A MULTI-CENTRE EFFORT AIMED AT IMPROVING MATCHING CRITERIA IN BONE MARROW AND RENAL TRANSPLANTATION

Key words
Transplantation, histocompatibility, mismatches, alloreactivity.

Objectives
1 To help define the role played by HLA-class II loci in transplantation.
2 To correlate number and positions of HLA-class II mismatches with functional tests aimed at quantifying the level of *in vivo* donor-recipient alloreactivity.
3 To refine and adapt rapid HLA typing techniques based on heteroduplexes analysis to the screening of donor-recipient compatibility and to apply theoretical models to the construction of computer programs aimed to predict the electrophoretic behaviour of heteroduplexes.

Brief description
Selection of donor-recipient pairs
DNAs from cells of donor and recipient pairs both from bone-marrow and renal transplantation will be collected at the Hammersmith Hospital in London (England), at Dept. of Immunohematology and Blood Bank in Leiden (Holland) and at policlinico Umberto I in Rome (Italy) and send to Rome for HLA-class II molecular typing.

HLA-class II typing:
DNA molecular typing will be performed by heteroduplexes analysis and the position and the type of mismatches will be correlated to the quantitative analysis of alloreactivity and to the outcome of transplantation.

Evaluation of the level of in vivo donor-recipient alloreactivity:
For HLA-matched unrelated bone marrow transplants (BMT) combinations, the frequency of donor anti-recipient alloreactive cells will be measured. For renal transplant patients, the frequency of recipient anti-donor Th cells will be quantitated. BMT patients will be followed up for a period of 100 days - this is the period during which acute graft versus host disease (GVHD) occurs. The severity of acute GVHD will be graded according to standard criteria.

Theoretical models:
Electrophoretic mobility changes of DNA heteroduplexes due to the presence of mismatches along the sequence will be analyzed adopting a theoretical model early proposed for predicting the electrophoretic manifestations of sequence dependent DNA curvature. The time schedule of this program comprises 30 months of research.

Project leader:
Dr. R. SORRENTINO
Dipartimento di Biologia Cellulare e dello Sviluppo,
Università "La Sapienza"
Via degli Apuli 1
IT 00185 Roma
Phone: +39 6 49 15 16
Fax: +39 6 49 91 75 94
Contract number: CT921781

Participants:
Dr. Robert LECHLER
Dept. of Immunology,
Royal Postgraduate Medical School,
Hammersmith Hospital
Du Cane Road
UK London W12 0NN
Phone: +44 81 743 2030
Fax: +44 81 740 3034

Dr. Frans H.J. CLAUS
Tissue Typing and Transplantation Immunology,
University Hospital Building 1, E3-62
P.O. Box 9600
NL 2300 RC Leiden
Phone: +31 71 263 801
Fax: +31 71 216 751

Dr. P. DE SANTIS &
dr. Antonio PALIESCHI
Dipartemento di Chimica,
Università di Roma "La Sapienza"
Piazzale Aldo Moro 5
IT 00185 Roma
Phone: +39 6 445 3827
Fax: +39 6 490 631

Dr. Elvira RENNA MOLAJONI
Laboratorio di Immunologia, Servizio Trapianti,
Seconda Clinica Chirurgica, Policlinico
Umberto I, Univ La Sapienza
Viale Regina Margherita
IT 00185 Roma
Phone: +39 6 4450 741
Fax: +39 6 4463 667

CHANGES IN GLIAL CELLS WITH AGEING: IN-CULTURE STUDIES

Key words
Ageing, glial cells, neurotrophin receptors.

Objectives
Introduction and Specific Aims:
1 Responsiveness of astrocytes derived from newborn and aged mouse brain to in vitro micro-environment: Substrata and Neurotrophins.
2 Comparison of neurotrophin receptor binding sites in astrocytes derived from newborn and aged mouse brain.
3 Changes in cell surface of astrocytes with aging.

Project Methodology:
- Culture Systems.
- Preparation of primary mixed glial-cell cultures.
- Preparation of substrata.
- Preparation of brain fibroblast substratum.

Brief description
This project will focus on comparative changes occurring in cultured glial cells derived from newborn mouse brain as tested by their responsiveness to:
1 Culture substrata and neurotrophins added to the culture medium; the responsiveness will be tested: (a) biochemically, using the activity of glutamine synthetase, an astrocyte enzyme; (b) the expression of neurotrophin receptors assayed biochemically and immunocytochemically.
2 Changes in cell membrane function testing: (a) ionic fluxes an membrane enzyme Na^+ K^+ ATPase; (b) adenylate cyclase and ß-adrenergic receptors.

Project leader:
Professor A. VERNADAKIS
Academic Research Institute
of Mental Health,
Eginition Hospital
Vas Sophias Avenue 74
GR 115 28 Athens
Phone: +30 1 721 77 83
Fax: +30 1 724 39 05
Contract number: CT921159

Participants:
Prof. Alain PRIVAT
Plasticité et Vieillisement
de Système Nerveux
Place Eugene Bataillion, Case
Courrier 106
FR 34095 Montpellier
Phone: +33 67 14 33 86
Fax: +33 67 14 33 18

Prof. Giorgio RACAGNI
Centro di Studio e Recercadi
Neuropharmacologia, Univer-
sita degli studi di Milano
Via Balzaretti 9
IT 20133 Milano
Phone: +39 2 204 48831
Fax: +39 2 294 04961

Prof. Arne SCHOUSBOE
Dept. of Biological Sciences,
Danmarks Farmaceutiske
Hojskole
Universitetsparken 2
DK 2100 Copenhagen
Phone: +45 31 37 08 50
Fax: +45 35 37 57 44

Prof. Klaus UNSICKER
Dept. of Anatomy and
Cell Biology,
University of Marburg
Robert-Koch-Strasse 6
DE 3550 Marburg
Phone: +49 64 21 28 40 30
Fax: +49 64 21 28 70 66

UNDERSTANDING AND PREVENTION OF INHERITED POLYCYSTIC RENAL DISEASE: DOES EARLY TREATMENT POSTPONE RENAL FAILURE?

Key words
Polycystic kidney, genetic disease, genetic mapping.

Objectives
The general objective is to develop a programme, started under the CA *Towards prevention of renal failure caused by inherited polycystic kidney disease*, that will encourage collaboration between European clinicians and geneticists with the twin aims of identifying the genes responsible for autosomal dominant polycystic dikney disease (ADPKD) and the clinical factors associated with the development of renal failure and formation of cerebral aneurysms.
Specific objectives are:
1 Hypertension: Identify whether hypotensive drugs with particular mechanisms of action have advantages in delaying the rate of deterioration of renal function.
2 Cerebral aneurysm: Determine the risk of development or growth of another intra-cranial aneurysm (ICA) in patients surviving a first ICA rupture.
3 Genetic mapping of PKD3 genetic mapping and clinical studies of PKD3 families: Identify further large kindreds unlinked to markers on chromosome 16 that are suitable for mapping PKD3 gene(s).

Brief description
Autosomal dominant polycystic kidney disease (EDPKD)is a common condition, in which the development of cysts within the kidney often leads to hypertension and renal failure. The project combines clinical and genetic approaches aimed at understanding the genetic mutation responsible for development of ADPKD and clinical factors associated with the progression of renal impairment.
The clinical component aims to coordinate and develop a series of studies on aspects of hypertension and the development of cerebral aneurysms. Particular emphasis will be placed on two studies:
- the first compares two different types of drugs for long-term treatment of hypertension and aims to determine whether selection of one particular drug type benefits renal function in the long term.
- the second explores the natural history of further cerebral aneurysm formation in patients who have already suffered an episode of ruptured cerebral aneurysm.

The genetic component aims to coordinate efforts to map the gene locus of PKDI (i.e. linked to chromosome 16) by collecting data on affected families throughout Europe. New recombinants will be sought with the aid of microsatellite markers and linkage studies undertaken to identify linkage disequilibrium. Finally efforts will be made to identify further large kindreds with polycystic kidney disease unlinked to chromosome 16 (PKD2).

Project leader:
Professor M.L. WATSON
Medical Renal Unit, University of Edinburgh
Royal Infirmary
UK Edinburgh EH3 9YW
Phone: +44 31 229 24 77
Fax: +44 31 229 99 73
Contract number: CT921094

Participants:

Dr. Martin BREUNING
NL Leiden

Dr. Peter CHANG
NL Leiden

Dr. Alan F. WRIGHT
UK Edinburgh

Dr. S.M.M.J. CASTEDO
PT 4200 Porto

Dr. Ama GONZALO
ES 28034 Madrid

Dr. F. MORENO
ES 28034 Madrid

Dr. C. BOULTER
UK Cambridge CB2 1QR

Dr. Ian FENTON
UK Cardiff CF4 4 XN

Dr. A.M. FRISCHAUF
UK London

Dr. Neta P. MALLICK
UK Manchester M13 9WL

Dr. Peter HARRIS
UK Oxford OX3 9DU

Dr. M. CARMODY
IE Dublin 9

Dr. David T. CROKE
IE Dublin 2

Dr. F. AJMAR
IT Genova

Dr. A. SESSA
IT 20059 Vimercate Milan

Dr. G. ROMEO
IT 16148 Genoa

Dr. A. CARBONARA
IT 10126 Turin

Dr. M. MARTINS PRATA
PT 1600 Moniz (Lisbon)

Dr. P. WILLEMS
BE 2610 Wilrijk

Dr. C. VERELLEN-
DUMOULIN
BE 1200 Brussels

Dr. Yves PIRSON
BE 1200 Brussels

Dr. S. NORBY
DK 2100 Copenhagen 0

Dr. M. SCHWARTZ
DK 1200 Copenhagen
OB02610

Dr. H. DANIELSEN
DK 8000 Aarhus C.

Dr. Jean Pierre GRUNFELD
FR 75743 Paris Cedex 15

Dr. Micheline LEVY
FR 75016 Paris

Dr. P. SIMON
FR 22023 St. Brieuc

Dr. E. RITZ
DE 6900 Heidelberg

Dr. Norbert GRETZ
DE 6800 Mannheim 1

Dr. K. ZERRES
DE 5300 Bonn 1

Dr. R. KLINGEL
DE 6500 Mainz

Dr. D. LOUKOPOULOS
GR 155 27 Athens

Dr. D. PAPADOPOULOU
GR 54639 Thessaloniki

Dr. P. DUHOUX
LU 1210 Luxembourg

Dr. H. KAARIASINEN
FI 00100 Helsinki

Dr. L. PULKKINEN
FI 70210 Kuopio

Dr. P. COUCKE
BE 2610 Wilrijk

Dr. Martyn ZEIER
DE 6900 Heidelberg 1

Dr. M. FEAD
UK Dundee DD1 9SY

Dr. F. MACDONALD
UK Birmingham B9 5PX

Dr. S. JEFFREY
UK London SW17 0RF

Dr. L. SENNO
IT Urmario Ferrara

Dr. F. CONTE
IT 20059 Vimelcare (Milan)

Dr. J. OLIVIERA
PT 4200 Porto

Dr. J. LAVINHA
PT 1699 Lisboa Codex

Dr. J. MILLARS
ES 28034 Madrid

ASSESSMENT AND COST-EFFECTIVENESS APPRAISAL OF VIDEOREFRACTIVE TECHNIQUES IN PAEDIATRIC VISION SCREENING PROGRAMMES

Key words
Videorefraction, screening, paediatric visual defects, refractive errors, strabismus, amblyopia.

Brief description
The Concerted Action has three main objectives:
1 the harmonization of infant vision screening protocols, using videorefraction;
2 the establishment of a common data base on screening and outcome, and;
3 cost effectiveness evaluation of these programmes across health systems in different
   EC countries.
The project will coordinate programmes in six European centres for population screening of infants and young children for visual problems. New videorefractive techniques, devised by the collaborators, will be used to detect refractive errors in infancy, which are known to be precursors of strabismus and amblyopia.
In particular, hyperopia and anisometropia will be detected along with manifest orthoptic problems.
The project will establish common protocols for videorefractive and orthoptic screening and follow-up.
It will bring together into a common data base results from these programmes on the incidence, progression, and outcome of infant refractive errors.
The numbers of children studied in this multi-centre trial will increase statistical reliability over those possible in a single centre, and the range of populations and social conditions in these centres will strengthen the generality of the findings.
The project will include a cost-effectiveness evaluation of this paediatric vision screening method, against the baseline of results from general surveillance in primary health care.
This evaluation will examine the comparative aspects of introducing such screening programmes, and their relative cost-effectiveness, in the context of the different systems of paediatric health care delivery existing in the different participating European countries.

Project leader:
Dr. Janette ATKINSON
Visual Development Unit,
University of Cambridge
Trumpington Street 22
UK Cambridge CB2 1QA
Phone: +44 223 33 35 73
Fax: +44 223 33 39 31
Contract number: CT931589

Participants:
Dr. M. ANGI
Università di Padova,
Clinica Oculistica
IT 35121 Padova
Phone: +39 49 875 23 50
Fax: +39 49 875 23 84

Dr. S. ATKINSON
Wessex Regional Health
Authority, Highcroft
Romsey Road
UK Winchester SO22 5DH
Phone: +44 962 86 35 11
Fax: +44 962 84 94 12

Dr. F. VITAL-DURAND
Unité 371 INSERM,
Cerveau et Vision
16 Av. du Doyen Lepine
FR 69500 Bron Lyon
Phone: +33 78 54 65 78
Fax: +33 72 36 97 60

Prof. A. CASTANERA
DE MOLINA
Instituto Castanera, Unidad
de Oftalmologia Pediatrica y
Estrabismo, Freixa
ES 08021 Barcelona
Phone: +34 3 202 18 81
Fax: +34 3 202 12 81

Dr. O. ALVES DA SILVA
Santa Maria Hospital, Dept.
Strabismology
Urbanizacao de Portela
PT 2685 Sacavem Lisbon
Phone: +351 1 943 10 11
Fax: +351 1 943 10 11

MANIPULATION OF OLIGOSACCHARIDE: ASSOCIATED INFLAMMATORY MECHANISM TO TREAT ARTHRITIS

Key words
Oligosaccharide, inflammation, arthritis, glycoprotein, immunology, acute phase, glycosyltransferase, cell adhesion.

Objectives
To capitalise upon arthritis oligosaccharide changes in glycoproteins and on cell surfaces to develop novel therapeutic strategies in the treatment of arthritis and increase our understanding on the pathogenic mechanisms causing disease.

Brief description
Oligosaccharides are integral to the physiology of all body systems and maybe associated with inflammation and arthritis by causing variation in glycoprotein function (eg. immunoglobulin G) or cell adhesion (eg. the selectins).

This proposal details concerted research on a broad basis aimed at elucidating the mechanisms whereby oligosaccharides exert their action within the inflammatory process and how these mechanisms may be inhibited to bring about improvement of the inflammation process resulting in arthritis.

The European laboratory formed by this concerted action will focus upon the following four areas of glycobiology:
- Gluconproteins (immunoglobulin G and acute phase proteins);
- Oligosaccharide molecular modelling;
- Cell adhesion molecules;
- The glycosyltransferases.

Chronic arthritis is of major public health importance to the European Community and this concerted action will bring together laboratories to form a cohesive unit that will be able to carry out the research proposal described to tackle arthritis.

Project leader:
Dr. John S. AXFORD
Academic Rheumatology Unit,
Division of Immunology,
St George's Hospital & Medical School
Cranmer Terrace
UK London SW17 ORE
Phone: +44 81 672 99 44
Fax: +44 81 784 26 49
Contract number: CT931607

Participants:

Dr. Barry BRESNIHAN
Univ College of Dublin, Dept. of Rheumatology,
St Vincent's Hospital
Elm Park
IE Dublin 4
Phone: +353 1 269 4533
Fax: +353 1 283 8123

Dr. Elisabeth HOUNSELL
MRC Clinical Research Centre
Watford Road
UK Harrow Middlesex
HA1 3UJ
Phone: +44 81 864 3232
Fax: +44 81 423 1275

Dr. Jim van DIJK
Vrije Universiteit, Faculty of Medicine,
Dep of Med Chemistry
Van der Boechorststraat 7
NL 1081 BT Amsterdam
Phone: +31 20 548 2067
Fax: +31 20 642 8555

Dr. Keith GUY
Univ of Strathclyde,
Dept. of Immunology
Taylor Street 31
UK Glasgow G4 ONR
Phone: +44 41 552 4400
Fax: +44 41 552 6674

Prof. Frank C. HAY
St. George's Hospital Medical School,
Dep of Cellular & Molecular Sciences
Cranmar Terrace
UK London SW17 ORE
Phone: +44 81 672 9944
Fax: +44 81 784 2649

Prof. Pierre YOUINOU
Centre Hospitalier Regional et
Universitaire de Brest
Avenue Foch 5
FR 29609 Brest
Phone: +33 98 223 384
Fax: +33 98 801 076

Prof. Roy JEFFERIS
Univ of Birmingham, Dept. of Immunology
UK Birmingham B15 2TT
Phone: +44 21 414 4063
Fax: +44 21 414 3599

BIOCHEMICAL PREDICTION OF HIP FRACTURE:

A Centralised Laboratory facility for the BIOMED-1 funded Concerted Action
'EPOS' (European Prospective Osteoporosis Study)

Key words
Osteoporosis, hip fracture, epidemiology, vertebral fracture, bone biochemical markers.

Objectives
The overall objectives are:
- to analyze changes of markers of resorption and formation in elderly who subsequently sustained a hip or vertebral fracture compared to 3 age-matched controls.
- to determine the predictive value of bone markers, alone or in combination with bone densitometry, in the evaluation of the risk of osteoporotic fracture.

Brief description
The European Prospective Osteoporosis Study has as its primary objective the need to explain the growing epidemic of hip and spine fractures with which Europe is confronted.

Although fracture rates seem to have been growing nearly everywhere, there are still wide geographical differences in rates between countries, with much smaller variations within countries.

In France and Britain, for example, the annual hospital costs exceed 15 ECU per head of population. Extrapolating this to the whole European Union, these costs amount to ECU 5.5 billion per year, and will rise to ECU 11 billion (at 1985 prices) in 10-20 years due entirely to the ageing of the population.

However, in many European countries there has been a rising secular trend in the age-specific incidence, which has doubled in 20-30 years.

If this trend to increased vulnerability continues, costs will rise even more steeply and thereby jeopardise the achievement of other health targets in the Community.

EPOS involves 26 clinical centres in the EC and COST countries and 5 additional centres in Eastern and Central European countries. Fifteen of these which are expecting over 65% of the total number of hip fractures are collecting blood and urine samples.

Within a case-control design, each case of hip fracture will be matched to 3 controls to evaluate the predictive power of selected biochemical markers. Their predictive power in relation to the different prevalence of hip fracture in the various populations will be compared.

In all centres standardised bone densitometry will be performed and biochemistry and densitometry combined in a search for multi-variable predictors of fracture. This study will be powerful and comprehensive in its search for environmental and life-style causes of the current epidemic of osteoporotic fractures and has the potential to provide future guidance to public health authorities seeking to reduce the impact of osteoporosis on the people of Europe and guide the future choice between targeting whole populations or at risk groups with new prevention strategies.

Project leader:
Professor P. DELMAS
INSERM, U 234, Hôpital E. Herriot,
Pavillon F   -
FR 69003 Lyon Cédex 03
Phone: +33 72 34 48 06
Fax: +33 72 35 05 57
Contract number: CT931448

Participants:
Prof. Alan SILMAN
ARC Epidemiology Research Unit,
University of Manchester, Stopford Building
Oxford Road
UK Manchester M 13 9PT
Phone: +44 61 275 5040
Fax: +44 61 275 5043

Dr. Jonathan REEVE
Institute of Public Health, University Forvie Site
Robinson Way
UK Cambridge CB2 2SR
Phone: +44 223 330 302
Fax: +44 223 330 399

Prof. Dieter FELSENBERG
FU Berlin-Universitätsklinikum Steglitz,
Abtlg. Röntgendiagnostik
Hindenburgdamm 30
DE 1000 Berlin 45
Phone: +49 30 798 3040
Fax: +49 30 798 4141

Prof. Pierre J. MEUNIER
INSERM Unit 403, Pavillon F,
Hôpital E. Herriot
FR 69437 Lyon Cedex 03
Phone: +33 72 34 48 06
Fax: +33 72 35 05 57

Mr. Nigel GARRAHAN
Dept. of Pathology,
University of Wales, College of Medicine
Heath Park
UK Cardiff CF4 4XN
Phone: +44 222 742 702

ESTABLISHMENT OF A EUROPEAN NETWORK FOR PREVENTION, DIAGNOSIS AND TREATMENT OF PRIMARY IMMUNODEFICIENCIES

A Proposal from European Group for Immunodeficiencies (EGID)

Key words
Primary immunodeficiency diseases, gene, immunoglobulins, bone marrow transplantation, gene therapy, prenatal diagnosis.

Objectives
1 Set up a European registry of primary immunodeficiencies as a basis for genetic and therapeutic studies.
2 Coordination of therapeutic trials including immunoglobulins, bone marrow transplantation and gene therapy.

Brief description
About 80 different primary immunodeficiencies (ID) have been described. Many are rare diseases that can not be properly studied by individual centers.
We therefore propose to set up a functional network of clinical and research centers involved in the study and treatment of primary immunodeficiencies.
The first goal will be the establishment of an European registry that will give information on the prevalence of the different IDs, so to be used as a basis for further genetic and therapeutic studies within usage guidelines.
The recent identification of ID genes such as X-linked agammaglobulinemia (XLA) or X-linked hyper IgM syndrome (HIGM1) will provide the basis for collaborative work defining genotype/phenotype correlations for these diseases.
Similar studies will be conducted for the different chronic granulomatous diseases (CGD) and adenosine deaminase deficiency (ADA).
Specimens collection from patients with rare diseases and their families - such as Chediak Higashi syndrome - will provide material for gene localization.
Our goal is to also coordinate therapeutic trials such as comparison of subcutaneous and IV administration of immunoglobulins in hypogammaglobulinemic patients, long term effect of G-CSF in patients with congenital neutropenia and itraconazole preventive effect against aspergillus in patients with CGD.
The European network will provide the number of patients required for these studies.
Retrospective evaluation of bone marrow transplantation (BMT) - the sole curative therapy for ID so far notably its long term effects, as well as prospective evaluation of extension of BMT using donors other than HLA identical siblings will be analyzed.
Finally, first application of gene therapy for ADA deficiency will be coordinated and evaluated.
All of these studies will contribute through publication and meeting reports to the education of European physicians in charge of patients with ID.
Genetic studies will also lead to the constitution of a prenatal diagnosis laboratories directory, available to the whole medical European Community.

Project leader:
Professor A. FISCHER
INSERM U. 132, Hôpital
Necker, Enfants Malades,
Pavillon Kirmisson
Immunologie-Hématologie/
Pédiatrie
Rue de Sèvres 149
FR 75743 Paris Cédex 15
Phone: +33 1 42 73 83 02
Fax: +33 1 42 73 28 96
Contract number: CT931321

Participants:
A. ARNAIZ-VILLENA
Hopital 12 de Octubre,
Immunologia
ES 28041 Madrid

Helen CHAPEL
Dept. of Immunology,
John Radcliffe Hospital
UK Oxford OX3 9DU
Phone: +44 865 22 17 69
Fax: +44 865 74 21 80

Teresa ESPANOL
Institut Catala de la Salut,
Clutat Sanitaria i
Universitaria
Valle Hebron
ES 08035
Fax: +34 3 428 1012

Wilhelm FRIEDRICH
Dept. of Paediatrics,
University of Ulm
Prittwitzstrasse 43   '
DE 7900 Ulm
Fax: +49 731 502 7789

Claudio BORDIGNON
Ospedale San Raffaelle
Via Olgettina
IT Milan
Phone: +39 2 2643 2351
Fax: +39 2 2643 2640/4827

Marthe EIBL
Institut für Immunologie
der Universitat Wien
Borschkegasse 8a
AT 1090 Wien
Fax: +43 1 408 109 113

E.J.A. GERRITSEN &
J. VOSSEN
Dept. of Paediatrics,
University Hospital
Rijnsburgerweg 10
NL Leiden
Phone: +31 71 26 24 94
Fax: +31 71 21 31 52

Lennart HAMMARSTROM
& Carl E. SMITH
Dept. Clinical Immunology,
Huddinge Hospital
SE 14186 Huddinge
Phone: +46 8 746 1000
Fax: +46 8 746 6869

Roland LEVINSKY &
Gareth MORGAN
The Institute of Child Health,
University of London,
Dept. of Immunology,
Molecular Immunology,
Host Defence Units
30 Guilford Street
UK London WCIN
Phone: +44 71 242 9789
Fax: +44 71 831 4366

Luigi NOTARANGELO
Dept. of Paediatrics,
University of Brescia
c/o Spedali Civili
IT 25123 Brescia
Phone: +39 30 399 5715
Fax: +39 30 303 658

Jose REGUEIRO
Dept. of Immunology,
Hospital 12 de Octubre
ES 28041 Madrid
Phone: +34 1 390 8315
Fax: +34 1 392 8399

Christine KINNON
The Institute of Child Health,
University of London,
Dept. of Immunology,
Molecular Immunology,
Host Defence Units
30 Guilford Street
UK London WCIN
Phone: +44 71 242 9789
Fax: +44 71 831 4366

Roberto PAGANELLI
Dept. of Clinical
Immunology,
University La Sapienza
Viale Universita 37
IT 00185 Roma
Phone: +39 6 445 49415
Fax: +39 6 444 0806

Dirk ROOS
Central Laboratory of the
Netherlands Red Cross Blood
Transfusion Service
Plesmanlaan 125
NL 1066 CX Amsterdam
Phone: +31 20 523 3317
Fax: +31 20 512 3310

Anthony SEGAL
Dept. of Medicine,
University Collge London,
The Rayne Institute
5 University Street
UK London WC1E 6JJ
Phone: +44 71 380 9837

Dinko VALERIO
TNO Division of Health
Research, Institut of
Applied Radiobiology
and Immunology
P.O. Box 5815
NL 2280 HV Rijswijk
Fax: +31 15 84 39 98

Reinhard SEGER
Dept. of Immunology/
Haematology, University
Children's Hospital
Steinwiesstrasse 75
CH 8032 Zurich
Phone: +41 1 266 7311
Fax: +41 1 266 7171

R.S. WEENING
Emma Kinderziekenhuis,
Academic Medical Center
Meibergdreef 9
NL 1105 AZ Amsterdam
Phone: +31 20 5669 111
Fax: +31 20 6911 7735

NEW DEFINITION OF ALPORT SYNDROME BASED ON MOLECULAR GENETICS, AND TOWARDS THE PREVENTION OF END STAGE RENAL FAILURE DUE TO ALPORT SYNDROME

Key words
X-linked Alport's syndrome, autosomal Alport's syndrome, collagen type IV, oesophageal leiomyomatosis, anti-GBM glomerulonephritis.

Objectives
1 Collect and characterize the phenotype of most European families affected with Alport syndrome (AS).
2 Identify the mode of transmission of the disease in each family. Characterize the phenotypes of autosomal forms of AS.
3 Characterize the gene defect in each family and organize COL4A3-6 mutation analysis at the European level as a diagnostic tool.
4 Establish valid correlations between genotypes and phenotypes, based on the analysis of a large series of AS kindreds.
5 Construct the mutation map of each AS gene to identify possible genetic markers of severe renal and extra-renal forms of the disease, and of patients at risk of developing anti-GBM glomerulonephritis after transplantation.

Brief description
Alport syndrome (AS) is a severe hereditary disease leading young affected males and some affected females to the double handicap of renal failure and deafness. The AS gene frequency is estimated to be 1/5000.

Most cases of AS are X-linked, and mutations in the COL4A5 gene located at Xq22 and coding for the $\alpha5$ chain of type IV collagen have now been detected in 10 to 15% of investigated families. A second collagen IV gene (COL4A6) also located at Xq22, has just been identified and is a 2nd candidate gene for X-linked AS.

In addition, it has become clear that autosomal inheritance does exist. Autosomal dominant transmission seems to be rare whereas the incidence of autosomal recessive inheritance is probably higher than previously thought and has to be reconsidered. The candidate genes for autosomal AS are COL4A3 and COL4A4 coding for the $\alpha3$ and $\alpha4$ chains of collagen IV respectively, and located head to head on chromosome 2. The first mutations in COL4A3 have just been detected in a 2 patients from the European Community.

In Europe, a large number of AS families has been identified, which is a prerequisite for valuable family studies. Our objectives are to progress rapidly in the identification in each family of the gene defect responsible for this condition, to allow accurate and early diagnosis, identification of healthy female carriers, precise genetic counselling and, if necessary prenatal diagnosis. Analysis of a large number of AS kindreds could also allow the establishment of correlations between genotypes and phenotypes and the identification of possible environmental factors associated with rapid progression to ESRF. In addition, establishment of correlations between varying gene defects, deduced changes in a(IV)-chains structure and type IV collagen molecule organization, and expression of the disease, may provide useful informations about the interaction of the a(IV)-chains and the structure and functions of type IV collagen.

Treatment of ESRF in the European Community is costing at least 2 billions ECU a year and according to dialysis-transplantation registries, AS is recognized as the cause of End Stage Renal Failure (ESRF) in 0.6 to 2.3 of patients. About 4% of men treated for ESRF (most often from the age of 15-34 years) are affected with AS. The final goal of the project should be the prevention of ESRF due to AS.

Project leader:
Dr. M.C. GUBLER
INSERM, U. 192, Hôpital Necker,
Enfants Malades
Rue de Sèvres 149
FR 75743 Paris Cedex 15
Phone: +33 1 44 49 40 00 (95101)
Fax: +33 1 44 49 02 90
Contract number: CT931052

Participants:
Karl TRYGGVASON
Dept. of Biochemistry,
University of Oulu,
Biocenter Oulu
Linnanmaa
FI 90570 Oulu
Phone: +358 81 553 1150
Fax: +358 81 553 1151

Yves PIRSON
Centre de Génétique
Médicale, Cliniques
Universitaires Saint-Luc,
Université Catholique
de Louvain
Avenue Hippocrate 10
BE 1200 Bruxelles
Phone: +32 2 7641 855
Fax: +32 2 7642 836

Michale HERTZ
Dept. of Clinical Genetics,
Institute of Human Genetics,
The Bartholin Building,
University of Aarhus
DK 8000 Aarhus C
Phone: +45 8942 1668
Fax: +45 8612 3173

Manfred WEBER
Medizinische Klinik IV m
Poliklinik
Krankenhausstr. 12
DE 91054 Erlangen
Phone: +49 9131 859 002
Fax: +49 9131 859 209

Hubert SMEETS
Dept. of Human Genetics,
University Hospital
P.O. Box 9101
NL 6500 HB Nijmegen
Phone: +31 80 61 37 99
Fax: +31 80 54 21 51

Maria F. CARVALHO
Laboratoire de Morfologia
renal, Servico de Nefrologia,
Hospital de Curry Cabral
Rua de Bebeficiencia 8
PT 1000 Lisboa
Phone: +351 179 33080
Fax: +351 179 69515

Juan SAUS
Citologia Molecular y
Cultivo de Tejidos
Amadeo de Saboya 4
ES 46010 Valencia
Phone: +34 6 369 8500
Fax: +34 6 360 1453

Martin BOBROW
Div. of Med. and Mol.
Genetics, Guy's and
St. Thomas's Hospitals,
7th & 8th Floors,
St. Thomas's Street
UK London SE1 9RT
Phone: +44 71 955 4456
Fax: +44 71 955 4644

Jörgen WIESLANDER
Dept. of Nephrology,
University Hospital
SE 221 85 Lund
Phone: +46 46 173 541
Fax: +46 46 184 493

Mario DE MARCHI
Dipartimento di Scienze
cliniche e biologiche,
Universita di torino
Regione Gonzole 10
IT 10043 Orbassano
Phone: +39 577 263 259
Fax: +39 577 263 302

STRATEGIES TO PREVENT INTRACELLULAR ACCUMULATION OF THE Z-ALPHA-I-ANTITRYPSIN VARIANT

Key words

Alpha 1-antitrypsin genetics, alpha 1-antitrypsin chemistry, alpha 1-antitrypsin metabolism, alpha 1-antitrypsin ultrastructure, liver diseases genetics, models, molecular.

Objectives

1 Unravel the mechanisms of Z α_1-antitrypsin accumulation in the endoplasmic reticulum of the hepatocyte.
2 Open up strategies to prevent this phenomenon.

Brief description

α_1-Antitrypsin (α_1-AT) is a major hepatic secretory protein and the most abundant serine protease inhibitor in the plasma. Several lines of evidence suggest that leukocyte elastase is the major target for α_1-AT (Carrell et al, 1982). The entire amino acid sequence of normal (M) human α_1-AT is known (Bollen et al, 1983) as is the sequence of the Z variant which contains a Glu to Lys substitution at residue 342 (Jeppson JO, 1976) that hinders its secretion from hepatic cells (Sifers et al, 1989).

The Z allele is found in approximately one in 25 Northern Europeans resulting in about one in 2000 ZZ homozygotes (Sveger, 1976). α_1-AT deficiency associated pathology consists mainly of panlobular emphysema but homozygote individuals carrying the Z allele suffer also from hepatic cirrhosis due to PiZ α_1-AT accumulation in the hepatocyte (Carlson et al, 1989).

The pathogenesis of the secretion defect of the PiZ al-AT remains controversial.

According to Lomas et al (1992), it could result from a change of conformational or physico-chemical properties of the protein; other authors (Ciccarelli et al, 1993) suggest, to the contrary, that the mutation generates a specific signal for retention in the endoplasmic reticulum (ER).

Our laboratories, each studying α_1-Antitrypsin for more than 10 years, want to join their efforts to elucidate the mechanisms involved in PiZ retention and accumulation in the ER and to open the way to therapeutical or preventive strategies intended to reduce or suppress the associated pathology. To achieve these aims, we will combine the protein structural and conformational studies which is the expertise of the Cambridge Laboratory, and the study of the secretion pattern of in vitro constructed variants and mutants expressed in transformed mammalian cells in the presence of various drugs, which is the expertise of the Nivelles Laboratory. Hypotheses about the mechanisms involved in retention and about the means to circumvent the problem will emerge from both experimental approaches and will synergistically improve the design of the following experiments, finally leading to novel therapeutical or preventive strategies.

Project leader:
Dr. P. JACOBS
Applied Genetics, ULB
Rue de l'Industrie 24
BE 1400 Nivelles
Phone: +32 2 67 28 77 64
Fax: +32 2 67 28 77 77
Contract number: CT931592

Participants:
Prof. Robin W. CARRELL
Haematology, MRC Center,
University of Cambridge
Hills Road
UK Cambridge CB2 2QH
Phone: +44 223 336 788
Fax: +44 223 336 827

PROLONGED COGNITIVE DYSFUNCTION: A PREVENTABLE POSTOPERATIVE COMPLICATION IN ELDERLY PATIENTS

Key words

Age, anaesthesia, cognitive function, hypoxemia, complication, postoperative, psychologic test, risk factor.

Objectives

The objectives are to test the hypothese that:

1 Anaesthesia and surgery in the elderly patients can cause a prolonged cognitive dysfunction.

2 The incidence of measurable prolonged postoperative cognitive dysfunctions increases with age.

3 Hypoxaemia is one of the major and preventable causes of prolonged postoperative cognitive dysfunction. The proposed methodology: A multicenter study of 2000 elderly patients tested for cognitive function before and after major operations. Oxygen saturation of blood will be surveyed intra- and for four days post-operatively.

Brief description

Clinical experience and literature suggest that many elderly patients suffer from protracted cognitive deficits after major operations. Preventable postoperative hypoxaemia is thought to be one of the risk factors responsible.

Psychologists from The Netherlands and UK will in cooperation with physicians from Denmark, Germany, Greece, France, Spain, The Netherlands, and UK develop parallel forms for the psychometric tests. Anaesthesiologists from these seven countries will collect data. Data handling will be centralized in Eindhoven (The Netherlands). Data will be analyzed for a correlation between prolonged cognitive dysfunction and perioperative hypoxaemia as well as several other risk factors.

The team will be lead by Dr. J.T. Moller (anaesthesiologist from Denmark), Dr. P. Rabbitt (psychologist from U.K.), and Dr. J.E. van Beneken (engineer from the Netherlands).

The first 6 months will be devoted to finalize details of the protocol and procedures (meetings and training sessions for all researchers and technicians) followed by 18 months of data collection and 6 months for analysis and preparation of reports and publications.

The study will generate a reference data base on an EC-level that can be applied by member States to enhance the quality of health care.

Project leader:
Dr. J.T. MOLLER
Department of Anaesthesia,
Rigshospitalet,
University of Copenhagen
Blegdamsvej 9
DK 2100 Copenhagen
Phone: +45 35 45 34 74
Fax: +45 35 45 29 50
Contract number: CT931290

Participants:

Dr. B. C. JÖRGENSEN
Dept. of Anaesthesia,
Herlev Hospital,
Univ of Copenhagen
DK 2730 Herlev
Phone: +45 44 53 53 00
Fax: +45 44 53 53 32

Dr. B. RIOU
Dept. of Anaesthesia,
Groupe Hosp.
Pitie Salpetriere
47-83 Boulevard de l'Hôpital
FR 75651 Paris
Phone: +33 1 42162259
Fax: +33 1 42162269

Dr. Ch.D. HANNING
Dept. of Anaesthesia,
Leicester General Hospital
Gwendolen Road
UK Leicester LE5 4PW
Phone: +44 533 584 602
Fax: +44 533 584 611

Dr. F. CHUNG
Dept. of Anaesthesia, Toron-
to Western Div. Hospital
399 Bathurst Street
Toronto, Ontario M5T 2S8
Phone: +1 416 369 5118
Fax: +1 416 369 6494

Dr. H. ASKITOPOULOU
Dept. of Anaesthesiology,
Univ Hospital of Iraklion
P.O. Box 1352
GR Iraklion 711 10
Phone: +30 81 269 413
Fax: +30 81 269 413

Dr. H. MENZEL
Senner Helweg 5
DE 33659 Bielefeld
Phone: +49 521 491 199
Fax: +49 521 491 199

Dr. H. VAN BEEM
Dept. of Anaesthesiology,
Nijmegen Univ Hospital
P.O. Box 9101
NL 6500 HB Nijmegen
Phone: +31 80 61 45 53
Fax: +31 80 54

Dr. J. CANET
Dept. of Anaesthesia,
Hospital Universitari;
Germans Trias i Pujol
Badalona
ES 08916 Barcelona
Phone: +34 34 651 200\299
Fax: +34 33 955 711

Dr. J.S. GRAVENSTEIN
Dept. of Anesthesiology,
Univ of Florida,
College of Medicine
P.O. Box 100254
US Gainesville, Florida
Phone: +1 904 392 3441
Fax: +1 904 392 7029

Dr. L. RASMUSSEN
Dept. of Anaesthesia,
National Univ Hospital,
Righospitalet
9 Blegdamsvej
DK 2100 Copenhagen
Phone: +45 35 45 34 74
Fax: +45 35 45 29 50

Dr. SMETS
Dept. of Anaesthesiology,
Academical Hospital
Maastricht
P.O. Box 5800
NL 6202 AZ Maastricht
Phone: +31 43 877 467

Dr. S. BLACK
Dept. of Anesthesiology,
Univ of Florida,
College of Medicine
P.O. Box 100254
US Gainesville Florida
Phone: +1 904 392 3441
Fax: +1 904 392 7029

Dr. T. JOHNSON
Dept. of Anaesthesia,
Hope Hospital
Eccles Old Road
UK Salford M6 8HD
Phone: +44 61 787 5108
Fax: +44 61 787 5072

G. BLOM
Dept. of Anaesthesia,
National Univ Hospital,
Righospitalet
9 Blegdamsvej
DK 2100 Copenhagen
Phone: +45 35 45 34 74
Fax: +45 35 45 29 50

L.T. SKOVGAARD
Statistical Research Unit,
Univ of Copenhagen
Blegdamsvej 9
DK 2200 Copenhagen N
Phone: +45 35 32 79 16
Fax: +45 35 32 79 07

Prof. J. JOLLES
Dept. of Psychiatry &
Neuropsychology,
Rijksuniversiteit Limburg
Postbus 616
NL 6200 MD Maastricht
Phone: +31 43 882 222
Fax: +31 43 671 096

Prof. J.E.W. BENEKEN
Eindhoven Univ of
Technology, Dept. of
Electrical Engineering
P.O. Box 513
NL 5600 MB Eindhoven

Prof. P. RABBITT
Age and Cognitive
Performance Research
Centre, Univ of Manchester
Oxford Road
UK Manchester M13 9PL

Prof. P.J.M. CLUITMANS
Eindhoven Univ of
Technology, Dept. of
Electrical Engineering
P.O. Box 513
NL 5600 MB Eindhoven

Prof. P.M. LAUVEN
Dept. of Anaesthesia,
SKA Bielefeld-Mitte
Teutoburgerstr. 50
DE 33604 Bielefeld

INTERACTIONS BETWEEN HLA-CLASS II AND PEPTIDES:

Definition of Functionally Important Epitopes Implicated in the Susceptibility to Chronic Autoimmune Diseases

Key words

Autoimmunity, t cell clones, l transfectansts., anti HLA monoclonals (MAbs), EBV transformed B cells (LCLs), HLA defective mutants, Juvenile Rheumatoid Arthritis (JRA), Multiple Sclerosis (MS), Insulin Dependent Diabetes (IDDM).

Objectives

The main objective of this project is the molecular characterisation of the HLA-Class II epitopes that seem to be implicated in the development of three very common autoimmune diseases - Juvenile rheumatoid Arthritis (JRA), Multiple Sclerosis (MS) and Insulin Dependent Diabetes (IDDM).

Brief description

Chronic autoimmune diseases have a high medical, economical and social impact in developed countries.

The interaction between certain T cells and some HLA-Class II molecules play a crucial role in the development of the aforementioned diseases.

The main objective of this project is the molecular characterisation of the HLA-Class II epitopes that seem to be implicated in the development of three very common autoimmune diseases (Juvenile Rheumatoid Arthritis, Multiple Sclerosis (MS) and Insulin Dependent Diabetes). In the generation of these epitopes not only the $\alpha 1$ and $\beta 1$ domains of some Class II molecules, but also the peptides enclosed in their clefts are involved.

For the study of these epitopes, a collection of B-LCL mutants defective in HLA Class II expression, as well as some HLA chimeric molecules and others modified by means of 'site directed' mutagenesis are generated.

A set of monomorphic and allele specific monoclonal antibodies are also available.

Other tools will be developed, namely T cell clones restricted by the HLA molecules (plus peptides) responsible for the individual's susceptibility to some of the aforementioned autoimmune diseases.

The use of B-LCL and L cell transfectants as well as peripheral blood cells from controls and patients will permit the identification of the determinants responsible for the reactivity of the aforementioned T cells.

Our main goal is therefore to make an indepth study of DR, DQ and DP in the context of autoimmune disease susceptibility. This kind of study may lead to the identification of potential targets for pharmacological action.

Furthermore, a grater knowledge about the interactions between T cell receptors and HLA-Class II molecules (plus peptides) would permit a better understanding of the regulation of the specific immune response, with the corresponding benefits for the design of better vaccines, or the control of the graft versus host disease, which is one of the mayor problems after bone marrow transplantation.

Project leader:
Professor M. SANCHEZ PEREZ
Departamento de Microbiologia II,
Facultad de Farmacia, Universidad Complutense
Ciudad Universitaria
ES 28040 Madrid
Phone: +34 1 394 17 44
Fax: +34 1 394 17 45
Contract number: CT931722

Participants:
Dimitros MONOS
Lab. of Human Biology & Genetics,
Democritus University of Thrace
Demokritus 17
GR 69100 Komotini-Thrace
Phone: +30 5 31 27017
Fax: +30 5 31 26660

Hubert KALBACHER
Medizinisch-Naturwissenschaftliches
Forschungszentrum
Ob dem Himmelreich 7
DE 7400 Tübingen
Phone: +49 7071 295212
Fax: +49 7071 87815

EUGERON: AGEING, HEALTH AND COMPETENCE

Key words
Ageing, health, competence, longitudinal studies, gerontology.

Objectives
1 Develop a knowledge base about the conditions of health and functioning that promote or inhibit the independent living in relation to age.
2 Develop a cross-national data base about the relative contribution of biophysiologic and pschosocial determinants of changes in competence across the life-span.

Brief description
The objective of the proposed EC concerted action on Gerontology (EUGERON) is to develop a knowledge base about the conditions of health and functioning that promote or inhibit the independent living in relation to age.

This knowledge is necessary to develop realistic public policy in ageing societies and to guide the enhancement of competence and quality of life of ageing persons in different geographic and socio-economic European settings.

EUGERON is designed as a cross-sectional, base-line study in longitudinal perspective. The central research question concerns the relation between age (independent variable) and competence (dependent variable), and the extent to which intervening factors, i.e., sociodemographic, environmental, psychosocial, biophysiologic and life-style factors, are related to the observed differences with age.

In order to answer this question a field survey of the home visit type will be conducted on a representative community based sample of around 3,000 individuals, aged 35-84 per participating country. The survey will be split up in a (semi) structured interview (1 hr. max.) on the total sample, and an instrumental examination (1,5 hour max.) on a smaller subsample (N=600).

The EUGERON project is scheduled for 36 months of research, and will be conducted in three phases on the basis of workshops and expert meetings: (1) develop research protocol, including manual of operations, (2) conduct pilot study, (3) conduct base-line survey. Project results will be disseminated in reports, journals and proceedings of the planned *European Conference on Ageing, Health and Competence*. After the end of the project, the study will be continued as a longitudinal investigation.

Project leader:
Dr. J.F. SCHROOTS
European Research Institute
on Health and Ageing,
University of Amsterdam
Roetersstraat 15
NL 1018 WB Amsterdam
Phone: +31 20 525 68 30
Fax: +31 20 639 02 79
Contract number: CT931165

Participants:
Prof. R. FERNANDEZ-
BALLESTEROS
Universidad Autonoma de
Madrid, Facultad de
Psichologia, Ciuadad
Universiatria de Cantoblanco
ES 28049 Madrid
Phone: +34 1 3975 181
Fax: +34 1 3975 5215

Prof. G. RUDINGER
Psychologische Institut
der Universität Bonn
Römerstrasse 164
DE 53117 Bonn I
Phone: +49 228 550 352
Fax: +49 228 550 350

EUROPEAN COLLABORATIVE RESEARCH ON MOSAICISM IN CVS (EUCROMIC)

Key words
Prenatal diagnosis, Chorionic villus sampling, CVS, Discrepancy, Chromosomal Mosaicism, Uniparental disomy, Genetic Counselling, Guidelines.

Objectives
1 Improve the effectiveness and efficiency of prenatal diagnosis.
2 Provide data for the harmonisation of clinical decisions and genetic counselling after prenatal diagnosis by CVS and new techniques.
3 Monitor the development of CVS for prenatal diagnosis in Europe and the implications of new techniques, e.g. early amniocentesis, on the use of CVS.
4 Facilitate access to information on controversial prenatal diagnoses for ancillary studies.
5 Determine the significance of controversial prenatal diagnoses for pre- and postnatal development.
6 Evaluate the association between a prenatal diagnosis of mosaicism and UPD.

Brief description
The present European collaboration on CVS and mosaicism is expanded and participation offered to European genetic centres in general. The goal is collection and interpretation of data on controversial diagnoses detected by CVS and upcoming methods for prenatal diagnosis in Europe.

Periodical information from the centres constitutes the basis for a database on sampling techniques, cytogenetic methods, controversial diagnoses, confirmatory investigations, and outcome of pregnancy. Th esurvey provides information on changes in use of present techniques, introduction of new techniques, and the type and rate of controversial diagnoses.

Coordinate collection of DNA and molecular analyses for uniparental disomy (UPD) detection in spontaneous/induced abortions and liveborn children after a prenatal diagnosis of mosaicism. When the techniques are not established as routine methods at the referring centre, tissue and blood samples are analyzed in special laboratories.

Coordinate collection of data on outcome of pregnancy and clinical information on children following a prenatal diagnosis of mosaicism.

The EUCROMIC database provides the basis for fu rther collaborative research on cytogenetics in prenatal diagnosis.

Coordination and data evaluation will be managed at the EUCROMIC secretariat. The present ancillary projects on Uniparental Disomy (UPD) and Clinical Follow-up after CVS Mosaicism are conducted in collaboration with Dr. C.D. Delozier-Blanchet, Geneva, Switzerland. The core elements of the project are: (1) the network of European genetic departments for data on prenatal diagnoses (2) single centres or groups of centres selected for specialized techniques, e.g. analysis for UPD.

Project leader:
Dr. L.O. VEJERSLEV
The John F. Kennedy
Institute, Dept. of
Medical Genetics
Gl. Landevej 7
DK 2600 Glostrup
Phone: +45 42 45 22 28
Fax: +45 43 43 11 30
Contract number: CT931673

Participants:
Dr. Johanne HAHNEMANN
DK 2600 Glostrup

Dr DELOZIER-BLANCHET
CH 1211 Geneve 4

Prof. N.J. LESCHOT
NL 1105 AZ Amsterdam

Dr. Nina GREGSON
UK Wiltshire SP2 8BJ

Prof. Albert SCHINZEL
CH 8001 Zürich

Prof. CASSIMAN
BE 3000 Leuven

Dr. M. MOLDAN-FREUND
BE 1200 Bruxelles

Prof. I. LIEBARES
BE 1090 Brussel

Dr. Esther VAMOS
BE 1020 Bruxelles

Dr. Peter K.A. JENSEN
DK 8000 Aarhus C

Prof. Maj HULTEN
UK Birmingham B9 5PX

Dr. GIRARD ORGEOLET
FR 75014 Paris

Dr. MORICHON-
DELVALLEZ
FR 75015 Paris

Dr. Caroline PIQUET
FR 13385 Marseille Cedex 5

Dr. Antje WIRTZ
DE 80336

Dr. Konstantin MILLER
DE 30625 Hannover

Dr. Werner SCHEMPP
DE 79106 Freiburg i. Br.

Prof. KENNERKNECHT
DE 89073 Ulm / Donau

Dr. Iris BARTELS
DE 37073 Göttingen

Prof. SCHWINGER
DE 25358 Lübeck

Dr. Rolf D. WEGNER
DE 14059 Berlin

Prof. METAXOTOU
GR 11527 Athens

Mrs. J.M. DE PATER
NL 3501 CA Utrecht

Dr. TAN-SINDHUNATA
NL 9713 AW Groningen

Dr. Lamberto CAMURRI
IT 42100 Reggio Emilia

Dr. Leda DALPRA
IT 20133 Milano

Dr. Gianfranco NOCERA
IT 20129 Milano

Dr. Silvana GUERNERI
IT 20122 Milano

Dr. Giorgio GIMELLI
IT 16148 Genova

Prof. B. DALLAPICCOLA
IT 00157 Roma

Dr. BRICARELLI
IT 16128 Genova

Dr. Elisabeth LENZINI
IT 35128 Padova

Dr. Gordon LOWTHER
UK Glasgow G3 8SJ

Dr. Ana CARRIO
ES 08036 Barcelona

Dr. Maria G. TIBILETTI
IT 21100 Varese

Dr. John WOLSTENHOLME
UK Newcastle upon Tyne
NE2 4AA

Dr. Robert SAURA
FR 33076 Bordeaux Cedex

Prof. Claude STOLL
FR 67091 Strasbourg Cedex

Prof. Christine GOSDEN
UK Liverpool L69 3BX

Dr. P.A. IN 'T VELD
NL 3000 DR Rotterdam

Dr. Ulf KRISTOFFERSSON
SE 22185 Lund

Prof. G. SZEMERE
HU 6720 Szeged

Dr. András TOTH
HU 1389 Budapest

Dr. Harriet V. KOSKULL
FI 00290 Helsingfors 29

THE ROLE OF MEMBRANES IN LENS AGEING AND CATARACT

Key words
Lens ageing, cataract, crystalline, cell membranes.

Objectives
1 Study of the electrophysiological, biochemical, molecular biological and morphological properties of membranes in animal and non-cataractous aged human lenses.
2 Identification of the adverse effects of Ca++, free radicals, UV and x-irradiation on lens membranes in animal experiments.
3 Unravelling of aberrant membrane properties in inherited and induced animal cataracts and in human cataractous lenses.
Operationally, this Concerted Action aims to optimalize collaboration between the eight European Cataract Research groups involved by making mutually available the various cataract models and by sharing the advanced equipment and techniques present in each group. Annual workshops, site visits and exchange of personnel are planned to identify the collaboration.

Brief description
There is no doubt that the advance in life coincides with a gradual decline in the functional abilities of cells, organs and organisms. It seems an attractive idea that age-related diseases as e.g. senile dementia, senile macular degeneration and cataract are terminal stages of this continuous process of deterioration. However, catastrophic events, accumulation of errors, insufficient DNA repair or genetic programming have also been postulated as main causes of senescent diseases.
The number of theories of senescence exceeds, however, the 'facts' available to support them. The lens is a simple organ, as compared to the brain or retina, consisting of life-long mitotic active epithelial cells, which may undergo catastrophic events at the DNA level. At the fibre cells level, accumulation of post-translational changes throughout the whole life span of the individual takes place. Moreover, 'normal' and diseased aged human lenses ans animal lenses, showing specific aspects of the 'natural' age-related deteriorations, are readily available. Hence the lens allows the study of all aspects of ageing and can be considered as an excellent tool for the study of senescence.
The present Concerted Action is meant to accumulate new 'facts' for cataract. It has recently been emphasized that membranes are crucial in maintaining lens transparency and that disturbed membranes are a major factor. Membranes are complex cell organelles consisting of a fluid bilayer of phospholipds and cholesterol studded with intrinsic channel proteins, associated enzymes and receptors, cytoskeletal scaffolding proteins and communicating gap junctional proteins.
To unravel the precise properties of membranes and the adverse effects of risk factors as Ca++ and free radicals and the eventual genesis of cortical cataract a multidisciplinary and multimodel approach is necessary.
A network of European lens researchers is the way par excellence to realize this by a formalized and financially supported sharing of expertise, equipment and model systems and by exchange of knowledge on an annual base. The aim to be addressed is to find an alternative for surgical cataract treatment by reducing the number of cataract patients or delay of cataract progression, to the benefit of both the aged individuals and the health care budgets.

Project leader:
Professor G.F.J.M. VRENSEN
The Netherlands Ophthalmic Research Institute,
Department of Morphology
P.O. Box 12141
NL 1100 AC Amsterdam
Phone: +31 20 566 44 28
Fax: +31 20 69 65 21
Contract number: CT931620

Participants:
Dr. A. WEGENER
Abt. für Experimentelle Ophthalmologie,
Universität Bonn
Sigmund-Freud-Strasse 25
DE 53105 Bonn 1

Dr. M.C. MOTA
Servicos de Oftalmologia,
Universidade de Coimbra
PT 3049 Coimbra

Dr. H. BLOEMENDAL
Afd. Biochemie,
Katholieke Universiteit Nijmegen
Postbus 9101
NL 6500 HB Nijmegen

Dr. G. DUNCAN
School of Biological Sciences,
University of East Anglia
UK Norwich NR4 7TJ

Dr. HARDING & A.J. BRON
Nuffield Laboratory of Ophthalmology,
University of Oxford
Walton Street
UK Oxford OX2 6AW

Dr. I. DUNIA
Institut Jacques Monod, Centre National
de Recherches Scientifique
2 Place Jussieu-Tour 43
FR 75251 Paris Cedex 05

Dr. G. MARAINI
Istituto di Oftalmologia,
Universita di Parma
Via Gramsci 14
IT 43100 Parma

THE HUMAN HAEMATOPOIETIC STEM CELL

Key words
Human Haematopoiesis, stem cells, cell surface molecules, purification, assays, cell cycle, transplantation, gene therapy, stem cell assays, stem cell purification, stem cell for clinical purposes, stem cell regulation.

Objectives
There are 4 closely integrated objectives for the Concerted Action:
1 Stem cell assays.
2 Stem cell purification.
3 Stem cell for clinical purposes.
4 Stem cell regulation.

Brief description
Haematopoietic Stem Cells are rare cells that have enormous developmental potential allowing both the production of all haematological cell lineages and supporting stromal cell elements.

A previous concerted action of human bone marrow stem cells has made major efforts in the long scale purification, characterization, assay and use for transplantation of this cell.
The proposed Concerted Action will develop:
1 in vitro assays for the lymphomyeloid stem cell;
2 new antibodies to select stem cell subsets;
3 cord blood and stem cell banks for clinical use including transplantation;
4 new vectors to correct haematopoietic genetic disorders in gene therapy protocols;
5 the regulation of stem cell Go phase controls to assist gene-therapy and transplantation of the non-cycling stem cell;
6 successful transplantation with purified stem cells, with or without gene therapy, with or without the addition of cytokines or other purified cell populations.

The availability of purified stem cells for transplantation coupled with gene transfer studies will provide major advances for clinical treatments of serious diseases such as leukaemia, other forms of cancer, immunodeficiency diseases, myelodysplasia, AIDS and genetic inherited diseases that occur in children, young adults or the elderly.

This has major social implications with cord blood stem cell banks potentially providing treatments for these diseases to all groups including ethnic minorities and patients without HLA matched donors.

The present Concerted Action will provide a means for quick exchange of information and allow multidisciplinary scientific cooperation in Europe.

A great diversity of scientists and clinicians is required for this interactive project.

These include: cell biologists (cytokines, receptor expression, cell cycle control); molecular biologists (gene regulation, cloning and therapy); immunobiologists (cell surface markers, tolerance, graft versus host disease); clinicians (haematology, cancer, aids, ageing); industry (production of new cytokines and antibodies, stem cell purification devices, culture systems), health administrators and lawyers (choice of stem cell banks, European patent policy).

Such expertise is generally not available in a single European laboratory. The programme is therefore of tremendous importance for the future management and control of diseases which involve haematopoietic and immune systems.

Project leader:
Dr. Suzanne WATT
Institute of Molecular
Medicine,
The John Radcliffe Hospital
UK Oxford OX3 9DU
Phone: +44 865 222 632
Fax: +44 865 222 500
Contract number: CT931424

Participants:
Dr. R. James MATTHEWS
UK Cardiff CF4 4XN

Dr. Ian B. PRAGNELL
UK Glasgow G61 1BD

Prof. David WEATHERALL
UK Oxford OX3 9DU

Prof. Walter KNAPP
AT 1090 Vienna

Prof. Michel SYMANN
BE 1200 Bruxelles

Dr. VAN BOCKSTAELE
BE 2650 Edegem

Dr. Ebbe DICKMEISS &
dr. Arne SVEJGAARD
DK 2100 Copenhagen

Dr. Kari ALITALO
FI 00014 Helsinki

Dr. Daniel BIRNBAUM
FR 13009 Marseille

Dr. Pierre CHARBORD
FR 25000 Besancon

Prof. Eliane GLUCKMAN
FR 75010 Paris

Dr. Jacques HATZFELD
FR 94801 Villejuif Cedex

Dr. Patrice MANNONI
FR 13009 Marseille

Dr. Bruno PEAULT
FR 94736 Nogent sur Marne
Cedex

Dr. Francoise PFLUMIO
FR 94805 Villejuif Cedex

Prof. VAINCHENKER
FR 94805 Villejuif Cedex

Dr. Hans-Jörg BUHRING
DE 72076 Tübingen

Prof. Axel A. FAUSER
DE 55743 Idar-Oberstein

Dr. HANDGRETINGER
DE 72070 Tübingen

Dr. Lothar KANZ
DE 7800 Freiburg

Prof. Wolfram OSTERTAG
DE 20246 Hamburg

Dr. Karl WELTE
DE 3000 Hannover 61

Prof. Axel R. ZANDER
DE 20246 Hamburg

Dr. Vassilis GEORGOULIAS
GR 71110 Heraklion, Crete

Dr. Shaun MCCANN
IE Dublin 8

Prof. A. Massimo GIANNI
IT 20133 Milani

Dr. Giovanni MIGLIACCIO
& dr Anna R. MIGLIACCIO
IT 29900161 Rome

Dr. Sergio OTTOLENGHI
IT 20133 Milano

Dr. Antonio TABILIO
IT 06100 Perugia

Dr. Isabel L. BARBOSA
PT 4200 Porto

Prof. J.E.T.E. GUIMARAES
PT 4200 Porto

Dr. Javier HORNEDO
ES 28041 Madrid

Dr. Federico GARRIDO
ES 18014 Granada

Prof. R.E. PLOEMACHER
NL 3015 GE Rotterdam

Dr. J.H.F. FALKENBURG
NL 2300 RC Leiden

Prof. Frank G. GROSVELD
NL 3000 DR Rotterdam

Prof. Bob LOWENBERG
NL 3015 GE Rotterdam

Prof. Dinko VALERIO
NL 2280 GG Rijswijk

Dr. Jan W.M. VISSER
NL 2333 AL Leiden

Prof. Ben A. BRADLEY
UK Bristol BS10 5NB

Prof. Alan K. BURNETT
UK Cardiff CF4 4XN

Prof. T. Michael CEXTER
UK Manchester M20 9BX

Dr. N. TESTA
UK Manchester M20 9BX

Prof. M.F. GREAVERS
UK London SW3 6JB

Dr. Jill M. HOWS
UK Bristol BS10 5NB

Prof. George JANOSSY
UK London NW3 2QG

Prof. Roland J. LEVINSKY
UK London WC1 1EH

CHONDRODYSPLASIAS: INHERITED GROWTH DEFECTS WITH CRIPPLING CONSEQUENCES

Key words
Chondrodysplasia, growth defect, growth plate, cartilage, chondrocyte, extracellular matrix, arthrosis, gene mutation.

Objectives
- To improve recognition and classification of chondrodysplasias.
- To help prevent complications of these chronic conditions and to provide better genetic counselling.
- To analyze candidate chondrodysplasias for mutations in cartilage specific genes.
- To establish genotype-phenotype correlations.
- To characterize new genes with growth plate and articular cartilage specific functions.
  To understand the cellular and molecular mechanisms underlying the development of osteoarthrosis and degenerative vertebral disease.

Brief description
The proposal represents a collaboration between eight clinical centres and research laboratories to study the human chondrodysplasias, a diverse group of more than 150 rare, usually severe inherited disorders affecting the growing cartilage.

Prominent clinical manifestations are progressive deformation and defective growth of the skeleton. Impaired cartilage function may be severe and as consequence most chondrodysplasias are crippling disorders developing osteoarthrosis. The clinical problems and their progress closely resemble those of degenerative changes of ageing but are more severe and occur prematurely. Therefore as long term objective, research on these individually rare conditions are expected to reveal principles on modes of treatment and prevention in degenerative processes in general.

The short term objectives for this project include:
- a better clinical and radiological recognition and classification and exact data about the natural course of the diseases, to prevent complications of these chronic conditions and improve genetic counselling;
- mapping of mutations in the cartilage-specific type II collagen gene COL2A1, which is known to be responsible for a group of severe chondrodysplasias and primary arthrosis with the aim to establish a genotype-phenotype correlation for COL2A1 defects;
- analysis of candidate chondrodysplasias for mutations in other cartilage specific genes and application of new molecular strategies to identify genes involved in skeletal development;
- establishment of in vitro systems to analyze degenerative processes and their influences on chondrogenesis.

Project leader:
Professor Dr. B. ZABEL
Children's Hospital, University of Mainz, Molecular Genetics Section
Langenbeckstraße 1
DE 55131 Mainz
Phone: +49 613 117 20 20
Fax: +49 613 117 66 10
Contract number: CT931316

Participants:

A. SUPERTI-FURGA
Univ of Zürich, Dept. of Pediatrics,
Div of Metabolism
Steinwiesstr. 75
CH 8032 Zürich

G. CETTA
Universita di Pavia,
Centro per lo Studio della
Malattie del TessutoConettivo,
Dip Biochimica
Via Taramelli 3/B
IT 27100 Pavia

G.A. WALLIS
Univ of Manchester, Dept. of Biochemistry &
Molecular Biology
Oxford Road
UK Manchester M13 9PT

I. KAITILA
Helsinki Univ Hospital,
Dept. of Clin Genetics
Tukholmankatu 8 F
FI 00290 Helsinki

J. BONAVENTURE
CNRS URA 584 Clinique M. Lamy,
Hopital Necker
Rue de Sèvres 149
FR 75743 Paris Cedex 15

L. ALA-KOKKO
Univ of Oulu, Biocentre and
Dept. of Med Biochemistry
Kajaanintie 52A
FI 90220 Oulu

P. FREISINGER
Children's Hospital,
Technical Univ of München
Kölner Platz 1
DE 8000 MÜNCHEN 40

BARRIERS AND INCENTIVES TO PRENATAL CARE IN EUROPE

Key words
Prenatal care, prenatal visits, health services, health status.

Objectives
a To measure the proportion of women with no care, late care or less than 3 prenatal visits;
b To identify barriers to care (e.g. financial barriers, waiting lists, distance, cultural barriers);
c To describe existing incentives to care (e.g. financial incentives) and to evaluate their impact.

Brief description
Poor attendance to prenatal care is a matter of concern because there is strong evidence that mothers who do not use the services are those who have the worst outcomes. In contrast with the United States there is a lack of information about prenatal care utilization in Europe.

Each participating country will be asked to provide a detailed description of the prenatal care delivery system, including existing incentives. An area based survey of women during their post-partum period will be performed. During one year in each area, the health personnel in charge of the deliveries will inquire about the time of the first prenatal visit and the number of visits for each women. All women with no prenatal care, and representative samples of women with late care and of a control group of women with adequate care will be interviewed or asked to fill in a questionnaire in the post-partum period. The total number of deliveries in each area involved in the study should be at least 1600. Questions will deal with barriers and incentives to prenatal care, socio-demographic characteristics of women, medical complications during pregnancy, women views on prenatal care and social networks available to the pregnant women. The frequency of no or late prenatal care, and the numbers of prenatal visits will be derived from the data collected for each delivery.

Further analysis will describe each of the groups interviewed and compare them. The impact of incentives for care will be evaluated comparing areas as similar as possible, among countries with different policies, and adjusting for confounding factors whenever possible.

Project leader:
Dr. Pierre BUEKENS
Lab. d'Epidémiologie et de Médecine Sociale,
Université Libre de Bruxelles
Route de Lennik 808
BE 1070 Brussels
Phone: +32 2 5554018
Fax: +32 2 5554049
Contract number: CT941169

Participants:

Dr. Sophie ALEXANDER
Lab. d'Epidémiologie et
de Médecine Sociale,
Université Libre de Bruxelles
Route de Lennik 808
BE 1070 Brussels
Phone: +32 2 555 4018/4046
Fax: +32 2 555 4049

F. BORLUM-KRISTENSEN
University Dept. of
General Practice
Blegdamsvej 3
DK 2200 Copenhagen
Phone: +45 3532 7942
Fax: +45 3532 7946

Béatrice BLONDEL
INSERM, Unité 149
16 avenue P. Vaillant
Couturier
FR 94807 Villejuif cedex
Phone: +33 1 4559 5096
Fax: +33 1 4559 5089

Helen VALASSI-ADAM
Institute of Child Health,
Dept. of Social Pediatrics
M. Asias 76
GR 11527 Athens
Phone: +30 1 7701 557
Fax: +30 1 7701 557

Peter BOYLAN
Dept of Obstetrics
and Gynecology,
National Maternity Hospital
1 Holles Street
IE Dublin
Phone: +353 16 610 277
Fax: +353 16 766 623

Elina HEMMINKI
National Research and
Development Centre for
Welfare and Health,
Health Services
Research Unit
P.O. Box 220
FI 00531 Helsinki
Phone: +358 0 3967 2307
Fax: +358 0 3967 2485

Leiv BAKKETEIG
Dept. of Health Society,
National Institute of
Public Health
Geitmyrsveien 75
NO 0462 Oslo 4
Phone: +47 22 04 22 00
Fax: +47 22 35 36 05

Geir JACOBSEN
University Medical Centre,
Community Medicine and
General Practice
NO 7005 Trondheim
Phone: +47 73 59 88 75
Fax: +47 73 59 87 89

Bjorn BACKE
Norwegian Institute of
Hospital Research
Strindveien 2
NO 7034 Trondheim NTH
Fax: +47 73 59 63 61

Sergio NORDIO
Istituto per l'Infanzia
Via del Istria 65/E
IT 34137 Trieste
Phone: +39 40 3785356
Fax: +39 40 3785210

Paolo PINTO
Istituto di Ginecologia
e Ostetricia,
Ospedale San Martino
Viale Benedetto XV,
10 Pad. 1
IT 16132 Genoa
Phone: +39 10 353 7709
Fax: +39 10 353 7645

Lya DEN OUDEN
N.I.P.G. - T.N.O.,
PERINET
P.O. Box 124
NL 2300 AC Leiden
Phone: +31 71 18 16 51
Fax: +31 71 17 63 82

Maria ARAUJO
Dept. Maternal Health
Alameda D. Alfonso
Henriques 45
PT 1056 Lisboa codex
Phone: +351 1 847 5515
Fax: +351 1 847 6639/6455

Antonio GONZALES
Allendesalazar 8
ES 28043 Madrid
Fax: +34 1 729 2808

Linda DE CAESTECKER
Greater Glasgow
Health Board
112 Ingram Street
UK Glasgow G1 1ET
Phone: +44 41 552 6222
Fax: +44 41 552 0945

Itsvan BERBIK
Dept. Obstetrics
and Gynecology,
Vaszary Kolos Hospital
HU 2500 Esztergom
Phone: +36 33 311 199
Fax: +36 33 311 950

MOLECULAR GERONTOLOGY: THE IDENTIFICATION OF LINKS BETWEEN AGEING AND THE ONSET OF AGE-RELATED DISEASES

Key words
Ageing, age-related diseases, molecular gerontology, ageing processes, molecular markers.

Brief description
Ageing is a highly complex multifactorial biological process characterized by the progressive loss of the ability of organs and cells to maintain biochemical functions.

Hence ageing is usually accompanied by an increase in the appearance of several diseases, such as atherosclerosis, amyloidosis, cataract, chronic renal failure, dementia, diabetes, osteoporosis, osteoarthrosis, and cancers of most types.

The importance of the connection between the ageing process and the incidence of age-related diseases is largely underestimated. It is often wrongly assumed that each age-related disease has its own particular cause distinct and separate from the cause of another disease. The development of major new molecular biological technologies during the past decades have opened the way for major advances in the study of the ageing process and its relationship with the origin of diseases of old age. It is now possible to identify major mechanisms of ageing. Among these (and not exclusively) are: genetic programming; somatic cell mutation, error accumulations; molecular instability, molecular crosslinking, generation/scavenging of free radicals etc.; decrease in protein activity; mitochondrial DNA mutations; bioenergetic decrease. All of these processes contribute to cell organ pathology, senescence and death.

We aim to identify elements of these processes which are potentially subject to modification and amelioration in order to lead to improved quality of life by preventing the early onset of major age-related diseases.

Organisms are exposed continuously to a variety of endogenous and exogenous insults.

In order to maintain organismal integrity cells are equipped with biological systems for protection and repair.

Elucidation of the underlying molecular mechanism involved in ageing will be aided by the identification of molecular markers of biological ageing. Furthermore, in order to distinguish successful ageing from the situation in age-related disease we plan to characterize normal ageing and accelerated ageing.

Both genetic and biochemical molecular markers will be evaluated in model systems and in human systems involving successful ageing (centenarians) and accelerated ageing (Werner's syndrome and Down's syndrome). These markers will be identified using state of the art molecular and cell biology techniques.

This approach will benefit of the work of the 12 cooperating research groups which have been chosen for the application of their various advanced complementary expertises in the field of ageing.

European added value will be achieved by cost effective efficient collaboration instead of fragmented uncoordinated efforts. In our cooperative network we plan to identify the common molecular mechanisms which are at the basis of systemic ageing and the onset of age-related diseases.

Diagnosis, prevention and therapy of major age-related diseases will also be facilitated by the determination of reliable biomarkers of ageing within our joint project.

Project leader:
Professor Brian F.C. CLARK
Dept. of Chemistry, Aarhus University
Langelandsgade 140
DK 8000 Aarhus
Phone: +45 86 12 46 33
Fax: +45 86 19 61 99
Contract number: CT941710

Participants:
Dr. Sidney SHALL &
dr. John SHEPHERD
Genetics & Development
Group, School of Biological
Sciences,
University of Sussex
Falmer
UK Brighton BN1 9QG
Phone: +44 273 606 755
Fax: +44 273 678 335

Dr. Heinz OSIEWACZ
Deutsches Krebs-
forschungszentrum,
Abt. Molekularbiologie
der Alterungsprozesse
Postfach 101949
DE 69009 Heidelberg
Phone: +49 6221 424 657
Fax: +49 6221 424 822

Prof. José REMACLE
Facultes Universitaires,
Notre-Dame de la Paix,
Lab. de Biochimie Cellulaire
Rue de Bruxelles 61
BE 5000 Namur   ,
Phone: +32 81 724 321
Fax: +32 81 724 135

Dr. D.L. KNOOK &
dr. Eline SLAGBOOM
TNO, Inst. of Ageing &
Vascular Research
P.O. Box 430
NL 2300 AK Leiden
Phone: +31 71 181 433/406
Fax: +31 71 181 900

Dr. Francois SCHACHTER
7 dr. Daniel COHEN
Human Polymophism,
Study Center
27 Rue Juliette Dodu
FR 75010 Paris
Phone: +33 1 424
99850/50417
Fax: +33 1 401 80155

Dr. Claudio FRANCESCHI
Institute of General
Pathology,
University of Modena
Via Campi 287
IT 41100 Modena
Phone: +39 59 360044
Fax: +39 59 362206

Dr. Paolo GIACOMONI
L'Oreal,
Lab. de Recherche
Fondamentale
90 rue du General Roquet
FR 92583 Clichy Cedex
Phone: +33 1 47 567 732
Fax: +33 1 47 564 527

Dr. Tom KIRKWOOD
School of Biological
Sciences,
University of Manchester,
3.614 Stopford Building
Osford Road
UK Manchester M13 9PT
Phone: +44 61 275 6851
Fax: +44 61 275 5640

Dr. Alexander BURKLE
Deutsches Krebsforschungs-
zentrum, Abt. 0610
Postfach 101949
DE 69009 Heidelberg
Phone: +49 6221 42 4613
Fax: +49 6221 42 4962

Dr. Dimitri STATHAKOS
Dept. of Biology,
Nuclear Research Center
Demokritos
GR 15310 Athens
Phone: +30 1 65 13111
Fax: +30 1 65 11767

Dr. Christine BRACK
Biozentrum,
University of Basel
Klingelbergstrasse 70
CH 4056 Basel
Phone: +41 61 267 2057
Fax: +41 61 257 2078

Dr. Suresh I.S. RATTAN
Dept. of Chemistry,
Aarhus University
DK 8000 Aarhus C
Phone: +45 89 42 33 33
Fax: +45 86 19 61 99

QAMC: QUALITY ASSURANCE IN MATERNITY CARE

Key words
Quality assurance, health services research, perinatal care, maternity care, pregnancy outcome, public health.

Objectives
QAMC has four principle objectives:
1 To develop an agreed set of 'Adverse Pregnancy Outcomes' covering the ante-natal, intra-partum and post-natal periods, which will serve as measures of the quality of pregnancy-care.
2 To collect and collate minimum prospective datasets, from pregnancies delivered at multiple European maternity centres, such minimum datasets being designed to predict high risk of certain specific, well-defined 'Adverse Pregnancy Outcomes' (from 1).
3 To investigate the use of various neural network paradigms in predicting from the minimum prospective datasets which pregnancies will end up with an adverse pregnancy outcome.
4 To establish a small number of randomized controlled clinical trials in order to evaluate the use of such neural networks in improving perinatal outcome.

Brief description
QAMC (Quality Assurance in Maternity Care) is a Concerted Action proposal involving 13 countries (the Member States and Turkey).
It is aimed at Health Services Research in the field of Perinatal Medicine, and involves the extensive use both of Quality Indicators and of Neural Networks.

These four objectives of QAMC, taken together, will meet all four of the objectives set out in the BIOMED-1 Work-Plan, under the heading of Health Services Research (1.4):
1.4.1a To emphasize the harmonization of methodologies and protocols in Health Services Research, including Public Health.
1.4.1b To provide information, and especially scientific data, necessary for improving the effectiveness and efficiency of health care and the ways in which health care systems are organized, managed and financed.
1.4.1c To improve the research methods available to provide this information.
1.4.1d To develop coordinated networks providing for adequate collection and interpretation of data on health status and health systems.
The QAMC project is innovative in exploring the potential of neural networks, as applied to the quality assurance of perinatal care, and also the potential of using such new technology in Health Services Research.
QAMC will be managed using formal project management methodology known as FRINCE, and Cambridge will serve both as the Project's Coordinating Centre and as its Data Processing Centre.

Project leader:
Dr. Kevin J. DALTON
Perinatal Research
Group/Obstetrics,   -
University of Cambridge,
Rosie Maternity Hospital Addenbrooke's Hospital
UK Cambridge CB2 2QQ
Phone: +44 223 410250
Fax: +44 223 215327
Contract number: CT941113

Participants:

Prof. Robert DEROM
Katholieke Universiteit
Herestraat 49
BE 3000 Leuven
Phone:+32 16 28 36 55
Fax:+32 16 29 18 55

Prof. Tom WEBER
Hvidovre Hospital
Kettegard 30
DK 2650 Copenhagen
Phone:+45 36 32 36 32
Fax: +45 31 47 39 41

Prof. S. SCHMIDT
Universitats Frauenklinik,
University of Bonn
Sigmund Freudstrasse 25
DE 5300 Bonn
Phone:49 228 280 2450
Fax: +49 228 280 3091

Prof. H. SELBMANN
Eberhard-Karls-
Universitat Tubingen
Westbahnhofstrasse 55
DE 7400 Tubingen 1
Phone:49 7071 295 218
Fax: +49 7071 295 219

Prof. J.M THOULON
Hopitaux de Lyon,
Service de Ob/Gyn
Hotel Dieu
FR 69288 Lyon Cedex 2
Phone: +33 78 371840
Fax: +33 78 922051

Dr. Gerard BREART
123 BD. de Port-Royal
FR 75014 Paris
Phone: +33 1 4326 0046
Fax: +33 1 4326 8979

Prof. A.J. ANTSAKLIS
Vas. Sofia 80
GR 611 Athens
Phone: +30 1 770 8749
Fax: +30 1 771 9271

Prof. C. O'HERLIHY
National Maternity Hospital
Holles Street
IE Dublin 2
Phone: +353 1 651
Fax: +353 1 610277

Prof. G.C. DI RENZO
Policlinico Monteluce
IT 06100 Perugia
Phone: +39 75 62552
Fax: +39 75 29271

Prof. E. COSMI
Via Monte Madonna 23
IT 00060 Formello - Rome
Phone: +39 6 446 0507
Fax: +39 6 446 9128

Dr. Jacques ARENDT
Centre Hospitalier
de Luxembourg
4 rue Barbie
LU 1250 Luxembourg
Phone: +352 441 13230
Fax: +352 441 13227

Prof. PEREIRA LEITE &
dr. J. BERNARDES
PT 4200 Porto
Phone: +351 2 487 151
Fax: +351 2 498 119

Prof MARQUES DE SA
University of Porto
Rua dos Bragos
PT 4099 Porto Cedex
Phone: +351 2 317 105
Fax: +351 2 319 280

Dr. R. PRAGER &
dr. M. NIRANJAN
Rosie Maternity Hospital
UK Cambridge
CB2 2SW
Phone:+44 223 332 771
Fax: +44 223 332 662

Dr. Philip BANFIELD
Dept. Obstetrics &
Gynaecology, Norfolk &
Norwich Hospital
UK Norwich - Norfolk

Dr. Susan COLES
Information & Statistics
Division, Common Services
Agency of the Scottish Health
Service, Trinity Park House
South Trinity Road
UK Edinburgh EH5 3SQ
Phone: +44 31 552 625
Fax: +44 31 551 1392

Prof. M. S. BEKSAC
Perinataology & Bio-Medical
Engineering Unit, Division of
Materno-Fetal Medicine,
Dept. of Obstetrics,
Hacettepe University
TR Ankara
Phone: +90 4 310 3545
Fax: +90 4 310 5552

ACE INHIBITION VERSUS CORTICOSTEROIDS IN MEMBRANOUS NEPHROPATHY (ACIMEN)

Key words
Membranous nephropathy, clinical trials, angiotensin-converting-enzyme (ACE)-inhibitors.

Brief description
Renal diseases, especially those with loss of proteins in the urine often progress with age to complete failure of the kidneys.

Such a worsening of renal function may also occur in patients with a well defined type of renal disease: membranous nephropathy.

Treatment to prevent such a progression is available but heavily debated. One of the best ways to end this debate is to perform a large study involving most of the expert clinicians in the field.

To achieve this goal the current proposal plans to evaluate two promising but debated treatment regimens to prevent progression of renal function loss.

The first treatment involves rather aggressive immunosuppressive agents; the second comprises a rather new class of antihypertensive drugs, called angiotensin-converting-enzyme (ACE)-inhibitors.

For a proper evaluation of the effects of these drugs we will need a large group of patients with membranous nephropathy (n=150).

Given the fact that one single European country would not be able to recruit enough of such patients in a short period of time, we chose to make this a European trial in different nephrology units, in order to obtain a scientific valid and by all accepted answer to the question on the best anti-progression therapy. If the treatment indeed will help to prevent a progressive renal failure less patients will in the future need hemodialysis and renal transplant programs.

This multicenter trial in 8 European countries will be coordinated by the Division of Nephrology in Groningen.

The coordinator together with a trial monitor from the same unit will be assisted by a project coordinating team.

This team will be formed by one scientist (nephrologist) from each participating country.

They will give expert advice to the participating nephrology units in their country (2 to 10 per country, up to a total of 40).

Project leader:
Professor Paul E. DE JONG
Div. of Nephrology, Dept. of Medicine,
Groningen Institute Drug Studies
Oostersingel 59
NL 9713 EZ Groningen
Phone: +31 50 612621
Fax: +31 50 613474
Contract number: CT941128

Participants:

Dr. M.G. KOOPMAN
Meibergdreef 9
NL 1105 AZ Amsterdam

Dr. J. V.D. MEULEN
De Boelelaan 1117
NL 1081 HV Amsterdam

Prof. W. WEIMAR
Dr. Molewaterplein 40
NL 3015 GD Roteerdam

Dr. J.F.M. WETZELS
Postbus 9101
NL 6500 HB Nijmegen

Dr. C. HALMA
Mr. P.J. Troelstraweg 78
NL 8917 CR Leeuwarden

Dr. J.J.G. OFFERMAN
Groot Wezenland 20
NL 8011 JW Zwolle

Dr. BLOM VAN
ASSENDELFT
Dr. van Heesweg 2
NL 8025 AB Zwolle

Dr. A.J.J. WOITTIEZ
Zilvermeeuw 1
NL 7609 PP Almelo

Dr. J.G.M. JORDANS
Ariensplein 1
NL 7511 JX Enschede

Dr. R. M. VALENTIJN
Sportlaan 600
NL 2566 MJ Den Haag

Dr. G.M.Th. DE JONG
V.d. Steenhovenplein 1
NL 3317 NM Dordrecht

Prof. VAN RENTERGHEM
Herestraat 49
BE 3000 Leuven

Prof. N.H. LAMEIRE
De Pintelaan 185
BE 9000 Gent

Dr. M. JADOUL
Av. Hippocrate 10
BE 1200 Bruxelles

Dr. G. ROSTOKER
Lattre De Tassigny
FR 94010 Creteil

Dr. I. ETIENNE
FR Bois Guillaume

Prof. A. FOURNIER
FR 80030 Amiens

Prof. D. CHEVET
FR 21034 Dijon

Dr. C.D. SHORT
UK Manchester M13 9WL

Dr. D.J. O'DONOGHUE
Dept. of Renal Medicine,
University of Manchester,
Hope Hospital
Eccles Old Rd
UK Salford M6 8HD

Prof. J. WALLS
Dept. of Nephrology,
Leicester Gen. Hosp.
Gwendolen Road
UK Leicester LE5 4PW

Dr. J.D. WILLIAMS
Dept. of Renal Medicine,
Royal Infirmary
Newport Road
UK Cardiff CF2 1SZ

Prof. G.R.D. CATTO
University of Aberdeen
Dean's Office, Polworth
Building/Medical School
Foresterhill
UK Aberdeen AB9 2ZD

Prof. J.F.E. MANN
VI Med. Abteilung, Städt
Klin. Schwabing
Kölner Platz
DE 8000 Munchen

Prof. C.A. BALDARNUS
Dept. of Nephrology,
Med. Klin. V,
University Hospital Cologne
J. Stelzmannstrasse 9
DE 50931 Köln

Dr. M. AURELL
Dept. of Nephrology,
Sahlgrenska Sjukhuset
SE 41345 Göteborg

Dr. I. ODAR-CEDERLOF
Dept. of Med/Nephrology,
Karolinska Hospital
SE 10401 Stockholm

Dr. U. BACKMANN
Dept. of Medicine,
University Hospital
SE 75185 Uppsala

Dr. S. STRANDGAARD
Dept. of Med. & Nephrol.,
B109 Herlev Hospital
DK 2730 Herlev

Dr. T. RING
Med. Dept. C,
Aalborg Hospital South
DK 9100 Aalborg

Dr. H. DIEPERINK
Dept. of Nephrology,
Odense University Hospital
Sdr. Boulevard 29
DK 5000 Odense

Dr. B. NIELSEN
Dept. of Nephrology,
Hvidovre Hospital
Kettegard allé 30
DK 2650 Hvidovre

Dr. P. FAUCHALD
Medical Dept. B:
Rikshospitalet
NO 0027 Oslo 1

Dr. L.M. RUILOPE
Dept. of Nephrology,
Hospital Universitario
12 de Octubre
ES 28041 Madrid

Dr. M. PRAGA
Dept. of Nephrology,
Hospital Universitario
12 de Octubre
ES 28041 Madrid

DEVELOPMENT OF A EUROPEAN QUALITY ASSURANCE PROGRAM OF DIAGNOSTIC ANALYTICAL METHODS USED FOR THE NEONATAL AND SELECTIVE SCREENING OF INHERITED DISORDERS OF METABOLISM: AN INTER-LABORATORY REPRODUCIBILITY STUDY (E.R.N.D.I.M.)

Key words
Quality amirance, neonatal screening, inborn errors of metabolism.

Brief description
On a national level, the individual countries of the EC have a broad experience in the diagnosis and the treatment of Inborn Errors of Metabolism (IDM). However, final conclusions about the best diagnostic and therapeutic approaches cannot be drawn on national level. In order to gain synergy the expertise of each individual member state should be combined on an European level.

To reach this aim, harmonization of diagnostical approaches is of primary importance. The benefits of the proposed inter-laboratory reproductibility study for the individual IDM laboratories will be:

- standardization and optimization of diagnostical analytical procedures, availability of generally accepted and quality-controled reference values of metabolites in physiological fluids, leading to improvement of the reliability of IDM diagnostics and of the analytical follow-up in treatment protocols; quality assesment is a necessity for allowing comparable criteria.
- improvement of the laboratory performance in detection of new metabolic disorders.

The specific knowledge and the laboratory capabilities of the different contractors are gathered in one integrated project. All participants of this study are actively involved in clinical research. A survey of the results of this inter-laboratory reproductibility study will be important for the maintenace and improvement of the diagnostical procedures in all participating IDM laboratories in the EC.

Project leader:
Dr. Baudouin FRANCOIS
Dr. L. Willems Instituut VZW,
Universitaire Campus
BE 3590 Diepenbeek
Phone: +32 11 26 9321
Fax: +32 11 26 9412
Contract number: CT941074

Participants:
Prof. P. KAMOUN
Lab. de Biochimie Génétique,
Hopital Necker
Rue de Sèvres 149
FR 75743 Paris Cedex 15
Phone: +33 1 4273 8812
Fax: +33 1 4273 0659

Dr. J. WILLEMS
SKZL, St Radboudziekenhuis,
afdeling Clin. Chemie
P.O. Box 9101
NL 6500 HB Nijmegen
Phone: +31 80 614 441
Fax: +31 80 541 743

Dr. J.R. BONHAM
Dept of Chemical Pathology,
Children's Hospital
UK Sheffield S10 2TH
Phone: +44 742 761 111
Fax: +44 742 766 205

Dr. A. VAN GENNIP
A.M.C., Lab Procreatie FO 224
Meibergdreef 9
NL 1105 AZ Amsterdam
Phone: +31 20 566 5958
Fax: +31 20 566 4440

Dr. P. DIVRY
Service de Biochimie,
Hopital Debrousse
FR 69322 Lyon Cedex
Phone: +33 72 385 709
Fax: +33 72 385 884

Prof. F. TRIJBELS
Kindergeneeskunde afdeling,
St. Radboud Ziekenhuis
P.O. Box 9101
NL 6500 HB Nijmegen
Phone: +33 80 613 986
Fax: +33 80 540 576

Prof. J.L. DHONDT
Laboratoire de Biochimie,
Hopital St. Philibert
FR 59160 Lomme
Phone: +33 20 22 50 50
Fax: +33 20 22 50 11

Dr. L. SPAAPEN
Dept of Genetics
P.O. Box 1475
NL 6201 BL Maastricht
Phone: +31 43 875 842
Fax: +31 43 877 877

Prof. C. BACHMANN
Laboratoire Central de Chimie Clinique, CHUC
CH 1011 Lausanne
Phone: +41 21 314 5238
Fax: +41 21 314 5266

Dr. B. FOWLER
Kinderspital
Römergasse 8
CH 4005 Basel
Phone: +41 61 692 6555
Fax: +41 61 692 6555

EUROPEAN CONCERTED ACTION ON THE IMMUNOGENETICS OF SYSTEMIC LUPUS ERYTHEMATOSUS

Key words
Immunogenetics, Systemic Lupus Erythematosus, autoimmune disorders, biological markers.

Brief description
Systemic Lupus Erythematosus (SLE) is a multisystemic autoimmune disorder of unknown etiology with different patterns of presentation and evolution. Genetic and/or ethnic predisposing factors are probably involved in the etiopathogenesis of the disease and in its clinical expression.

The aims of our project are first to test in a large series of SLE Patients, of different ethnic origin, the hypothesis that the clinically and/or serologically defined subsets of the disease show more consistent association with the HLA alleles and then to study the influence of ethnic factors on the HLA-SLE association.

For the present study a cohort of 720 SLE patients and an equal number of ethnically matched healthy controls will be enrolled. Patients and controls will come from 6 different European countries. In all patients the HLA study and the search of specific circulating auto-antibodies will be performed. An accurate clinical chart will be filled out for each patient in order to obtain clinical and epidemiological information to be correlated with the genetic and the immunological features.

At the end of the three years study it is expected to obtain information on the identification of clinically, serologically and genetically defined subsets of SLE, which might be responsive to different therapeutic approaches, and on the identification of biological markers, either genetical or serological, of prognostic value for susceptibility to different clinical aspects of the disease.

Project leader:
Dr. Mauro GALEAZZI
Institute of Rheumatology,
University of Siena
Via Tufi 1
IT 53100 Siena
Phone: +39 577 288 132
Fax: +39 577 404 50
Contract number: CT941260

Participants:
Prof. Alessandro MATHIEU
Il Cattedra di Reumatologia,
Istutito di Clinica Medica, Università di Cagliari
Via S. Giorgio 12
IT 09124 Cagliari
Phone: +39 70 660 211
Fax: +39 70 660 213

Prof. Raffaella SCORZA
Laboratory of Cellular
Immunology and Immunogenetics,
University of Milano
Via F. Sforza 35
IT 20122 Milano
Phone: +39 2 5511 958
Fax: +39 2 5519 2842

Dr. Frédéric HOUSSIAU
Dervice du Rhumatologie, Cliniques Univ.
Saint-Luc, Université Catholique
de Louvain
Avenue Hippocrate 10
BE 1200 Bruxelles
Phone: +32 2 7645 390
Fax: +32 2 7645 394

Prof. Jean-Charles PIETTE
Service Medecine
Interne Godeau: CHU Pitie-Salpetriere
83 Boulevard de l'Hopital
FR 75013 Paris
Phone: +33 1 4570 3408
Fax: +33 1 4570 6353

Dr. Ch. PAPASTERIADES
Dept.of ImmunologyHistocompatibility,
Evangelismos Hospital
45-47 St. Ipsilantou
GR 10676 Athens
Phone: +30 1 7248 312
Fax: +30 1 7291 808

Prof. Helmuth DEICHER
Division of Immunology and Blood Transfusion
Medicine, Dept. of Medicine, Medizinische
Hochschule Hannover
Konstanty-Gutschow-Str. 8
DE 3000 Hannover
Phone: +49 511 531/532
Fax: +49 511 532 5648

Dr. FERNANDEZ-NEBRO
Dept. of Medicine, Section Lupus Unit, Univ.
Hospital, University of Malaga
Campus de Teatinos s/n
ES 29080 Malaga
Phone: +34 5 2131 615
Fax: +34 5 2131 511

Dr. DE RAMON GARRIDO
Servicio de Medicina Interna, Unidad de
Enfermedades Autoimmunes Sisteemicas, Hospital Regional del SAS
Av. da Carlos Haya s/n
ES 29016 Malaga
Phone: +34 5 2287 340
Fax: +34 5 2288 349

Dr. Ricard CERVERA
Servei de Medicina Interna General,
Hospital Clinic y Provincial,
Facultat de Medicina, Universitat de Barcelona
Villarroel 170
ES 08036 Barcelona
Phone: +34 3 4546 000
Fax: +34 3 4515 272

Prof. Licinio CONTU
Dept. of Medical Genetics, Istituto di Clinica
Medica, University of Cagliari
Via S. Giorgio 12
IT 09124 Cagliari
Phone: +39 70 6028 315
Fax: +39 70 6596 27

Prof. G. Battista FERRARA
Immunogenetics Laboratory, Istituto Nazionale
per la Ricerca sul Cancro
Viale Benedetto XV n. 10
IT 16132 Genova
Phone: +39 10 302754/300767
Fax: +39 10 352999

Dr. Luisa BRACCI
Immunochemistry Unit,
Dept. of Molecular Biology, University of Siena
Viale Mario Bracci
IT 53100 Siena
Phone: +39 577 263 229

Prof. P. ANNUNZIATA
Istituto di Scienze Neurologiche,
Università di Siena
Viale Mario Bracci
IT 53100 Siena
Phone: +39 577 290 111
Fax: +39 577 403 27

Dr. A. JEDRYKA-GORAL
Dept. of Connective Tissue Diseases,
Institute of Rheumatology,
University of Warsaw
Spartanska 1
PL 02637 Warsaw
Phone: +48 2244 5726
Fax: +48 2244 9522

PRENATAL ADMINISTRATION OF THYREOTROPIN RELEASING HORMONE TO REDUCE THE HUMAN AND HEALTH SERVICE BURDEN OF NEONATAL IMMATURITY

Key words
Thyrotropin releasing hormone, neonatal immaturity, prenatal care, clinical trials.

Brief description
The smallest 1% of babies carry substantial human and economic costs for EC Member States. Sequelae of neonatal immaturity require prolonged hospitalization and commonly cause death and serious morbidity. Nevertheless, such babies are not seen commonly in individual hospitals, or even in some smaller EC countries, and reliable evaluation of prevention strategies requires multicentre, ideally international, collaboration. Extensive laboratory research and five small controlled trials in human pregnancy suggest that thyrotropin releasing hormone (TRH) given to a mother before the birth of her immature baby will substantially reduce these risks.

This Concerted Action will harmonise on-going and planned research on TRH within the EC. One (or possibly several parallel) placebo-controlled trials will be facilitated, aiming to confirm (or refute) the clinical and cost effectiveness, and safety of TRH. By bringing together research groups throughout Europe, the Concerted Action will ensure that TRH is evaluated promptly and reliably before its unevaluated use becomes widespread.

Clinical centres in each participating country will be represented by a national co-ordinator on the project steering group. This organisation is based on previous successful European collaborative perinatal trials coordinated by the project leader.

The research within individual countries will be assisted by a major Belgian pharmaceutical company. This arrangement will also ensure European commercial exploitation if the Concerted Action demonstrates TRH's effectiveness and safety.

The structure of the Concerted Action will allow efficient dissemination of the results and its impact will be evaluated by questionnaire survey at the conclusion of the project.

Project leader:
Dr. Adrian GRANT
Perinatal Trials Service,
National Perinatal Epidemiology Unit,
Radcliffe Infirmary, University of Oxford
UK Oxford OX2 6HE
Phone: +44 865 22 41 33
Fax: +44 865 72 63 60
Contract number: CT941373

Participants:
Dr. ELBOURNE
Perinatal Trials Service,
National Perinatal Epidemiology Unit,
Radcliffe Infirmary, University of Oxford
UK Oxford OX2 6HE
Phone: +44 865 22 41 33
Fax: +44 865 72 63 60

Dr. Heracles DELLAGRAMMATICAS
2nd Dept of Pediatrics,
Athens University,
Aglaia Kyriakou Children's Hospital
GR 11527 Athens
Phone: +30 1 778 7196

Prof. J. RIGO
Neonatal Unit, Hospital de la Citadelle
BE 4000 Liège
Phone: +32 41 26 47 47
Fax: +32 41 25 65 54

Dr. Luis JANUARIO
Dept. of Neopathology,
Hospital Pediatrico de Coimbra,
Centro Hospitalar de Coimbra
Av Bissaya Barreto
PT 3000 Coimbra
Phone: +351 39 484 163
Fax: +351 39 484 464

Dr. Joke K. KOK
Pediatrician-Neonatologist,
Dutch TRH Trial, Academic Medical Center
Meibergdreef 9
NL 1105 AZ Amsterdam
Phone: +31 20 566 3969
Fax: +31 20 696 5099

Dr. Olivier CLARIS
Service de Neonatologie et Reanimation
Neonatale, Hopital E Herriot
5 Place d'Arsonval
FR 69374 Lyon Cedex 03
Phone: +33 7234 4658
Fax: +33 7211 1050

Dr. Niels Jorgen SECHER
Dept of Obstetrics and Gynaecology,
University Hospital,
Arhus Kommunehospital
37-39 Norrebrogade
DK 8000 Arhus C
Phone: +45 86 125 555
Fax: +45 86 197 413

Prof. James NEILSON
Dept Obstetrics & Gynaecology,
University of Liverpool,
Royal Liverpool University Hospital
Prescor Street
UK Liverpool L7 8XP
Phone: +44 51 706 2000/4100
Fax: +44 51 706 5993

Dr. Carlos BROTONS
Clinical Epidemiology Department,
Sabadell Hospital
ES Barcelona
Phone: +34 3 723 1010
Fax: +34 3 716 0646

CONCERTED ACTION ON GENETIC SERVICES IN EUROPE (CAGSE) RELATED TO INDIVIDUAL NATIONAL CHARACTERISTICS AND NEEDS

Key words

Health service research, medical genetics, genetic counselling, networking, genetic diagnosis.

Brief description

This Concerted Action, involving collaborators in all EC and COST countries, is concerned with the reactions of health services to the challenges of human genome analysis and increased public awareness. Our preliminary surveys on behalf of the European Society of Human Genetics (ESHG) show that most countries do not yet recognise medical genetics as a specialty and we know little about how genetic services are provided, organised and delivered, nor how they relate to special national epidemiological, economic, social, ethical, and other characteristics.

By developing our established ESHG network, we will investigate the structure, workloads and quality of genetic services and the different responses made by each country to these challenges. We will assess the contribution made by specialist doctors, by other health care workers and by those from other fields of medicine. We will investigate the extent to which non-geneticists and health officials are coming to recognise the increasing influence of genetics in health care. By cooperation between collaborators we will encourage the evolution of medical genetics services in a manner which is consistent with the special needs of each country and the explicit wishes of consumers.

This CA will complement other proposed initiatives designed to investigate the specific ethical issues raised by human genome analysis.

Project leader:
Professor Rodney HARRIS
Dept. of Medical Genetics,
St. Mary's Hospital
Hathersage Road
UK Manchester M13 0JH
Phone: +44 612766262
Fax: +44 612488308
Contract number: CT941557

Participants:
Dr. L. KOCH
Institute of Social Medicine,
University of Copenhagen,
Panum Institute
Blegdamsvej 3
DK 22000 Copenhagen
Phone: +45 31 35 7900
Fax: +45 31 35 1181

Prof. J.F. MATTEI
Centre de Diagnostic
Prenatal, C.R.E.B.I.O.P.,
Hopital d'Enfants
de la Timone
FR 13385 Marseille Cedex 5
Phone: +33 91 49 32 37
Fax: +33 91 49 41 94

Prof. M. MIKKELSEN
John F. Kennedy Institute
GL. Landevej 7
DK Glostrup
Phone: +45 4245 2228
Fax: +45 4343 1130

Prof. M. NIERMEIJER
Dept. Clinical Genetics,
Erasmus University/
University Hospital Dijkzigt
P.O. Box 1738
NL 3000 DR Rotterdam
Phone: +31 10 463 4307
Fax: +31 10 408 7213

Prof. G. ROMEO
Instituto Giannina Gaslini,
Laboratory of Molecular
Genetics
IT 16148 Genova Quarto
Phone: +39 10 56 36 400
Fax: +39 10 39 12 54

Dr. D. STEMERDING
Centre for Studies of Science,
Technology & Society,
University of Twente
NL Enschede
Phone: +31 53 89 33 48
Fax: +31 53 35 06 25

IMPROVEMENT OF ORGAN TRANSPLANTATION BY INCREASE OF THE EXTRACORPOREAL LIFE-TIME AND BY IMPROVEMENT OF THE FUNCTIONAL QUALITY OF THE TRANSPLANT, USING CONTINUOUS PERFUSION OF OXYGEN CARRYING FLUIDS BASED ON FINE EMULSIONS OF FLUOROCARBONS

Key words
Organ transplantation, organ storage, ischemia, membrance lipoperoxidation, free radicals, fluorocarbon emulsions, oxygen.

Brief description
The success of organ transplantation is actually still limited by the difficulties encountered after a too long organ storage in hypothermic and ischemic conditions. During this storage, the organ is submitted to ischemia with structural and functional alterations which are aggravated at reperfusion when the return of oxygen leads to free radical production and membrane lipoperoxidation.

Our objective is to prolonge the lifetime of the harvested organ by its continuous perfusion at room temperature with oxygen carrying fluorocarbon emulsions. Fluorocarbon emulsions will be prepared, optimized for particle size, fluidity and stability, and adapted for biological use by addition of appropriate nutrients. These emulsions will be tested on cultured human endothelial cells (viability, conservation of morphological characteristics and multiplication capacity). Osmolality will be controlled and oncotic pressure will be adjusted by addition of macromolecules. The anti-oxidant and antiradicalar potency of these emulsions will be tested and increased by addition of appropriate agents in order to avoid lipoperoxidation. The possibility of a free radical production in these emulsions will be tested (electronic paramagnetic resonance). According to the results obtained on cell culture, the emulsions will be enriched with appropriate protective molecules.

The final emulsions will be used in animal models of pancreas conservation and transplantation (rabbit and inbreed rat). The structural and functional integrity of the organ will be tested after variable periods of conservation and after transplantation and reperfusion. The production of free radicals (in blood and tissue) will be investigated and the antioxidant status of the graft will be measured in the rabbit model. In the inbreed rat model (in which rejection phenomenons are suppressed) the preservation of endocrine and exocrine functions of the graft will be tested. Functional integrity of the isolated mitochondria will also be examined.

Project leader:
Professor Maurice LAMY
Centre for the Biochemistry of Oxygen,
Centre Hospitalier Universitaire
Domaine du Sart Tilman B 35
BE 4000 Liege
Phone: +32 41 66 71 79
Fax: +32 41 66 76 36
Contract number: CT941249

Participants:

C. DEBY
Centre de Biochimie de l'Oxygène (C.B.O.) B6,
Centre Hospitalier Universitaire B35
Domaine de Sart Tilman
BE 4000 Liège
Phone: +32 41 667179/563360
Fax: +32 41 667636/563366

Jean RIESS
Unité de Chimie Moléculaire,
Faculté des Sciences,
Université de Nice, Sophia Antipolis
28 Avenue de Valrose
FR 06108 Nice
Phone: +33 9352 9839
Fax: +33 9352 9352/9020

Francis SLUSE
Laboratoire de Bioénergétique,
Institut de Chimie B6
Domaine du Sart Tilman
BE 4000 Liège
Phone: +32 4156 3587

Michel MEURISSE
Centre de Transplantation,
Centre Hospitalier Universitaire B35
Domainde Universitaire du Sart Tilman
BE 4000 Liège
Phone: +32 4188 2428
Fax: +32 4166 7517

Milbhor D'SILVA
The Liver and Hepatobiliary Unit,
The Queen Elizabeth Hospital Centre
Edgbaston
UK Birmingham
Phone: +44 21 47 21 311
Fax: +44 21 62 72 497

ISLET RESEARCH EUROPEAN NETWORK (IREN): MOLECULAR AND CELLULAR BIOLOGY APPROACHES FOR THE PREVENTION AND TREATMENT OF DIABETES MELLITUS

Key words
Diabetes mellitus, prevention, gene therapy, B-cells.

Brief description
Diabetes mellitus is a metabolic disorder with an enormous socio-economic impact affecting up to 5% of the population in the various European countries. The disease is becoming increasingly common in the older age groups and is associated with severe late complications. In many patients with diabetes (both, type I and type II) insulin deficiency due to a loss and/ or to glucose insensitivity of the insulin-secreting pancreatic B-cells is a major underlying cause.

During recent years the basic mechanisms underlying stimulus-secretion coupling in pancreatic B-cells have been elucidated, and European islet diabetes research groups have provided the major contribution. Molecular biology is a potent new tool in islet diabetes research. It now permits the generation of novel insulin-producing tissue culture cell lines in which the structures essential for stimulus-secretion coupling can be modified in a well defined manner and compared with B-cells from normal and diabetic animals. This will allow characterisation of molecular structures essential for stimulus-secretion coupling and the involvement of defective insulin secretion. The result will be the possibility to design rational approaches for the therapy of pancreatic B-cell dysfunction in diabetic patients. This approach will provide also the basis for gene therapy of diabetes or alternatively the generation of insulin-secreting cells from pluripotent donor cells which can be transplanted into diabetic patients to counteract insulin deficiency.

In this proposal for a leading European islet diabetes network researchers have been brought together to provide all cellular and molecular biology methods required to make it successful. The proposal has a significant innovation potential and represents a great opportunity to provide novel methods for the prevention, treatment and cure of diabetes. Such an achievement would have a substantial impact upon general health in Europe.

Project leader:
Professor Sigurd LENZEN
Medizinische Hochschule Hannover,
Institut für Klinische Biochemie
Konstanty Gutschow Straße 8
Postfach 610180
DE W-30625 Hannover 1
Phone: +49 511 532 65 25
Fax: +49 511 532 35 84
Contract number: CT941285

Participants:

Prof. H.P.T. AMMON
DE 72076 Tübingen

Dr. Steven J.H. ASHCROFT
UK Oxford OX3 9DU

Dr. Clifford J. BAILEY
UK Birmingham B4 7ET

Prof. Tatiana BANI SACCHI
IT 50139 Firenze

Dr. Dominique BATAILLE
FR 34094 Montpellier
Cedex 5

Dr. Francisco BEDOYA
ES 41009 Sevilla

Dr. Leonard BEST
UK Manchester M13 9WL

Dr. Patrik RORSMAN
SE 41390 Göteborg

Prof. Janove SEHLIN
SE 90187 Umeå

Dr. Kurt WEBER
AT 8036 Graz

Prof. Adrian BONE
UK Brighton BN2 4GJ

Dr. Bernadette BREANT
FR 75571 Paris Cedex 12

Dr. Kirsten CAPITO
DK 2200 Copenhagen N

Dr. Mark J. DUNNE
UK Sheffield S10 2TN

Prof. Peter R. FLATT
UK Coleraine BT52 1SA

Dr. Maie-Hélène GIROIX
FR 75251 Paris Cedex 05

Dr. Irene C. GREEN
UK Brighton BN1 9QG

Prof. Dietrich GRUBE
DE 30623 Hannover

Prof. Lieselotte HERBERG
DE 40225 Düsseldorf

Prof. André HERCHUELZ
BE 1070 Brussels

Dr. Peter JONES
UK London W8 7AH

Dr. Klaus-Dieter KOHNERT
DE 17495 Karlsburg

Prof. Willy MALAISSE
BE 1070 Brussels

Dr. Noel MORGAN
UK Keele ST5 5BE

Dr. Jens H. NIELSEN
DK 2820 Gentofte

Prof. Uwe PANTEN
DE 37075 Göttingen

Dr. P. PETIT
FR 34060 Montpellier Cedex

Dr. Andreas PFEIFFER
DE 44789 Bochum

Prof. Sotos RAPTIS
GR 11510 Athens

Dr. Luis M. ROSARIO
PT 3049 Coimbra Codex

Prof. Bernat SORIA
ES 03080 Alicante

Prof. Jorge
TAMARIT-RODRIGUEZ
ES 28040 Madrid

Dr. Isabel VALVERDE
ES 28040 Madrid

Prof. Eugen J. VERSPOHL
DE 48149 Münster

Dr. Gerrit H.J. WOLTERS
NL 9713 BZ Groningen

Prof. Hartmut ZUHLKE
DE 17489 Greifswald

Dr. Per-Olof BERGGREN
SE 10401 Stockholm

Prof. Jon FLORHOLMEN
NO 9037 Tromsö

Dr. Erik GYLFE
SE 75123 Uppsala

Dr. Timo OTONKOSKI
FI Helsinki

Prof. Philippe HALBAN
CH 1211 Geneva 4

Dr. Paolo MEDA
CH 1211 Geneva 4

Prof. Claes B. WOLLHEIM
CH 1211 Geneva 4

THE RETINAL ANGIOGRAPHY WITH SODIUM FLUORESCEIN AND GREEN INDOCYANINE IN THE DETECTION OF SUBRETINAL NEOVASCULAR MEMBRANE IN THE SECOND EYE OF PATIENTS WITH WET AGE-RELATED MACULAR DEGENERATION

Key words

Age-related macular degeneration, angiography clinical trial, subretinal neovascularization, fluorescein angiography, indocyanine green angiography.

Brief description

This project will study patients with Age-Related Macular Degeneration (ARMD) with subretinal neovascular membrane (SRNVM) in one eye. Due to the unknown pathophysiology no therapy for prevention of progression of ARMD has been proven to be efficient. Laser treatment is the only well established therapy in cases with neovascular membranes. Nevertheless laser therapy allows only destructive treatment of subretinal membrane and the overlying retina. The larger is the lesion produced either by natural history or by laser treatment, the worse is the capacity of good prognosis. Therefore prevention of subretinal neovascularization would improve visual prognosis.

The study is divided in two parts. The first part consists of the observation of the second eye of patients affected by wet ARMD with traditional fluorescein angiography (FA) and indocyanine green angiography (ICG).

The second part provides a randomized clinical trial for treatment of neovascular membranes in the patients who have developed a SRNVM. At this point the patients will be randomized and divided in two groups:

- the first group will have photocoagulation of SRNVM detected with ICG angiography according to the Macular Photocoagulation Study Group protocol;
- the second group (the control group) will not receive any treatment until the SNRVM is identified with FA; at this point current therapeutic procedure will be applied.

Patients will be recruited at the Outpatients' Department of University Eye Clinics of Milan, Aachen and Nijmegen.

For the angiographic study the Scanning Laser Ophthalmoscope or a fundus camera prepared to perform ICG and FA is utilized. Each patient undergoes an angiographic examination with indocyanine green and sodium fluorescein every six months.

The objective of our project is to evaluate if the ICG is more useful for the early diagnosis of SRNVM compared to FA. Moreover we want to verify if early treatment could be useful for the visual outcome.

Project leader:
Dr. Nicola ORZALESI
Clinica Oculistica, Istituto di Scienze Biomediciche Ospedale San Paolo
Università'degli Studi di Milano
Via di Rudini' 8
IT 20142 Milano
Phone: +39 2 8139221
Fax: +39 2 8139221
Contract number: CT941263

Participants:

Dr. Giovanni STAURENGHI
Istituto di Scienze Biomediche
Ospedale San Paolo
Via Di Rudinì 8
IT 20142 Milan
Phone: +39 2 8139221
Fax: +39 2 8139221

Dr. Monica ASCHERO
Istituto di Scienze
Biomediche Ospedale San Paolo
Via Di Rudinì 8
IT 20142 Milan
Phone: +39 2 8139221
Fax: +39 2 8139221

Dr. Maria Cristina CARRARO
Istituto di Scienze Biomediche
Ospedale San Paolo
Via Di Rudinì 8
IT 20142 Milan
Phone: +39 2 8139221
Fax: +39 2 8139221

Dr. Annunciata LA CAPRIA
Istituto di Scienze Biomediche
Ospedale San Paolo
Via Di Rudinì 8
IT 20142 Milan
Phone: +39 2 8139221
Fax: +39 2 8139221

Prof. M. REIM
Rheinisch-Westfälische
Technische Hochschule Aachen,
Medizinische Fakultät,
Dept. of Ophthalmology
Pauwelstrasse 30
DE 5100 Aachen
Phone: +49 241 8088351
Fax: +49 241 875992

Dr. Sebastian WOLF
Rheinisch-Westfälische
Technische Hochschule Aachen,
Medizinische Fakultät,
Dept. of Ophthalmology
Pauwelstrasse 30
DE 5100 Aachen
Phone: +49 241 8088351
Fax: +49 241 875992

Dr. Karen SCHULTE
Rheinisch-Westfälische Technische
Hochschule Aachen, Medizinische Fakultät,
Dept. of Ophthalmology
Pauwelstrasse 30
DE 5100 Aachen
Phone: +49 241 8088351
Fax: +49 241 875992

PATHOPHYSIOLOGY OF IMPAIRED PLACENTAL TRANSFER IN INTRAUTERINE GROWTH RETARDED (IUGR) PREGNANCIES: CORRELATION BETWEEN IN VIVO AND IN VITRO STUDIES

Key words
Intrauterine growth retardation, pathophysiology, placental transfer, perinatal care.

Brief description
The aim of this project is to study the causes of intrauterine growth retardation, which represents one of the most important causes of perinatal morbidity and mortality.

Comparisons will be made between clinical studies of the placental circulation (by Doppler waveform analysis of the umbilical and uterine arteries), *in vivo* studies of amino acid placental transfer and metabolism (by stable isotope methodologies at the time of fetal blood sampling) and morphological and *in vitro* functional studies of the placenta from the same pregnancies, in order to establish whether there is a strong relationship between a specific placental abnormality and the clinical findings on the fetus.

Particular focus will be met on the pathophysiology of impaired placental transfer of amino acids as a specific cause of IUGR.

The clinical studies will be performed in Milano, in Torino and in Glasgow. Studies will involve both pregnancies carrying fetuses appropriate for gestational age (AGA) and IUGR fetuses.

IUGR will be defined by standard ultrasound parameters of fetal growth and will be confirmed at birth according to standards developed for the population under study.

The studies have been approved by the ethical committees of the institutions involved.

These groups will perform complete studies of the utero-placental circulation by Doppler waveform analysis of the uterine and umbilical arteries, collection of blood samples for amino acid analysis and collection of placental samples.

In vivo studies of amino acid transfer and metabolisn by stable isotope methodologies will be performed prior to fetal blood sampling under untrasound guidance in Milano and analysis of enrichments by Gas Chromatography Man Spectromrtry (GCMS).

Placental samples will be collected and prepared for:

1 morphometric studies using 3-dimensional methods on human placental cotyledons obtained from normal and IUGR pregnancies, prepared by perfusion fixation and examined by scanning electron microscopy, and;

2 amino acid transport studies on vesicles isolated from the microvillous plasma membrane of the syncytiotrophoblast of placentae from normal and IUGR pregnancies.

Project leader:
Professor Giorgio PARDI
Dept. of Obstetrics and Gynecology,
Istituto di Scienze Biomediche,
San Paolo
Via A. Di Rudini 8
IT 20142 Milano
Phone: +39 28 18 45 06
Fax: +39 28 13 56 62
Contract number: CT941715

Participants:

Dr. Colin SIBLEY
Dept. of Child Health,
University of Manchester,
St. Mary's Hospital
Hathersage Road
UK Manchester M13 OJH
Phone: +44 61 2766 484
Fax: +44 61 2241 013

Prof. Peter KAUFMANN
Anatomisches Institut,
University of Aachen
DE 5100 Aachen
Phone: +49 241 8089 190
Fax: +49 241 8044 13

Dr. John KINGDOM
Dept. of Obstetrics and Gynecology,
Royal Infirmary,
Queen Elizabeth Building
UK Glasgow G31 2ER
Phone: +44 55 23535
Fax: +44 55 31367

Dr. Tullia TODROS
Istituto de Ginecologia e
Ostetricia,
Università di Torino
Via Ventimiglia 3
IT 10126 Torino
Phone: +39 11 6396 401
Fax: +39 11 6647 910

Dr. Roberto FANELLI
Istituto di Ricerche
Farmacologiche Mario Negri
Via Eritrea
IT 20157 Milano
Phone: +39 2 3901 4498
Fax: +39 2 3900 1916

MOLECULAR BIOLOGY OF IMMUNOSENESCENCE

Key words
Immunosenescene, molecular genetics, lymphocytes-T, immunology, immunogenetics.

Brief description
Immunosenescence results in deterioration of immune function in elderly individuals as well as in individuals with premature ageing syndromes. Dysfunction of the immune system, particularly the T cells even in apparently healthy individuals, may be involved in the increased susceptibility to infection, autoimmunity and cancer of the elderly. Certain genes have been found to be transcribed only or preferentially in senescent non-lymphoid cells and some of these have been shown to have a direct anti-proliferative activity. If this was the case also with lymphocytes, molecular approaches to modulate lymphocyte Senescence genes might improve immune function in ageing.

Research in the proposed concerted action will resolve the question of whether immuno-senescence of lymphocytes-T is partially or totally caused by the active upregulation of new genetic programmes involving the participation of senescence-inducing and/or growth arrest-specific genes. The expression of such genes will be examined on lymphocytes-T which have been aged in tissue culture, compared with those aged in vivo, as well as in non-lymphoid tissues and tumour cells. It will be explored whether any of such genes are tissue-specific, particularly T cell-specific, or even T cell subset-specific, and their relationship to tumour suppressor genes will be established. The activation state of any such gene candidates will be investigated in healthy aged, clinic aged, prematurely aged, and in young healthy controls, as well as in long-term culture systems.

Attempts will be made to manipulate gene expression in cultured cells and in ex vivo material in order to construct a model for modifying processes resulting in immuno-senescence, which could be eventually applied *in vivo*. To meet the goals outlined above, this Concerted Action will collect/generate and screen candidate genes for their specific expression in aged T cells and their causative role in immunosenescence and make such probes available to participants for testing on their patient materials.

The coordinator's laboratory will act as well as central facility to provide gene probes and antisense technology as well as molecular genetic backup, teaching and expertise, and quality control by partial duplication of participants experiments with their cellular materials.

Project leader:
Dr. Graham PAWELEC
Medizinische Universitäts- und Poliklinik
Otfried Müller Straße 10
DE W-7400 Tübingen
Phone: +49 70 71 29 28 05
Fax: +49 70 71 29 44 64
Contract number: CT941209

Participants:

Prof. C. BARTOLONI
Laboratorio di Immunulogia Clinica,
Istituto di Clinica Medica Generale
e Terapia Medica,
Università del Sacro Cuore
IT 00168 Rome
Phone: +39 6 3015 4900
Fax: +39 6 3054 481

Dr. R. SOLANA
Dept. Immunologia, Facultad de Medicina,
Hospital Reina Sofia
ES 14004 Córdoba
Phone: +34 57 202 094
Fax: +34 57 218 229

Dr. E. MARIANI
Istituto di Ricerca Codivilla Putti,
Laboratorio di Immunologia e Genetica
Via di Barbiano 1/10
IT 40136 Bologna
Phone: +39 51 63 66 803
Fax: +39 51 63 66 807

Dr. G.M. TAYLOR
Immunogenetics Laboratory,
St. Mary's Hospital
Hathersage Road
UK Manchester M13 0JH
Phone: +44 61 276 6472
Fax: +44 61 224 1013

Prof. S. SHALL
Cell and Molecular Biology Laboratory,
University of Sussex Biology Building
UK Brighton BN1 9QG
Phone: +44 273 678 303
Fax: +44 273 678 335

Dr. C. PARASKEVA
Dept. of Pathology and Microbiology,
School of Medical Sciences,
University of Bristol
University Walk
UK Bristol BS8 1TD
Phone: +44 272 3031
Fax: +44 272 303497

Dr. G. LIGTHART
Dept. Pathology, Section of Gerontology,
University of Leiden
P.O. Box 9603
NL 2300 RC Leiden
Phone: +31 71 276 638
Fax: +31 71 276 640

Dr. V. SORRENTINO
European Molecular Biology Laboratory
Postfach 102209
DE 6900 Heidelberg
Phone: +49 6221 3871
Fax: +49 6221 387306

THE ASSESSMENT OF DRUG RELATED PROBLEMS IN THE ELDERLY AND THE EVALUATION AND HARMONISATION OF PREVENTATIVE Strategies ON A EUROPEAN BASIS

Key words

Elderly, prevention, drug-related problems, hospital care, gerontology.

Objectives

- to monitor hospital admissions of patients over 65 years for an 8 month period in order to identify for each of the participating centres drug-related morbidity in the elderly associated with inappropriate and ineffective use of medicines in the local community.
- to evaluate the total data obtained in order to agree and implement harmonised preventive strategies.
- to test these strategies by remonitoring hospital admissions for an 8 month period to determine whether the identified problems have been reduced or eliminated.
- to assess for each centre the economic benefits associated with preventing drug related morbidity in the community.
- to share and spread good practice by producing reports, convening meetings with physicians and pharmacists, presenting the research findings at conferences and publishing in refereed journals.

Brief description

Iatrogenic disease is a particular risk in older patients due to their altered pharmacodynamics and the altered pharmacokinetics of many drugs with age. In addition the elderly take a great number of medicines and suffer from multiple disease states. They may also have impaired hearing, loss of vision, and increasing loss of dexterity and mobility which may affect compliance with treatment regimes.

Each objective provides the opportunity to obtain valuable information which is no t at present available in a European context and which will be of great interest to all participants. All centres follow the same methodology on the basis of a common research protocol. This protocol will involve the determination, by means of structured interviews of those patients, aged 65 years and over, being admitted into a particular hospital over an eight month period because of drug related problems. The patient screening will again be carried out for an eight month period after harmonised preventative strategies have been put into practice. In addition to collecting useful comparative data of drug prescribing practices, patient compliance and the incidence of adverse drug reactions, the knowledge gained will be used to harmonise protocols, affect the management of the healthcare workforce and systems and develop methodology of research into prevention of drug related problems.

Project leader:
Professor R.M.E. RICHARDS
Head of School of Pharmacy, The Robert Gordon University
Schoolhill
UK Aberdeen AB9 1FR
Phone: +44 22 42 62 500
Fax: +44 22 46 26 559
Contract number: CT941664

Participants:

Prof. E. MARINO
Faculty of Pharmacy; University of Barcelona
Avenida Joan XXII
ES Barcelona
Phone: +34 3330 7961
Fax: +34 3490 8279

Prof. J. CROMARTY
Clinical Pharmacy Practice Unit;
School of Pharmacy;
The Robert Gordon University
Schoolhill
UK Aberdeen AB9 1FR
Phone: +44 224 262 541
Fax: +44 224 626 559

Dr. R. WALKER
Medicines Research Unit;
Welsh School of Pharmacy; University of Wales
P.O. Box 13
UK Cardiff CF1 3XF
Phone: +44 222 874 783
Fax: +44 222 874 149

Dr. A DE BOER
Faculty of Pharmacy; Utrecht University
P.O. Box 80082
NL 3508 TB Utrecht
Phone: +31 30 536 990
Fax: +31 30 517 839

Prof A.L. WAN PO
School of Pharmacy;
The Queen's University of Belfast
97 Lisburn Road
UK Belfast BT9 7BL
Phone: +44 232 330 505
Fax: +44 232 247 794

CALCIUM INTAKE AND PEAK BONE MASS: A EUROPEAN MULTI CENTRE STUDY (CALEUR)

Key words
Osteoporosis, calcium intake, peak bone mass, peidemiology, risk factors.

Brief description
Epidemiological studies indicate that the bone mass at young adult age is a critical parameter for the risk of osteoporosis at old age. The effect of different levels of calcium intake on bone development during adolescents, the critical period for bone growth, is actually unknown. It is likely that a threshold level exists beyond which calcium intake no longer influences peak bone mass.

The aim of the study is to answer the following questions:

1 Does a positive relation exist between calcium intake and the attainment of peak bone mass?
2 Does a threshold level exist beyond which a positive relation between calcium intake and peak bone mass no longer exists?

The answers will be obtained in a cross-sectional study in five countries, being Finland, Denmark, the Netherlands, France and Italy. These countries are selected because of the existence of a north-south gradient in calcium intake, thus providing a wide range of calcium intake levels across Europe.

In each centre calcium intake and bone mass will be assessed in two selected subgroups of adolescent girls and young adult women, according to a strictly standardized protocol. The subgroups are classified as being either at the lower or at the higher region of the calcium intake range.

Bone mass confounding variables and effect modifiers will be analysed by the centralized facility.

Results in the five centres can be compared directly. Data in each centre will be processed separately and a pooled analysis across the centres will be done by the co-ordinating centre.

Project leader:
Dr. Gertjan SCHAAFSMA
TNO Toxicology and Nutrition Institute, Department
of Human Nutrition
P.O. Box 360
NL 3700 AJ Zeist
Phone: +31 3404 44 144
Fax: +31 3404 57224
Contract number: CT941523

Participants:
Dr. G. VAN POPPEL
TNO Nutrition and Food
Research
P.O. Box 360
NL 3700 AJ Zeist
Phone: +31 3404 44754
Fax: +31 3404 57952

Dr. P. CHARLES
Dept. of Endocinology and
Metabolism,
Aarhus Universiteitshospital
DK 8000 Aarhus C
Phone: +45 86 12 68 66
Fax: +45 86 19 30 75

Dr. H.K. VAANANEN
Dept. of Anatomy,
University of Oulu
Kajaanintie 52A
FI 90220 Oulu
Phone: +358 81 537 5011
Fax: +358 81 537 5172

Dr. M. ROTILY
Centre Hospitalier,
Univ de Grenoble
B.P. 217
FR 38043 Grenoble cedex 09
Phone: +33 76 76 54 58
Fax: +33 76 76 56 02

Prof. S. ANDO
Universita degli Studi
delle Calabria
Centro Sanitario
IT 87030 Arcavata di Rende
Phone: +39 984 839 624
Fax: +39 984 493 160

THE PHARMACOLOGICAL AND SOCIOCULTURAL RESPONSE TO ASTHMA IN CHILDREN: A HEALTH PROMOTION CONCERTED ACTION PROJECT

Key words
Asthma, childhood asthma, health promotion, therapy, prevention.

Brief description
Research teams from five EC countries will participate in the proposed project on the pharmacological, educational and sociocultural responses to childhood asthma.
Their objectives will be to:
1 identify cultural similarities and differences in responses to childhood asthma in the EC;
2 evaluate the pharmacological treatment of childhood asthma and its medication within children's sociocultural context;
3 evaluate asthma health promotion among children, five to ten years of age, and their families;
4 investigate the pharmacological and sociocultural responses to treating childhood asthma among minorities and/or recent immigrants to EC countries.

In each participating research team, the study population will consist of three groups of fifty asthmatic children and their families (in each group):
1 health promotion intervention group;
2 matched control group (for age, gender, educational level of parents, and residence: e.g., high/low pollution areas);
3 high risk group according to sociocultural and environmental variables related to their minority and/or immigrant status.

The project will include four stages:
1 pilot study;
2 collection of retrospective data from all study groups (socio-economic, biomedical, etc);
3 implemention of the health promotion intervention;
4 evaluation of results (e.g., comparisons between intervention and control groups, and between totals.

The results will be presented at the project level in comparative publications including a consensus report regarding the pharmacological, educational and sociocultural management of childhood asthma. At the local levels, culturally specific health promotion packages will be produced for use among asthmatic children and their families by doctors and other health professionals involved in the management of childhood asthma.

Project leader:
Dr. Deanna TRAKAS
Institute of Child Health, Aghia Sophia Children's Hospital
GR 11527 Goudi, Athens
Phone: +30 17 701557
Fax: +30 17 700111
Contract number: CT941399

Participants:
Dr. Chrysoula BOTSI
Institute of Child Health,
Aghia Sophia Children's Hospital
GR 15527 Goudi - Athens
Phone: +30 1 7701 557
Fax: +30 1 7700 111

Dr. Emilio J. SANZ
Dept. of Pharmacology,
Faculty of Medicine,
University of La Laguna
ES 38971 La Laguna
Phone: +34 22 603 477
Fax: +30 22 655 995

Dr. Tuula VASKILAMPI
Dept. of Community Health and
General Practice, University of Kyopio
PO Box 1921
FI 70210 Kyopio
Phone: +358 71 162 988
Fax: +358 71 162 937

Dr. Rolf WIRSING
Fachbereich Sozialwezen,
Hochschule fur Technik und Wirtschaft
Zittall/Gorlitz
Goethestrasse 5
DE 08900 Gorlitz
Fax: +49 3581 406344

Pia HAUDRUP CHRISTENSEN
DSHSD, Dept. of Human Sciences,
Brunel: The University of West London
UK Uxbridge UB8 3PH Middlesex
Phone: +44 895 27 4000

Dr. Alan PROUT
Dept. of Sociology and Social Anthropology,
Centre for Medical School,
Keel University
UK Keele - Staffordshire
Phone: +44 782 583 364
Fax: +44 782 613 847

Dr. Else-Lydia TOVERUD
Section of Social Pharmacy,
Institute of Pharmacy
PG 1068 University of Oslo
NO 0316 Blindern

Dr. Zolton RONAI
Dept. of Paediatric Pulmonology,
Hospital for Chest Diseases
Phone: +82 377055
Fax: +82 377029

Dr. Milan KRISKA
Dept. of Pharmacology,
Faculty of Medicine,
Commenius University
Sasinkove 4
SK 81108 Bratislava

Dr. Piotr GUTKOWSKY
Lung Function Unit, Child's Health Center,
Memorial Hospital
Al Dzeici Polskich 20
PL 04736 Warszawa-Miedzylesie
Phone: +48 22 151 703
Fax: +48 22 151 703

Dr. Patricia J. BUSH
Children's Health Promotion, 415 Kober Cogan
Building, Georgetown University
School of Medicine
3750 Reservoir Road NW
US Washington DC 20007

PROVISION OF PRIMARY HEALTH CARE FOR THE PROMOTION OF CHILDREN'S EARLY PSYCHOSOCIAL DEVELOPMENT

Key words
Primary care, child health, psychosocial development, health services research.

Brief description
The objective of the project is the provision of primary health care for the promotion of children's early psychosocial development.
In this project a multilevel approach is designed concerning the following:
A   training of Primary Health Care Workers (PHCWs);
B   the holding, by PHCWs, of three semi-structured interviews with mothers at three stages from pregnancy up to 3 months, from 3 to 12 months, and from 12 to 24 months of the child's life.

The programme includes an evaluation component regarding the skills gained by the PHCWs and the benefits to the mothers and their children.
The program was launched by the WHO, Regional Office for Europe, Division of Mental Health and is being developed and applied in Greece, England, Portugal and Turkey (as a COST Country).
The innovative aspects of the present project are: it is thoroughly preventive action, implemented within existing primary Health Care Services, and it does not depend upon additional resources, it is being cost effective. A basic element of this project is the use of a problem solving approach encouraging families to draw on their own resources.

Project leader:
Professor John TSIANTIS
Aghia Sophia Children's
Hospital, Dept. of
Psychological Paediatrics
Thivon and Mikras Asias
GR 11527 Athens
Phone: +30 17 798748
Fax: +30 17 797649
Contract number: CT941161

Participants:
Dr. Thalia DRAGONAS
Dept. of Pre-school
Education,
33 Hippocrates Str.
GR 10680 Athens
Phone: +30 1 3617922
Fax: +30 1 8084875

Prof. H. MCGURK
Thomas Coram Research
Unit, Institute of Education
27-28 Woburn Sq.
UK London WC1 HOAA
Phone: +44 71 6126957
Fax: +44 71 6126927

Dr. Nese EROL
United Medical and Dental
Schools of Guy's and St.
Thomas' Hospital,
Bloomfield Clinic,
Guy's Hospital
UK London SE1 9RT
Phone: +44 71 9554697
Fax: +44 71 9554898

Dr. Pedro CALDEIRA
Departtamento de
Pedopsiquiatria e Saude,
Mental Infantil e
Juvenil do Hospital
de D. Estefania
PT Lisbon
Phone: +351 1 653544

Dr. Veronica ISPANOVIC
Institute for Mental Health
37 Palmoticeva
SI 11000 Belgrade
Phone: +38 11 334 610
Fax: +38 11 331 333

Dr. Anica COS
Svetovalni Center
Gotska
SI 61000 Ljublajana
Phone: +38 61 575 195

Prof. A. Cox
Dept. of Child Psychiatry,
School of Medicine,
Ankara University
TR Ankara
Phone: +90 4 4671998

EUROPEAN BLADDER DYSFUNCTION STUDY IN CHILDREN: A CONTROLLED PROSPECTIVE THERAPEUTIC TRIAL AND EPIDEMIOLOGICAL SURVEY

Key words
Bladder disfunction, clinical trial, urge syndrome, urinary tract infection, reflux nephropathy, urodynamics.

Brief description
The complex of bladder/sphincter dysfunction and recurrent urinary tract infections is common in school-age children, especially in girls. Both parts of the complex cause considerable morbidity, from incontinence and infections, from toddler-age to adolescence. The prevalence in children with this complex of reflux nephropathy is high, and does not correlate with the grade of vesicoureteral reflux. World wide, reflux nephropathy accounts for 20% of all cases of end-stage kidney failure under age 16, and is a well known cause for hypertension.
Pediatric urodynamics revealed the pathophysiology behind the signs of bladder/sphincter dysfunction, which can be classified now in two main categories: urge syndrome, with idiopathic detrusor instability, and dysfunctional voiding, with detrusor-sphincter dyscoordination. Pediatric urodynamics also provided a very effective therapy: cognitive bladder rehabilitation, with the actual voiding as bio-feedback. The reported succes rate of this approach to bladder/sphincter dysfunction in neurologically normal children is as high as 60%: incontinence is cured, urinary infections do not recur anymore, and the vesicoureteral reflux regains its normal resolution rate.
In retrospect, this approach has so many potential benefits economically and socially that a prospective randomized trial is justified. To obtain a sufficient number of patients, and to rule out personal practice as a key factor to succes, a multi-center trial is mandatory. The office of the International Reflux Study in Children (Essen, Germany), with 12 years of experience in a multi-center study in the fields of urinary infection and reflux, provides the centralized facility for the proposed project, including data acquisition, statistical analysis and coordination. Full urologic coverage will be given to the project by two centres with an internationally accepted reference function in the field of pediatric urodynamics: Aarhus (Denmark) and Utrecht (The Netherlands).
Apart from the clinical trial, the project aims to standardize definitions and terminology for bladder sphincter dysfunction in children, to be approved by the International Continence Society. This will help to shorten the time children with bladder sphincter dysfunction spend in medical channels, and prevent unnecessary morbidity.

Project leader:
Dr. M.D. VAN GOOL
Pediatric Renal Centre,
University Children's Hospital,
Het Wilhelmina Kinderziekenhuis
P.O. Box 18009
NL 3501 CA Utrecht
Phone: +31 30 32 09 11
Fax: +31 30 33 48 25
Contract number: CT941006

Participants:

Dr. M.D. DE GROOT
Pediatric Renal Centre,
University Children's Hospital,
Het Wilhelmina Kinderziekenhuis
P.O. Box 18009
NL 3501 CA Utrecht
Phone: +31 30 32 09 11
Fax: +31 30 33 48 25

Dr. T.P.V.M. DE JONG
Dept. Pediatric Nephrology
and Pediatric Urology,
Pediatric Renal Center,
University Children's Hospital
NL 3501 CA Utrecht

Prof. H. OLBING & prof. H. RUBBEN
Dept. Pediatrics,
University Children's Hospital
DE 4300 Essen 1

Dr. J. DJURHUUS, dr. T.M. JORGENSEN,
dr. E. NATHAN
Departments Urology and Pediatrics,
Institute of Experimental Clinical Research,
University of Aarhus, Skejby Hospital
DK 8200 Aarhus N

Dr. R. WALCH & dr. R. VETTER
Departments of Pediatrics and Urology,
Kinderklinik der Medizinische Akademie
DE 5080 Erfurt

Prof. J. MISSELWITZ
Dept. Pediatrics, Universitäts-Kinderklinik
'Jussuf Ibrahim'
DE 6900 Jena

Dr. R. BEETZ & dr. S. MULLER
Departments Pediatrics and Urology,
Universitäts-Kinderklinik
DE 6500 Mainz

Dr. O. KOSKIMIES & dr. S. WIKSTROM
Departments Pediatric Nephrology and Urology
(Pediatric Surgery), Children's Hospital,
University of Helsinki
FI 00290 Helsinki 29

Dr. J. SEPPANEN & dr. N.P. HUTTUNEN
Departments Pediatrics and Urology (Pediatric
Surgery), Oulun Yliopistollinen Keskussairaala,
University of Oulu
FI 90220 Oulu 22

Prof. K. HJALMAS & prof. U. JODAL
Departments Pediatric Nephrology and Pediatric
Urology, Ostra Sjukhuset, University of
Göteborg
SE 41685 Göteborg

Prof. A. APERIA & dr. K. TULLUS
Pediatric Nephrology, Pediatric Urology
SE 11281 Stockholm

Area III

HUMAN GENOME ANALYSIS

III. HUMAN GENOME ANALYSIS

Introduction

The world-wide design and coordination of genome projects has existed since the mid 80's. Particularly the ambitious "Human Genome Project", and its impact on mankind and specifically the expected medical benefits were a major dimension of this endeavour. This debate on "Big Science" since its start has received great public attention. Fears and anxieties about misuse of the new knowledge have existed since the beginning, along with new hopes, especially for people suffering from diseases where no cure is yet available. These arguments and initiatives were taken up by scientists and politicians in Europe, and eventually led to the European Commission being charged with developing a separate "Human Genome Analysis Programme" (HGAP) under the Second Framework Programme to be implemented during the years 1990 to 1992.

During a preparatory phase of two years an "Ad Hoc Working Party on Human Genome Research" was established, which itself set up six study groups on (1) genetic (linkage) mapping, (2) physical mapping, including ordered clone libraries, (3) data handling and databases, (4) advanced genetic technologies, (5) training, and (6) ethical, social and legal aspects. This eventually materialized in the first programme, which was then adopted on 29 June 1990 with a budget allocation of 15 million ECU. Compared to the medical and health research programme, where most projects are concerted actions, the Human Genome Analysis Programme should be implemented through shared-cost projects, i.e. financial contribution to research rather than coordinated through concerted actions. This was an important decision since one of the main objectives of this programme was to set up an infrastructure and make resources available to allow for a substantial European contribution to human genome research. A "Research evaluation - Report N° 59" on this first programme was recently published by the European Commission (EUR 15706 EN).

One of the four research areas of the ongoing BIOMED I programme is related to human genome analysis. This "Area III" is the successor to the first "Human Genome Analysis Programme". A budget of 25 million ECU are spent for activities in the field of human genome analysis, which now emphasizes closer coordination in areas such as (1) the integration of physical and genetic linkage maps, (2) mapping cDNAs on YACs and cosmids in view of better understanding of diseases, their development and possible treatment, and (3) improvement of data handling and analysis. A total of 41 projects focusing on fundamental research are now being supported by this programme area:

Area III.1 Genetic (linkage) mapping,
  III.2 Physical mapping,
  III.3 DNA sequencing,
  III.4 Handling of genetic data and databases,
  III.5 Technology development and applications of human genome analysis.

In the mid-term evaluation report of this programme it is stated, that "the European Commission activity in human genome analysis is a driving force in the field of European human genome research". In addition to national programmes like those in France or United Kingdom the Commission initiative furthers "European collaboration and allows smaller research units a transfer of knowledge and access to sophisticated technologies".

Dr. Manuel Hallen

EUROGEM: THE EUROPEAN HUMAN GENETIC LINKAGE MAPPING PROJECT

Key words
High resolution map, resource centres, genetic map, physical map, transcriptional map.

Brief description
The aim of the EUROGEM project is to provide high resolution maps of all the human chromosomes. These maps and the resources used in their construction will form the basis for future human genetics projects aimed at locating and isolating specific disease causing genes. This project will be of long term benefit to all workers in the field of human genetics wishing to locate the region in which a specific defective gene may lie, and will help speed the process of the final identification of the gene and the mutations responsible for the disease phenotype.

The project has two resource centres, one providing DNA from forty of the CEPH families for use in genotyping and the other providing other resources, for example markers for genetic and physical mapping. The mapping is carried out by a selection of 23 Network laboratories based throughout the European Union. These laboratories are all linked by a computer network and data transfer and analysis is conducted using this electronic system.

The Network laboratories are expected to participate in the work plan and to share their data freely. The outcome of this project will be the publication of detailed genetic, physical and transcriptional maps of each human chromosome.

Project leader:
Dr. N.K. SPURR
Human Genetic Resources,
Imperial Cancer Research Fund,
Clare Hall Laboratories
Blanche Lane
South Mimms
Potters Bar
UK Herts EN6 3LD
Phone: +44 71 269 3846
Fax: +44 71 269 3802
Contract number: CT930101

Participants:
Dr. S. ADAMS
University of Leicester
UK Leicester

Dr. E. BAKKER
Leiden University
NL Leiden

Dr. J. BECKMANN
CEPH
FR Paris

Prof. Dr. C.H.C.M. BUYS
University of Groningen
NL Groningen

Dr. H. CANN
CEPH
FR Paris

Prof. J.J. CONTU
University of Cagliari
IT Cagliari

Dr. M. DIXON
University of Manchester
UK Manchester

Dr. X. ESTIVILL
Hospital Duran i Reynals
PT Barcelona

Prof. M.A. FERGUSON-SMITH
University of Cambridge
UK Cambridge

Prof. Dr. K.H. GRZESCHIK
University of Marburg
DE Marburg

Prof. I. HANSMANN
Institut für Humangenetik
DE Göttingen

Dr. T.A. KRUSE
Aarhus University
DK Aarhus

Dr T. McCARTHY
University College Cork
IE Cork

Dr. F. MORENO
Hospital Ramon y Cajal
ES Madrid

Dr. N. MOSCHONAS
IMBB
GR Heraklion

Dr. M.S. POVEY
University College London
UK London

Dr. G. ROIZES
CRBM du CNRS
FR Montpellier

Prof. L. TERRENATO
University of Rome
IT Rome

Dr. G. VERGNAUD
Labratoire de Génétique de Espèces
FR Nantes

Dr. J. WEISSENBACH
Généthon
FR Evry

Prof. R. WILLIAMSON
St. Mary's Hospital Medical School
UK London

Dr. A. WRIGHT
MRC Human Genetics Unit
UK Edinburgh

RESOURCE CENTRE 1 FOR THE EUROPEAN HUMAN GENETIC LINKAGE MAPPING PROJECT (EUROGEM)

Key words

Human genetic map, microsatellites, CEPH reference families.

Brief description

This project is in fact the obvious continuation of the EUROGEM work performed from March 1991 to July 1993. Its first objective is to establish a Human Genetic Map with informative markers spaced every 5 cM. Its aim is clearly to offer to the scientific community a new precise tool useful for all studies of gene disease localisations. This *innovative* project created the first European network of scientific laboratories, approved the establishment of resource centres and the organisation by a coordinator. Obviously, all participants wanted to take advantage of the most informative markers available to be the most efficient, i.e. the nearest markers on the map.

VNTR (variable number tandem repeat), microsatellites, (CA)n repeats, cosmids, genomic or cDNA cloned probes revealing RFLPS were both tested. The CEPH, as resource centre 1, supplied all participants with DNA for PCR-typing of the 40 large reference families and more than 5500 filters of digested DNAs for RFLP analysis. In July 1992, mid-way in the project, more than 300 new markers had already been tested. At the same time, a new generation of highly polymorphic markers, i.e. microsatellites with more than 70% heterozygosity, was appearing. They are abundant and ubiquitous throughout the genome and so could be exploited for genetic mapping if they are assayed by PCR (Polymerase Chain Reaction). Already genotyped on 8 reference families, they offer the opportunity to reach a high resolution Human Genetic Linkage Map with markers spaced every 1 to 2 cM. EUROGEM, even before the results of its first session were completed, could plan to perform these essential studies with more than 3000 microsatellites on the reference extended pedigrees. This will basically be organised as for the first session, with CEPH as resource centre for DNA and ICRF for markers.

Project leader:
Professor D. COHEN
C.E.P.H.B., I.G.M. Institut de Génétique Moléculaire
27 Rue Juliette Dodu
FR 75010 Paris
Phone: +33 1 42 49 98 50
Fax: +33 1 42 06 16 19
Contract number: CT930078

RESOURCE CENTRE 2 FOR THE EUROPEAN HUMAN GENETIC LINKAGE MAPPING PROJECT (EUROGEM)

Key words
Genetic linkage mapping, genetic markers, microsatellites.

Brief description
This centre will provide DNA markers and the necessary expertise to build high resolution genetic linkage maps of each chromosome. The aim will be to extend the work started in the first round of the project. The Resource Centre will supply PCR formatted DNA markers of high heterozygosity to each of the Network laboratories to genotype. These markers will form the framework of the genetic maps. Up to 1500 marker equivalents will be supplied in 24 months for genotyping by the Network laboratories. They will consist of markers obtained from the Genethon project, markers published in the literature, as well as a range of tri-tetra nucleotide repeat markers isolated by the resource centre. Many of these will be targeted to fill gaps which exist in the current maps. Also, to help enhance the existing maps, PCR markers detecting variations within, or close to known genes will be distributed. This will help us to create landmarks on the maps and they will be important resources for the future integration of these markers into the physical maps and for screening on the YAC and cosmid libraries.

As well as supplying and distributing markers we also aim to assist with the necessary computing problems associated with map building. We will offer a service to the Network laboratories to help with database and networking problems and to collaborate in the construction of the multi-point linkage maps of each chromosome. We will also extend this analysis to produce meiotic breakpoint maps of each chromosome. These will be of enormous value for the future of genetic mapping and will reduce the number of samples to be genotyped on each chromosome and should speed the process of assigning markers to specific chromosome intervals. Another important by-product of this work will be the ability to define a set of markers suitable for use in genome searching for linkage to a particular disease.

We also aim to offer a number of training opportunities for scientists and technicians from the Network laboratories. Training in laboratory techniques and also in the use of computer software for the construction of the multi-point linkage maps and the databases for the genotyping data will be given.

Project leader:
Dr. N.K. SPURR
Imperial Cancer Research Fund,
Human Genetic Resources,
Clare Hall Laboratories
Blanche Lane
South Mimms
Potters Bar
UK Herts EN6 3LD
Phone: +44 71 269 3846
Fax: +44 71 269 3802
Contract number: CT930077

RESOURCE CONSORTIA FOR cDNA LIBRARIES
FOR PHYSICAL MAPPING

Key words
cDNA, cDNA libraries, partial cDNA sequencing, est, ests, subtractive libraries, subtractive cloning, partial sequence tags.

Brief description
The present cDNA consortia, supported by the European Commission (EC), has successfully developed a number of libraries and improved the technology for generating cDNA fragments. The substantial data generated by the consortia has been placed in publicly accessible databases. Wide use is now being made of this information for gene identification purposes and the physical mapping programmes.

With EC support we have recently instituted a series of small grants to test a number of novel methods for adding both physical and biological value to the cDNA fragments generated under the programme. High density grids of large numbers of cDNA fragments are now being made available to the physical mapping community in Europe and some worldwide centres. In addition to generating additional cDNA fragments, greater emphasis will now be placed on improving the technology, making high density gridded libraries available to a wider mapping community and adding biological value to the cDNA fragments. Data generated from the libraries is fed back to a database that can be accessed by anyone wishing to use the data so that it can be analyzed and comparison made between the various libraries. The precise nature of the proposed studies on the biological value of the fragments will need to be determined when the results of the first round of small grant projects is completed later.

The success of the present EC sponsored cDNA consortia has led to a greater collaboration within the physical mapping community. We plan to meet as a consortia at least twice a year, one meeting just with consortia members to plan the evolving strategy, and another with the wider community involved in cDNA studies.

Project leader:
Dr. K.I. GIBSON
HGMP Resource Centre
Clinical Research Centre
Watford Road
UK Harrow HA1 3UJ
Phone: +44 81 869 3446
Fax: +44 81 869 3807
Contract number: CT930089

Participants:
Professor C. AUFFRAY
Généthon, Centre de Recherche sur le Génome Humain
Rue de l'Internationale 1
FR 91002 Evry Cedex
Phone: +33 1 69 47 28 00
Fax: +33 1 60 77 86 98

Professor H. DOMDEY
Ludwig-Maximilians-
Universität München
Laboratorium für Molekulare
Biologie, Genzentrum
Am Klopferspitz 18A
DE 82152 Martinsried
Phone: +49 89 85 78 39 92
Fax: +49 89 85 78 37 95

Dr. H. LEHRACH
Imperial Cancer
Research Fund
44 Lincoln's Inn Fields
UK London WC2A 3PX
Phone: +44 71 269 33 08
Fax: +44 71 269 30 68

Prof. G. TOCCHINI-
VALENTINI
Istituto di Biologia Cellolare
Viale Marx 43
IT 00137 Roma
Phone: +39 6 827 46 42
Fax: +39 6 827 32 87

MAINTENANCE AND EXPANSION OF THE CENTRALIZED FACILITY ON COSMID LIBRARIES FOR A EUROPEAN CONSORTIUM ON ORDERED CLONE LIBRARIES

Key words
Cosmid libraries.

Brief description
The maintenance and expansion of the existing centralised facility is proposed to give access to uniform, well characterised and documented cosmid library material enabling researchers to accelerate their genome research. The expansion includes: the construction of two additional single human chromosome cosmid reference libraries, the preparation and expansion of use of four more human chromosome reference cosmid libraries constructed during the last year, the construction of a gridded NotI linking clone library covering the whole genome, the ability to satisfy requests for screening membranes and positive cosmid clones for 10 (ten) different human chromosome libraries, the upgrading of the density of storage and spotting of clones as well as the expansion of the central database.

The facility has been successfully running for several years. For the last two years it had been partly funded by the European Commission (EC) and this covered the construction of cosmid libraries for the human chromosomes 11 and 17 and the distribution of high density membranes and clones for these two as well as chromosomes X and 21. The objectives of the previous project have been achieved and in addition four new cosmid libraries have been constructed for human chromosomes 6, 13, 18 and 22, and the start of the successful use of the chromosome 13 and 22 libraries as reference libraries has been demonstrated. Here we propose to construct new human chromosome cosmid reference libraries for the chromosomes 1 and 7, and to bring to full reference library stage the chromosome 6, 13, 18 and 22 libraries. We further propose to act as the central cosmid reference facility for the EC for ten human chromosomes (1, 6, 7, 11, 13, 17, 18, 21, 22 and X) and provide the users within the EC with at least 100 library membrane sets per year as well as up to 3,000 positive cosmids per year. These are total numbers taking all chromosomes together.

Project leader:
Dr. H. LEHRACH
Genome Analysis Laboratory
Imperial Cancer
Research Fund
44 Lincolns Inn Fields
UK London WC2A 3PX
Phone: +44 71 269 3308
Fax: +44 71 269 3068
Contract number: CT930062

Participants:
Dr. A. POUSTKA
Deutsches Krebs-
forschungszentrum
Angewandte Tumorvirologie
Im Neuenheimer Feld, 596
DE 69120 Heidelberg
Phone: +49 6221 42 34 09
Fax: +49 6221 47 03 33

Dr. D. NIZETIC
University of London
School of Pharmacy
28-29 Brunswick Square
UK London WC1N 1AX
Phone: +44 71 753 58 00
Fax: +44 71 278 06 22

SCREENING AND DISTRIBUTION OF YAC LIBRARIES

Key words
YAC, Human Genome.

Brief description
C.E.P.H. offers its whole YAC library for screening at Pavia, Harrow and Leiden, including the new MegaYAC library. This new library, because of its very big insert size (megabase range), will greatly improve the physical mapping efforts of laboratories in the European Union and the characterisation of new genes implicated in hereditary diseases. YAC clones will be sent by the aforementioned screening centres to the EC applicants for further study. The achievement and target of this project can be easily monitored in terms of probes tested and number of clones characterised.

Past experience indicates that well over 1,000 screenings will be performed for other laboratories during the course of the project.

Project leader:
Professor D. COHEN
C.E.P.H.B.
I.G.M. Institut de Génétique Moléculaire
27 Rue Juliette Dodu
FR 75010 Paris
Phone: +33 1 42 49 98 50
Fax: +33 1 42 06 16 19
Contract number: CT930005

PROVISION OF A EUROPEAN YAC RESOURCE THROUGH A COORDINATED CONSORTIUM

Key words
YACs, YAC library, YAC screening, PCR screening, hybridisation screening, library screening, mega YACs, mega YAC library.

Brief description
The coordinated consortium is made up of groups who are already sponsored by the European Commission (EC) for individually providing such a service, plus additional members whose skills will enhance the range of possible options. Providing a YAC screening source in this way will allow for greater interchange between groups providing the resource. This in turn will ensure the best methods are being used in the most effective places, that data is pooled and widely disseminated, and that fluctuations in levels of demand can be accommodated by sharing screenings and facilities.

All four major YAC libraries (CEPH megayac, ICI, ICRF and St. Louis) plus some chromosome specific libraries (1p, 17, 19q, Xp), prepared by the Dutch group, will be made available for screening. Screening can be by PCR or by hybridisation to high density grids. Grids will be provided as large or small arrays. PCR will be performed at the resource centres or in users' own laboratories using pools provided by the resource centres. Hybridisation screening will also be performed in one of the resource centres using probes supplied by users. Opportunity will be provided for users to work to a limited extent in the resource centres, to perform activities which are too specialised to be offered as a general service or are applications of isolated YACs.

Data will be collected centrally, placed into the ICRF reference library database and made available publicly on-line. Users will be able to request clones that have been previously characterised. Data will be used to construct a physical map which will be used to complement other genome maps and will also be made publicly available.

Project leader:
Dr. K.I. GIBSON
HGMP Resource Centre
Clinical Research Centre
Watford Road
UK Harrow, Middlesex HA1 3UJ
Phone: +44 81 869 3446
Fax: +44 81 869 3807
Contract number: CT930088

Participants:
Dr. H. LEHRACH
Imperial Cancer Research Fund
Lincoln's Inn Fields 44
UK London WC2A 3PX
Phone: +44 71 269 33 08
Fax: +44 71 269 30 68

Dr. D. TONIOLO
Istituto di Genetica Biochemica
ed Evoluzionistica
Via Abbiategrasso, 207
IT 27100 Pavia
Phone: +39 3 82 54 63 40
Fax: +39 3 82 42 22 86

Professor G.J. VAN OMMEN
Department of Human Genetics
Sylvius Laboratory
State University Leiden
Wassenaarseweg 72
NL 1015 LW Leiden
Phone: +31 71 27 60 65
Fax: +31 71 27 60 75

CONSTRUCTION OF A HIGH RESOLUTION MAP OF CHROMOSOME 21 INTEGRATING GENETIC, PHYSICAL, OVERLAP AND TRANSCRIPTIONAL DATA

Key words
Chromosome 21, high resolution map.

Brief description
The chromosome 21 is serving as a prototype for the European human genome analysis programme. The purpose of the consortium is to reach a level of resolution unprecedented for a chromosome map. This will be possible by using the recent progress made by the preceding CHR21 consortium and the CEPH-Généthon programme and by bringing together 12 participants who have a large experience in CHR21 analysis and who have developed new skills for mapping of genomic DNA and YACs DNA. This should permit a large improvement in:
- the linkage map (one marker every 200 kb with a relation between genetic distances and physical distances)
- the physical map (one marker every 200 kb or less)
- the YACs map (continuum of unrearranged YACs, physically mapped)
- the cosmids map (large contigs with the order of each cosmid)
- the transcriptional map (40 genes only are cloned out of a total of 500-1000)
- the identification of candidate genes such as: gene(s) responsible for the morphological features of DS, the mental retardation, heart defect (DS type), transient leukemia; gene(s) responsible for specific features of monosomy 21; the gene mutated in familial amyotrophic lateral sclerosis, the gene involved in progressive myoclonic epilepsy.

Project leader:
Dr. J.M. DELABAR
CNRS, URA 1335, Hôpital Necker
Rue de Sèvres, 149
FR 75743 Paris   ,
Phone: +33 1 42 73 09 60
Fax: +33 1 42 73 06 59
Contract number: CT930015

Participants:
Dr. X. ESTIVILL
Molecular Genetics Department, Cancer
Research Institut, Hospital Duran i Reynals
Autovia Castelldefels KM 2,7
18907 Hospitalet Llobregat
ES 08907 Barcelona
Phone: +34 3 335 7152
Fax: +34 3 263 2251

Dr. C. BRAHE
Istituto di Genetica Medica
Università Cattoglica Sacro
Cuore Facoltà di Medicina e Chirurgia
Largo F. Vito 1
IT 00178 Roma
Phone: +39 6 30 15 49 27
Fax: +39 6 30 50 031

Dr. E. FISHER
The Imperial College of Science Technology and
Medicine, Department of Biochemistry and
Molecular Genetics
Norfolk Place
UK London W2 1PG
Phone: +44 71 723 12 52
Fax: +44 71 706 32 72

Dr. H. LEHRACH
Imperial Cancer Research Fund
Lincoln's Inn fields 44
UK London WC2A 3PX
Phone: +44 71 269 33 08
Fax: +44 71 269 30 68

Dr. R. OLIVA
Molecular Genetics Research Group,
Faculty of Medicine, University of Barcelona
Calle Diagonal, 643
ES 08028 Barcelona
Phone: +34 3 339 78 85
Fax: +34 3 490 93 46

Dr. D. NIZETIC
Istituto Nazionale per la Ricerca Sol Cancro
Via Benedetto XV 10
IT 16132 Genova
Phone: +39 1 03 53 41
Fax: +39 1 03 52 999

Dr. M.B. PETERSEN
The John F. Kennedy Institute,
Department of Medical Genetics
Gl. Landevej, 7
DK 2600 Glostrup
Phone: +45 42 45 22 28
Fax: +45 43 43 11 30

Dr. G. ROIZÈS
UPR 9008 CRBM, Institut de Biologie
Bd Henri IV
FR 34060 Montpellier Cedex
Phone: +33 67 66 35 54
Fax: +33 67 60 94 78

Dr. C. VAN BROECKHOVEN
Laboratory Neurogenetica,
Department Biochemie
Universiteitsplein, 1
BE 2610 Antwerpen
Phone: +32 3 820 26 01
Fax: +32 3 820 25 41

Professor S.E. ANTONARAKIS
Centre Médical Universitaire,
Division de Génétique Médicale
Avenue de Champel, 9
CH 1211 Geneve 4
Phone: +41 22 702 57 08
Fax: +41 22 702 57 06

Dr. M.C. POTIER
Institut Alfred Fessard,
Centre National de la Recherche Scientifique
FR 91198 Gif-sur-Yvette
Phone: +33 1 69 82 34 40
Fax: +33 1 69 82 43 43

CONSTRUCTION OF A PHYSICAL, GENETIC AND TRANSCRIPT MAP OF HUMAN Xq21.1-q21.3

Key words
Human, Xq21, physical map, genetic map, transcript map.

Brief description
An integrated physical, genetic and transcript map will be constructed for the Xq21.1-Xq21.3 region on the long arm of the human X chromosome. This region encompasses approximately 15-20 megabases (Mb) of the physical length of the X chromosome. The physical map will be constructed with Yeast artificial chromosome (YAC) contigs isolated using over 30 DNA probes and genes located in the Xq21.1-Xq21.3 region and 33 STSs defining the X/Y homology region. The ICRF and other human YAC libraries will be screened by both hybridisation and PCR and bidirectional chromosome walks will be used to fill in the gaps. YACs will be tested by FISH on normal chromosomes for chimeric inserts and on a subset of cell-lines derived from female patients with X; autosome translocations and males with deletions breaking in this region to define the physical relationship of YACs to the breakpoints. All genes, DNA Probes, STSs, YAC end-probes, and new microsatellite markers generated in this project will be tested by PCR analysis or hybridisation on a series of 9 translocation hybrid cell-lines derived from females with X; autosome translocations, and 17 lymphoblastoid cell-lines from males with deletions and duplications that break the Xq21 region into 19 intervals. To develop new genetic markers in this region, YACs will be either hybridised to the ICRF human X chromosome cosmid grids or subcloned into cosmid and smaller insert sublibraries and short tandem repeat polymorphisms (microsatellites) will be isolated and tested in standard CEPH pedigrees. The transcript map of the region will be constructed using cosmid contigs generated from the YAC clones in each contig. Genes will be identified mostly using 1) Exon amplification of cosmids and 2) cDNA selection procedures using hybridisation of PCR amplified cDNA library inserts to pooled biotinylated cosmid DNA. Transcribed sequences isolated from the region will be further analyzed for tissue distribution of expression and related to several disease loci mapping in deletion intervals in this region (X-linked deafness, mental retardation and clef lip and palate).

Project leader:
Dr. A.P. MONACO
Imperial Cancer Research Fund, Human Genetics Laboratory,
Institute of Molecular Medicine,
John Radcliffe Hospital
UK Oxford PX3 PDU
Phone: +44 865 222371
Fax: +44 865 222431
Contract number: CT930022

Participants:
Professor H.H. ROPERS
Department of Human Genetics
University Hospital
P.O. Box 9101
NL 6500 HB Nijmegen
Phone: +31 80 61 40 17
Fax: +31 80 54 04 88

Professor G.S. GERMAINE
Laboratoire de Génétique
Avenue de Bourgogne
FR 54511 Vandoeuvre les Nancy Cedex
Phone: +33 83 44 62 62
Fax: +33 83 44 60 46

PHYSICAL, GENETIC AND FUNCTIONAL MAP OF Xp22 (AND APPLICATION TO IDENTIFICATION OF DISEASE GENES)

Key words
Human, Xp22, physical map, genetic map, functional map, disease genes.

Brief description
The objective of this project is to provide an integrated physical, genetic and functional map of a large region of the human X chromosome, which corresponds roughly to the Xp22 band (15 to 20 Mb). At present, there is very little physical map information: no YAC contigs or PFGE maps have been reported, few chromosomal breakpoints were available for ordering markers until very recently. Partial genetic maps have been published, but they have a low density and all available markers have not been integrated in a single genetic map. Although general mapping efforts, as developed in GENETHON, are likely to provide, within the next two years, YAC contigs and genetic maps over the whole genome, these maps will not have the precision, completeness and validation that are needed to identify disease genes or as a prerequisite for sequencing regions of interest.

Our goal is to provide complete coverage in validated YAC contigs of the region, to map its CpG islands and estimate gene density, and to identify expressed genes in regions of special interest. A high density genetic map will be constructed and the polymorphic markers integrated in the YAC contig map. A common database format will be used that will allow efficient integration of the results generated by the collaboration in public databases. This study includes some more specific aims of biological and medical interest. The analysis of inactivation status of genes in the Xp22.3 region will determine whether genes that escape inactivation are clustered and show a clear boundary with genes that are subject to X inactivation, or whether there is interspersion of the two types of genes. Members of the collaboration have important patients and family material that should allow precise mapping and identification of several disease genes which notably include: retinoschisis (an important cause of severe visual impairment), Coffin-Lowry syndrome (a pleiotropic disorder with mental retardation and severe skeletal deformations), x-linked hypophosphataemic rickets (a defect in the control of phosphate metabolism and the most common form of vitamin-D resistant rickets) and a gene implicated in sex determination, the function of which appears uniquely sensitive of dosage.

Project leader:
Professor J.L. MANDEL
U184/INSERM, LGME du CNRS,
Institut de Chimie Biologique,
Faculté de Médecine
11 Rue Humann
FR 67085 Strasbourg Cedex
Phone: +33 88 37 12 55
Fax: +33 88 37 01 90
Contract number: CT930027

Participants:

Professor J. O'RIORDAN
University College, The Middlesex Hospital
Mortimer Street
UK London W1N 8AA
Phone: +44 71 380 93 73
Fax: +44 71 636 31 51

Dr. G. CAMERINO
Dipartimento di Patologia Umana ed Ereditaria
Sezione di Biologia Generale e Genetica Medica
Via Forlanini, 14
IT 27100 Pavia
Phone: +39 3 82 39 25 19
Fax: +39 3 82 52 50 30

Professor J. HOUGHTON
Cytogenetics Unit, Department of Microbiology
University College Galway
University Road
IE Galway
Phone: +353 9 15 03 84
Fax: +353 9 12 57 00

Dr. H. LEHRACH
Imperial Cancer Research Fund
Lincoln's Inn Fields, 44
UK London WC2A 3PX
Phone: +44 71 269 33 08
Fax: +44 71 269 30 68

Dr. C. PETIT
Institut Pasteur, Unité de Génétique
Moléculaire Humaine, CNRS URA 1445
Rue du Docteur Roux, 25
FR 75015 Paris
Phone: +33 1 45 68 88 50
Fax: +33 1 45 68 87 90

Dr. C. FARR
University of Cambridge, Dept of Genetics
Downing Street
UK Cambridge CB2 3EH
Phone: +44 223 33 39 99
Fax : +44 223 33 39 92

PHYSICAL MAPPING OF THE LONG ARM OF CHROMOSOME 10q24-q26. A RESOURCE TO IDENTIFY GENES INVOLVED IN MALIGNANCY AND IN DISEASE SUSCEPTIBILITY

Key words
Chromosome 10, genetic and physical mapping.

Brief description
This project aims to construct a detailed physical and transcriptional map of the region q24-q26 on the long arm of chromosome 10. Our primary objective is the construction of an overlapping contig of the region based on YACs identified using STSs and DNA probes already localised using other techniques, for example genetic linkage mapping.

The aim of this will be to integrate both genetic and physical map data and to use this as a base for the isolation and mapping of new cDNAs and the preparation of a transcription map of the region. This resource will be of value in the search for genes involved in malignance and disease susceptibility that have been located in this region. A number of lines of evidence indicate that this region contains genes involved in tumour suppression and progression.

For example, allele loss studies have indicated that a tumour suppressor gene involved in prostate cancer maps to the band 10q24. Also mapping to this chromosome band are three cytochrome P450 loci of which mutations in two genes in these loci have been associated with susceptibility to cancer and differences in abilities to metabolise certain classes of drugs. The objectives can be summarised as follows:

1 The construction of an overlapping YAC contig based on PCR formatted STSs.
2 Quality checking of the YAC contig for chimeras and rearrangements.
3 Screening of YACs for tri- and tetra-nucleotide repeats and the development of new markers for genetic mapping.
4 Mapping and ordering of all known markers in this region including the development of a long range restriction map to assist in the identification of CpG islands.
5 Isolation of cDNAs using the YACs and also cosmids cloned from regions close to known CpG islands to construct a transcription map.
6 Detailed mapping of the three cytochrome P450 loci to determine the number of active genes.

This resource would be freely available to those interested in identifying the disease associated genes in this region.

Project leader:
Dr. N.K. SPURR
Human Genetic Resources,
Imperial Cancer
Research Fund,
Clare Hall Laboratories
Blanche Lane
South Mimms, Potters Bar
UK Herts EN6 3LD
Phone: +44 71 269 3846
Fax: +44 71 269 3802
Contract number: CT930032

Participants:
Dr. D.C. MONTEIRO
Department of Genetics
Faculty of Medical Sciences
Rua da Junqueira, 96
PT 1300 Lisbon
Phone: +351 1 364 50 83
Fax: +351 1 362 20 18

Dr. C. NOBILE
Institute di Genetica
Molecolare del CNR
Viale San Pietro 438
IT 07100 Sassari
Phone: +39 7 922 84 64
Fax: +39 7 921 23 45

MAPPING CHROMOSOME 1 WITH TELOMERE BREAKAGE HYBRIDS

Key words
Chromosome 1, cDNA, YACs, contigs, deletion hybrids.

Brief description
As a project of a European research programme we have established the use of cloned telomere to produce single chromosome hybrids containing terminal deletions of the long arm of the X chromosome (TACF, Nature Genetics 2 275). These hybrids are stable, easily propagated and can provide a source of additional mapped markers for the chromosome being deleted.

Rapid progress in genome analysis has resulted in almost complete YAC Contig maps of two small chromosomes, a large fraction of the human genome present in unassigned contigs, a rapidly improving genetic map and many thousands of anonymous cDNA partial sequences. Assembly of this data into an integrated whole is the next stage of the process. For small chromosomes much of this task can be accomplished on YAC contigs of the whole chromosome. In the case of larger chromosomes our technology of chromosome fragmentation, producing a distributable resource of terminally deleted chromosomes, will provide a means of giving a chromosomal order to YAC or cosmid contigs assembled by comparison of their restriction profiles. Southern blots of such hybrid cell panels can also be used to provide map locations for cDNAs without the intricacies of in situ hybridisation or the expense of PCR primer synthesis. Our approach to the creation of hybrids is particularly necessary in the case of chromosome 1 because of a dearth of existing hybrid lines.

In a rodent/human hybrid line we will target +/- selectable markers to the angiotensinogen locus in 1q42-43 and to the G418 gene present on distal chromosome 1p. This will provide counterselectable markers on both arms of the chromosome. Following back selection, broken chromosomes will be rescued and stabilised by the introduction of cloned telomere. The products of breakage will be analyzed by in situ hybridisation to check the chromosomal integrity of each cell line.

In cooperation with Genethon we will select YACs using previously genetically mapped CA repeat sequences and use in situ hybridisation to map them within the panel of deletion hybrids. These YACs, selected to be unrearranged, will then provide anchor and orientation sites for YAC contigs developed by others. Southern blots for panels of hybrids will be made and used for mapping cDNAs to establish the utility of this approach.

Project leader:
Dr. H. COOKE
MRC Human Genetics Unit, Western General Hospital
Crewe Road
UK Edinburgh EH4 2XU
Phone: +44 31 343 2620
Fax: +44 31 332 2471
Contract number: CT930039

Participants:

Dr. C. FARR
University of Cambridge
Department of Genetics
Downing Street
UK Cambridge CB2 3EH
Phone: +44 223 33 39 99
Fax: +44 223 33 39 92

Dr. D. TONIOLO
Istituto di Genetica Bio-
chimica ed Evoluzionistica
Via Abbiategrasso, 207
IT 27100 Pavia
Phone: +39 3 82 54 63 40
Fax: +39 3 82 42 22 86

Dr. C. PETIT
Unité de Génétique
Moléculaire Humaine
Rue du Dr. Roux, 25
FR 75015 Paris
Phone: +33 1 45 68 88 50
Fax: +33 1 45 68 87 90

PHYSICAL MAPPING OF THE SHORT ARM
OF HUMAN CHROMOSOME 16

Key words
Chromosome 16, physical map, transcriptional map, gene, cosmid, YAC, contig.

Brief description
The overall aim of the project is to complete a physical map of the short arm of chromosome 16. The project will allow the extension of ongoing work of the participating laboratories and will also build on, rather than duplicate, the results obtained by other laboratories with whom the groups already collaborate.

The construction of the physical map of 16p divides into three stages. The first is to connect existing contigs of cloned genomic DNA by isolating intervening genomic clones. The second is to construct a detailed physical map of the assembled contigs to allow the identification, and filling in, of any gaps. The third is to identify and map genes on to the physical map generated in the project.

Several simultaneous approaches will be used to achieve the aim. Sequence tagged sites (STSs) from the length of the short arm will be used as multiple nucleation sites to screen human genomic libraries in yeast artificial chromosomes (YACs). Isolated clones will be assembled into contigs by identifying regions of overlap. End clones will be derived from the YACs delimiting each contig and, if necessary, new markers will be isolated from gaps between contigs, to allow further rounds of chromosome walking. Libraries of smaller genomic clones, such as cosmids, will be screened if any regions are unstable as large clones. To avoid duplication of effort, contigs generated as a direct result of the project will be merged with contigs assembled by other laboratories.

Long range restriction mapping will be used to locate CpG islands and hence potential genes. Suitable genomic clones will be used in the systematic screening of cDNA libraries to identify new genes which will then be located on the map. The map generated in this project will be linked to the genetic map using existing genetic markers, and genes which have already been identified will be located on the map.

Four laboratories will be participating in this project. Three will be directly involved in isolating genomic clones and assembling a map of adjacent regions. Two will use their existing expertise to act as resource centres for the project. By combining and coordinating our efforts we will make a substantial contribution to the human genome mapping effort by completing a physical map of the short arm of chromosome 16.

Project leader:
Dr. S.E. MOLE
Department of Paediatrics, The Rayne Institute,
University College London Medical School
University Street
UK London WC1E 6JJ
Phone: +44 71 387 9300 ext. 5059
Fax: +44 71 380 9681
Contract number: CT930040

Participants:

Dr. I. CECCHERINI
Istituto 'Giannina Gaslini'
Laboratory of Molecular
Genetics
Largo Gerolamo Gaslini, 5
IT 16147 Genova
Phone: +39 1 056 36 40
Fax: +39 1 039 12 54

Dr. P. HARRIS
Molecular Haematology Unit
Inst. of Molecular Medicine
University of Oxford
John Radcliffe Hospital
Headington
UK Oxford OX3 9DU
Phone: +44 865 22 23 91
Fax: +44 865 22 25 00

Dr. M.H. BREUNING
Leiden University
Dept of Medical Genetics
P.O. Box 9503
NL 2300 RA Leiden
Phone: +31 71 27 60 48
Fax: +31 71 27 60 75

CONSTRUCTION OF A PHYSICAL, GENETIC AND TRANSCRIPT MAP IN REGION q32-qTER OF HUMAN CHROMOSOME 5 AND RELATION TO A CRANIOSYNOSTOSIS LOCUS

Key words
Chromosome 5 (q32-qter), physical map, genetic map, transcript map, craniosynostosis locus.

Brief description

An integrated physical, genetic and transcript map will be constructed for the distal portion of the long arm of human chromosome 5 (q32-qter). This region encompasses approximately 70 cM or 23% of the genetic length of chromosome 5. The physical map will be constructed with yeast artificial chromosome (YAC) contigs isolated using genes and DNA probes located in the 5q32-qter region including polymorphic markers that have been applied to the construction of the genetic map. The ICRF and other human YAC libraries will be screened by both hybridization and PCR and bidirectional chromosome walks will be used to fill in the gaps. To develop new genetic markers in this region, nonchimeric YACs (determined by FISH) will be subcloned into cosmid and smaller insert sublibraries and short tandem repeat polymorphisms (STRPS or microsatellites) will be isolated. Linkage analysis will be performed in standard CEPH pedigrees and in a large family with autosomal dominant craniosynostosis (skull deformities resulting from abnormal development of the calvarial sutures). The craniosynostosis locus has recently been linked to D5S211 in 5q33.3-qter with a maximum LOD score of Zmax=4.8 at theta=0, with no linkage found with markers 25.2 cM proximal in 5q22-q22.3. The transcript map of the region will be constructed using cosmid contigs generated from the nonchimeric YAC clones in each contig. Genes will be identified using:
1) Exon amplification of cosmids, 2) cDNA selection procedures using hybridization of PCR amplified cDNA library inserts to pooled biotinylated cosmid DNA, 3) CpG island identification and 4) Searching for sequences conserved during evolution. Transcribed sequences isolated ·from the region delimiting the craniosynostosis locus will be further analyzed for tissue distribution of expression and for abnormalities in patients with craniosynostosis.

Project leader:
Professor Dr. U. MÜLLER
Institute of Human Genetics,
Justus-Liebig-Universität Giessen
Schlangenzahl 14
DE 35392 Giessen
Phone: +49 641 702 4145
Fax: +49 641 702 4158
Contract number: CT930050

Participants:
Dr. A.P. MONACO
Imperial Cancer Research Fund,
Human Genetics Laboratory,
Institute of Molecular Medicine
UK Oxford OX3 9DU
Phone: +44 865 22 23 71
Fax: +44 865 22 24 31

CONSTRUCTION OF A BIOLOGICALLY INTEGRATED MAP OF THE HUMAN CHROMOSOME 11 SHORT ARM

Key words
Chromosome 11p, physical map, YAC contig map, cosmid contig map, PFGE map.

Brief description
We propose constructing a physical map of the short arm of human chromosome 11 (11p) that will comprise a YAC contig map of the whole region, a cosmid contig map of a substantial proportion and a PFGE map of selected regions. The work programme will incorporate clones from several major external mapping projects, integrating and expanding these data.

The physical map location of all 67 genes known to map to 11p will be established and a systematic program to identify new genes initiated. Over 100 chromosomal breakpoints have been identified on 11p and the locations of these will be established on the physical map by in situ hybridisation of cosmid clones that we have shown define breakpoint intervals.

This programme of work will establish an integrated physical, genetic and biological "map" of 11p that combines most or all of the known genetic and biological data in a coherent fashion.

The integrated set of data will be stored and distributed in a computerised form.

The potential use of clones for diagnostic application to WAGR, Usher type 1, long QT and BW syndromes will be an active area of interest. The technical methods to achieve these goals are by construction of contigs at the YAC level by hybridisation overlap analysis of YAC filters (LONICRF) and by YAC Alu PCR fingerprinting (LONICSTM) and at the cosmid level by fingerprint analysis and YAC hybridisation probing of cosmid libraries (LONICSTM, LONICRF).

WAIHG will position YAC and cosmid clones and contigs on the chromosome by in situ analysis of fractional length positions and breakpoints and will contribute to the PFGE analysis of 11p15.

PARINS and MRCHGU will concentrate on the breakpoint analysis and relationship to disease states of 11p1S and 11p14-cen respectively and will use a collection of approximately 30 somatic cell hybrids to localise the 30 genetic (recombination) markers from Genethon in a continuing program. PARINS, for 11p15, and later MRCHGU, for 11p14-cen, will initiate a systematic search for coding sequences by cDNA PCR methods and establish the sequences of these clones LONICRF and LONICSTM, will establish an integrated database that will contain YAC and cosmid clones and contigs, breakpoints, PFGE maps, downloaded GDB data and some DNA sequences.

Project leader:
Dr. P. LITTLE
Biochemistry Department,
Imperial College of Science,
Technology and Medicine
Imperial College Road
UK London SW7 2AZ
Phone: +44 71 225 8259
Fax: +44 71 823 7525
Contract number: CT930057

Participants:
Dr. C. JUNIEN
INSERM UR 73
Château de Longchamp
FR 75016 Paris
Phone: +33 1 42 24 13 57
Fax: +33 1 46 47 95 01

Dr. V. VAN HEYNINGEN
Medical Research Council
Human Genetics Unit
Crewe Road
UK Edinburgh EH4 2XU
Phone: +31 332 24 71
Fax: +31 343 26 20

Dr. M. MANNENS
Institute of Human Genetics
Meibergdreef, 15
NL 1105 AZ Amsterdam
Phone: +31 205 66 51 11
Fax: +31 206 91 86 26

Dr. H. LEHRACH
Imperial Cancer Research Fund
Lincoln's Inn Fields, 44
UK London WC2A 3PX
Phone: +44 71 269 33 08
Fax: +44 71 269 30 68

MOLECULAR ANALYSIS FROM X(q27.3 TO qTER)

Key words
Chromosome X(q27.3 to qter), clone library, cosmid library, P1 library, mouse YACs.

Brief description
We propose to complete the establishment of overlapping clone libraries of the end of the long arm of the human X chromosome, the region between the position of the fragile site and the telomere, and to compare the structure of the regions to that in the mouse. The size of this region as determined by pulsed field gel analysis is between 8.5 to 9.5 megabases (Poustka et al., 1991). This area has the highest density of mutations associated with human genetic diseases and has therefore been analyzed intensely in a number of laboratories by different techniques and large amounts of information and resources have been generated. This region can thus serve as a prototype for the further analysis of larger regions of the human genome. In previous work we have constructed overlapping clone coverage of a major fraction of this area, based on the integration of YAC, cosmid and linking clone contigs. In extension to this work we propose to close the remaining gaps in the YAC clone coverage by hybridisation of additional probes to YAC filter grids of additional YAC libraries (which have not been screened yet). As yet unassigned cosmid and linking clone contigs will be positioned on the physical map of the region by hybridisation of Alu PCR products of gel-purified rare cutter restriction fragments to the gridded clone libraries (Poustka, A., 1991). To complete the complementary coverage of the entire region in bacterial cloning systems, we will screen high density filters of a cosmid library of the entire X chromosome and a P1 library of the entire genome. In parallel, we plan to construct a complementary coverage of the region in mouse YACs, to allow a detailed comparison of this region in these two species and easy access to conserved sequences.

This work will complete the clone coverage of Xq28 in both yeast and bacterial cloning systems, and will serve as the basic material in the establishment of a gene and transcript map of this area, and the determination of the complete genomic sequences of this region, planned in collaboration with the groups of John Sulston (Sanger Institute, Cambridge, UK) and Andre Rosenthal (Jena, Germany), as well as other groups in the US and Europe.

Project leader:
Dr. A. POUSTKA
Deutsches Krebsforschungszentrum
Angewandte Tumorvirologie
Im Neuenheimer Feld 280
DE 69120 Heidelberg
Phone: +49 6221 42 34 09
Fax: +49 6221 47 03 33
Contract number: CT930058

Participants:
Dr. H. LEHRACH
Imperial Cancer Research Fund
P.O. Box 123
UK London WC2A 3PX
Phone: +44 71 269 33 08
Fax : +44 71 269 30 68

SEARCH FOR PUTATIVE TUMOUR SUPPRESSOR GENES WITHIN THE q23-32 CRITICAL REGION OF HUMAN CHROMOSOME 5

Key words
5q-syndrome, chromosome 5, leukemogenesis, tumour suppressor genes, Yeast Artificial Chromosomes (YAC), cDNA libraries, physical mapping, band-specific libraries, microdissection, fluorescence *in situ* hybridization (FISH).

Brief description
Several informative cases of leukemia patients with translocations instead of deletions of the 5q region, have suggested that the putative tumour suppressor gene is within the 5q31 band. Therefore, as a first step an attempt will be made to cover the region which flanks this breakpoint by generating a contig assembly of YAC clones. These YAC clones will be initially derived by screening of human genomic YAC libraries using the cloned genomic fragments of interleukin 3 and GM-CSF genes, as probes.

Following the establishment of a complete pulse-field map using YAC clones and genomic DNA digests encompassing the two clusters, the YAC clones will be used as probes to screen two cDNA libraries in Agt11:1) a human bone marrow library and 2) a Chinese hamster x human cell hybrid library containing chromosome 5 as the only human chromosome. The above approach will lead to the detection of novel genes which may include putative tumour suppressor expressed sequences, either in hemopoietic-specific (human bone marrow cDNA library) or in a constitutive (CHO x human cell hybrid cDNA library) fashion. To increase the sensitivity of the screening process for the identification of transcribed sequences within the region, three alternative cDNA screening approaches will be employed, that have been successfully tried recently, including a) cDNA selection techniques, b) recombination based techniques and c) exon trapping.

The approach for more accurate identification of the region and for the generation of the YAC contigs, will be considerably facilitated by the utilization of a very informative patient with myelodysplastic syndrome undergoing leukemic transformation and exhibiting in his bone marrow DNA a deletion of one GM-CSF allele and rearrangement of the other, with no rearrangements of the IL-3 gene, which resides 9 kb upstream of the GM-CSF gene. Thus, this mutant is extremely informative and suggests that the putative tumour suppressor gene is included within the deletion region between the GM-CSF gene and the 3 juxtaposed sequences, normally residing downstream of the GM-CSF gene, that have been fused with the GM-CSF gene. Using this approach, and cloning the abnormal bridging fragment from this patient, several informative YAC clones that cover the region between the GM-CSF gene and the 3 breakpoint of the deletion that might contain the putative tumour suppressor gene could be isolated and characterized.

The region of interest will be expanded by generating more YAC clones using a powerful technique of band-specific microdissection and mircocloning. Two overlapping microdissection libraries will be constructed encompassing the 5q23.2-31.2 and the 5q23.3-32 regions respectively. The identification of new microclones mapping within this 'critical region' and their use in isolating YAC clones is anticipated to contribute to the construction of a contiguous physical map of this 5q region. The isolated cDNA clones derived from the employment of the above described procedures, will be characterized and those which will be shown to represent novel genes will be further tested functionally for their capacity to confer suppression of the neoplastic phenotype by transfection of transformed cells using eukaryotic expression vectors. This experimental approach is based on the assumption that a single gene is responsible for the suppression of the neoplastic phenotype, which can be transferred to the recipient cells in a functional unit by DNA transfection. Those novel genes which do not exhibit any tumour suppressor activity will be further characterized structurally and functionally. It is anticipated that this approach will reveal novel genes within this region. Alternatively, the transfer of the entire YAC clones by cell fusion into the transformed cell will be attempted, by inserting a neomycin-resistance gene into the vector. This approach has been recently shown to be feasible and will permit the rapid screening of large segments of the 5q23-32 region containing genes along with their flanking regulatory sequences that can confer dominant phenotype. The advantage of a functional assay is based on the fact that it allows the detection and isolation of functional clones without the prior knowledge of their mechanism of action. further structural analysis of the human DNA sequences will be carried out in order to define their precise organisation as well as their transcriptional unit and other regulatory elements of the putative tumour suppressor gene(S) contained within these fragments. The tissue and developmental specificity of the putative suppressor gene or the other novel genes will be investigated by the analysis of total cellular mRNAs from a series of cell lines or tissues that exhibit various developmental programmes. The above strategies are expected to provide novel insights of the understanding of the chromosomal structure and function of genes regulating haemopoiesis and/or leukaemogenesis and identify all the possible genetic components that maintain normal haemopoiesis or lead to the early steps of leukaemogenesis.

Project leader:
Professor N.P. ANAGNOU
Institute of Molecular Biology
and Biotechnology (IMBB)
P.O. Box 1527
GR 711 10 Heraklion
Phone: +30 81 313 676/210 091
Fax: +30 81 312 377/230 469
Contract number: CT930070

Participants:
Professor R. SCHÄFER
University of Zurich
Institute of Pathology
Division of Cancer Research
Schmelzbergstr. 12
CH 8091 Zürich
Phone: +41 1 255 34 43
Fax: +41 1 255 45 08

Professor U. CLAUSSEN
Klinikum der Friedrich-Schiller Universität Jena
Institut für Humangenetik und Anthropologie
Kollegiengasse 10
DE 07740 Jena
Phone: +49 3641 63 17 13
Fax: +49 3641 42 50 39

Dr. I. RAGOUSSIS
United Medical and Dental Schools of Guy's and
St. Thomas's Hospitals
Division of Medical and Molecular Genetics
Guy's Hospital
London Bridge
UK London SE1 9RT
Phone: +44 71 955 44 38
Fax: +44 71 955 46 44

PHYSICAL MAPPING OF HUMAN CHROMOSOME 6: DETAILED ANALYSIS OF CERTAIN REGIONS INCLUDING THE MAJOR HISTO-COMPATIBILITY COMPLEX

Key words
Chromosome 6, physical map, major histo-compatibility complex (MHC).

Brief description
This project is designed to coordinate efforts of thirteen laboratories, from 5 countries of the European Union, on physical mapping of human chromosome 6. All of these laboratories have an interest either in large scale chromosome mapping or in detailed analysis of a region of the chromosome. Tools will be constructed to enable local short range maps to be integrated into a larger scale map which will be assembled and refined by continued cooperation and consultation between the participants.

These tools include radiation-fusion hybrids (RFH), YAC libraries and gridded cosmid libraries from flow sorted chromosome 6. Most of these facilities are already in place.

The initial fragmentary physical map will be frequently updated and will be integrated, where possible, with the genetic map.

On a smaller scale, several of the cooperating groups are involved in investigating key regions of the chromosome. These include: the MHC, where considerable effort is going into locating all of the genes, for haemochromatosis for example, and the sequencing of some regions in their entirety.

Another region of interest is 6p23, the location of spinocerebellar ataxia (SCA).

At the other end of the chromosome (6p27) there is evidence of a tumour suppressor gene involved in a range of tumours including ovarian cancer.

Three year goals:
1 Isolation of all genes with the MHC (4Mbp)
2 Complete sequence of the Class II region of the MHC
3 Complete physical map of chromosome 6

Project leader:
Dr. J. TROWSDALE
Human Immunogenetics Laboratory
Imperial Cancer Research Fund
Lincoln's Inn Fields 44
UK London WC2A 3PX
Phone: +44 71 269 3209
Fax: +44 71 831 6786
Contract number: CT930075

Participants:
Dr. P. BRULET
Unité d'Embryologie
Moleculaire
Institut Pasteur
FR 75724 Paris Cedex 15
Phone: +33 1 45 68 84 70
Fax: +33 1 40 61 31 16

Dr. R. CAMPBELL
Department of Biochemistry
South Parks Road
UK Oxford OX1 3QU
Phone: +44 865 27 52 63
Fax: +44 865 27 52 59

Dr. J. BOYLE
Paterson Institute for Cancer Research
Christie Hospital (NHS) Trust
Wilmslow Road
UK Manchester M20 9BX
Phone: +44 61 446 31 62
Fax: +44 61 446 31 09

Dr. D. NIZETIC
Istituto Nazionale per la Ricerca Sol Cancro
Via Benedetto XV 10
IT 16132 Genova
Phone: +39 1 03 53 41
Fax: +39 1 03 52 999

Dr. I. RAGOUSSIS
United Medical and Dental Schools of Guy's
and St. Thomas's Hospitals
Division of Medical and Molecular Genetics
Guy's Hospital
Tower London Bridge
UK London SE1 9RT
Phone: +44 71 955 44 38
Fax: +44 71 955 46 44

Dr. Y. EDWARDS
MRC Human Biochemical Genetics Unit
The Galton Laboratory
University College London
Stephenson Way, 4
UK London NW1 2HE
Phone: +44 71 387 70 50
Fax: +44 71 387 34 96

Professor J.Y. LE GALL
Centre National de la Recherche Scientifique,
UPR 8291, Centre de Recherches sur le Poly-
morphisme Génétique des Populations Humaines
Avenue de Grande Bretagne
FR 31300 Toulouse Cedex
Phone: +33 61 49 60 80
Fax: +33 61 31 97 52

Dr. P. PONTAROTTI
Centre National de la Recherche Scientifique,
UPR 8291, Centre de Recherches sur le Poly-
morphisme Génétique des Populations Humaines
Avenue de Grande Bretagne
FR 31300 Toulouse Cedex
Phone: +33 61 49 60 80
Fax: +33 61 31 97 52

Dr. F. GALIBERT
Laboratoire d'Hematologie Experimentale
UPR 41
Vellefaux, 1
FR 75475 Paris Cedex 10
Phone: +33 1 42 02 16 05
Fax: +33 1 42 06 02 50

Professor J. PAPAMATHEAKIS
Institute of Molecular Biology and
Biotechnology Foundation for Research
PO Box 1527
GR 71110 Heraklion, Crete
Phone: +30 81 21 03 64
Fax: +30 81 23 04 69

Dr. A. ZIEGLER
Freie Universität Berlin
Institut für Experimentelle Onkologie
und Transplantationsmedizin
Spandauer Damm, 130
DE 14050 Berlin
Phone: +49 30 35 34 18
Fax: +49 30 35 37 78

Professor L. TERRENATO
Università degli Studi di Roma 'Tor Vergata'
Via della Ricerca Scientifica
IT 00133 Roma
Phone: +39 6 72 59 43 20
Fax: +39 6 202 35 00

Dr H. CANN
Centre d'Etude du Poly-morphisme Humain
Rue Juliette Dodu, 27
FR 75010 Paris
Phone: +33 1 42 49 98 70
Fax: +33 1 40 18 01 55

Dr. M. FRONTALI
Istituto di Medicina
Sperimentale del CNR
Via Marx, 15
IT 00137 Roma
Phone: +39 6 86 09 03 39
Fax: +39 6 82 22 03

NEW TECHNIQUE FOR FINE STRUCTURE DNA ANALYSIS USING HYBRIDIZATION WITH A SET OF MODIFIED OLIGONUCLEOTIDES

Key words
DNA analysis, genetic diagnosis, DNA sequencing, nucleic acids hybridization.

Brief description
The major part of the programs of fine structure analysis of the human genome is mainly dealing with direct DNA sequencing, which involves a number of rather complicated manipulations including loading samples onto a gel and reading sequences after separation of DNA fragments. Electrophoresis is the bottleneck for large scale analysis.

This project will explore a method for DNA sequencing based on the hybridization of the DNA fragment of interest to every oligonucleotide of a complete set (i.e. all possible sequences of a given length). The suggestion is to immobilize each of the oligonucleotides at an individual dot of a 2-D matrix, thus allowing all the hybridizations to be processed in parallel, with the DNA fragments serving as a probe.

This procedure requires a reduction of the influence of base composition and sequence on the stability of short DNA hybrids (to be able to discriminate fully annealed hybrids from hybrids with mismatches). Our approach consists of designing modified oligonucleotides that will form hybrids with DNA sequences, whose stability will not depend on base content, but only on hybrid length and presence of a mismatch.

Suitable modifications, solid supports and sample preparation methods will be explored. Applications will not only include fast large scale DNA sequencing, but also fast identification of genetic variability, e.g. diagnosis of genetic and infectious diseases.

Project leader:
Dr. D. DUPRET
Appligene SA
Laboratory for Molecular Biology Application
FR 67402 Illkirch Cedex
Phone: +33 88 67 22 67
Fax: +33 88 67 19 45
Contract number: CT930009

Participants:
Dr. N. THUONG
Centre de Biophysique Moleculaire
CNRS, UPR 4301
Avenue de la Recherche Scientifique 1A
FR 45071 Orleans 02
Phone: +33 38 51 55 97
Fax: +33 38 63 15 17

Dr. F. GANNON
University College Galway
National Diagnostic Center
IE Galway
Phone: +353 91 66 559
Fax: +353 91 66 570

Dr. D. NUSSBAUMER
Sartorius AG
Weender Landstr. 94-108
DE 37070 Göttingen
Phone: +49 551 308 312
Fax: +49 551 308 510

IMPROVEMENTS IN SINGLE-STRANDED DNA SEQUENCING BY PULSED FIELD GEL ELECTROPHORESIS. COMPREHENSION OF THE IMPLIED MOLECULAR MECHANISMS AND INVESTIGATION OF NEW ADAPTED TYPES OF GELS

Key words
Pulsed field gel electrophoresis, PFGE, DNA sequencing, gels with mixed-bed matrices, videomicroscopy, 2-D DNA typing, electric birefringence, molecular dynamics in gels.

Brief description
This proposal aims at the improvement of the sequencing techniques of DNA by determining, then by using, the optimal experimental conditions of Pulsed Field Gel Electrophoresis (PFGE). This technique, used with agarose gels, allowed to enhance the limit of separability in length of double stranded DNA by a factor greater than 100 (up to several millions of base pairs). It is quite realistic to transpose our knowledge of the separation mechanism of double stranded DNA to perform separation of longer single stranded DNA (several thousands of base pairs). To achieve this goal, a detailed study of the dynamics of single stranded DNA in a gel after turning the electric field on or off will be undertaken in order to allow a correct extrapolation of the parameters which are well known with double stranded DNA. Otherwise, the influence of herniae that the DNA molecule is constantly forming when it is migrating in the gel matrix pulled by the electric field is still not well known and its importance has been underestimated. In order to precise the general model of migration that governs the separation of polyelectrolytes according to their lengths, the study of the DNA chain behaviour and, in particular, the formation of herniae will be examined thoroughly under different electric field programs. These experiments will be done with double stranded DNA for experimental convenience, using the electric birefringence technique (Strasbourg) and fluorescence videomicroscopy (Soeborg). The study of model polyelectrolytes will also be addressed. The possibility to use the best separation condition for single stranded DNA will then lead to prepare new types of gels, the apparent pore sizes of which will be intermediate between acrylamide and agarose gels (mixed-bed matrices). The Milan team will synthesize these new gels which will be characterized and tested in Milan and in Strasbourg by techniques which are well mastered by these teams. The sequencing itself will then be tested and the optimal pulse trains for PFGE determined, in particular by using the video image processing and the software of Soeborg which permit to analyze electrophoregrams in real time. At the same time, the study of the molecular mechanism taking place in PFGE with double stranded DNA of a few kbp will be carried out using the same techniques and the same gels; it should lead to a resolution extended to higher lengths for performing 2-D DNA typing (Leiden).

Project leader:
Dr. J. STURM
Institut Charles Sadron (CRM-EAHP)
CNRS-ULP
6, rue Boussingault
FR 67083 Strasbourg Cedex
Phone: +33 88 41 40 39
Fax: +33 88 41 40 99
Contract number: CT930024

Participants:

Dr. C.H. BROGREN
National Food Agency of Denmark
Ministry of Health
Moerkhoej Bygade, 19
DK 2860 Soeborg
Phone: +45 39 69 66 00
Fax: +45 39 66 01 00

Dr. M. CHIARI
Istituto di Chimica degli Ormoni
Via Mario Bianco, 9
IT 20131 Milano
Phone: +39 2 284 77 37
Fax: +39 2 284 19 34

Dr. E. MULLAART
Department of Genetic Diagnostics
Ingeny B.V.
P.O. Box 685
NL 2300 AR Leiden
Phone: +31 71 21 45 75
Fax: +31 71 21 02 36

DEVELOPMENT OF AN INTEGRATED INFORMATION MANAGEMENT SYSTEM FOR HUMAN GENOME DATA (IGD)

Key words
Information systems, software design, databases, genome, Integrated Genomic Database (IGD).

Brief description
The aim is to develop an open software system to handle human genome data. The system, called IGD, will integrate information from many genomic databases and experimental resources into a comprehensive target-end database (IGD TED). Users will use front-end client systems (IGD FRED) to download data of interest to their computers and merge them with their own local data. FREDs will provide persistent storage of and instant access to retrieved data, friendly graphical user interface, tools to query, browse, analyze and edit local data, interface to external analysis, and tools to communicate with the outside world.

The TED will be implemented using both relational and object-oriented technologies in parallel; it will be accessible over the network (online and offline) as a read-only resource for multiple clients. Tools will be developed for automated updating of the TED from its resource databases and data sets, which include major databases for nucleotide and protein sequences and structures, genome maps, experimental reagents, phenotypes, and bibliography, and sets of raw data produced at genome centres and laboratories.

Besides character-based access via Gopher, WAIS, FTP, and several query language interfaces to the TED, we will develop a specialized front-end client, IGD FRED, with its own database manager, based on the ACEDB program. The FRED will support graphical display methods for sequence feature maps, chromosomal genetic and physical maps, and for experimental objects like clone grids, etc. FRED data will be coupled with rules and knowledge via PROLOG interface. FRED will also provide interface to important analysis software packages, and tools to submit data to external databases in their own format.

The IGD schema will model objects and processes in considerable detail, so that scientists will be able to use the FRED as a laboratory notebook. At the same time, and in the same environment, they will link their experimental data to public reference data coming from the TED. This permits the use of FRED as a single editorial interface to multiple genomic databases at once.

The power of the IGD approach is in using general tools rather than ad hoc solutions to accomplish concrete tasks. The open design will simplify rapid evolution and incorporation of new features and resources provided by third parties.

Project leader:
Dr. O. RITTER
Deutsches Krebsforschungszentrum
Im Neuenheimer Feld 280
DE 69120 Heidelberg
Phone: +49 6221 422332
Fax: +49 6221 422333
Contract number: CT930003

Participants:
Dr. N. SPURR
Imperial Cancer Research Fund
Clare Hall Laboratories
Blanche Lane
South Mimms
Potters Bar
UK Herts EN6 3LD
Phone: +44 71 269 38 46
Fax: +44 71 269 38 02

Dr. J. THIERRY-MIEG
Centre de Recherches de Biochimie
Macromoleculaire
Route de Mende BP 5051 1919
FR 34033 Montpellier 1
Phone: +33 67 61 33 24
Fax: +33 67 52 15 59

Dr. D.V. MARKOWITZ
Lawrence Berkely Laboratory
Cyclotron Road, 1
US Berkely, CA, 94720
Phone: +1 510 486 68 35
Fax: +1 510 486 40 04

Dr. M. BISHOP
Human Genome Mapping Project
Resource Centre
Clinical Research Centre
UK Harrow HA1 3UJ
Phone: +44 81 869 38 04
Fax: +44 81 869 38 07

Dr. H. LEHRACH
Imperial Cancer Research Fund
Genome Analysis Laboratory
44 Lincoln's Inn Fields
UK London WC2A 3PX
Phone: +44 71 269 33 08
Fax: +44 71 269 30 68

EUROPEAN DATA RESOURCE FOR HUMAN GENOME RESEARCH

Key words
Genome, informatics support, Integrated Genomic Database (IGD).

Brief description
Within the framework of this project, a data resource centre is made available to provide informatics support for the European human genome research community in the acquisition, management, and analysis of human genomic data. The resource centre should provide on-line access to the most important databases in the field of genome mapping, sequencing and analysis, network services and general information retrieval tools. It will have to install up-to-date software for the scientific evaluation of genomic data and make available specific compute servers in Heidelberg for the efficient processing of those data by a large user community through network. The staff of the data resource should support the users by telephone hotlines, electronic-mail, a regular newsletter, database and software documentation, training workshops, technical courses and scientific meetings. They will have to host specific developers' workshops on new aspects of genome computing and provide scholarships at post-doctoral and senior scientist levels, to promote collaborative European research projects whose developments will be installed at the resource centre and made available for all its users. The centre will have to contribute to the core activities of GDB by implementing curators, a nomenclature node, aliterature scanning functionality, a Unix programmer, and funding of visiting scientists to GDB.

The data resource will develop a locally-editable version of GDB in close collaboration with the Baltimore group and based on the IGD technology (using the ACEDB DBMS) and its implementation for GDB editors and Single Chromosome Workshop organisers. It should contribute to the further integration of data into the Integrated Genomic Database (IGD), to the maintenance of the central IGD server, to cooperate with and support further national IGD server nodes in Europe. It will implement and support new developments as specified in the research plan of the IGD consortium.

Project leader:
Dr. S. SUHAI
Deutsches Krebsforschungszentrum,
Department of Molecular Biologies
Im Neuenheimer Feld, 280
DE 69120 Heidelberg
Phone: +49 6221 422369
Fax: +49 6221 422333
Contract number: CT930006

Participants:
Dr. S. AYMÉ
Service Commun N° 11 'Gene Mapping and
Clinical Research', INSERM SC11
Faculté de Médecine 45
FR 75270 Paris Cedex 06
Phone: +33 1 47 03 39 47
Fax: +33 1 47 03 38 88

Dr. M. BISHOP
Human Genome Mapping Project
Clinical Research Centre
UK Harrow HA1 3UJ
Phone: +44 81 869 38 04
Fax: +44 81 869 38 07

DEVELOPMENT OF A EUROPEAN INTEGRATED DATABASE OF IMMUNOLOGICAL INTEREST

Key words
Integrated Database, interconnection of data, immunological molecular data.

Brief description
The main objective of the project is the development of a database of immunological interest that combines nucleotide and protein sequences of immunoglobulins, T-cell receptors and HLA proteins and their genes, detailed expert annotation of these sequences, mapping data and the results of comparative sequence analysis, i.e. sequence alignments. This database will provide immunologists with an integrated tool that allows them to manage and analyze the complex information they are interested in.

Genes and proteins of immunological interest are not appropriately covered by the existing molecular biological databases. General databases such as EMBL, Swiss-prot or GDB cannot store all information important to immunologists. Moreover, data from sequences, mapping and other databases are not interconnected. Here we propose to establish a new European database that overcomes most of these short-comings by using state-of-the-art database technology combined with expert knowledge to integrate sequence information, annotation, sequence alignments and mapping data, diagnosis and treatment of many diseases such as autoimmune diseases or leukemia which depend heavily on the kind of information provided by a database as proposed here. Such an integrated database of immunological molecular data would be of immense value for biomedicine as well as the European pharmaceutical industry and would considerably help to strengthen Europe's role in these areas.

The mapping of genes and the elucidation of gene sequences is important for the analysis of the human and other genomes. However, for an understanding of the accumulating data, special databases are necessary that sort, arrange and most importantly interpret the collected information. The interpretation of the data related to immunologically important genes and proteins is perhaps one of the most complex problems, and considerable expert knowledge is required. The proposed project is therefore an important contribution in the area of "Human Genome Research".

Project leader:
Dr. R. FUCHS
European Molecular Biology
Laboratory
Meyerhofstrasse 1
DE 69117 Heidelberg
Phone: +49 6221 387258
Fax: +49 6221 387519
Contract number: CT930038

Participants:
Dr. M.P. LEFRANC
Lab. d'Immunogénétique
Moléculaire URA CNRS1191
101 Place Eugène Bataillon
FR 34095 Montpellier
Phone: +33 67 61 36 34
Fax: +33 67 14 30 31

Dr. J. BODMER
Tissue Antigen Laboratory
Imp. Cancer Research Fund
Lincoln's Inn Fields, 44
UK London WC2A 3PX
Phone: +44 71 269 33 95
Fax: +44 71 831 67 86

Dr. W. MÜLLER
Institut für Genetik
Abt. Immunbiologie
Weyertal, 121
DE 50931 Köln 41
Phone: +49 221 470 45 86
Fax: +49 221 470 51 85

SRS: AN OBJECT-ORIENTED SOFTWARE ENVIRONMENT TO SEARCH AND ANALYZE MULTIPLE AND NETWORKED MOLECULAR BIOLOGICAL DATABASES RESIDING IN LOCAL AND REMOTE SITES

Key words

Molecular biology, molecular sequence data, software, information systems -information services, database management systems, computer communication networks, data display, artificial intelligence.

Brief description

The primary aim of this proposal is the creation of a computer package (SRS for *S*equence *R*etrieval *S*ystem) that will allow scientific users to search and analyze many molecular biological databases from their home site.

A recently developed computer language (ODD for Object Design and Definition) will be significantly expanded to integrate easily all flat-file databases regardless of format and information type.

The SRS framework for the algorithmic modules will be object-oriented.

Data read (ROB) and analysis (SOB) objects will be specifically created.

Interface modules will allow communication with file servers at remote computer sites to extract and search databases for query-requested information, analyze the resulting data with remote or local program engines, and present transparently the results to the user at the local site.

Data analysis can also be performed through a local or remote BATCH environment permitting usage of specially architectured computers (eg massively parallel).

A comprehensible and easily understood query language will be developed for users.

It is intended that the SRS package will be user-friendly, connect a local client to a worldwide server network for information and algorithmic resource sharing, and operate on several computer systems.

Project leader:
Professor P. ARGOS
European Molecular Biology Laboratory
Meyerhofstrasse 1
DE 69117 Heidelberg
Phone: +49 6221 38 72 75
Fax: +49 6221 38 75 17
Contract number: CT930043

Participants:
Dr. E. TROIANO
AITEK S.R.L.
Via Pisa 12/1
IT 16146 Genova
Phone: +39 1 031 51 80
Fax: +39 1 031 48 73

Dr. R. DOELZ
Biozentrum der Universität Basel
Biocumputing
Klingelbergstrasse 70
CH 4056 Basel
Phone: +41 612 67 22 47
Fax: +41 612 67 20 78

DATA ANALYSIS ALGORITHMS FOR
GENOME MAPPING AND SEQUENCING

Key words
DNA, image processing, data analysis, physical mapping, genetics, sequencing by hybridisation.

Brief description
The aim of this project is to develop computer algorithms for the analysis and classification of hybridisation data.
Specifically, the areas covered by the project are:
Image analysis of hybridisation filters.
Reconstruction of physical genome maps from hybridisation data.
Normalisation of cDNA libraries.
Reconstruction of sequence order from oligonucleotide hybridisations.
Characterisation of DNA and protein sequences from hybridisation data.
Design of experiments to optimise data rates.

Project leader:
Dr. H. LEHRACH
Imperial Cancer Research Fund, Genome Analysis Laboratory
44 Lincoln's Inn Fields
UK London WC2A 3PX
Phone: +44 71 269 3308
Fax: +44 71 269 3068
Contract number: CT930061

Participants:
Dr. G. ZANETTI
Centro di Ricerca, Sviluppo e Studi Superiori in Sardegna
Via Nazario Sauro 10
IT 09123 Cagliari
Phone: +39 7 02 79.61
Fax: +39 7 02 79 62 16

Professor K. CONRADSEN
The Institute of Mathematical Statistics
and Operations Research
Building 321
DK 2800 Lyngby
Phone: +45 42 88 14 33
Fax: +45 42 88 13 97

MANAGEMENT AND COORDINATION OF
SINGLE CHROMOSOME WORKSHOPS

Key words
Human Genome Project, Single Chromosome Workshops, Chromosome Maps.

Brief description
An important aspect of the European approach to the Human Genome project has been its commitment to international collaboration and its support for the Human Genome Organisation (HUGO) in its role in coordinating the international effort. In recent years, one of the chief approaches of HUGO to the co-ordination of genome projects and the construction of detailed genetic and physical maps has been the organisation of international Single Chromosome Workshops (SCW). At each SCW participants update the genetic and physical maps relating to a specific chromosome, resolve inconsistencies between data sets and arrange collaborations including the sharing of materials. During 1992, CEC have provided core funding for SCWs held in Europe and assistance from European scientists attending SCWs elsewhere. The European Commission's (EC) support has included coordination of SCWs and the development of guidelines for participation and organisation. The contribution of the EC to the success of recent SCWs is widely acclaimed. The present contract extends core support for SCWs and their management for a further 30 months and travel costs to SCWs for participants from European countries without a national genome programme.

Project leader:
Professor M.A. FERGUSON-SMITH
HUGO
Park Square West One
UK London NW1 4LJ
Phone: +44 71 935 8085
Fax: +44 71 935 8341
Contract number: CT930002

INTEGRATION OF GENE AND GENOME MAPS BY MULTICOLOUR-FISH AND DNA-HALO HYBRIDISATION

Key words

cDNAs, genes, genome, chromosomes, fluorescence, in situ hybridisation, molecular cytogenetics, microscopy, automation.

Brief description

In the genome project, the first step of gene analysis has been the ongoing construction of contiguous genetic and physical maps and the large scale accumulation of partial cDNA sequences to provide a working resource to the community. The next logical step is to integrate the gene and genome maps. Further research will then be needed to elucidate the functions of the encoded proteins, to unravel their potential role in genetic diseases and to develop diagnostic and therapeutic approaches. The work of the first step is well under way in many places. This project aims to contribute to the next step, the integration of genome and gene maps by fluorescence in situ hybridisation (FISH).

Subproject I aims at high-throughput multicolour chromosomal FISH-mapping of cDNAs, generated by the GenExpress program at Genethon. It will lead to a steady flow of cytogenetic cDNA localisation data that will be disseminated to the Human Genome Analysis Community via existing central databases. To increase throughput, we will continually integrate the results of parallel research and development into microscope automation and digital image analysis techniques under development in separate projects.

Subproject II entails research and development to establish, validate and apply the high resolution "DNA-halo" FISH methodology to gene mapping and distance determination of genomic contigs under investigation in Leiden and Villejuif (e.g. 1p13, 4q35, 11p13, 12p13, 16p13 and Xp22). It will yield a novel generally applicable method for high resolution gene tracing by FISH on YAC contigs, generated by the genome project.

Project leader:
Professor Dr. G.J.B. VAN OMMEN
Department of Human Genetics
P.O. Box 9503
NL 2300 RA Leiden
Phone: +31 71 276065
Fax: +31 71 276075
Contract number: CT930004

Participants:
Dr. C. AUFFRAY
Centre National de la Recherche
UPR 420 Génétique Moléculaire et Biologie du Développement
Rue Guy Moquet, 7, BP 8
FR 94801 Villejuif Cedex
Phone: +33 1 49 58 11 11
Fax: +33 1 49 58 11 22

NEW ELECTROPHORETIC STRATEGIES FOR FASTER SEQUENCING, MAPPING AND DNA ASSAY

Key words
Electrophoresis, DNA sequencing, genome mapping, capillary electrophoresis, pulsed electrophoresis, polymer solutions.

Brief description
The project proposes a strategy aimed at increasing by an important factor the output of electrophoretic sequencing, mapping and DNA-probe genetic diagnosis, by consistently integrating innovations in different fields in which the proposers have specific competences.

The most important of these innovations, each of which represents a valuable intermediate target, are:
- New improved permanent and non-permanent sieving matrices for sequencing and duplex DNA separation
- Design of an automated capillary array electrophoresis apparatus able to load from Microtiter plates, and to perform constant-field and pulsed-fields electrophoresis.
- Alternative strategies using neutral molecules or particles bound to DNA to increase band separation.
- Improved injection protocols for capillary electrophoresis to avoid prepurification steps and increase automation.
- Comprehensive predictive models to accelerate the optimization of sequencing and DNA assay using pulsed-fields and/or polymer solutions.
- Theoretical modelling and computer simulations.
- Extensive studies of molecular migration mechanisms and of collective behaviour by fluorescence microsopy.

This approach, which requires multiple acute competences but no dramatic and hypothetical technological breakthrough, would provide a rather secure and short route to accelerated sequencing and mapping, and automatized diagnosis.

The chances of success of the project are maximised by exploring several parallel solutions for the most critical aspects (e.g. sieving matrices, increase of resolution).

Project leader:
Professor J. L. VIOVY
E.S.P.C.I.
10, rue Vauquelin
FR 75231 Paris Cedex 05
Phone: +33 1 407 94600
Fax: +33 1 407 94731
Contract number: CT930018

Dr. W. MARTIN
University of Manchester
Institute of Science and Technology
Sackville Street
UK, MANCHESTER M60 1QD
Phone: +44 61 200 42 26
Fax: +44 61 236 04 09

Participants:
Dr. G. RIGHETTI
University of Milano
Dept of Biomedical Sciences and Technologies
Via Celoria, 2
IT 20133 Milano
Phone: +39 2 23 64 288
Fax: +39 2 23 62 288

Dr. L. SALOMÉ
Centre de Recherche Paul Pascal
Avenue Albert Schweitzer
FR 33600 Pessac
Phone: +33 56 84 56 08
Fax: +33 56 84 56 00

CHROMOSOMAL DISTRIBUTION AND BIOLOGICAL FUNCTION OF HUMAN ENDOGENOUS RETROVIRAL ELEMENTS

Key words

Human endogenous retroviral elements, retrotansposons, insertion mutagenesis, chromosome rearrangements, chromosome-specific markers, cDNA, regulation of gene expression, evolution, tumour markers.

Brief description

Human endogenous retroviral elements (HERHVs) comprise about 0.6% of the human genome. They are thought to have acted as a constructive driving force in evolution and contributed in shaping the human genome by intracellular transposition and by generating hot spots of recombination. Furthermore, some of these elements have acquired cellular function, e.g. in regulation of gene expression. In addition, HERVs represent a reservoir of possibly pathogenic retroviral genes and are believed to be involved in insertion metagenesis and chromosome rearrangements. In this project we will examine the chromosomal distribution and expression of HERVs in order to obtain information on their biological function and pathogenic potential. Furthermore, we expect to obtain more insight in the architecture of the human genome and the role of HERHVs in shaping it.

We will isolate HERV sequences that are expressed in normal and malignant human tissues. These will be characterized by sequence analysis and assigned to HERV families. Comparison of various HERV sequences will allow us to understand the phylogeny of HERV families and assist in developing a more definite nomenclature. The chromosomal location of specific HERV sequences and banding profiles of distinct HERV families will be determined and used to develop chromosome-specific markers. We further plan to use HERV sequences for physical mapping of chromosome regions of special interest, e.g. for regions involved in chromosome rearrangements associated with human cancer. HERV cDNAs with open reading frames will be expressed in appropriate vectors and antibodies will be generated. The possibility of diagnostic application and the use of these sequences as tumour markers will be evaluated. This project is a joint effort of the major European groups working on HERHVs and will cover all important types of HERV elements analyzed to date.

Project leader:
Dr. C. LEIB-MÖSCH
Forschungszentrum für Umwelt und Gesundheit GmbH
Inst für Molekulare Virologie
Ingolstädter Landstrasse 1
DE 85758 Neuherberg
Phone: +49 89 31 87 46 09
Fax: +49 89 31 87 33 29

Participants:
Professor Dr. R. KURTH
Paul-Ehrlich-Institut
Federal Agency for
Sera and Vaccines
Paul-Ehrlich-Str. 51-59
DE 63225 Langen
Phone: +49 6103 77 10 01
Fax: +49 6103 77 123

Professor J. BLOMBERG
Lab. of Clin. Microbiology
Section of Virology
Sölvegatan, 23
SE 22362 Lund
Phone: +46 46 17 32 75
Fax: +46 46 18 91 17

Dr. G. LA MANTIA
Dip. di Genetica, Biologia
Generale e Molecolare
Università di Napoli
Via Mezzocannone, 8
IT 80134 Napoli
Phone: +39 8 15 52 62 08
Fax: +39 8 15 52 79 50

Dr. M. BOYD
Chester Beatty Laboratories
Institute of Cancer Research
237, Fulham Road
UK London SW3 6JB
Phone: +44 71 352 81 33
Fax: +44 71 352 32 99

DEVELOPMENT OF A HIGH THROUGHPUT (250-350 KB) AUTOMATED DNA SEQUENCING SYSTEM AND SEQUENCING OF HUMAN cDNA AND POLYMORPHIC MICRO-SATELLITE DNA CLONES

Key words
Automated DNA sequencing, human cDNA, polymorphic micro-satellite DNA clones.

Brief description
The objective and result of this collaboration among European scientists will be the development and improvement of advanced technologies which will facilitate the physical mapping and sequencing of the human genome. The sequencing system of the next generation should have a potential throughput of 250-350 kb per device per run. The number of simultaneously used different fluorescent dyes will be expanded to four, increasing further the on-line per day throughput of the system and approaching the potential capacity of the off-line multiplex methods. Longe gel readings will improve dramatically the efficiency of DNA sequencing. Sequence accuracy will be further improved as compared to existing devices. The low error rate, already achieved in the EMBL system, is a key prerequisite for efficient sequencing with lowest possible (2-3 times) redundancy. A novel sequencing strategy will involve direct sequencing from large vectors, increase the efficiency and lower the cost per finished base. Human cDNAs and polymorphic microsatellite DNAs will be sequenced to demonstrate the function and applicability of the newly designed equipment and developed methodologies for human genome analysis. Analysis of polymorphic microsatellite clones will be focused on human chromosome 21, using an ordered YAC Contig covering the region 21q22.1 to refine further the existing map of this region. In addition, the linkage between microsatellites and coding regions will be investigated.
Because of the innovative design and the original ideas implemented in this research proposal, the information derived from this project will have many implications for basic research in biology as well as in clinical research and medicine. Other laboratories in Europe and worldwide will benefit from the more efficient equipment and technical protocols resulting from this project.

Project leader:
Dr. W. ANSORGE
European Molecular Biology Laboratory
Meyerhofstrasse 1
DE 69117 Heidelberg
Phone: +49 6221 387355
Fax: +49 6221 387306
Contract number: CT930037

Participants:
Professor. J. CELIS
Institute of Medical Biochemistry
Ole Worms Alle, Building 170
DK 8000 Aarhus
Phone: +45 86 12 93 99
Fax: +45 86 13 11 60

Dr. X. ESTIVILL
Molecular Genetics Department
Cancer Research Institut
Hospital Duran y Reynals
ES 08907 Barcelona
Phone: +34 3 335 71 52
Fax: +34 3 263 22 51

FURTHER DEVELOPMENT OF 2-D DNA TYPING: APPLICATION IN THE ANALYSIS OF GENETIC LINKAGE AND SOMATIC MUTATION

Key words

DNA, genome mapping, genetic disease, tumour, trinucleotide, genetic linkage analysis, 2D DNA typing.

Brief description

One of the goals of mapping the human genome is to determine the genetic basis for disease. Chromosomal areas harbouring disease-related genes can be identified by genetic marker analysis, i.e. scanning the genome at many sites for genetic variation associated with the disease. In a previous project supported by the European Commission (EC) the two-dimensional (2-D) DNA typing technique has been evaluated for its potential to measure DNA sequence variation at many sites in the genome simultaneously. The method is based on hybridization analysis of a 2-D separation pattern of a genomic DNA restriction enzyme digest using micro- and minisatellite core probes which detect many highly informative VNTRs. Major applications of 2-D DNA typing including analyzing somatic genetic instabilities, eg. occurring in tumorigenosis, and linkage analysis of genetic diseases. In the first phase of the proposed project 2-D DNA typing will be used (1) to further analyze CEPH pedigrees to develop more genetic markers, and (2) to develop a 2-D spot variant database which will be linked to databases containing physical mapping information. To facilitate the 2-D DNA typing procedure a newly developed apparatus will be used in which the first and second electrophoretic separation can be run in a single gel without manual interference. Subsequently, the 2-D method will be applied to compare tumour DNA with normal DNA from patients with cancer. 2-D DNA typing allows detection of allelic imbalance due to deletion and/or amplification at many chromosomal sites. This approach will identify genetic markers and corresponding YAC clones to map chromosomal regions most likely containing tumour associated genes. In addition, 2-D DNA typing will be used to analyze genomic DNA of patients with diseases with genetic anticipation (Myotonic Dystrophy and fragile X), using core probes for (CNG) motifs. Expansion of (CNG) repeats 5' and 3' of these disease genes has been shown to correlate with severity of the disease. Screening genomic DNA of patients with similar disease by 2-D DNA typing with microsatellite core probes might identify genomic regions associated with these diseases. Finally, 2-D DNA typing will be used for pedigree analysis to detect genetic linkage with a disease gene. The expected results of the project include VNTR genetic markers, DNA markers for genetic diseases including cancer, and an optimized 2-D DNA typing protocol for analyzing human genomic DNA.

Project leader:
Dr. E. MULLAART
Genetic Diagnostics
Ingeny B.V.
P.O. Box 685
NL 2300 AR Leiden
Phone: +31 71 21 45 75
Fax: +31 71 21 02 36
Contract number: CT930041

Professor Dr. L. BOLUND
Institute of Human Genetics
DK 8000 Aarhus
Phone: +45 86 13 97 11

Professor T.A. KRUSE
Institute of Human Genetics
DK 8000 Aarhus
Phone: +45 86 13 97 11
Fax: +45 86 12 31 73

Dr. H. LEHRACH
Genome Analysis Laboratory
Lincoln's Inn Fields, 44
UK, LONDON WC2A 3PX
Phone: +44 71 269 33 08
Fax: +44 71 269 30 68

TOWARDS CONSTRUCTION OF A COMPLETE PHYSICAL MAP OF THE MOUSE GENOME: INTEGRATION OF YAC CLONE RESOURCES WITH THE EUROPEAN COLLABORATIVE INTERSPECIFIC BACKCROSS (EUCIB)

Key words
Mouse genome, genetic mapping, physical mapping.

Brief description
The European Collaborative Interspecific Backcross (EUCIB) is a major collaborative European effort to provide resources for the high resolution genetic mapping of the mouse, an important model organism in the Human Genome Project. A 1,000 animal backcross has been anchor mapped across the genome providing DNAs to allow users to map new markers to a resolution of 0.3 cM. EUCIB is also supported by a sophisticated database.

In collaboration with the Mouse Genome Center in the US, EUCIB is being used for the construction of a high resolution genetic map of 6,000 microsatellites across the mouse genome, a prelude to the STS (sequence tagged site) based YAC contiging of the mouse genome. EUCIB aims to map 3,000 of the proposed 6,000 microsatellites.

This program will take a major proactive role in the provision of YAC clones covering a major portion of the mapped microsatellites and thus contribute in a substantial way to the construction of the mouse physical map. Two mouse YAC libraries have been constructed in Europe and are being widely and successfully used. We propose to screen both these libraries for 1,750 genetically mapped microsatellites over the next three years laying down YACs that will cover up to one-third of the mouse genome.

Project leader:
Dr. S.D.M. BROWN
Dept. of Biochemistry and Molecular Genetics
St. Mary's Hospital Medical School
University of London
UK London W2 1PG
Phone: +44 71 723 1252 Ext. 5484
Fax: +44 71 706 3272
Contract number: CT930046

Participants:
Dr. J. L. GUENET
Institut Pasteur
Unité de Génétique des Mammifères
Rue du Docteur Roux 25
FR 75724 Paris
Phone: +33 1 45 68 85 55
Fax: +33 1 45 68 86 39

Dr. P. AVNER
Généthon
BP60
FR 91002 Evry Cedex
Phone: +33 1 69 47 28 00
Fax: +33 1 60 70 86 98

Dr. R. SIBSON
Human Genome Mapping Project
Resource Centre
Clinical Research Centre
UK Harrow HA1 3UJ
Phone: +44 81 869 38 03
Fax: +44 81 869 38 07

HEMIZYGOSITY OF CHROMOSOME 22q11
AND HUMAN BIRTH DEFECTS

Key words
Chromosome deletion, congenital heart defect, chromosome 22, immunodeficiency, Shprintzen syndrome, DiGeorge syndrome, CATCH22, mutation.

Brief description
Hemizygosity for a region of chromosome 22q11 causes a wide range of congenital defects including DiGeorge syndrome, Shprintzen (velo-cardiofacial syndrome) and congenital heart disease. There are now several well characterised DNA probes that can detect these deletions, and the saturation cloning of the region is proceeding. The aim of this proposal is to conduct a multi-centre analysis of this group of birth defects. The project has several goals. We wish to determine the range of birth defect and phenotypic variability associated with deletions of chromosome 22q11. With specific abnormalities, such as congenital heart defects, we will estimate the proportion of cases in which hemizygosity within 22q11 is causative. On the basis of our current data we predict that congenital heart defect will be the major cause of morbidity and mortality secondary to this chromosome abnormality. These experiments will allow us to refine our shortest region of overlap map for the genes which have a haploinsufficient phenotype, and detect any correlation between size/position of deletion and resulting phenotype. This will facilitate efforts to isolate candidate cDNAs. The deletion screening experiments will identify those patients with no apparent chromosome 22 abnormality who would be candidates for having intragenic mutations. Appropriate candidate genes will be screened for such mutations. Subsidiary goals include comparative mapping between mouse and man, and mapping of chromosome deletion breakpoints.

Project leader:
Dr. P.J. SCAMBLER
Institute of Child Health
Molecular Medicine Unit
30 Guilford Street
UK London WC1N 1EH
Phone: +44 71 242 9789
Fax: +44 71 831 0488
Contract number: CT930053

Participants:
Dr. J. GOODSHIP
University of Newcastle
Dept. of Human Genetics
Claremont Place
UK Newcastle-upon-Tyne
Phone: +44 91 222 73 86
Fax: +44 91 222 71 43

Dr. C. MEIJERS
Cell Biology and Genetics
P.O. Box 1738
NL 3000 DR Rotterdam
Phone: +31 10 408 81 40
Fax: +31 10 436 02 25

Professor M. VEKEMANS
Hôpital Necker,
Enfants Malades
Laboratoire Histologie
Embryologie Cytogénétique
Rue de Sèvres 149
FR 75743 Paris 15
Phone: +33 1 42 73 88 51
Fax: +33 1 44 49 01 47

Dr. X. ESTIVILL
Molecular Genetics Dept.
Cancer Research Institut
Autovia Castelldefels KM 2,7
Hospitalet Llobregat
E, 08901 Barcelona
Phone: +34 3 335 71 52
Fax: +34 3 363 22 51

Professor N. PHILIP
Unité de Recherche
INSERM U.242 Physio-
pathologie Chromosomique
Faculté de Médécine 27
FR 13385 Marseille Cedex 5
Phone: +33 91 38 66 36
Fax: +33 91 49 41 94

Prof. B. DALLAPICCOLA
Cattedra di Genetica Umana
Dipart. di Sanita Pubblica
e Biol. Cell.
Università "Tor Vergata"
di Roma
Via Ramazzini, 15
IT 0100 Roma
Phone: +39 6 65 74 12 13
Fax: +39 6 65 74 11 83

DEVELOPMENT OF DIAGNOSTIC MULTICOLOUR IN SITU HYBRIDIZATION PROBE SETS

Key words
Fluorescence, in situ hybridization, comparative genomic hybridization, microdisection, molecular cytogenetics, diagnostic DNA probes, chromosome region specific DNA libraries.

Brief description
1 Diagnostic probes will be combined according to the clinical needs resulting in cytogenetic tools on different levels, i) to differentiate between different types of leukemias, and ii) to differentiate within a particular leukemia type by means of molecular cytogenetics:
Following optimization of single probes, diagnostic probe combinations are designed for acute lymphatic and myeloid leukemias as well as for chronic lymphopid leukemias and other types of malignant lymphomas.

2 Comparative genomic hybridization (CGH) will be used to analyze the genomic imbalances in these leukemias on a new level. Aberrations which are found newly or at higher frequencies will lead to the redesigning and optimization of the combined probe pools:
Genomic DNA from cell populations enriched in tumour cells is hybridized in situ to metaphase chromosome spreads from normal individuals. Above a general chromosomal staining (and in comparison to signals from cohybridized normal DNA), DNA sequences overrepresented in the tumour genome result in stronger and underrepresented sequences in a weaker staining of the corresponding region. For the aberrations newly defined by CGH, DNA probes will be included in the disease specific probe combinations. The diagnostic potential of these probe sets will then be tested using cytogenetically characterized patient cells followed by a blind study.
The optimal probe sets should provide a basis for the automated analysis of chromosomal aberrations in leukemias and lymphomas.

3 The ideal probe for the detection of a deletion would consist of the whole genomic DNA present in the targeted chromosomal region. We propose to elaborate techniques for a new strategy which would allow the generation of region specific DNA probe pools suitable for the diagnosis of even microdeletions: Highly extended chromatin fibers prepared from normal individuals will be used for CGH to develop a technique for the delineation of disease specific deletions at a very high resolution. It is planned to elaborate a microdisection technique allowing physical isolation of the corresponding genomic material from such fibers. Following amplification by universal PCR, these sequences could be used i) to probe for the corresponding aberration in patients, ii) to be integrated as an optimized probe into the multicolor probe sets and iii) to probe YAC and cDNA libraries in order to isolate the complete sequences from this genomic region or disease candidate genes, respectively.

This technology development will be conducted using DNA from renal cell carcinomas with well defined deletions in 3 p and could be extended using DNA from leukemia cells.

Project leader:
Dr. P. LICHTER
Angewandte Tumorvirologie
Deutsches Krebsforschungszentrum
Im Neuenheimer Feld 280
DE 69120 Heidelberg
Phone: +49 6221 42 46 09
Fax: +49 6221 42 46 39
Contract number: CT930055

Participants:
Dr. U. BERGERHEIM
Karolinska Hospital
Department of Urology
Solnavägen 60500
SE 10401 Stockholm
Phone: +46 8 729 22 30
Fax: +46 8 30 81 43

Dr. H. DOEHNER
Cytogenetics Laboratory
Medizinische Klinik und Poliklinik
University of Heidelberg
Hospitalstrasse, 3
DE 69115 Heidelberg
Phone: +49 6221 56 80 63
Fax: +49 6221 56 38 13

Professor Dr. A. HAGEMEIJER-HAUSMAN
Erasmus University Rotterdam
Institute of Genetics
Molenwaterplein, 50
NL 3015 JI Rotterdam
Phone: +31 10 408 71 96
Fax: +31 10 436 02 25

GENOMIC STUDIES OF EXPANDED UNSTABLE TRINUCLEOTIDE SEQUENCES IN RELATION TO HEREDITABLE DISORDERS

Key words
Genetics, trinucleotide repeats, hereditary disease, anticipation.

Brief description
Six important inherited disorders have recently been explained at the molecular level by the discovery that expanded trinucleotide repeat sequences disrupt the normal function of a gene. Fragile-X mental retardation (FRAXA and FRAXE), myotonic dystrophy, spinocerebellar atrophy (SCA1) and Kennedy-disease (spino-bulbarmuscular atrophy) and Huntingtons chorea are caused by this new class of mutations.

This finding implies that multiple disorders of great social and economic impact may depend on this disease mechanism. We have consequently developed a novel genome wide analysis method, Repeat Expansion Detection (RED). Using this method we have already identified some novel expanded repeats in the genome. This application is aimed at developing the system to rapidly elucidate the molecular mechanism behind numerous inherited disorders. To this end it is important to collect large family material from multiple sites within Europe.

Determining the involvement of trinucleotide instability in human genetic disease

We will use a novel technique called repeat expansion detection (RED) to screen human genetic disorders. This method allows a genome wide screening for mutational analysis. The driving force has been the observation that general methods may be very cost effective relative to traditional isolation and cloning of single genes.

Converting RED to a procedure applicable for routine use

Once trinucleotide expansion is found in correlation to a particular disease, the new method also provides the tools necessary for direct cloning approaches. Non-radioactive RED and Locus specific RED will be developed.

Developing cloning procedures for expanded trinucelotide repeats.

Three approaches will be undertaken to clone the sequences surrounding the repeats:
1 Selection of cloned DNA by RED.
2 Purification of expanded repeat containing DNA prior to cloning.
3 Cloning expanded repeats from RNA.

Project leader:
Dr. F. BAAS
Neurology, AMC
Meibergdreef 9
NL 1105 AZ Amsterdam
Phone: +31 20 56 65 998/3325
Fax: +31 20 56 64 440
Contract number: CT930060

Participants:
Dr. M. SCHALLING
Department of Clinical Genetics
Karolinska Hospital
PO Box 60500
SE 10401 Stockholm
Phone: +46 8 729 39 28
Fax: +46 8 327 734

Dr. J. DE BELLEROCHE
Charring Cross and Westminster Medical School
Department of Biochemistry
Fulham Palace Road
UK London W6 8RF
Phone: +44 81 846 70 52
Fax: +44 81 846 70 99

ISOLATION, MAPPING AND PARTIAL SEQUENCING OF POTENTIAL CODING SEQUENCES FROM THE HUMAN X-CHROMOSOME

Key words
Chromosome X, potential coding sequences.

Brief description
The work proposed here has as its goal the establishment of a map of potential coding sequences of the human X chromosome, which will be constructed in concert with the rapidly progressing physical map. To identify potential gene sequences, we plan to rely on three different strategies, the identification of exons by an exon amplification protocol, the isolation of cDNA sequences by a selection/amplification protocol, and the isolation of evolutionarily conserved sequences by a similar technique, as well as combinations of these techniques with the goal of establishing sublibraries of these different types of candidate sequences from the entire X chromosome, as well as from subregions defined from X chromosome contigs. Libraries will be picked by a robotic device developed at the ICRF, and will be used to construct high density filter grids (up to 40,000 clones per filter) by a high throughput, high accuracy spotting robot to generate filter grids, which can be provided to other laboratories. In parallel, we plan to amplify the insert sequence from 10,000 clones from each library by PCR with flanking primers in a high throughput PCR robot, and to use a 'sequencing by hybridisation' strategy developed by us and other groups to identify corresponding clones in each library, and to select one clone for each gene on the X chromosome, followed by hybridisation of permuted pools of clones from this gene catalogue to high density filter grids of X chromosome libraries.

Project leader:
Dr. H. LEHRACH
Imperial Cancer Research Fund
Lincoln's Inn Fields 44
UK London WC2A 3PX
Phone: +44 71 269 3308
Fax: +44 71 269 3068
Contract number: CT930066

Participants:
Dr. A. POUSTKA
Deutsches Krebsforschungszentrum
Angewandte Tumorvirologie
Im Neuenheimer Feld 280
DE 69120 Heidelberg
Phone: +49 6221 42 34 09
Fax: +49 6221 47 03 33

A NEW METHOD FOR THE CONSTRUCTION OF A HIGH RESOLUTION MAP OF THE WHOLE HUMAN GENOME

Key words
Human genetics, gene mapping, somatic cell hybrids.

Brief description
Irradiation and fusion gene transfer (IFGT, also known as "radiation hybrids") has been used to construct high resolution genetic maps of defined regions of the human genome. The current methods for producing IFGT maps have the drawback of requiring "single chromosome" hybrids as donors, furthermore, between 100 and 200 radiation hybrids are required for each human chromosome mapped. To construct a map of the whole genome up to 5,000 hybrid cell lines would be needed. The original idea for IFGT technique was suggested by Pontecorvo and was pioneered by Goss and Harris. Instead of "single chromosome hybrids" the latter authors used human cells as donors. We have repeated these early experiments and have found that non-selected markers are retained at frequencies sufficiently high that the same set of hybrids can be used to map the whole genome. A set of 200 hybrids should be capable of generating a map with an average marker spacing of less than 500kb. Based on this observation and by combining the skills of the Cambridge laboratory in somatic cell genetics with the expertise of Genethon in marker testing, we propose to create a high resolution map of the whole human genome. This map will have different biases from the recombination map and will be particularly useful for constructing YAC contigs of the human genome. In the future, we propose to extend this technology to map the genomes of other large mammals.

Project leader:
Professor P. GOODFELLOW
University of Cambridge
Department of Genetics
Downing Street
UK Cambridge CB2 3EH
Phone: +44 223 333999
Fax: +44 223 333992
Contract number: CT930067

Participants:
Dr. J. WEISSENBACH
Généthon
Boîte Postale 60
FR 91002 Evry Cedex
Phone: +33 1 69 47 28 00
Fax: +33 1 60 70 86 98

A TRANSGENIC RAT MODEL FOR ALZHEIMER'S DISEASE

Key words
Transgenic rat, Alzheimer's Disease, neurology, mutation, immunohistochemistry, amyloid precursor protein, β-amyloid protein.

Brief description
Development of transgenic rat model for Alzheimer's disease:

1 Isolation of the normal and mutant human APP gene and development of the appropriate DNA construct for the microinjection by molecular biological techniques including YAC gene construction.

2 Development of transgenic rats by the introduction of the DNA construct to the fertilized rat eggs.

3 Determination of the expressed normal and mutant human APP gene by molecular biological techniques including Northern blot analysis, PCR, ELISA, Western blot analysis, immuno-cytochemistry and in situ hybridization.

4 A comprehensive innate and learned behavioral analysis of the transgenic rats including locomotion and exploration, social interaction, anxiety and fear, habituation learning, passive avoidance, place position, spatial learning and operant conditioning.

5 Biochemical analysis for cholinergic and glycolytic system in the brain and peripheral nerve tissues of transgenic rats. Detection of the early gene expression (c-fos) in transgenic rats.

6 Development of the primary neuronal cell cultures from transgenic rate embryo or progeny.

7 Cross-breeding of the established transgenic rat line with hypertensive rate to examine the pathophysiological effects of hypertension on Alzheimer's disease.

Project leader:
Professor Dr. D. GANTEN
Max-Delbrück-Centrum für Molekulare Medizin
Robert-Rössle Strasse 10
DE 13125 Berlin
Phone: +49 30 9406 3278
Fax: +49 30 949 7008
Contract number: CT930076

Participants:
Professor B. WINBLAD
Alzheimer's Disease Research Center
Department of Geriatric Medicine
Karolinska Institute
SE 14186 Huddinge
Phone: +46 8 746 36 13
Fax: +46 8 711 17 51

Professor L. AMADUCCI
Dept of Neurological and Psychiatric Sciences
University of Florence
Morgagni, 85
IT 50134 Firenze
Phone: +39 55 41 26 34
Fax: +39 55 41 36 03

Professor K. FUXE
Karolinska Institutet
Department of Histology and Neurobiology
SE 1000 Stockholm
Phone: +46 8 728 64 00
Fax: +46 8 833 79 41

THE SIGNIFICANCE OF ALLELIC VARIATION FOR THE PHENOTYPIC DIVERSITY OF PHENYLKETONURIA EXAMINED BY APPLICATION OF A NEW AND FAST MUTATION DETECTION ASSAY AND BY THE DEVELOPMENT OF A EUROPEAN DATA BASE

Key words
Phenylketonuria, phenotypic diversity, mutation detection assay, European database.

Brief description
The primary goal is to study the significance of allelic variation for the various biological phenotypes of phenylketonuria (PKU) in order to improve diagnosis and treatment of the disease in Europe.

The study involves the development of a European database correlating mutant alleles with biological phenotypes and includes the application of a new technique for fast, simple and reliable detection of mutations in all coding regions and flanking intronic sequences of the gene.

The new mutation detection assay has enabled us to detect and identify a molecular lesion in 99% of Danish PKU alleles.

The approaches available so far are based on detection of previously identified mutations and the applicability is generally hampered by a large number of mutations. Until now, approximately 100 different mutations causing PKU have been identified. The proportion of mutations detected for a population has, however, not exceeded 30-70%. We have established unified conditions for mutation analysis of the entire coding sequence of the gene, and the resulting assay offers a simple and reliable methodological entity that can be applied to rapid detection of the mutant alleles in any individual, irrespective of the frequency and distribution of mutations in the population.

The results obtained by this European study will establish whether the new assay system is marketable in its present form. Neonatal screening programmes followed by therapy for PKU introduced within the first weeks of life were implemented in Europe 20 years ago. Within recent years, however, the effectiveness and adequacy of dietary therapy have been questioned by an increasing number of reports demonstrating learning disabilities, neurological abnormalities, psychological problems, and white matter changes detectable by MRI even in patients treated early. These findings stress the importance of intensified research on the genetic basis for the pathobiological function.

To initiate a better coordination of the research within the European Union on the genetic basis for PKU, Professor Jean Rey organised a Symposium in Paris in November 1990. The participants agreed to establish a database in Europe on the various mutant alleles and their relation to different biological phenotypes of PKU. A European database has not yet been established due to lack of financial support and in the meantime a database on mutant alleles has been established in Montreal.

The establishment of this database only stresses the need for the development of a European database which strengthens the coordination of the Member States' research on allelic variation in PKU, particularly related to the genetic basis for the biological diversity of the disease.

With the establishment of a European database relating allelic genotype to biological phenotype, knowledge about the genotype of the hyperphenylalaninemic neonate will provide information regarding the severity of the disorder. This will permit an earlier implementation of dietary therapy better tailored to each individual patient and thus may provide a more favourable prognosis.

The project benefits PKU patients in Europe and in turn the economic and social implications of the disease.

Finally, the new method for mutation detection surpasses previous methods and all Member countries will benefit from this method. It should be added that due to continuous budget cutbacks the Kennedy Institute cannot establish a European database without EC-support.

Project leader:
Dr. F. GÜTTLER
Department of Inherited Metabolic Diseases
and Molecular Genetics
University of Copenhagen
The John F. Kennedy Institute
Gl. Landevej, 7
DK 2600 Glostrup
Phone: +45 43 96 86 12
Fax: +45 43 43 11 30
Contract number: CT930081

Participants:
Professor B. FRANÇOIS
Dr. L. Willems-Instituut v.z.w.
Universitaire Campus
BE 3590 Diepenbeek
Phone: +32 1 126 92 11
Fax: +32 1 126 93 12

MASS SPECTROMETRY OF POLYNUCLEOTIDES BY MATRIX-ASSISTED LASER DESORPTION/IONISATION (MALDI-MS)

Key words
Laser-desorption, mass-spectrometry, MALDI-MS, polynucleotides.

Brief description
Based on the results of a pilot project this project aims at exploring and establishing the potential of Matrix-Assisted Laser Desorption/Ionisation Mass Spectrometry (MALDI-MS) for the mass spectrometric analysis of polynucleotides and the routine, large scale sequencing of DNA. Even in the most advanced automated instruments for the Sanger technique separation of the polynucleotides on a gel is generally considered the limiting step, which could prohibit routine sequencing of the Human Genome in reasonable time. One of the promising alternative approaches towards this goal is to replace the separation on a gel by mass spectrometry, which in principle has a comparable sensitivity, but is much faster, has a superior absolute accuracy in terms of the exact definition of the polynucleotide (by absolute molecular weight) and is better suited for integration into a fully automated system and data analysis. Before the advent of MALDI-MS mass spectrometry of nucleic acids had been limited to relatively small oligonucleotides and sensitivity had been very low. Results obtained during the pilot phase have shown that with MALDI-MS polydeoxyribonucleotides with up to 20 bases give very good results. Between 20 and 30 bases spectra deteriorate significantly, no useful spectra could be recorded for DNA molecules with more that 30 bases. For polyribonucleotides, which generate more stable ions, spectra of molecules with up to 100 bases have been recorded. The results suggest that there is still considerable room for further improvement and that the technique indeed holds a potential for sequencing of polynucelotides, if chemical and physical conditions and parameters are optimized. Accordingly, this project therefore has the following goals: (1) to extend the mass range for the analysis of deoxyribonucleic acids beyond the currently accessible range of ca. 30 bases, (2) to establish the optimum parameters for the analysis of ribonucleotide acids with at least 100 bases, (3) analyze without further purification polynucleotide mixtures as obtained routinely from sequencing solutions and (4) demonstrate the potential of the technique for a prototype clinical application by sequencing of (relatively short) well defined DNA-segments in search of point mutations.

Project leader:
Professor Dr. F. HILLENKAMP
Institut für Medizinische Physik und Biophysik,
University Münster
Robert-Koch Strasse 31
DE 48149 Münster
Phone: +49 251 83 5103
Fax: +49 251 83 5121
Contract number: CT930082

Participants:
Dr. P. ROEPSTORFF
Department of Molecular Biology,
Odense University
Campusvej 55
DK 5230 Odense M
Phone: +45 6 615 86 00
Fax: +45 6 593 27 81

CONSTRUCTION OF ORDERED CLONE LIBRARIES
OF THE HUMAN GENOME

Key words
Yeast artificial chromosome, contig maps, integrated genome maps.

Brief description
The project aims at establishing a physical map of the human genome based on a set of ordered YAC clones, and to integrate this with information on chromosomal location and indicators for the positions of genes. Clones will be selected from YAC libraries constructed at CEPH (Albertsen et al., 1990) (to be enlarged to give a twenty fold coverage of the human genome) a library constructed at the ICRF (Larin et al., 1991) and a library constructed at the ICI (Anand et al., 1990).

Different types of complementary information will permit the identification of overlapping clones and the assembly of contigs:

1 Iterative hybridisation of high-density filter grids presenting ordered arrays of YAC clones (Larin et al., 1991; Ross et al., 1992a) or YAC inter-Alu polymerase chain reaction (PCR) products (Chumakov et al., 1992a; Meier-Ewert et al., 1993).

2 STS (including microsatellite sequence) content mapping of YACs (Chumakov et al., 1992b).

3 Medium-repeat restriction fragment fingerprinting of YAC clones (Bellanné-Chantelot et al., 1992).

By combining these data with information on insert size and chromosome origin of YAC clones, and with results of hybridisation of cDNA probes and other indicators of expressed genes, physical maps covering the human genome and containing information on gene position can be established.

Project leader:
Dr. H. LEHRACH
Imperial Cancer Résearch Fund
Lincoln's Inn Fields 44
UK London WC2A 3PX
Phone: +44 71 269 3308
Fax: +44 71 269 3068
Contract number: CT940079

Participants:
Professor D. COHEN
Centre d'Etudes du Polymorphisme Humain
Rue Juliette Dodu, 27
FR 75010 Paris
Phone: +33 1 42 49 98 50
Fax: +33 1 42 06 16 19

Area IV

RESEARCH ON BIOMEDICAL ETHICS

IV. RESEARCH ON BIOMEDICAL ETHICS

Introduction

Research on Biomedical Ethics address general standards for the respect of human dignity and the protection of the individual in the context of biomedical research and its clinical applications. This area is also concerned with the evaluation of the social impact of the BIOMED 1 programme and any risks which might be associated with it.

Research projects are aiming at analyzing the problems raised by the application of new therapy technologies in the health services like medically assisted procreation, organ transplantation, and occupational health screening with an emphasis on genetic screening.

The ethical questions raised by medical decision making especially with specific patients (patients in persistent vegetative state or with impaired capacities for instance) are also considered, as well as the social, legal and ethical aspects of disease with major social impact like AIDS, and the problem of resources allocation and access to health care.

Dr. Christiane Bardoux

MARKETING BLOOD?: AN ETHICAL ANALYSIS AND LEGAL REVIEW OF THE TENSION BETWEEN A COMMERCIAL AND NON-COMMERCIAL BLOOD DONATION SYSTEM IN THE COMMON MARKET

Key words
Medical ethics, health law, blood donation.

Objectives
1 To provide an ethical analysis of the arguments in favour of a self-sufficient European market for blood products based on a system of non-remunerated blood donation.
2 To provide a review of the legal consequences of the availability of both commercially and non-commercially supplied blood products on a common European market with regards to product liability. Indeed, should it be shown that a non-remunerated system is safer than a commercial one, then liability within the latter will increase.
3 To produce a review of the existing regulations in EC countries for the collection and distribution of blood products.
4 To review materials produced by experts in the field on the safety and efficiency of blood products in order to get a picture of the actual safety and sufficiency of non-commercial systems (existing in the Netherlands and the United Kingdom) as compared to more or less commercialized systems (existing in Germany).

Brief description
For both ethical and clinical reasons, the present system of collecting and distributing blood and blood products in several European countries is based on two principles: non-remunerated donation and self-sufficiency. Most experts in the field maintain that in a self-sufficient system based on non-remunerated donation, blood products are more safe, less scarce and more carefully used than in a commercialized system.

In the near future, it is to be expected that, as a result of medical and technological innovations, the need for blood and blood products will continue to increase. Furthermore, it is to be expected that before long the national regulations of countries participating in the European community will give way to a common European market. Although a self sufficient system of non-remunerated donation is encouraged on European levels, a common European market is expected to result in a mixed system of both non-remunerated and commercially supplied blood. This expectation is based on three considerations.

First of all, current national systems of non-remunerated donation are occasionally mixed with a system of commercially supplied products.

Second, a European system of non-remunerated donation does not everywhere meet the demand for some blood products (e.g. Factor VIII).

Third, the current national regulations concerning collection and distribution of human blood diverge considerably amongst EC countries, throwing serious doubts on the possibility of a uniform European system. For these reasons we expect that Europe will soon be facing hard choices about marketing blood.

The results of an initial exploration of ethical dilemmas were recently published. t is the aim of the project to elaborate this exploration into an extensive ethical analysis and a legal review. The concerted action will cover 4 member States, some of them representing the system based on non-remunerated donation, others the commercialized system.

Project leader:
Dr. M.A.M. DE WACHTER
Institute for Bioethics (IGE)
P.O. Box 778
NL 6200 AT Maastricht
Phone: +31 43 21 75 75
Fax: +31 43 25 63 73
Contract number: CT920787

Participants:
R. BERGHMANS & I. RAVENSCHLAG
Institute for Bio-ethics (IGE)
P.O. Box 778
NL 6200 AT Maastricht
Phone: +31 43 21 75 75
Fax: +31 43 25 63 73

J. KEOWN & P. BARRISTER
Centre for Health Care Law
UK Leicester LE1 7RH
Phone: +44 533 52 23 66/70 19 06
Fax: +44 533 52 22 00

H. VON SCHUBERT
Ev. Beratungsstelle für Erziehungsberatung
Bugenhagenstrasse 21
DE 2000 Hamburg 1
Phone: +49 40 33 44 22 46/33442247
Fax: +49 40 33 44 23 00

L. LÉRY & N. LÉRY
Dept Ethique et Santé, Univ de Lyon
8 Av. Rockefeller
FR 69008 Lyon
Phone: +33 78 77 71 61
Fax: +33 78 77 71 60

A EUROPEAN MULTICENTRE STUDY OF TRANSPLANTATION OF ORGANS FROM LIVING DONORS: THE ETHICAL AND LEGAL DIMENSIONS (EUROTOLD)

Key words

Ethics, Living donor transplantation, law.

Objectives

1 To acquire an understanding of the interaction of ethical values, cultural traditions and social customs in the practice of living donor transplantation (LDT).
2 To assess the legal and ethical acceptability of LDT in general and of 'marginal' donors in particular.
3 To develop a fuller appreciation of the effect of legal factors on professional attitudes to the use of living organ donors.
4 To assess the importance of donor age in the context of LDT.

Brief description

The Eurotold project will be carried out by the management group in close collaboration with members of participating centres. The commonly used modality of interim meetings, workshops, site and contact visits will be used to develop a network for the dissemination of material and information generated by the project through the whole of Europe. The principle methods used are summarised below:

a *Attitudes survey:* Investigation of attitudes of professionals (clinicians and coordinators), patients (including families) and community through questionnaires, follow-up interviews and personal communications (involving overseas visits) as outlined below:
(i) a preliminary questionnaire to identify the key personnel, to determine the routine donor work-up protocol, to determine previous experience at a particular centre,
(ii) visits and interviews to provide background information and verify responses where necessary and, (iii) a problem orientated questionnaire based on a series of clinical scenarios to explore the limits of attitudes to LDT.

b *Donor Health Registry:* This database will house information on the postoperative physical well-being of donors assessed in terms of psychological and mental, as well as physical factors. Data on these items will be collected from all countries participating in the study.

c *Legisearch:* This database will contain a registry of laws regulating LDT across Europe. A substantial amount of data has already been collected but requires collation and categorisation for accessibility. It is anticipated that an E-Mail system will enable direct access to much of this data during the period of the project.

Project leader:
Professor P.K. DONNELLY
Department of Surgery,
Leicester General Hospital
Gwendolen Road
UK Leicester LE5 4PW
Phone: +44 533 588080
Fax: +44 533 490064
Contract number: CT921841

Participants:
Dr. A JAKOBSEN
Dept. of Surgery, Rikshospitalet
NO 0027 Oslo 1
Phone: +47 2 20 10 50

Prof. G. OPELZ
Inst. für Immunologie der
Universität Heidelberg
Im Neuenheimer Feld 305
DE 6900 Heidelberg
Phone: +49 6221 56 40 13
Fax: +49 6221 56 42 00

Prof. G. BENOIT
Service d'Urologie, Univ Paris-Sud
FR Paris
Phone: +33 1 45 21 36 99
Fax: +33 1 45 21 36 94

Prof. S. LINDKAER JENSEN
Kirurgisk afdeline L, sektion AAS,
Aarhus Univ. Hospital
DK Aarhus
Phone: +45 86 12 55 55
Fax: +45 86 18 52 39

Mr. D. MURPHY
Transplantation Unit, Beaumont Hospital
IE Dublin 1
Phone: +353 1 37 77 55

Dr. H. AKVELD
Faculteit der Rechtsgeleerdheid,
Erasmus Universiteit
NL Rotterdam
Phone: +31 10 408 23 48/16 47
Fax: +31 10 453 29 16

Prof. M.Y. TÜLBEK
Dept. of Nephrology,
Gata Haydarpasa Training Hospital
Haydarpasa 18327
TR istanbul
Phone: +90 1 527 67 72

Dr. R. HENDERSON
Dept. of mathematics,
Univ of Newcastle upon Tyne
UK Newcastle upon Tyne
Phone: +44 91 232 85 22
Fax: +44 91 261 11 82

Mr. D. PRICE
Dept. of Law, Leicester Polytechnic
UK Leicester
Phone: +44 533 57 71 75
Fax: +44 533 57 71 86

THE ETHICAL QUALITY ADJUSTED LIFE YEARS (QALY): AN INVESTIGATION OF THE ETHICAL IMPLICATIONS OF MEASURES OF QUALITY OF LIFE APPLICABLE TO A RANGE OF DISEASES AND HEALTH STATES FOR USE IN THE ALLOCATION OF RESOURCES IN PREVENTION, DIAGNOSIS AND TREATMENT

Key words

QALY, health indexes, quality of life, resource allocation, ethics.

Objectives

1 To investigate the ethical issues that arise in the derivation of QALYs and the ethical consequences of existing methods used in the construction of QALY scales, in terms of potential injustice in the representation of different groups, through:
- consideration of the temporal aspects of quality of life valuation;
- consideration of the use of discounting in quality of life calculations;
- investigation of the conceptualisation of health in existing quality of life measurement-scales;
- consideration of the nature of the valuations used in the construction of quality of life measurement-scales.
2 To identify the ethical problems arising from the application of QALYs in the distribution of health care resources, through investigation of the rational planning of health care and the use of quality of life measures in the context of such planning by:
- considering the geographical patterns for preference for the rational planning of health care within Europe;
- considering the divergences between the approaches to rational planning in the participating countries;
- considering the desirability of rational planning with specific reference to the weighted QALY, and the possibility that weighting may reflect potentially unjust social preferences.

Brief description

The proposed Concerted Action contributes primarily to the tasks of the programme stated in section IV.2., and also concerns the ethical implications of the objectives stated under 1.4. QALYs are widely employed in the planning and allocation of health care resources, and specifically in improving the effectiveness and efficiency of health care, and the improvement of research methods available to provide information for the organisation of health care.

The Project stems from the urgent need to determine priorities in health care. Scarcity of resources in most western societies has resulted in the objective of improving the health of the population to the maximum extent within given resources. This in turn leads to a need to prioritize services, taking into account both benefits produced and costs incurred. The QALY is an attempt to describe dimensions of health in a way which can be utilised as a prioritization mechanism.

Methodologically, the project has two elements: initially to consult experts in relevant fields to compile data to provide scenarios for the description of ethical dilemmas arising from the allocation of health care resources; and consequently a range of normative ethical theories will be examined along with the ethical considerations assumed implicitly or explicitly in the existing use of QALYS and other methods of health care allocation currently used in the EC.

The time schedule is 24 months.

Project leader:
Dr. A. EDGAR
Centre for Applied Ethics,
University of Wales, College of Cardiff
P.O. Box 94
UK Cardiff CF1 3XB
Phone: +44 222 87 40 25
Fax: +44 222 87 42 42
Contract number: CT921388

Participants:
Dr. Robin ATTFIELD
Centre for Applied Ethics,
Philosophy section, University of Wales
P.O. Box 94
UK Cardiff CF1 3XB
Phone: +44 222 87 40 25
Fax: +44 222 87 42 42

Mr. David COHEN
Dept. of Management Studies,
Polytechnic of Wales
Pontypridd
UK Mid Glamorgan CF37 1DL
Phone: +44 443 48 23 61
Fax: +44 443 48 22 22

Prof. Anne FAGOT-LARGEAULT
115-117 rue Saint Antoine
FR 75004 Paris

Dr. Ian HARVEY & Dr. D. SHICKLE
Centre for Applied Public Health Medicine,
Temple of Peace and Health
Cathays Park
UK Cardiff CF1 3NW
Phone: +44 222 23 10 21
Fax: +44 222 23 86 06

Prof. hent TEN HAVE
Dept. of Ethics Philosophy and
History of Medicine,
Faculteit der Medische Wetenschappen
P.O. Box 9101
NL 6500 HB Nijmegen
Phone: +31 80 61 53 20
Fax: +31 80 54 18 62

Prof. J. HUSTED
Aarhus University
Universitetsparken
DK 8000 Aarhus
Phone: +45 86 13 67 11
Fax: +45 86 19 16 99

Prof. Spyros G. MARKETOS
Dept. of History of Medicine,
Univ of Athens
20 Patr. Ioakeim St
GR 10675 Athens
Phone: +30 1 364 1 972

FERTILITY, INFERTILITY AND THE HUMAN EMBRYO ETHICS, LAW AND PRACTICE OF HUMAN ARTIFICIAL PROCREATION

Key words

Assisted reproduction, IVF, infertility, human embryo, law, ethics, gamete donation, rights, children.

Objectives

1 To analyze the conceptual issues involved in human artificial procreation.
2 To compare the predominant conceptual views in various Member States and to establish the extent of possible consensus.
3 To analyze the ethical issues involved in human artificial procreation.
4 To compare the predominant ethical views in various Member States and to establish the extent of possible consensus.
5 To analyze the legal issues involved in human artificial procreation.
6 To compare the predominant legal views in various Member States and to establish the extent of possible harmonisation of those States' laws and regulations.
7 To make recommendations concerning harmonisation or approximation of Member States' laws and regulations concerning human artificial procreation, and to recommend material which could be made available as guidance for practitioners in the various Member States.

Brief description

The proposed research is a multi-disciplinary, multi-location investigation into the law, ethics and practice, in a variety of Member States, regarding the conditions known medically as infertility and the variety of treatments developed to address those conditions. The investigation recognises the pertinence of a number of key questions, for instance: Is the condition of infertility to be regarded as a genuine health need simply because we have the medical means to circumvent it? In treating infertility and in providing assisted conception services are we meeting needs which are clinical, or social? Similar confusion surrounds the question of the status of the human foetus. Is it a human being with all the rights and interests people are generally thought to have? Is it a proper subject for experimentation? Is it someone's property?

Following the investigation of these questions, and of predominant ethical and legal responses to them as these responses affect clinical practice in the Community Member States concerned, the Project aims to make Recommendations to the Commission concerning the possibility and desirability of harmonisation or law and practice, concerning human artificial procreation, within the Community.

Project leader:
Dr. D. EVANS
Centre for Philosophy & Health Care,
University of Wales, College of Swansea
Singleton Park
UK Swansea SA2 8PP
Phone: +44 792 29 56 12
Fax: +44 792 29 57 69
Contract number: CT921276

Participants:
Derek MORGAN
Centre for Philosophy &
Health Care,
College of Swansea
Singleton Park
UK Swansea SA2 8PP
Phone: +44 792 29 56 12
Fax: +44 792 29 57 69

Erwin BERNAT
Inst für Burgerliches Recht,
Karl Frangens Univ
Heinrichstasse 22
DE 8010 Graz

Christian BYK
Council of Europe,
Directorate of Legal Affairs
FR Srasbourg

Flavio CRUCIATTI &
Guido GERIN &
Anton REVEDIN
Inst International for the
Study of Human Rights
10 Rue Cantri
IT 34127 Triest

Erwin DEUTSCH
Juristisches Seminar de
Universität Go Huiger
Platz de Gottinger Sieben 6
DE 3400 Gottinger

Peter HARPER
Inst. of Genetics,
Univ of Wales Hospital
Health Park
UK Cardiff CF 4 4XN

Soren HOLM
Neurofysiologisk Institut,
Panum Institut
Blegdamsvej 3c
DK 2200 Copenhagen N

Elena MANCINI
Policlinico Umberto 1
Viale Regina Elena 324
IT 00161 Roma

Jean MARTIN
Service de la Santé Publique
Cite Devant
CH 1014 Lausanne

Alex MAURON &
Marie THEVOZ
Foundatio Louis,
Jeantet de Medicine
P.O. Box 277
CH 1211 Geneve 17

Marian MENGARELLI
Ricerca ed Inndagini
Sociologische
Via L. Stefano 101
IT 40125 Bologna

Maurizio MORI
Politeia
Via Cosimo Del Fante 13
IT 20122 Milano

Demitrio NERI
Inst di Filosofia
'Galvano della Volpe',
Univ di Messina
IT Messina

Linda NIELSEN
Det Retsvidenskabelige
Institut C
Studiestraede 6
DK 1455 Copenhagen

John PARSONS
Dept. of Assisted
Conception,
Kings College Hospital
Denmark Hill
UK London

Neil PICKERING &
Zbigniew SZAWARSKI
Centre for Philosophy &
Health Care,
College of Swansea
Sigleton Park
UK Swansea SA2 8PP
Phone: +44 792 29 56 12
Fax: +44 792 29 57 69

Frances PRICE
Child Care and Development
Group, Univ of cambridge
Free School Lane
UK CA2 3RF Cambridge

Gian DI RENZO
Policlinico Umberto 1
Viale Regina Elena 324
IT 00161 Roma

Knut W. RUYTER
Center for Medical Ethics
Guastadalleen 21
NO 371 Oslo

Hartwig VON SCHUBERT
Diakonisches Werk
Bugenhagen Strasse 21
DE 2000 Hamburg 1

Carmine VENTIMIGLIA
Instituto de Sociologia, Universita Degli studi de Parma
IT Parma

Dalla VORGIA
Dept. of Hygiene and
Epidemiology,
School of Medicine,
University of Athens
GR Athens

Paulo ZATTI
Inst di Scienze Guiridicfie
Via del Santo 77
IT 35123 Padova

FAMILY FUNCTIONING AND CHILD DEVELOPMENT IN FAMILIES CREATED BY THE NEW REPRODUCTIVE TECHNOLOGIES

Key words
In vitro fertilization, donor insemination, adoption parenting, child development.

Objectives
The objective of the proposed research is to obtain standardized data on the quality of parent-child relationships and the social and emotional development of children in families created as a result of the new reproductive technologies. While such data is currently being collected in a study in the UK by the project coordinator (funded by the Medical Research Council), extending this research to include other European countries will allow us to compare culturally determined attitudes towards the new reproductive technologies, and to examine the influence of attitudes to human artificial procreation on family functioning and child development.

Brief description
A sample of 25 families in which one child was conceived by in vitro fertilization (IVF) and a sample of 25 families where one child was conceived by donor insemination (DI) will be obtained through each centre. In each country, these children and their families will be compared with a sample of 25 families which include a child who was adopted at birth, and a sample of 25 families with a naturally conceived child. All of the children will be aged between 4 and 8 years. The adoptive families will be recruited through adoption agencies which work with babies, and the normally conceived children will be obtained through the department of Obstetrics & Gynaecology at each participating clinic. The IVF families will be randomly selected and the families in the other groups will be made comparable by matching overall for the age and social class of the parents and the presence of siblings.

The quality of parenting will be assessed using a standardised interview with the mother, and mothers and fathers will complete questionnaire measures of stress associated with parenting, marital satisfaction, and emotional state. Data on the presence of behavioral and emotional problems in the children will also be obtained by standardised interview with the mother, and by questionnaires completed by the mother and the children's teachers. The children will be administered the Separation Anxiety Test to provide a measure of security of attachment to parents, the Family Relations Test to assess feelings towards the parents and the Pictorial Scale of Perceived competence and Social Acceptance.

Project leader:
Professor S.E. GOLOMBOK
Clinical & Health Psychology Research Centre, City University
Northampton Square
UK London EC1V 0HB
Phone: +44 71 477 85 14
Fax: +44 71 477 85 82
Contract number: CT920023

Participants:

Prof. Eylard VAN HALL
Dept. of Gynaecology & Reproductio,
Leiden University ,
Rijnsburgersweg 10
NL 2333 AA leiden
Phone: +31 71 26 33 32
Fax: +31 71 91 96 29

Prof. Ettore CITTADINI
Dept. of Obstetrics & Gynaecology,
Inst. Materno Infantil
Via Cardinale Rampolla
IT 90142 Palermo
Phone: +39 91 54 63 04
Fax: +39 91 58 95 08

Prof. Santiago DEXEUS
Dept. of Obstetrics & Gynaecology,
Inst. Dexeus
PO Bonanova 67
ES 08017 Barcelona
Phone: +34 34 18 65 00
Fax: +34 34 18 78 32

AIDS: ETHICS, JUSTICE AND EUROPEAN POLICY

Key words
AIDS, HIV, ethics, legislation, public policy, social planning, discrimination, AIDS serodiagnosis, partner notification, education.

Objectives
The chief aim of the project is to identify basic principles of and sketch a framework for European social and legislative policy on AIDS. This will complement and build upon existing national policy, and will help create a climate in which the scientific and technological research efforts to contain the spread of HIV/AIDS may be enhanced and consolidated.

Brief description
Ethics: The HIV seropositive individual has often been the object of discrimination and has been denied civil rights, but it may be that the persisting animosity and prejudice shown the HIV seropositive individual may be diffused by the recognition of their clear duties to others and to society. One focus of the project will thus be the question of what moral duties the HIV seropositive individual has towards his/her sexual partner(s), those he/she shares syringes with in drug use, to health care professionals, and towards society generally. In particular, whether the seropositive individual has a moral duty to disclose his/her HIV status, and what the likely social impact of such a duty would be, will be investigated. We shall be interested in the question of whether some HIV seropositive individuals, such as health care professionals, have special duties in this regard.

It is our intuition that we should think in terms of a reciprocity of obligations, that is, in terms of a reciprocity between obligations *to* the seropositive individual and obligations *of* the seropositive individual. It should be confirmed that HIV seropositive individuals be treated with the respect they are due as persons, and that they remain fully integrated within society and are not ostracised, stigmatised or labelled. It is unrealistic to hope for HIV seropositive individuals' serious recognition of a duty to disclose their serostatus if to do so is to open those individuals to discrimination.

If this positive effect for HIV seropositive individuals could be confirmed, further likely positive outcomes for society would include greater and more accurate information on the spread of HIV/AIDS. It is likely that many carry the virus in ignorance and for fear of ostracism do not undergo testing. Greater openness with a concomitant promise of equitable treatment could result in greater voluntary testing and even in a decrease in the spread of the disease among the non-infected population.

Law: If there is a moral duty to disclose HIV status, should it be ratified in law? How could such a legal duty be reconciled with jurisdictions such as the United Kingdom which protects medical confidentiality? How would such a duty affect confidentiality of medical records? How could a legal duty to disclose be enforced effectively at the legislative level? In some jurisdictions it is a criminal offence to transmit knowingly the disease. Should European policy move in the direction of criminalising or decriminalising cognisant transmission?

Social Policy: The duty to disclose seems to presuppose an individual's certain knowledge of his/her HIV status. If this was the case, the duty to disclose might raise questions about mandatory HIV testing for all citizens. Ethically, mandatory testing poses many problems, for example the challenge to personal autonomy and the violation of the right to refuse medical 'laying on of hands', a right which is legally protected in many jurisdictions. Moreover, doubts have been raised about the practicability and economic viability of establishing a system of mandatory testing. The duty to disclose falls on all those who have reason to suspect, as well as those who know, they are HIV sero-positive. One responsibility of the former is, a priori, to undergo testing. Insomuch as such testing is not obligatory but relies on the rationality of the individual, it is voluntary. Such voluntary testing is motivated by conscience and would be facilitated by the reciprocity of obligations thesis.

If it can be established that there exists a duty on seropositive individuals to disclose their HIV status, could this be reconciled with citizens' civil rights? For example, it should somehow be ensured that such disclosure will not jeopardise employment, housing, insurance, access to health care.

Project leader:
Professor J. HARRIS
Centre for Social Ethics &
Policy,
University of Manchester
Oxford Road
UK Manchester M13 9PL
Phone: +44 61 275 34 14
Fax: +44 61 275 32 62
Contract number: CT920729

Participants:
Prof. Margaret BRAZIER
Centre for Social Ethics and
Policy, Univ of Manchester
Oxford Road
UK Manchester M13 9PL
Phone: +44 61 275 35 93
Fax: +44 61 275 35 19

Prof. Anthony O. DYSON
Centre for Social Ethics and
Policy, Univ of Manchester
Oxford Road
UK Manchester M13 9PL
Phone: +44 61 275 35 97
Fax: +44 61 275 35 19

Prof. Paola CATTORINI
Istituto di Ricovero e Cura
a Carrattere Scientifico,
H. San Raffaele
Via Olgettina 60
IT 20132 Milano
Phone: +39 2 26 43 27 65
Fax: +39 2 26 43 24 82

Dr. Gerald CORBITT
Regional virus lab.,
Booth Hall Hospital
UK Manchester M9 2AA
Phone: +44 61 741 52 00
Fax: +44 61 741 52 14

Dr Peter EXON
AIDS Unit, Room 219,
Friars house
157-168 Blackfriars Road
UK London SE1 8EU
Phone: +44 71 972 32 18
Fax: +44 71 972 30 31/3301

Dr. Caliope C.S. FARSIDES
Centre for Contemporary
Ethical Issues,
Keele University
UK Keele, Staffs ST5 5BG
Phone: +44 782 58 33 04
Fax: +44 782 58 33 99

Prof. Dieter GIESEN
Working Centre for german
& International Medical
Malpractise Law,
Freie Univ Berlin
Boltzmannstrasse 3
DE 1000 Berlin 33
Phone: +49 30 838 47 13
Fax: +49 30 838 47 09

Prof. Heta HAYRY
Dept. of Philosophy,
Univ of Helsinki
Unionkatu 40 B
FI 00170 Helsinki
Phone: +358 0 191 76 27

Dr. Soren HOLM
Neuropsykiatrisk Institut,
Rigshospitalet 6102
Blegdamsvej 9
DK 2100 Copenhagen

Dr Catherine MANUEL
Lab. de santé Publique,
Faculté de Médecine
27 Bd. Jean Moulin
FR 13385 Marseille Cedex 5
Phone: +33 91 38 75 83
Fax: +33 91 79 75 20

Prof. Mike MORAN
European Policy Review
Unit, Univ of Manchester
Oxford Road
UK Manchester M13 9PL
Phone: +44 61 275 48 89
Fax: +44 61 275 47 51

Dr Lorraine SHERR
Dept. of Clinical Psychology,
St. Mary's hospital
Praed street
UK London W2 1NY
Phone: +44 71 725 66 66
Fax: +44 71 721 62 00

Dr. Anton VEDDER
Centre for Bio-Rthics &
Health Law, Utrecht Univ
Heidelberglaan 2
NL 3584 CS Utrecht
Phone: +31 30 53 43 99
Fax: +31 30 53 32 41

BIOMEDICAL ETHICS IN EUROPE: INVENTORY, ANALYSIS, INFORMATION

Key words
Methodology, information.

Objectives
1 Drawing up a list of ethics methodologies by listing the typical cases encountered and the reasoning, values, disciplines and criteria involved in the analysis of biomedical situations and the ethical decision making process.
2 Identifying the basis for a new scientific discipline; setting up a database of biomedical ethics resource people in a directory.

Brief description
This project will include the organization of discussion conferences on for instance genetic screening, euthanasia, quality of life, AIDS, neurological diseases, and definition of private domain.

Project leader:
Dr. G. HUBER
Association Descartes
1, rue Descartes
FR 75231 Paris Cédex 05
Phone: +33 1 46 34 32 96
Fax: +33 1 46 34 33 40
Contract number: CT920169

Participants:
Teresa IGLESIAS
Dept. of Philosophy,
Univ College Dublin
IE Dublin
Phone: +353 1 269 32 44
Fax: +353 1 269 34 69

Lord Wayland KENNET
Office of Science and
Technology,
House of Lords
UK London SW1
Phone: +44 71 219 31 41
Fax: +44 71 219 59 79

Dr. Stelaa REITER-THEIL
Institut fur Geschichte
der medizin der
Georg-August-Univ
Humboldtallee 11
DE 3400 Göttingen
Phone: +49 55 139 96 80
Fax: +49 55 139 95 54

Prof. Paul SCHOTSMANS
Centrum voor Bio-Medische
Ethiek en Recht,
Kath. Univ Leuven
Kapucijnenvoer 35
BE 3000 Leuven
Phone: +32 16 21 69 51
Fax: +32 16 21 69 52

Prof. C.N. STEFANIS
Athens Univ Medical School,
dept. of Psychiatry
GR Athens
Phone: +30 1 72 17 763
Fax: +30 1 72 43 905

Dr. M. DE WACHTER
Inst. de Bioéthique,
St. Servaasklooster
NL 6299 AT Maastricht
Phone: +31 43 21 75 75
Fax: +31 43 25 63 73

F.S.J. ABEL
Institut Borja de Bioética
Llaseres 30
ES 08190 Sant Cugat
del Vallès
Phone: +34 367 447 66
Fax: +34 367 479 80

Prof. Svend ANDERSEN
Inst. for Etik og Religions-
filosofi, Aarhus Universitet
Hovedbygninden
DK 8000 Aarhus
Phone: +45 86 13 67 11
Fax: +45 86 13 04 90

Prof. Luis ARCHER
Autonoma de Biotecnologia,
Univ. Nova de Lisboa
PT 2825 M. Caparica

Guido GERIN
Inst. International d'Etudes
des Droits de l'Homme
IT 34127 Trieste
Phone: +39 49 551 399 680
Fax: +39 49 551 399 554

Prof. Erny GILLEN
Centre Jean XXIII
52 rue Jules Wilhem
LU 2728 Luxembourg
Phone: +352 43 60 51 24
Fax: +352 40 21 31 26

Prof. Gilbert HOTTOIS
Centre de Recherches Inter-
discilpinaires en Bioéthique,
Univ Libre de Bruxelles
145 avenue Adolphe Buyl
BE Bruxelles

ETHICAL, SOCIAL AND SCIENTIFIC PROBLEMS RELATED TO THE APPLICATION OF GENETIC SCREENING AND GENETIC MONITORING FOR EMPLOYEES IN THE CONTEXT OF A EUROPEAN APPROACH TO HEALTH AND SAFETY AT WORK

Key words
Ethical, social, scientific, genetic, screening, monitoring, occupational selection, surveillance.

Objectives
To evaluate the scientific relevance of the possible use of genetic screening and genetic monitoring as a means for the selection and surveillance of workers and to identify specific ethical and social problems at both industry and society level related to the application of these techniques in occupational settings.

To contribute to preserving current European social and ethical values by producing guidelines for all parties involved in decision making in the fields of ill-health prevention in the workplace and in social security.

Brief description
A series of current medical selection and health surveillance practices in occupational settings as well as possible future genetic ones will be analyzed regarding accuracy, relevance, necessity and consequences.

A susceptibility model relating exposure, susceptibility and health impairment will be developed and used for the analysis. Necessity will be studied with regard to the relationship between primary prevention, medical selection and surveillance. Consequences will be considered on the level of both the individual and society.

At the same time, a series of international declarations on human and workers' rights, the constitutional laws of western European countries and the concepts which form the basis of their social security systems will be analyzed in order to identify ethical principles directly or indirectly related to health at work. These principles will then be used to evaluate the ethical acceptability of current practices and future genetic ones regarding selection of workers and health surveillance.

Current practices and future genetic ones will be compared in this respect and possible specific problems related to the new genetic techniques will be identified.

The current legislation to workers' health protection will be checked for its accuracy in preserving the ethical values. Guidelines will be established with respect to ethical selection and surveillance techniques. These will be destined for all parties involved in regulatory activities on the subject.

Project leader:
Dr. K. VAN DAMME
European Trade Union Technical Bureau (TUTB)
Bd E. Jacqmain 155
BE 1210 Brussels
Phone: +32-2-224 05 60
Fax: +32-2-224 05 61
Contract number: CT921213

Participants:
Dr. Marja SORSA
Inst. of Occupational Health,
Dept. of Industrial Hygiene and Toxiology
Topeliuksenkatu 41 aA
FI 00250 Helsinki
Phone: +358 0 47 471
Fax: +358 0 413 691

Dr. Paola VINEIS
Dipartimento di Scienze Biomediche
e Oncologia Umana
Via Santana 7
IT 10126 Torino
Phone: +39 11 67 88 72
Fax: +39 11 63 52 67

Prof. Madeleine MOULIN
Univ Libre de Bruxelles,
Inst. de Sociologie
BE Bruxelles
Phone: +32 2 650 34 51
Fax: +32 2 650 33 35

Dr. Jean-Claude ZERBIB
INPACT, Dept. Recherches
4 Boulevard de la Villette
FR 75019 Paris
Phone: +33 1 42 06 40 50
Fax: +33 1 69 08 34 94

Dr. Nic VAN LAREBEKE
Fédération des Maisons Médicales
255 Chaussée de Waterloo
BE 1060 Bruxelles
Phone: +32 2 424 04 01
Fax: +32 2 424 02 94

Dr. Sakari KARJALAINEN
National Agency for Welfare and Health
Siltasaarenkatu 18 C, P.O. Box 220
FI 00531 Helsinki
Phone: +358 0 396 71
Fax: +358 0 761 307

Dr. P. JACQUES &
R. OWEN & R. BIBBINGS
TUC, Health and Safety, Congress House
Great Russell Street
UK London WC1B 3LS
Phone: +44 71 636 40 30
Fax: +44 71 636 06 32

John POULSEN
Salaries Employees and
Civil Servants Confederation
Niels Hemmingsensgade 12,
P.B. 1169
DK 1010 Copenhagen K
Phone: +45 3 315 30 22
Fax: +45 3 391 30 22

Gloria MALASPINA
CGIL
Corso d'Italia 25
IT 00198 Roma
Phone: +39 6 847 61
Fax: +39 6 884 56 83

GENETIC SCREENING AND PREDICTIVE MEDICINE: ETHICAL AND PHILOSOPHICAL PERSPECTIVES, WITH SPECIAL REFERENCE TO MULTIFACTORIAL DISEASES

Key words
Genetic screening, predictive medicine, multifactorial conditions, genetic predisposition.

Brief description
Human genome analysis will facilitate genetic screening on an unprecedented scale. Hitherto screening has largely followed the identification of an index case, but in the future we can anticipate mass carrier screening and the development of predictive medicine, with possibly undesirable consequences for individuals, relating to insurability, discrimination and stigmatisation. special problems concern screening for multifactorial conditions and testing children for late onset diseases.

The project will monitor the development of genetic screening in various countries in Europe and collect information on national social policies in participating countries. As a primarily philosophical project, its main objective will be to make recommendations on ethical criteria for the introduction, conduct and evaluation of genetic screening programmes, and to clarify concepts involved in genetic screening, such as health, disease and the notion of genetic predisposition. It will be an interdisciplinary study, however, involving history of medicine, genetics anthropology, law, nursing, public health medicine and theology.

The involvement of other disciplines will facilitate the examination of historical precedents, cultural context, and the desirability of legislation. special attention will be paid to the feasibility of raising public awareness of the issues.

Project leader:
Professor R. CHADWICK
Centre for Professional Ethics,
University of Central Lancashire
UK Preston PR1 2HE
Phone: +44 772 892 541
Fax: +44 772 892 942
Contract number: CT931348

Participants:
Dr. Angus CLARKE
Insitute of Medical Genetics,
Unversity of Wales College of Medicine
Heath Park
UK Cardiff CF4 4XN
Phone: +44 222 744052
Fax: +44 222 747603

Dr. Darren SHICKLE
Temple of Peace and Health
Cathays Park
UK Cardiff CF1 3NW
Phone: +44 222 231021
Fax: +44 222 238606

Dr. Dolores DOOLEY
Dept. of Philosophy
Lucan Place
IE Cork
Phone: +353 21 27 68 71
Fax: +353 21 27 28 36

Dr. Elisabeth ANIONWU
Mothercare Unit of Clinical Genetics and Fatal Medicine, Inst. of Child Health,
Univ of London
30 Guildford Street
UK London WC1N 1EH
Phone: +44 71 242 9789
Fax: +44 71 831 0488

Dr. Luca SINEO
Inst. of Anthropology, Univ of Florence
Via del Proconsolo 12
IT 50122 Florence
Phone: +39 55 23 98 065
Fax: +39 55 23 98 065

Dr. Rodriques de AREIA
Inst. of Anthropology, Univ of Coimbra
PT Coimbra
Phone: +351 39 29 051
Fax: +351 39 23 491

Dr. Sorby NORBY
Inst. of Forensic Genetics
P.O. Box 2713
DK 2100 Copenhagen
Phone: +45 35 32 61 21
Fax: +45 35 32 61 20

Mr. Andrew BELSEY
Centre for Applied Ethics,
Univ of Wales, College of Cardiff
P.O. Box 94
UK Cardiff CF1 3XB
Phone: +44 222 874025
Fax: +44 222 874242

Mr. Charles NGWENA
Cardiff Law School,
Univ of Wales, College of Cardiff
P.O. Box 427
UK Cardiff CF1 1XD
Phone: +44 222 874348
Fax: +44 222 874097

Prof. Brunetto CHIARELLI
Inst. of Anthropology, Univ of Florence
Via del Proconcolo 12
IT 50122 Florence
Phone: +39 55 23 98 065
Fax: +39 55 23 98 065

Prof. Dr. Gertrud HAUSER
Inst. of Histology and Embryology,
Univ of Vienna
Schwarzspanierstrasse 17
AT 1090 Vienna
Phone: +431 403 05 43

Prof. SCHROEDER-KURTH
Inst. fur Humangenetik und Anthropologie,
Ruprecht Karls Universitat
Im Neuenheimer Feld 328
DE 6900 Heidelberg 1
Phone: +49 6221 56 38 77
Fax: +49 6221 56 38 98

Prof. Henk ten HAVE
Dept. of Ethics, Philosophy and History
of Medicine Fac der Med Wetenschappen,
Kath Univ Nijmegen
P.O. Box 9101
NL 6500 HB Nijmegen
Phone: +31 80 61 53 20
Fax: +31 80 54 02 54

Prof. Ingmar PÖRN
Dept. of Philosophy, Univ of Helsinki
Unioninkatu 40 B
FI 00170 Helsinki
Phone: +358 0 19 17 627

Prof. Jorgen HUSTED
Dept. of Philosophy, Aarhus Univ
Universitetsparken
DK 8000 Aarhus C
Phone: +45 86 13 67 11
Fax: +45 86 19 16 99

Dr. Urban WIESING
Inst. for Theory and History of Medicine,
Westfälische Wilhelms Universität Münster
Waldeyerstrasse 27
DE 4400 Münster
Phone: +49 251 83 52 91
Fax: +49 251 83 53 39

PARENTS' INFORMATION AND ETHICAL DECISION-MAKING PROCESS IN NEONATAL INTENSIVE CARE UNITS: STAFF ATTITUDES AND OPINIONS

Key words
Decision-making, Neonatal Intensive Care, parents information.

Brief description
The aim of the Project is to study parents information and the ethical decision-making process in Neonatal Intensive Care Units (NICUs) from the health personnel perspective, in relation with the social, cultural, legal and ethical backgrounds of the various countries.

The Project is made up of two major parts:

1 A survey of the health personnel self reported practices, opinions and problems on the issues of parents information and ethical decision making for three main categories of patients: the extremely premature, the severely malformed, and the brain damaged one.

2 A survey of the existing legislation, as well as guidelines and/or recommendations issued by official bodies (National Ethics Committees, Medical Societies) on the problems at hand. In each participating country a random sample of NICUs will be asked to take part in the study.

Data about the NICUs, the staff self reported practices and opinions, and legislation will be collected by means of questionnaires.

The materials will be prepared by the Project coordinator, and finalized by the study group formed by researchers from different backgrounds: physicians, medical law experts, bioethicists, psychologists and sociologists.

The NICUs description questionnaire will be completed by the Head of the Units.

The staff questionnaire will be anonymous and self-administered, in order to guarantee confidentiality.

The informations about the legislation will be collected by the medical law experts of each country.

All the questionnaires will be sent to Trieste, Italy, for coding, computer storage and data analysis.

The findings of the study will be reported to all the participating NICUs, and will be the subject of presentations in scientific conferences, and papers to be published in medical, medical law, health policy and medical ethics journals.

Project leader:
Dr. M. CUTTINI
Istituto de Puericultura
Via dell'Istria 65/1
IT 34100 Trieste
Phone: +39 40 378 51 11
Fax: +39 40 378 52 10
Contract number: CT931242

Participants:

Dr. C. COLOMER
I.V.E.S.P.
Juan de Garay 21
ES 46017 Valencia

Dr. J. PERIS PERIS
Legal Advisor of the Official
College of Medical Doctors
of Valencia, Colegio Oficial
de Medicos
Avenida de la Plata 20
ES 46013 Valencia

Dr. M. GAREL
I.N.S.E.R.M. U. 149
16 Av. P. Vaillant-Couturier
FR 94807 Villejuif Cedex

Dr. M. REID
Dept. of Public Health,
Univ of Glasgow
2 Lilybank Gardens
UK Glasgow G12 8R

Dr. M. SCHROELL
Clinique Pédiatrique,
Centre Hospitalier de
Luxembourg
4 Rue Barblé 1210
LU Luxembourg

Dr. P. ROMITO
Istituto di Puericultura,
I.R.C.C.S. Burlo Garofolo
Via dell'Istria 65/1
IT 34100 Trieste

Dr. R. De LEEUW
Dept. of Neonatology,
Univ of Amsterdam
Meibergdreef 9
NL 1105 AZ Amsterdam

Dr. S. LENOIR
I.N.S.E.R.M. CJF 89-08,
Hopital de La Grave
FR 31052 Toulouse Cedex

Dr. S. SPINSANTI
Direzione Scientifica,
Ospedale Fatebenefratelli
Isola Tiberina
Piazza dei Ponziani 8
IT 00186 Roma

Prof. H.G. LENARD
Dept. of Neuropediatrics,
Heinrich Heine Universitat
Moorenstrasse 5
DE 4000 Dusseldorf 1

Prof. I. de BEAUFORT
Dept. of Medical Ethics,
Med. Fac. of Erasmus Univ
NL Rotterdam

Prof. P. CENDON
Istituto Giuridico,
Facoltà di Economia
e Commercio,
Università di Trieste
P.le Europa 1
IT 34100 Trieste

Prof. P.J.J. SAUER
Sophia Children's Hospital
Gordelweg 160
NE 3038 GE Rotterdam

Prof. R. SARACCI
Unit of Analytical
Epidemiology I.A.R.C.
150 Cours Albert-Thomas
FR Lyon

Prof. S. NORDIO
Istituto di Puericultura,
I.R.C.C.S. Burlo Garofolo
Via dell'Istria 65/1
IT 34100 Trieste

Prof. U. DE VONDERWEID
Istituto di Puericultura,
I.R.C.C.S. Burlo Garofolo
Via dell'Istria 65/1
IT 34100 Trieste

ETHICAL ASPECTS OF COERCIVE SUPERVISION AND/OR TREATMENT OF UNCOOPERATIVE PSYCHIATRIC PATIENTS IN THE COMMUNITY

Key words
Coercive supervision, health laws, mental patients.

Brief description
The focus of this proposal is on the moral issues that are involved in coercive supervision and/or treatment of mentally ill patients in the community. As a result of reforms in mental health care and developments in the mental health laws in several European countries, civil commitment of mental patients takes place in a modern, 'legalized' context. Criteria for involuntary psychiatric hospitalization in several countries have shifted from 'best interests' (or 'need for treatment') to 'dangerousness'. In the view of commentators, new statutory regulations often constrict practitioners in providing treatment or care they deem medically necessary for the patient. In the practice of mental health care, the unmotivated patient, who lacks insight in his or her mental illness, cannot be committed or treated, unless, as a result of the mental illness, his/her condition deteriorates to such a degree that he/she poses a(n) (imminent) danger to him/herself or others. The morally troubling issue is that some mentally ill patients who could, with treatment or supervi- sion, cope in the community may be left to deteriorate until they finally become a danger to themselves and/or society. Some may even suffer without ever becoming dangerous. In order to contribute to the assistance and management of uncooperative mentally ill patients in the community 'out-patient commitment' ('involuntary outpatient treatment'; 'community treatment/supervision order') has been proposed as a possibly fruitful alternative strategy in the field of mental health care. Coercion in the community, however, raises difficult and complex moral issues.

The goal of this proposed project is to clarify these moral issues, to analyze them from an ethical perspective, and to formulate recommendations regarding the moral status and feasibility of coercive measures in community mental health care.

The main benefit of this study for the EC is that it aims at clarifyinq strategies for change regarding specific problems that by many professionals in the field throughout Europe are regarded as a (by)product of changes in mental health care delivery and reforms in mental health law.

Project leader:
Dr. M.A.M. DE WACHTER
Institute for Bioethics, I.G.E.
P.O. Box 778
NL 6200 AT Maastricht
Phone: +31 43 21 75 75
Fax: +31 43 25 63 73
Contract number: CT931679

Participants:
Dr. Med. J. ZEILER
Medizinische Hochschule
Hannover, Abteilung
Klinische Psychiatrie
P.O. Box 610180
DE Hannover
Phone: +49 5115322492
Fax: +49 5115322415

E. MORDINI
Inst.o Psicoanalytico per
le Ricerche Sociali (I.P.R.S.)
Via Arenula 21
IT 00186 Roma
Phone: +39 6 6867495

Prof. R. BLUGLASS
The Univ of Birmingham,
Dept. of Psychiatry
Bristol Road South, Rubery,
Rednal
UK Birmingham B45 9BE
Phone: +44 21 4536161

DECISION MAKING AND IMPAIRED CAPACITY: THE ETHICS, LAW AND PRACTICE CONCERNING INCOMPETENT PATIENTS

Key words
Law, ethics, decision making, impaired capacity.

Brief description
The proposed research is a multi-disciplinary, multi-location investigation into law, ethics and practice regarding a variety of clinical conditions whose common feature is that they involve an impairment in the capacity of the patient to make decisions for him/herself, including decisions regarding his/her clinical care.

The investigation will bring together the insights and perspectives of four distinct academic disciplines, namely clinical medicine, law, philosophy, and history of medicine social history. It will encompass academics working within protestant, Roman Catholic and humanist perspectives from four European States: the Netherlands, Spain, Sweden and the United Kingdom.

The research will proceed in three study phases, each culminating in an interim report to the Commission. These stages and their associated interim reports will all concern the ethics, law and practice relating to decision making and impaired capacity; the first will concern identification and description of law and practice; the second will concern analysis and evaluation of law and practice; the third will concern the basis of recommendations concerning the harmonisation or approximation of law and practice. At the end of the third study period, the whole project will culminate in a final report to the Commission constituting final recommendations on law and practice in these areas.

Project leader:
Dr. D. EVANS
Centre for Philosophy & Health Care,
University of Wales, College of Swansea
Singleton Park
UK Swansea SA2 8PP
Phone: +44 792 295 612
Fax: +44 792 295 769
Contract number: CT931714

Participants:

Prof. Diego GRACIA
Dept. of History of Medicine
and Bioethics,
Faculty of Medicine
Complutense Univ,
Pabellon IV Bajo
Cuidad Universitaria
ES 28040 Madrid
Phone: +34 1 394 1414
Fax: +34 1 394 1415

Prof. Göran LANTZ
Ersta Institute for
Health Care Ethics
P.O. Box 4619
SE 11691 Stockholm
Phone: +46 8 714 6100
Fax: +46 8 641 6671

Prof. Henk ten HAVE
Dept. of Ethics,
Philosophy and History
of Medicine,
Catholic Univ of Nijmegen
P.O. Box 9101
NL Nijmegen 6500 HB
Phone: +31 80 615320
Fax: +31 80 540254

THE MORAL AND LEGAL ISSUES SURROUNDING THE TREATMENT AND HEALTH CARE OF PATIENTS IN ' PERSISTENT VEGETATIVE STATE

Key words
Ethics, law, persistent vegative state, medical decisions.

Brief description
The question of when, if ever, a medical practitioner may rightfully withdraw or withhold treatment arises in many different medical contexts.

The moral criteria for such decisions are notoriously difficult. Recent radical changes in legislative policy regarding non-treatment in some EC countries (most notably the United Kingdom and The Netherlands) lend urgency to the moral and social debate, if large disparities in policy are to be avoided.

This project is therefore necessarily interdisciplinary - involving research in ethics, national and international law and social policy as well as a consideration of the state of the art in neurological science and medical practice. It aims to identify, clarify and assess the moral principles which are thought to provide the justificatory basis for decisions to withdraw or withhold treatment, through a consideration of the very special difficulties presented by patients in persistent vegetative state. For this group of patients, unlike others for whom the withholding or withdrawing of treatment may sometimes be morally legitimate, are neither brain-dead nor dying, even though they may never regain consciousness and have little prospect of improvement. They therefore raise moral problems of a particularly fundamental kind.

However, a precise analysis of the moral issues depends on a clarification of the scientific and medical debate concerning persistent vegetative state, which is as yet only poorly understood. The project, therefore, involves a comparative study of medical opinion involving international experts in the field, and of different treatment options across Member States.

To further facilitate the ethical enquiry, and to provide a basis for recommending social policy, it is also necessary to conduct comparative analyses of existing national laws and regulations governing medical decisions to withhold or withdraw treatment, and their application to patients in persistent vegetative state, thereby providing a framework for European social and legislative policy in this area.

Project leader:
Mr. A. GRUBB
Centre of Medical Law and Ethics,
King's College
Strand
UK London WC2R 2LS
Phone: +44 71 873 2382
Fax: +44 71 873 2575
Contract number: CT931507

Participants:
Dr. Dolores DOOLY
Univ College
IE Cork

Dr. Hans Georg KOCH, Prof. A. ESER
Max-Planck-Inst. für Auslandisches und
Internationales Strafrecht
DE

Dr. Keith ANDREWS
Royal Hospital and Home
UK Putney London

Dr. M. de WACHTER
Instituut voor Gezondheidsethiek
NL Maastricht

Dr. Tina GARANIS
Athens School of Public Health
GR Athens

Prof. B. JENNETT
Inst. Neurological Sciences
UK Glasgow Scotland

Prof. LAMAU
Universite Catholique de Lille
FR Lille

Prof. L. HONNEFELDER
Friedrich-Wilhelms-Universität
DE Bonn

Prof. P. SCHOTSMANS
Katholieke Universiteit Leuven
BE Leuven

ETHICAL ISSUES IN BIOMEDICAL RESEARCH WITH COGNITIVELY IMPAIRED ELDERLY SUBJECTS

Key words

Cognitively impaired, elderly subjects, dementia, consent, non-therapeutic research.

Brief description

The focus of this study is on cognitively impaired, elderly subjects as potential candidates for participation in biomedical research. This implies that the project has special relevance for the field of dementia research.

Since there are no acceptable (animal) models for dementia, the necessary research into the causes, prevention and treatment of dementia must be done mainly with demented patients themselves. As a consequence of their disease, dementia patients gradually loose their ability to give valid consent to participate in biomedical research. As free and informed consent is a necessary condition for biomedical research with human persons, their participation in biomedical research raises difficult ethical questions. In most countries, proxy consent is legally obligatory. There exists, however, no international consensus about the role, responsibilities and authority of proxy decision makers. Besides the issue of informed consent, consensus is lacking about the participation of cognitively impaired elderly subjects in non-therapeutic research.

The goal of scientific progress in the cure of dementia will often demand the participation of demented subjects in research which will not benefit them immediatetely (but may benefit future patients). There is no international consensus with regard to the regulation of this issue too.

Our proposed project has three objectives:

1 Inventory and clarification of the specific moral issues that are raised by the participation of cognitively impaired elderly subjects in biomedical research;
2 Inventory and ethical analysis of laws, regulations and guidelines on the conduct of research with these subjects in several European countries, and;
3 Formulation of recommendations with regard to the process of informed consent and the assessment of risks and benefits regarding the participation of these subjects in biomedical research.

Advancement at the European level of ethical acceptable biomedical research with cognitively impaired elderly subjects is of great importance, because of the great societal need for strategies to diagnose, prevent and cure or alleviate the symptoms of dementia. Uniform regulation at the European level is also important, because of the practice of international multicenter trials.

Project leader:
Prof. R.H.J. TER MEULEN
Institute for Bioethics, I.G.E.
P.O. Box 778
NL 6200 AT Maastricht
Phone: +31 43 21 75 75
Fax: +31 43 25 63 73
Contract number: CT931701

Participants:
C.A. DEFANTI
Ospedali riuniti di Bergamo,
Neurologia 1
Largo Barozzi 1
IT 24100 Bergamo
Phone: +39 35 269466
Fax: +39 35 401563

H. HELMCHEN
Freie Universität Berlin,
Universitätsklinikum Rudolf
Virchow Psychiatrische
Klinik und Poliklinik
Eschenallee 3
DE 1000 Berlin 19
Phone: +49 30 3003700
Fax: +49 30 3003726

LIMITING ACCESS TO HEALTH CARE IN
VARIOUS EUROPEAN COUNTRIES

A Study of The Legitimacy of Government Control
and the Relevance of Consumer and Provider Preferences

Key words
Health care, priorities, resource, resource allocation.

Brief description
A major challenge to be met in the 1990s by the governments of Western European countries is containment of public expenditures to health care, without unduly curtailing consumers and providers liberties.

In terms of organization of health care, this means seeking an acceptable balance between the central planning- and the market-approach.

The aim of the proposed research is to collect data from the participating countries (N, NL, DK, D and GB) on limiting access to health care: which types of services are being rationed, how is this done, by whom, and which reasons are provided? Our focus will be on the institutional level.

As far as possible, we will aim at standardized data collection, to facilitate cross-country comparisons. Short-term exchange of researchers should also contribute to this aim.

The collected data will subsequently be analyzed, the central questions being: do the collected data allow us to determine what it is, that makes a health care service the appropriate object of public responsibility and concern? or: what is it, that justifies some curtailment of individual liberties, and that serves as a basis for solidarity? If successful, such an endeavour improves our understanding of morality, and should help to motivate each of the parties involved to strive for a morally better health care.

This over-arching issue will be addressed in a number of sub-questions, dealing with: accountability of governmental institutions; rationality of providers and consumers behaviour; decision procedures in setting priorities in health care which try to accommodate for different valuations of health states; how resource scarcity carries-over in individual resource allocation decisions; the impact of various ways of limiting access to health care on development, adoption, and diffusion of novel bio-medical technologies (as examplified by infertility treatments).

Such an analysis, and the sharing of this information should help each of the countries to identify areas in health care which are the appropriate target of public responsibility and concern, and those areas which are the appropriate target of private responsibility and concern.

Project leader:
Dr. G. J. VAN DER WILT
University of Nijmegen, Faculty of Medical Sciences,
Dept of Medical Information Science and Epidemiology
P.O. Box 9101
NL 6500 HB Nijmegen
Phone: +31 80 61 31 25
Fax: +31 80 61 35 05
Contract number: CT931393

Participants:
Andrew EDGAR
Centre for Applied Ethics, Univ of Wales
P.O. Box 94
UK Cardiff CF1 3XB
Phone: +44 222874025
Fax: +44 222874242

Evert van LEEUWEN
Faculty of Medicine,
Dept. of Metamedicine, Philosophy and
Medical Ethics, Vrije Universiteit
Van der Boechhorststraat 7
NL 1081 BT Amsterdam
Phone: +31 205483340

Hans-Martin SASS
Zentrum Medizinische Ethik, Ruhr Universität
P.O. Box 102148
DE 4630 Bochum
Phone: +49 2347002760
Fax: +49 2347094201

J. HARRIS
Univ of Manchester, Centre for
Social Ethics and Policy
Oxford Road
UK Manchester M13 9PL
Phone: +44 061 2753473
Fax: +44 061 2753519

Ole Frithjof NORTHEIM
Center for Medical Ethics
Gaustadalléen 21
NO 0371 Oslo 3
Phone: +45 22958780
Fax: +45 22698471

Peter ROSSEL
Inst. of Biostatistics and Theory of Medicine,
Faculty of Health Sciences, Univ of Copenhagen
Blegdamsvey 3
DK 2200 N Copenhagen
Phone: +45 35327931
Fax: +45 35327907

Soren HOLM
Inst. of Biostatistics and Theory of Medicine,
Faculty of Health Sciences, Univ of Copenhagen
Blegdamsvej 3
DK 2200 N Copenhagen
Phone: +45 35327931
Fax: +45 35327907

Susanne van de VATHORST
Dept. of Philosophy, Vrije Universiteit
De Boelelaan 1105
NL 1081 HV Amsterdam
Phone: +31 205483696

APAS[1] PHARMACEUTICALS RESEARCH

Dr. Giovanni N. Fracchia

On the decision by the European Parliament, a new budget line outside the third Framework Programme was opened for 1992 by the European Commission to identify areas in which it would be possible to develop more efficient treatments of diseases. The main aim was to facilitate, in coordination with the national health authorities and industries, pilot projects in the field of toxicity tests, multicentric clinical experimentation and safety tests related to new drugs.

Accordingly, a series of expert meetings were organised in 1992, with the aims of defining the needs and opportunities for research at Community level in these fields and of drafting recommendations for research priorities.

The invited experts were representatives from the pharmaceutical industry, senior officials in regulatory affairs and in CPMP[2], senior scientists from the academic world and officials of the EC (DG XII and DG III).

The recommendations for research priorities in each field have been published in different peer-reviewed international journals, as attached.

According to the priorities expressed by the experts, twenty-five pilot research projects have been conducted during 1993/1994 and are listed below.

These actions were instrumental in preparing future harmonisation of methodologies, in defining common terminologies and in bringing together at European scale a number of researchers which have prepared the basis for future action and establishment of networks in the different fields.

The results, which can be obtained directly from the project leader in the annexed list have stimulated ideas and suggestions for the work programme of the future Fourth Framework Programme.

---

[1] APAS stands for: Action de Promotion, Accompagnement et Soutien.

[2] CPMP stands for Committee for Proprietary Medicinal Products.

TASK FORCE ON BRAIN RESEARCH

A.-E. Baert, MD, PhD

An understanding of the function of the brain now represents one of the greatest intellectual and scientific challenges to mankind, and at the same time will bring far-reaching practical applications which may contribute to the solution of the major brainrelated medical and psychological problems. Science has just reached the point where the enabling technologies for this long-dreamed-of goal have been developed: neuroscience has undergone a major revolution in the last few years, based upon the new capabilities created by molecular biology and genetics, by space-age instrumentation and by information technology.

This situation is well understood in America and Japan, where vast new Governmentally-funded programmes have recently been inaugurated, investing heavily in research and development in neuroscience. Those countries have assessed the immense economic and social burdens created by high-prevalence mental illnesses; the alarming incidence of Alzheimer's dementia due to our increased longevity, stroke, motor disorders, epilepsy, and the other common neurological disabilities; mental retardation, addictive behaviour, and yet other brain-based disorders, The EC Member States are all bearing a major economic and social burden in caring for the large numbers with these afflictions, in the productivity losses the cause and the human problems and social tensions which they create.

Further, the USA and Japan have fully appreciated the industrial implications of the advance of neuroscience. Pharmaceutical industry of the early 21st century is confidently predicted to benefit substantially from the new drugs acting on the brain that the new era of neuroscience will develop. The supply of diagnostics and of instrumentation in this field likewise will become a major growth industry. The harnessing of the new knowledge of the human brain will contribute to the development of new robotics and revolutionary computer devices throughout industrial and daily life. These types of industries can add greatly to the wealth of the large and the small nations in Europe. Europe is playing a leading role in neuroscience today, however it needs new initiatives to maintain a key position in the world. Indeed, Europe is being left far behind by the lack of comparable investment here. Our young neuroscientists are being attracted away to the new centres being established on a massive scale elsewhere. The effort required is far-ranging, transnational, multi-disciplinary, industrially relevant and it will be science-led. For these reasons, only an initiative at the Community level can be effective in creating the resources needed.

The Services of the European Commission have set up a task force (list of members attached) to propose a thematic programme, with the human brain as a focus of attention and its projects a major investment in neuroscience research, resources, training and the intersectoral stimulation of relevant industrial research for developing new high technology in Europe.

The conclusions of the Task Force were useful in drafting the relevant brain research area of the second Biomedical and Health Research Programme, 1994-1998 (BIOMED 2), which will launch calls for research proposals in 1995 and 1996.

Appendix I

EC TASK FORCE MEMBERS
EUROPEAN DECADE OF BRAIN RESEARCH

Prof. L. Amaducci, Florence, Italy
Prof. P. Andersen, Oslo, Norway
Prof. E. Barnard, Cambridge, U.K.
Prof. Sir J.W. Black. London, U.K.
Prof. F. Boller, Paris, France
Dr. C. Bostock, Compton, U.K.
Dr. C. Braestrup, Malev, Denmark
Prof, F. Gerstenbrand, Innsbruck, Austria
Prof. W.H. Gispen, Utrecht, The Netherlands
Prof. F. Holsboer, Munich, Germany
Dr. S.Z. Langer, Paris, France
Prof. J.J. Lopez-Ibor, Madrid, Spain
Prof. J. Mendlewicz, Brussels, Belgium (chairman)
Prof. K. Poeck, Aachen, Germeany
Prof. G. Racagni, Milan, Italy
Prof. A. Ribeiro, Ociras, Portugal
Prof. B. Sakmann, Heidelberg, Germany
Prof. B. Samuelson, Stockholm, Sweden
Prof. W. Singer, Frankfurt, Germany
Prof. C. Sotelo, Paris, France
Prof. C. Stefanis, Athens, Greece
Ex Officio: Dr. A.E. Baert, CEC

COOPERATION IN SCIENCE AND TECHNOLOGY WITH CENTRAL AND EASTERN EUROPEAN COUNTRIES

'PECO': Pays d'Europe Centrale et Orientale

Manuel Hallen, MD

From the outset the European Union (EU) has supported the reforms in Central and Eastern Europe. It has inter alia provided humanitarian aid, given technical assistance, and contributed to reconstruction and development.

With regard to the reform of research systems in Central and Eastern Europe, the European Union has provided and is providing assistance and advice, albeit on a limited scale. Part of this is realised through activities undertaken in the framework of the association agreements and the agreements for trade and commercial and economic cooperation which the EU has signed with a number of countries in Central and Eastern Europe.

In 1990 the Research Council discussed the issue of scientific and technological cooperation between the EU and countries of Central and Eastern Europe. Special attention was paid to initiatives directed towards the creation of a pan-European research community. The twelve Ministers underlined the necessity to strengthen cooperation with Central and Eastern Europe.

The European Parliament has on many occasions discussed the issue of scientific and technological cooperation with Central and Eastern Europe. In 1990 and 1991 it adopted resolutions on initiatives in this area, which underlined the need for such cooperation.

In 1991 a limited number of preparatory actions related to science and technology were defined and implemented by the European Commission (EC), which have provided useful experience as a basis for the initiation of future actions.

On the initiative of the European Parliament, the 1992 EU budget foresaw three budget lines to allow additional preparatory and pilot actions: to support exploratory cooperation projects in the field of science and technology between the EU and countries of Central and Eastern Europe; to support the participation of organisations from Central and Eastern Europe in those specific Third Framework R&D programmes admitting such participation on a project-by-project basis; and to further participation in COST projects by such organisations.

The overall objective of the preparatory cooperation activities within the scheme was and still is to explore possibilities for contributing to the rehabilitation of industry, and to promote the quality of life in the societies concerned. It is seen as essential to establish durable contacts between researchers in the EU and those in Central and Eastern Europe, to develop research networks and to promote the preparation of joint research projects.

In the light of these broad objectives a number of modalities have been identified: first, the training and mobility of scientists; second, the development of networks; third, the organisation of scientific conferences and workshops; fourth, the promotion of joint research projects, whether on science and technologies of particular interest to the countries of Central and Eastern Europe, or through the cooperation of organisations from those countries in COST and in specific EU research programmes allowing such participation on a project-by-project basis. These modalities form the basis of the 1992 scheme for Cooperation in Science and Technology.

Priorities for cooperation have emerged from discussions with representatives from

Central and Eastern Europe, from fact-finding missions, from discussions in Council and the European Parliament, from conferences and workshops, and from expressions of interest in joint research projects received from countries of Central and Eastern Europe. The 1992 exercise has been made possible thanks to the cooperation of all interested parties in the EU and in Central and Eastern European countries. In this context the involvement of the European Research Councils, the Rectors Conference, EARCO and FEICRO is particularly noted, as well as the contribution of the contact persons of all the countries involved.

The exploratory cooperation scheme in 1992 covered an exceptionally wide range of scientific and technological endeavour, and involved not only the twelve Member States of the EU but also nine countries of Central and Eastern Europe (Albania, Bulgaria, Czechoslovakia, Estonia, Hungary, Latvia, Lithuania, Poland, Romania). In consequence of the breadth of the scheme, the exercise has been realised as an inter-service operation between two Directorates-General of the European Commission, DG XII and DG XIII. The EC staff involved in the call and the evaluation have been drawn from both Directorates-General.

The cooperation scheme was initiated using the same procedures as apply for EU programmes, that is, an open call for proposals and an assessment by independent experts on the basis of scientific and technological quality.

1992

A first Call for Proposals for Cooperation in Science and Technology with Central and Eastern European Countries was published in the Official Journal 92/C 111/06 on 30 April 1992 with a closing date of 7 August 1992. The call invited proposals within six major action lines, as follows:

A   Scientific and Technical Mobility, fellowships awards. This scheme fell into two parts, 'Go West' and 'Go East', the former for visits of in general three months by scientists of Central and Eastern European countries to institutions in EU Member States, the latter for generally shorter visits by EU scientists to institutions in Central and Eastern European countries.

B1 Pan-European Scientific Networks. This action provided for preparatory activities with a view to exploring the setting up of pan-European scientific networks.

B2 Conferences, Workshops and Seminars.

C   Joint Research Projects. This action promoted new joint research projects in priority areas, between organisations and enterprises, both public and private, of the EU and the countries of Central and Eastern Europe. The areas include the quality of life (environmental protection, health protection, social sciences and societal problems) and industrial technologies (information and communication technologies, materials and production, agro and food industries.)

D   Participation in EU Programmes. This action provided support for the participation of organisations and enterprises of Central and Eastern European countries in projects of specific existing and approved EU programmes for research and technological development which allow such participation on a project-by-project basis.

Organisations in Central and Eastern European countries were eligible under the Third Framework Programme to participate in programmes in the areas 'Biomedical and Health Research', 'Environment', 'Non Nuclear Energy', 'Nuclear Fission Safety' and 'Human Capital and Mobility'.

The Biomedical and Health Research Programme BIOMED 1 was involved in all action lines A to D of this rather ambitious exploratory scheme 1992. About 1,600 proposals were received in this area. In general the scientific quality of the proposals was good, and exceptionally excellent or poor.

With a few exceptions most fields of biomedical research were represented. Clinicians among the evaluators felt that the fundamental research projects were over-represented, while others considered the relative number of proposals in each sub-speciality to be fairly representative of the ongoing research activities of EU Member States.

Particular areas of biomedicine were found to be strikingly under-represented. This was the case for prevention of cancer and sexually transmitted diseases, gerontology and in particular human genetics and genome studies. Very few projects covered the social aspects of health care. The highest impact was found in action line A (fellowships) and D (participation of 28 research teams of Central and Eastern Europe in 25 out of 114 BIOMED 1 projects).

1993

In 1993 the European Commission opened again five of its specific Research and Technological Development programmes to research organisations and enterprises in Central and Eastern Europe. These programmes were again 'Biomedical and Health Research (BIOMED 1)', 'Environment', 'Non Nuclear Energy', 'Nuclear Fission Safety' and 'Human Capital and Mobility'.

The eligible countries to participate in this action were: Albania, Bulgaria, Czech Republic, Estonia, Hungary, Latvia, Lithuania, Poland, Romania, Slovakia, and Slovenia. The main objective was to enable scientists and researchers from these countries to participate in *ongoing* EU projects. The proposers were invited to contact directly the relevant BIOMED project coordinator. A complete list of all 114 ongoing projects in BIOMED 1 was attached to the Information Package. It was not possible to set up independent projects.

In BIOMED 1 a total of 139 application were received by the deadline of 2 July 1993 for participation in the 114 ongoing Concerted Actions selected at the first Call of this programme. 106 applications were sent in by the coordinators, 33 forms were received by applicants without prior contact of the coordinator. All 136 applications were for participation in 81 out of 114 ongoing Concerted Actions. Some applications asked for participation of one single team, others included up to 15 individual teams from the countries concerned. A total of 315 teams have thus applied requesting a financial contribution of almost 18.5 million ECU. 111 proposals have been selected for a total amount of 3.514 million ECU.

The inclusion of teams from Central and Eastern Europe did not propose for any increase of the available budget of the Concerted Action, but to enable the new partner to participate in the Concerted Action without using BIOMED funds.

1994

In 1994 the European Commission launched two types of activities with regard to Cooperation in Science and Technology with Central and Eastern European Countries, including for the first time, the New Independent States (NIS) of the former Soviet Union (Armenia, Azerbaijan, Belorus, Georgia, Kazakhstan, Kyrgyzstan, Moldova, Russia, Tajikistan, Turkmenistan, Ukraine, Uzbekistan):

COPERNICUS with an emphasis on new joint (East-West) research projects and concerted actions/networks in two targeted research sectors:

- Industrial technologies (information technologies; communication technologies; telematics; language engineering; manufacturing, production, processing and materials; measurement and testing) and;

- Life sciences (agro- and food industries; biotechnology).
In each research sector specific priority themes have been identified as being of particular importance. The deadline for submission of proposals was 2 May 1994.

'PECO 94' (Pays d'Europe Centrale et Orientale)
Like in 1993 the European Commission opened the same five specific Research and Technological Development programmes to research organisations and enterprises in Central and Eastern Europe, i.e. 'Biomedical and Health Research (BIOMED 1)', 'Environment', 'Non Nuclear Energy', 'Nuclear Fission Safety' and 'Human Capital and Mobility'. In the BIOMED programme 263 projects, including 149 new projects launched in 1993 and for the first time projects on Human Genome Analysis, were open for participation.
In BIOMED 1 a total of 178 proposals, including 456 teams from 17 countries have been proposed by the deadline 6 June 1994:

country	# teams
Albania	9
Bulgaria	20
Czech Republic	38
Estonia	26
Hungary	55
Latvia	14
Lithuania	43
Poland	47
Romania	36
Slovakia	20
Slovenia	21
Armenia	5
Azerbaijan	1
Belarus	2
Georgia	2
Russia	78
Ukraine	39
Total	456

Another 252 research teams from Central and Eastern Europe will join 118 projects in BIOMED 1 in addition to the already collaborating 139 researchers selected in 1992 and 1993.

Cooperation in science and technology with central and
eastern European countries BIOMED 1 - PECO 92, 93, 94

Action	N° of projects/teams	Budget 92+93 (ECU)
PECO 92:		
A: (Fellowships)	464	3,944,000
B1: (Networks)	7	630,000
B2: (Conferences)	18	574,654
C: (Joint research projects)	42	7,619,504
D: (Part. in BIOMED 1)	28	2,038,700
PECO 93:		
Participation in BIOMED 1	111	3,514,000
PECO 94:		
Participation in BIOMED 1	?	?
Total	670	18,320,858

Contact:
Dr. Manuel Hallen
European Commission
DG XII-E-4
Rue de la Loi 200
BE 1049 Brussels

THE BIOMEDICAL AND HEALTH RESEARCH NEWSLETTER
Dr. A.J.G. Dickens

The Biomedical and Health Research Newsletter has been published three times per year since June 1990 following a recommendation of the programme management committee of the Fourth Medical and Health Research Programme (MHR4, 1987-1991) of the European Union, the *CGC No. 9 Medical and Health Research*. The Commission was at that time advised on the way that information about the programme could be made available to:
- the European scientific community;
- the public authorities;
- the general public.

The programme management committee therefore recommended the creation of a programme newsletter providing early and complete information on both future developments and ongoing activities in the Medical and Health Research Programme.

Each Member State and third country participating in this research programme receives a predetermined package of copies for immediate distribution to crucial points, eg central libraries, bulletin boards of major research institutions, national authorities, EU-research interested scientists and scientific journals and periodicals carrying science news. Distribution to the European Parliament, the Council and other European bodies is carried out by the Commission Services.

The ultimate responsibility for the publication and its content rests with the European Commission. The editorial board is composed of members of the current programme committee, the *CAN-MED* (=Committee of an Advisory Nature - Biomedical and Health Research), and of the Commission Services. The editor is the head of the 'Medical Research Division'. The publication of such a newsletter is considered both by CAN-MED and by Directorate DG XII-E, *Life Sciences and Technologies*, as being fundamental to the success of the former programme MHR4 and the subsequent activities under the current BIOMED 1 programme in biomedical and health research.

This newsletter receives a very positive welcome not only from researchers in the Member States but also, since the recent political changes in Europe, from Central and Eastern Europe as well as countries further away. From initially 40,000 copies in 1990 the distribution has steadily grown to 50,000 copies in 1994; these are dispatched to national contact points in 30 European countries and to individual interested parties worldwide. This newsletter can be obtained free of charge through the relevant national contact point or from:

Medical Research Division, Directorate-General XII-E-4, European Commission, 200, rue de la Loi, BE 1049 Brussels, fax: +32-2-295 5365.

Editorial Board (1995)
Dr. V. O'Gorman, Ireland (Chairman)
Professor J. Cunha-Vaz, Portugal
Professor J. Huttunen, Finland
Dr. H. Lehmann, Germany
Dr. D. van Waarde, Netherlands
(past Chairman)
Professor G. Tobelem, France

Professor K. Vuylsteek, Belgium

European Commission
Editor: Dr. A.-E. Baert
Editorial Adviser: Dr. A.J.G. Dickens
Editorial Assistant: Dr. A. Vanvossel
Writer: Dr. K. Broman

KEY WORD INDEX

PROJECT LEADER INDEX